nnf6

Companion website

A free companion resources site for this book is available at:

www.neonatalformulary.com

The website lists each drug described in the book, with:

Updates and new material

New – Monographs on new drugs available since the publication of the book.

Updates – Revisions to monographs revised since the publication of the book.

Comments – Temporary postings, e.g. a change in usage.

Commentaries – Permanent website commentaries about a drug.

Web archive – Drug monographs for little-used drugs no longer included in the book.

Useful links

Cochrane reviews – Links to relevant Cochrane reviews for listed drugs.

UK guidelines – Links to UK management guidelines for listed drugs.

WHO – Identification of drugs classified as essential by the World Health Organisation.

E-mail alerting

Sign up for the e-mail alerting service and we will let you know whenever a new batch of updates is added to the site.

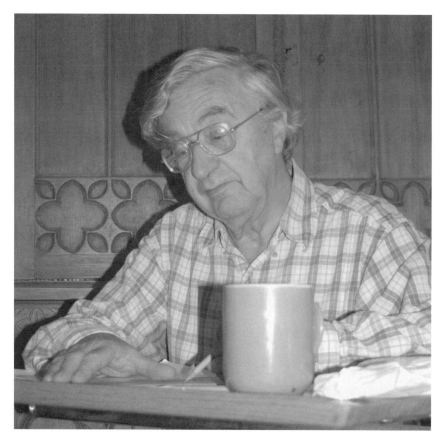

Edmund Hey, 1934–2009

Neonatal Formulary 6

Drug Use in Pregnancy and the First Year of Life

nnf6

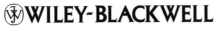
WILEY-BLACKWELL
A John Wiley & Sons, Ltd., Publication

BMJ|Books

This edition first published 2011, © 2007, 2003, 2000, 1998, 1996 by Edmund Hey

BMJ Books is an imprint of BMJ Publishing Group Limited, used under licence by Blackwell Publishing which was acquired by John Wiley & Sons in February 2007. Blackwell's publishing programme has been merged with Wiley's global Scientific, Technical and Medical business to form Wiley-Blackwell.

Registered office: John Wiley & Sons Ltd, The Atrium, Southern Gate, Chichester, West Sussex, PO19 8SQ, UK

Editorial offices: 9600 Garsington Road, Oxford, OX4 2DQ, UK
The Atrium, Southern Gate, Chichester, West Sussex, PO19 8SQ, UK
111 River Street, Hoboken, NJ 07030-5774, USA

All important amendments made to this regularly revised text after the present edition went to press can be found on the web at: www.neonatalformulary.com. Contact can be made with the team responsible for the current text and for keeping it up to date via the Pharmacy staff at the Royal Victoria Infirmary in Newcastle upon Tyne NE1 4LP, UK. Please use the following e-mail address for all such contact: drug.information@nuth.nhs.uk.

For details of our global editorial offices, for customer services and for information about how to apply for permission to reuse the copyright material in this book please see our website at www.wiley.com/wiley-blackwell.

Library of Congress Cataloging-in-Publication Data
Neonatal formulary 6: drug use in pregnancy and the first year of life / [compiled and edited by Edmund Hey]. – 6th ed.
       p. cm.
     "Nff6"
     Includes index.
     "This compendium was originally developed for use in the north of England, and sponsored for ten years by the Northern Neonatal Network. It continues to be compiled and edited by past and present members of this network" – Prelim.
     ISBN 978-1-4051-9660-4
     1. Newborn infants – Effect of drugs on.   2. Obstetrical pharmacology.   3. Pharmacopoeias – Great Britain.
I. Hey, Edmund.   II. Northern Neonatal Network (England).   III. Title: NNF6.
     RG627.6.D79N463 2011
     618.92'01–dc22
     2010024519

A catalogue record for this book is available from the British Library

ISBN 978-1-4051-9660-4

This book is published in the following electronic formats: ePDF 9781444329780; Wiley Online Library 9781444329773; ePub 9781444329797

Set in 8.5/10.5pt Frutiger condensed by Graphicraft Limited, Hong Kong
Printed and bound in Malaysia by Vivar Printing Sdn Bhd

01   2011

Contents

Companion website

A free companion resources site for this book is available at:

www.neonatalformulary.com

Updates – New drugs – Additional articles – Links to Cochrane – Guideline links

---

All substances are toxic; only the dose makes a thing not a poison.

Paracelsus (1493–1541)

Introduction

NNF6 has been designed to answer the growing need for compact and up to date, referenced, advice on the prescribing of drugs, and their safe and accurate nursing administration, during pregnancy, labour and the first year of life. While the book's main focus is on the baby, many drugs that are given to women during pregnancy are given with the baby's welfare in mind as much as the mother's. To exclude a drug simply because it is mostly given before birth rather than after birth would be to create an entirely artificial divide, so both receive attention in this compendium. Only limited information is provided, however, when the indications for use during pregnancy are essentially the same as at any other time in adult life in order to conserve space, and because this information is readily available in many other texts, including the *British national formulary* (BNF) and the important new parallel publication *BNF for children*.

The number of drugs used in late pregnancy and the first few weeks of life continues to rise rapidly, even though the manufacturers have not yet, in many cases, sought market authorisation to recommend neonatal use. One recent study in the UK found that more than 80% of neonatal prescriptions were for a product, or for a dose, formulation or purpose, that lacked licensed endorsement from the manufacturer. The situation in the rest of Europe is not dissimilar. While a lot of general information on these drugs is given in the manufacturer's Summary of Product Characteristics (SPC), advice on use in young children is often non-existent. Since advice in the SPC is all that has been seen and approved by the UK Committee on Safety of Medicines, and since the BNF normally limits itself, as a matter of policy, to summarising information that has been so validated, much drug use in the neonate occurs in a dangerous information vacuum. Much the same goes for the use of many drugs during pregnancy and lactation. All this makes it increasingly important for midwives and nurses, as well as pharmacists and doctors, to be able to put their hands on a pocket-sized reference text that summarises the scattered but extensive therapeutic and pharmacokinetic information that *is* available on the safe and appropriate use of these products. A number of other drugs that have a well-authenticated, if limited, therapeutic role are also reviewed – even though no commercial product is currently available.

Information on placental transfer and teratogenicity, and on the extent to which each drug appears in human milk (and the extent to which this matters), is provided for each drug. Where the text merely says that treatment during lactation is safe it can be taken that the dose ingested by the baby is likely to be less than 5% of the dose taken by the mother on a weight-for-weight basis, and that no reports have appeared suggesting that the baby could be clinically affected. Special attention has been paid to the rapid changes that occur in the renal and hepatic handling of some drugs in the first few weeks of life, and the impact of illness and severe prematurity on drug metabolism and drug elimination. The symptoms associated with overtreatment are summarised, and the management of toxicity is outlined. Information is also included on the best way to use the few drugs so far known to be of therapeutic benefit to the fetus.

NNF6 provides information on the main drugs used to modify the diet of babies with congenital enzyme deficiencies ('inborn errors of metabolism'), a short monograph on breast milk fortifiers and a monograph on the artificial milks ('formula' milks) most commonly used in the UK. However, no attempt has been made to list other dietary products – a need that was very comprehensively covered in *Medicines for children*, published by the Royal College of Paediatrics and Child Health in London, and is also covered, rather more briefly, by its successor *BNF for children*.

While the text reflects, in the main, practice in the UK, medicine is increasingly international in its scope. Every section of the text has been revised with this in mind by a wide range of local, national and overseas collaborators. A comprehensive range of journals have been searched in order to make the advice given in the latest revision as comprehensive and up to date as possible, and all relevant Cochrane reviews have been consulted. Input has also been sought from colleagues with a range of professional expertise in an attempt to ensure that the text reflects a distillate of current opinion. However, in deciding what should eventually find its way into print, it was the advice of those who could provide evidence to support their approach that carried most weight. A consensus driven text could, all too easily, merely reflect what most people are doing rather than what they ought to be doing! The references cited below each entry should make it easier for readers to make up their own minds on such issues.

The ***first*** part of the book contains important general information on drug storage, drug licensing and drug prescribing, with advice on drug administration, the care and use of intravascular lines, drug management in renal failure, and the recognition, management and reporting of adverse reactions. The information given on individual drugs in Part 2 needs to be interpreted in the light of this general advice. Readers skip this at their peril.

The ***second*** (and largest) part contains whole page monographs on 216 of the drugs most often used during labour and the first few months of life, listed in alphabetical order. Information on a number of blood products and vaccines is included. Each monograph lists the drug's main uses, and the most appropriate dose to give, both in the term and the preterm baby. The neonatal half life is noted where known, and a note made of those with an unusually large volume of distribution (V_D >1 l/kg). A brief summary of the drug's discovery and development is usually included. Advice is also provided on how to measure accurately the small volumes frequently required, and how to administer bolus and IV infusions safely. The advice given can, in general, be used to guide management throughout the first year of life. Significant interactions between drugs included in the main section of the compendium are outlined. Adverse effects commonly encountered in infancy, and their management, receive attention, but the SPC should be consulted in respect of other, less common, adverse effects. All the major multicentre clinical drug trials under development, or in progress, in the UK when the book went to press get a mention. Information under the heading 'supply' refers to the formulation most widely used in the UK. It is important to realise that other strengths and formulations may exist, and essential to check the label on the container before giving medicine to any patient. The stated cost is the basic net price (normally quoted in the BNF) when the book went to press, rounded to two significant figures. This information has been included in order to make clinicians more cost conscious, but should not be interpreted as representing the pricing policy of any particular hospital. Every monograph concludes with one or more recent key references to the obstetric, perinatal or neonatal literature (from which it is usually possible to identify other key reports).

The ***third*** part contains brief notes on a further 147 drugs, or groups of drugs, that are not infrequently taken by mothers during pregnancy, labour or the puerperium. The drugs mentioned include all the more commonly used products thought to affect the baby either because of placental transfer or because of excretion in human milk. Illicit drug use and legitimate self-medication both receive attention. Entries are almost always linked to two key references that can be used to access additional original studies and reports.

The ***index*** at the back of the compendium includes all the UK and US synonyms by which some drugs are occasionally known, and serves to identify more than 50 other drugs only referred to, in passing, within another drug monograph. Various common contractions are also spelt out.

A ***website*** was launched in January 2001 (www.neonatalformulary.com). New drugs continue to come onto the market at regular intervals, and further information relating to the use of many of the drugs already contained in the book continues to appear almost monthly. As a result, the text remains under semi-continuous review. The website also provides longer, more fully referenced, commentaries on some important products, direct access to abstracts of all the relevant Cochrane Reviews and link access to the UK Government's current vaccination policy guidelines. It also contains monographs on a number of drugs that were included in earlier editions of this book, but which do not appear in the present print version (although their existence can still be traced using the index) because they are no longer used as often as they once were. While the publishers plan to continue producing new editions of the paperback book approximately once every 3 years, the existence of this website makes it possible to alert readers to all the more important changes that get made to the text just as soon as they are issued.

Important advisory statement

While every effort has been made to check the veracity of the information in this compendium, those responsible for its compilation cannot accept responsibility for the consequences of any remaining inaccuracy.

The drugs included are, for the most part, those in current use in neonatal units in the United Kingdom, but the most recent updates have increasingly attempted to reflect international practice. Omission can not be taken as implying criticism of a particular drug's usefulness, but neither is inclusion necessarily a recommendation either. Indeed, a number of products are mentioned specifically to alert clinicians to some of the uncertainties or limitations associated with use in infancy. Personal preference and past experience must inevitably influence prescribing practice, and in neonatal practice, more than any other branch of medicine, it is better to use a limited number of carefully evaluated and widely used drugs knowledgeably than to use drugs with which the prescriber is not fully familiar.

It is also dangerous to go uncritically for the latest product to reach the market. Too many drugs of proven value in adult medicine have been widely and indiscriminately used in pregnancy and in the neonatal period over a number of years before the potential hazards associated with their use ever became apparent. If diethylstilbestrol had been tested for efficacy before being given to millions of women in an effort to prevent miscarriage and premature delivery, many children would have been saved from genital tract deformity, and several hundred from developing vaginal cancer. If the pharmacokinetics of chloramphenicol and the sulphonamides had been established before these drugs were first widely used in the neonatal period some 50 years ago, many hundreds of deaths could have been avoided. Hexachlorophene baths and vitamin K injections also killed several hundred babies before anyone realised what was happening. A worrying number of babies died in the early 1980s before it was realised that preterm babies cannot metabolise one of the bacteriostatic drugs commonly used to ensure the sterility of the water used to 'flush' the line every time a blood sample is taken or a drug is given (as described in the archived entry on benzyl alcohol).

Nor are such inadvertent drug tragedies merely a thing of the past. It took 10 years for people to realise that cisapride did little to reduce the incidence of troublesome reflux 'posseting', and that overenthusiastic use risked triggering a cardiac arrhythmia, and it then took another 8 years for many to realise that much the same could be true of domperidone. Evidence emerged some 12 years ago that the use of acetazolamide to control post-haemorrhagic hydrocephalus was doing more harm than good, and that the amount of aluminium that often gets infused when a baby is offered parenteral nutrition can cause permanent neuro-logical damage. The harm that was being done to these patients only finally came to light when these forms of treatment were eventually subjected to controlled trial scrutiny. In the same way concern over the near 'routine' use of insulin in babies thought to have an 'abnormally' high blood glucose level only surfaced, quite recently, when this strategy was also scrutinised for the first time in a controlled trial of meaningful size. Conversely, however, because all the early trials only focused on short-term outcomes, it took 20 years for the long-term benefits of early treatment with caffeine to be recognised.

The simultaneous use of several drugs increases the risk of harm from drug interaction. Examples include furosemide with an aminoglycoside, erythromycin with carbamazepine, and ibuprofen or indometacin with dexamethasone or hydrocortisone. Errors also more commonly creep into drug prescribing and drug administration when several products are in use at the same time. Almost all drugs are potentially harmful, and some of the drugs most frequently used in the neonatal period are potentially lethal when given in excess. It has been seriously suggested that every hospital drug cupboard should have the motto 'Is your prescription really necessary?' pinned on the door – sadly such a step would probably have little effect because, while doctors are responsible for the original prescriptions, they nearly always leave the hard and responsible work of drug administration to their nursing colleagues!

Many paediatric and neonatal texts provide tabular drug lists and dosage guidelines. While these can be a useful *aide mémoire*, they can give the false impression that all you need to know about a drug is how much to give. These reference tables should *never* be used on their own, except be somebody who is already fully familiar with all the drug's indications and contraindications, and with all aspects of the drug's pharmacokinetic behaviour (including its behaviour in the sick preterm baby). Information also becomes dated quite quickly, so any text that is more than 2 years old should be used with great caution.

Further reading

A lot of good books about drug use in children now exist, but detailed up to date neonatal information is harder to find. The world's first neonatal reference text published by Roberts in 1984 was never updated, while the slim American reference booklet by Young and Mangum is not widely available in the UK and only covers a limited range of drugs. The paediatric text by Taketomo is very comprehensive, and this is updated annually, but is only thinly referenced. *Martindale* remains a mine of useful information, and there is more specific information relating to pregnancy and the neonatal period available in the *British national formulary* (BNF and BNFC) than is generally realised (although the BNFC is the only text to include much information on dosage other than that suggested in the manufacturer's Summary of Product Characteristics). These books and the local formularies produced by the Hammersmith Hospital in London, by the Hospital for Sick Children in Toronto and by the Royal Women's Hospital in Melbourne were all consulted during the preparation of the latest edition of the present text. For books relating to drug use during pregnancy and lactation see p. 283.

Aronoff GR, Bennet WM, Berns JS, *et al.*, eds. *Drug prescribing in renal failure. Dosing guidelines for adults and children*, 5th edn. Philadelphia: American College of Physicians, 2007.
Guy's, St Thomas' and Lewisham Hospitals. *Paediatric formulary*, 7th edn. London: Guy's Hospital Pharmacy, 2005.
Isaacs D, ed. *Evidenced-based pediatric infectious diseases*. Oxford: BMJ Books, 2007.
Jacqz-Aigrain E, Choonara I, eds. *Paediatric clinical pharmacology*. Switzerland: FontisMedia SA, 2006.
Martin J, ed. *British national formulary for children (BNFC)*. London: BMJ Publishing Group, 2009.
Pagliaro LA, Pagliaro AM, eds. *Problems in pediatric drug therapy*, 4th edn. Hamilton, IL: Drug Intelligence Publications, 2002.
Pickering LK, ed. *Red book. 2009 report of the Committee on Infectious Diseases*, 28th edn. Elk Grove Village, IL: American Academy of Pediatrics, 2009.
Sweetman SC, ed. *Martindale. The complete drug reference*, 37th edn. London: Pharmaceutical Press, 2009.
Taketomo CK, Hodding JH, Kraus DM. *Pediatric dosage handbook*, 16th edn. Hudson, OH: Lexi-Comp Inc, 2009. (With international trade names index.)
Trissel L. *Handbook of injectable drugs*, 15th edn. Bethesda, MD: American Society of Health-System Pharmacists, 2008.
World Health Organisation. *WHO model formulary 2004*. Geneva: WHO, 2004.
Yaffe SJ, Aranda JV. *Neonatal and pediatric pharmacology. Therapeutic principles in practice*, 3rd edn. Philadelphia: Lippincott, Williams and Wilkins, 2005.
Young TE, Mangum B. *Neofax 2009. A manual of drugs used in neonatal care*, 22nd edn. Montvale, NJ: Thomson Reuters, 2009. (Also available in an electronic format.)
Zenk KE, Sills JH, Koeppel RM. *Neonatal medications and nutrition. A comprehensive* guide, 3rd edn. Santa Rosa, CA: NICU Inc, 2003. (Not since updated.)

Many drugs in common use have never been shown to achieve what is claimed for them. Others, when subjected to rigorous evaluation in a randomised controlled trial, have eventually been shown to cause unexpected adverse problems. An increasingly complete tally of all such studies and overviews is now available in *The Cochrane Library*, an electronic data base published for the international Cochrane Collaboration by John Wiley and Sons Ltd, and updated quarterly. For details contact John Wiley, Journals Fulfillment, 1 Oldlands Way, Bognor Regis, West Sussex PO22 9SA, UK (tel: +44 (0) 1243 843397). A ⬤ (Cochrane collaboration) symbol has been used to highlight those drugs or topics for which there is at least one review relating to use in pregnancy or the neonatal period. The whole text of these systematic reviews can now be viewed on the NNF6 website (www.neonatalformulary.com). The symbol **DHUK** identifies those drugs and vaccines for which there is a useful and relevant UK management guideline (documents that can also be accessed in the same way).

Part 1

Drug prescribing and drug administration

Staff should never prescribe or administer any drug without first familiarising themselves with the way it works, the way it is handled by the body, and the problems that can arise as a result of its use. Most of the essential facts relating to use in adults are summarised by the manufacturer in the 'package insert' or Summary of Product Characteristics (SPC). Many are also summarised in a range of reference texts, such as the *British national formulary* (BNF), and the related text *BNF for children* (BNFC). However, manufacturers seldom provide much information about drug handling *in infancy*, and although the BNFC now offers more advice on dosage in childhood than can be obtained from the manufacturer's package insert, it stresses that the use of any unlicensed medicine (or licensed medicine in an unlicensed manner) should only be undertaken by those who have also first consulted 'other appropriate and up-to-date literature'. The present book aims to summarise, and to provide a referenced guide, to that literature.

While many texts have long offered advice on the best dose to use in infancy – often in tabular form – very few provide much information on the idiosyncrasies associated with neonatal use. Such dosage tables can be a useful *aide mémoire*, but they should **never** be relied upon, on their own, to help the staff decide what to use when, what works best, or what potential adverse effects are commonly encountered during use in infancy. In addition, lists summarising common side effects and potential drug interactions are seldom of much help in identifying which problems are common or likely to be of clinical importance in the neonate, and access to this more detailed information is as important for the staff responsible for drug administration as it is for those prescribing treatment in the first place.

Similar challenges relate to the safe use of drugs during pregnancy and lactation because standard texts (such as the BNF) offer very little information as to what is, and is not, known about use in these circumstances. Such information is available in a range of specialised reference texts (see p. 283) and the Part 3 of this compendium summarises what is currently known about the use of most of the more commonly used drugs.

Never use anything except the most recent edition of this or any other reference text. Indeed copies of earlier editions should not be left where they might be used in error.

Terms, symbols, abbreviations and units

Postmenstrual age: The term postmenstrual age, as used in this book, refers to the child's total age in weeks from the start of the mother's last menstrual period. Thus a 7-week-old baby born at 25 weeks' gestation is treated as having a postmenstrual age of 32 weeks. The term 'postconceptional age' is sometimes used to describe this combination of gestational and postnatal age, although technically conception occurs about 2 weeks after the start of the last menstrual period.

Giving intravenous drugs: Intravenous (IV) drugs should *always* be given slowly, with a few notable exceptions. This universal good practice is not reiterated in each drug monograph. A simple way of achieving slow administration is described on p. 6. Where previous dilution or a particularly slow rate of infusion is important this is specified in the relevant drug monograph, and the reason given. Drugs should also be given separately. Where two different IV drugs have to be given at the same time, the best way to stop them mixing is described on p. 15. Intramuscular (IM) drugs should never be mixed, except as described in the individual drug monographs.

Continuous co-infusion: Special problems arise when it is necessary to give more than one drug continuously and vascular access is limited. Here terminal co-infusion (the mixing of two different infusates using a tap or Y connector sited as close to the patient as possible) is sometimes known to be safe. In the most frequently encountered situations where such co-infusion is safe, a comment to that effect occurs in the relevant monograph. In all other situations two different infusion sites should be used unless advice to the contrary has been obtained from the local hospital pharmacy. Advice relating to total parenteral nutrition (TPN) *only* applies to formulations similar to the one described in this compendium.

Drug names: Drugs are, in general, referred to by their non-proprietary ('generic') name, following the usage currently adopted by the *British national formulary* (BNF). Where, for clarity, a proprietary name has been used, the symbol ® has been appended the first time it is used. Where the British Approved Name (BAN) or the United States Adopted Name (USAN) differ from the International Non-proprietary Name (rINN), these alternatives are also given. All synonyms are indexed.

Symbols and abbreviations: Cross references between monographs are marked by the Latin phrase *quod vide* (contracted to q.v.). Drugs vary in the extent to which they are distributed within the body. Some only accumulate in the extracellular tissues. Others are taken up and concentrated in some or all body tissues, the total amount in the body being more than would be presumed from a measure of that present in the blood. This is referred to as the drug's apparent volume of distribution – summarised by the symbol V_D. References to a randomised controlled trial are marked [RCT]; those referring to a systematic review or meta-analysis are marked [SR]. Drugs for which the Cochrane Collaboration has produced a systematic review are marked with ![Cochrane logo], and vaccines for which one can access official UK guidance *via* this book's website are marked with **DHUK**. Other abbreviations have been kept to a minimum and are explained in the index.

UNITS

1 kilogram (kg)	=	1000 grams
1 gram (g)	=	1000 milligrams
1 milligram (mg)	=	1000 micrograms
1 microgram (µg)[†]	=	1000 nanograms
1 nanogram (ng)[†]	=	1000 picograms

A 1% weight for volume (w/v) solution contains 1 g of substance in 100 ml of solution

It follows that:
a 1:100 (1%) solution contains 10 milligrams in 1 ml
a 1:1000 (1‰)[†] solution contains 1 milligram in 1 ml
a 1:10,000 solution contains 100 micrograms in 1 ml

† These contractions are best avoided as they can easily be misread when written by hand.

Drug storage and administration

Mastering the art of safe drug administration is at least as important and substantial a challenge as mastering the art of safe and effective drug prescribing. Nurses and midwives shoulder responsibilities that are at least as onerous as their medical colleagues.

Neonatal prescribing: It is important to consider the practicalities of drug administration when prescribing, and to avoid prescribing absurdly precise doses that cannot realistically be measured. Such problems arise with particular frequency when body weight enters into the calculation. It is difficult to measure volumes of less than 0·05 ml even with a 1 ml syringe, and any doctor who prescribes a potentially dangerous drug without first working out how to give it must inevitably carry much of the responsibility if such thoughtlessness results in an administrative error. Guidance on this is given in the individual drug monographs, with advice on prior dilution where necessary.

Equal thought should also be given to the timing and frequency of drug administration. Because many drugs have a relatively long neonatal 'half life', they only need to be given once or twice a day. More frequent administration only increases the amount of work for all concerned, and increases the risk of error creeping in. Parents are also more likely to give what has been prescribed after discharge if they are not asked to give the medicine more than twice a day!

Length of treatment: Remembering to stop treatment can be as important as remembering to start it. Half the mothers on anticonvulsants booking into some maternity units seem to be taking medication merely because nobody ever told them they could stop! Neonatal antibiotic treatment seldom needs to be continued for very long. Treatment should always be stopped after 48 hours if the initial diagnosis is not confirmed. Babies with meningitis, osteitis and staphylococcal pneumonia almost always need 2–3 weeks' treatment, but 10 days is usually enough in septicaemia. Few babies need to go home on treatment; even anticonvulsants can usually be stopped prior to discharge (cf. the monograph on phenobarbital). Babies are often offered respiratory stimulants like caffeine for far longer than is necessary. Few continue to need such treatment when they are more than 32 weeks' gestation: it should, therefore, usually be possible to stop all treatment at least 3 weeks before discharge. In the case of some widely used nutritional supplements (such as iron and folic acid), there was probably never any indication for starting treatment in the first place given the extent to which most artificial milks are now fortified (cf. the monograph on milk).

Storage before use: Most drugs are perfectly stable at room temperature (i.e. at between 5 and 25°C) and do not require specialised storage facilities. Temperatures above 25°C can be harmful, however, and some drugs are damaged by being frozen, so special thought has to be given to transport and despatch. Some drugs are best protected from direct daylight, and, as a general rule, all drugs should be stored in a cupboard and kept in the boxes in which they were dispensed and despatched. Indeed, in a hospital setting, all drugs are normally kept under lock and key.

Hospital guidelines usually specify that drugs for external use should be kept in a separate cupboard from drugs for internal use. Controlled drugs, as specified in the regulations issued under the UK Misuse of Drugs Act 1971, must be kept in a separate cupboard. This must have a separate key, and this key must remain under the control of the nurse in charge of the ward at all times. A witnessed record must be kept of everything placed in, or taken from, this cupboard and any loss (due to breakage, etc.) accounted for. Medical and nursing staff must comply with identical rules in this regard.

Special considerations apply to the storage of vaccines. Many of these are damaged if they are not kept at between 4 and 8°C at all times – even during transit and delivery (no mean feat in many Third World countries). A range of other biological products, such as the natural hormones desmopressin, oxytocin, tetracosactide and vasopressin, need to be stored at 4°C. So to do the cytokines, such as erythropoietin (epoietin) and filgrastim, and some surfactant products of animal origin. The only other widely used neonatal drugs that need to be kept in a fridge at 4°C are amphotericin, atracurium, dinoprostone, soluble insulin, lorazepam and pancuronium, and even here the need to maintain such a temperature *all* the time is not nearly as strict as it is with vaccine storage. Many oral antibiotic preparations only have a limited shelf life after reconstitution. The same goes for a number of oral suspensions prepared for neonatal use 'in house'.

The 'shelf life' of all these preparations can be increased by storage at 4°C. Drugs that do not *need* to be kept in a ward refrigerator should *not* be so stored.

All the drugs mentioned in this compendium that require special storage conditions have their requirements clearly indicated in the relevant drug monograph – where no storage conditions are specified it can be taken that no special conditions exist.

Continued retention of open vials: Glass and plastic ampoules must be discarded once they have been opened. Drug vials can generally be kept for a few hours after they have been reconstituted, as long as they are stored at 4°C but, because they often contain no antiseptic or preservative, it becomes increasingly more hazardous to insert a fresh needle through the cap more than two or three times, or to keep any open vial for more than 6–8 hours. It is, therefore, standard practice to discard all vials promptly after they have been opened (with the few exceptions specifically mentioned in the individual monographs in Part 2).

Drug dilution: Many drugs have to be diluted before they can be used in babies because they were formulated for use in adults. In addition, dilution is almost always required when a drug is given as a continuous infusion. Serious errors can occur at this stage if the dead space in the hub of the syringe is overlooked. Thus if a drug is drawn into a 1 ml syringe up to the 0·05 ml mark the *syringe* will then contain between 0·14 and 0·18 ml of drug. If the syringe is then filled to 1 ml with diluent the syringe will contain **three times** as much drug as was intended!

To dilute any drug safely, therefore, draw some diluent into the syringe first, preferably until the syringe is about half full, and then add the active drug. Mix the drug and diluent if necessary at this stage by one or two gentle movements of the plunger, and then finally make the syringe up to the planned total volume with further diluent. In this way the distance between two of the graduation marks on the side of the syringe can be used to measure the amount of active drug added.

While this may be adequate for ten-fold dilution, it is not accurate enough where a greater dilution than this is required. In this situation it is necessary to use two syringes linked by a sterile 3-way tap. The active drug is drawn up into a suitable *small* syringe and then injected into the larger syringe through the side port of the tap. The tap is then turned so as to occlude the side port and diluent added to the *main* syringe until the desired total volume is reached.

Detailed guidance is given in Part 2 of this compendium on how to reconstitute each drug prior to administration, and how to handle drug dilution whenever this is called for. This can be found under the heading 'Supply' or 'Supply and administration' in each drug monograph.

Giving drugs by mouth: Oral medication is clearly unsuitable for babies who are shocked, acidotic or otherwise obviously unwell because there is a real risk of paralytic ileus and delayed absorption. Babies well enough to take milk feeds, however, are nearly always well enough to take medication by mouth, and many drugs are just as effective when given this way. Antibiotics that can be given by mouth to any baby well enough to take milk feeds without detriment to the blood levels that are achieved include amoxicillin, ampicillin, cephalexin, chloramphenicol, ciprofloxacin, co-trimoxazole, erythromycin, flucloxacillin, fluconazole, flucytosine, isoniazid, metronidazole, pyrimethamine, rifampicin, sodium fusidate and trimethoprim. Oral administration is often quicker, cheaper and safer than intravenous administration. Oral administration is also much more easily managed on the postnatal wards, and treatment can then be continued by the parents after discharge where appropriate.

Remember that if medicine is passed down an orogastric or nasogastric feeding tube much of it will be left in the tube unless it is then flushed through. It used to be standard practice to formulate drugs given by mouth so that the neonatal dose was always given in 5 ml aliquots (one teaspoonful), but this practice has now been discontinued. Dilution often reduced stability and shortened the drug's shelf life, while dilution with a syrup containing glucose threatened to increase the risk of caries in recently erupted teeth in later infancy. Small quantities are best given from a dropper bottle (try to avoid the pipette touching the tongue) or dropped onto the back of the tongue from the nozzle of a syringe.

Additives to milk: Vitamins are often added to milk. Sodium, phosphate and bicarbonate can also be given as a dietary supplement in the same way. It is important to remember that if only half the proffered feed is taken, only half the medicine is administered. Where possible all of a day's supplements should be added to the first feed of the day, so the baby still gets all that was prescribed even if feeding is later curtailed. The giving of any such dietary supplement must be recorded either on the feed chart or on the drug prescription sheet, and, to avoid confusion, each unit needs to develop a consistent policy in this regard.

IV drugs: Intravenous drugs should be given slowly and, where possible, through a secure established intravenous line containing glucose and/or sodium chloride. Drugs should never be injected or connected into a line containing blood or a blood product. Since the volume of drug to be given seldom exceeds 2 ml in neonatal practice, abrupt administration can be avoided by siting a 3-way tap so there is only 10–25 cm of narrow-bore tubing containing about 2 ml of fluid between the tap and the patient. Give the drug over about 5 seconds as described under the heading 'IV injections' below, but do not, except in special circumstances, flush the drug through. The adoption of this practice as a *routine* ensures that any 'bolus' of drug reaches the patient slowly over a period of 5–20 minutes after being injected into the fluid line without staff having to stand by the patient throughout the period of administration, or set up a special mechanical infusion system.

On the rare occasions when a small rapid bolus injection *is* called for (as, for example, when adenosine is used in the management of a cardiac arrhythmia) the drug infusion should be followed by a 2 ml 'chaser' of 0·9% sodium chloride from a second syringe in order to flush the active drug through the IV line as rapidly as possible. Do not flush the drug through by changing the basic infusion rate: several deaths have resulted from a failure to handle this manoeuvre correctly. Giving a routine chaser by hand ties up valuable senior nursing time, tends to result in over-rapid administration when staff time is at a premium, and can, if repeated frequently, result in the baby getting a lot of undocumented water, sodium or glucose.

Particular care must be taken not to mix potentially incompatible fluids. This issue is dealt with, in some detail, below in the section on 'Care and use of intravascular lines' (see p. 12). Staff must also remain alert to the very real risks of air embolism, infection, inflammation, thrombosis and tissue extravasation (as set out in the earlier parts of that section). They should also be familiar with the management of anaphylaxis (see p. 136).

IV injections: The standard procedure for using a 3-way tap to give a slow IV 'stat' dose is to:
- Connect the pre-loaded syringe to the free tap inlet.
- Turn the tap so the syringe is connected to the patient and give the injection.
- Turn the tap so the syringe is connected to the giving set, draw up about 0·2 ml of infusion fluid, turn the tap back so the syringe is reconnected to the patient, and flush this fluid through so that it just enters the giving set.
- Where two drugs are scheduled for simultaneous administration proceed as outlined on p. 15.

While the above method is adequate for most purposes, it always results in the administration of too much medicine because it causes the baby to get the medicine that was trapped in the hub of the syringe. A slightly more complex (and expensive) procedure that avoids this problem is preferable when the amount of drug to be given is less than 0·3 ml, and essential whenever a potentially toxic drug such as digoxin, chloramphenicol or an aminoglycoside is given intravenously. Proceed as above but modify the third of the three stages listed by using a second small syringe containing water for injection or 0·9% sodium chloride, instead of fluid from the drip line, and flush just 0·2 ml of fluid through the tap. Do not give more than this or you will end up giving the drug as a relatively rapid bolus.

Slow intermittent IV infusions: Drugs that need to be given by slow intermittent IV infusion (such as phenobarbital, sodium bicarbonate or THAM) can, if necessary, be given by hand through a 3-way tap as a series of 2 ml bolus doses every few minutes, but aciclovir, amphotericin B, ciprofloxacin, co-trimoxazole, erythromycin, fluconazole, flucytosine, phenytoin, rifampicin, sodium fusidate, vancomycin and zidovudine are best injected into an existing IV line through a 3-way tap using a programmable syringe pump. Slow infusion has been recommended for a range of other antibiotics without the support of any justificatory evidence. Manufacturers recommend slow aminoglycoside administration in North America, but not in Europe. Inconsistencies abound. The continued unquestioning acceptance of any time-consuming policy of this type without a critical review of its justification limits the time staff can give to other potentially more important tasks.

Continuous IV infusions: Drugs for continuous infusion such as adrenaline, atracurium, atosiban, diamorphine, dobutamine, dopamine, doxapram, enoximone, epoprostenol, glyceryl trinitrate, hydrocortisone, insulin, isoprenaline, Intralipid®, labetalol, lidocaine, magnesium sulphate, midazolam, milrinone, morphine, noradrenaline, nitroprusside, oxytocin, prostaglandin E, streptokinase, thiopentone and tolazoline should be administered from a second carefully labelled infusion pump connected by a 3-way tap into the main infusion line. Remember to readjust the total fluid intake. Great care is needed to ensure that patients never receive even a brief surge of one of the vasoactive drugs accidentally, and the same is true of many inotropes.

Never load the syringe or burette with more of the drug than is likely to be needed in 12–24 hours to limit the risk of accidental overinfusion. Also check and chart the rate at which the infusion pump is actually operating by looking at the amount of fluid left once an hour. The guidelines relating to the administration of intermittent IV injections also apply when a continuous infusion is first set up.

IM administration: Intramuscular medication is more reliable than oral medication in a baby who is unwell, but drug release from the intramuscular 'depot' is sometimes slow (a property that is used to advantage during treatment with naloxone, procaine penicillin and vitamin K). It may also be unreliable if there is circulatory shock. Bulky injections are also painful, but it should not necessarily be assumed that permanent attachment to an IV line is without its frustrations either, especially if this involves limb splinting. Prior cleaning of the skin is largely a token ritual. The main hazard of IM medication is the risk that the injection will accidentally damage a major nerve. Small babies have little muscle bulk and the sciatic nerve is easily damaged when drugs are given into the buttock, even when a conscious effort is made to direct the injection into the outer upper quadrant. The anterior aspect of the quadriceps muscle in the thigh is the *only* safe site in a small wasted baby, and this is the only site that should be used routinely in the first year of life. Try to alternate between the two legs if multiple injections are required. Multiple large injections into the same muscle can, very rarely, precipitate an ischaemic fibrosis severe enough to cause muscle weakness and a later disabling contracture. Intramuscular injection should also be avoided in any patient with a severe uncorrected bleeding tendency. A superficial injection may result in the drug entering subcutaneous fat rather than muscular tissue causing induration, fat necrosis, delayed drug release and a palpable subcutaneous lump that may persist for many weeks. An intradermal injection can also leave a permanent scar. With certain drugs, such as bupivacaine, the accidental injection of drug into a blood vessel during deep tissue infiltration is toxic to the heart, and it is essential to pull back the plunger each time the needle is moved to ensure that a vessel has not been entered. It is also wise to give any dose slowly while using a pulse oximeter in order to get early warning of any possible adverse cardiorespiratory effect.

Intradermal and subcutaneous administration: BCG vaccine has to be given *into* the skin (intradermally). The best technique for achieving this is outlined on p. 53. A number of other products, including insulin and the cytokines filgrastim and erythropoietin, are designed to be given into the fatty tissue just below the skin (subcutaneously). Vaccines were often given subcutaneously in the past, but it is now generally accepted that IM injection actually causes less pain at the time and less discomfort afterwards. IM injection also improves the immune response. It is wrong to assume that a long needle makes any injection more painful – there are many pain receptors just below the skin but relatively few in muscle tissue. Approach the skin vertically when giving an IM injection, and at 45° when giving a subcutaneous injection. Use a needle at *least* 15 mm long for any IM injection, even in the smallest baby.

Rectal administration: This can be a useful way of giving a drug that is normally given by mouth to a baby who is not being fed. Chloral hydrate, cisapride, codeine phosphate and paracetamol are sometimes given this way. So are some anticonvulsants such as carbamazepine, diazepam and paraldehyde. However, absorption is usually slower, often less complete, and sometimes less reliable than with oral administration. Suppositories have usually been used in the past but liquid formations are more appropriate in the neonatal period. Absorption is always more rapid and often more complete when a liquid formulation is used. It is also much easier to administer a precise, weight-related, dose. Half a suppository does not necessarily contain half the active ingredient even when accurately halved.

Intrathecal and intraventricular administration: Streptomycin was the first effective antituberculous drug. Because it does not cross the blood:brain barrier well, a policy of repeated intrathecal injection evolved to cope with the scourge of TB meningitis. It then quickly became common to treat other forms of meningitis the same way. Penicillin, in particular, was quite often injected into the cerebrospinal fluid (CSF), even though good levels can be achieved with high-dose IV treatment. This approach is now seldom adopted because a range of antibiotics are available that penetrate the CSF well. Gentamicin and vancomycin are, however, still occasionally injected into the CSF in babies with ventriculitis, particularly if the ventricles need to be tapped diagnostically, or therapeutically, because of obstructive hydrocephalus. Diagnostic needling of a thick-walled intracerebral abscess can also usefully be followed by the direct injection of a suitable antibiotic into the abscess cavity. The use of an intraventricular reservoir is often recommended when repeated intrathecal treatment is called for, but implanted plastic can increase the difficulty of eliminating bacterial infection because there is a strong risk of the catheter itself becoming colonised.

The intrathecal dose is always much smaller than the IV or IM dose because of the smaller volume of distribution. Gentamicin is still sometimes given into the cerebral ventricles, but the only published controlled trial has suggested that children so treated actually did worse than children given standard IV treatment. Many antibiotics are irritant and the preservatives even more so. Special intrathecal preparations of benzylpenicillin and gentamicin should always be used. Dilute the preparation before use, and check there is free flow of CSF before injecting the drug.

Intraosseous administration: This can be a valuable way of providing fluid in an emergency. Any drug that can be given IV can also be given by this route. Insert the needle into the upper end of the tibia a little below the tuberosity, using a slight screwing action, until marrow is entered. Point the needle obliquely and away from the knee joint. An 18 gauge bone marrow needle is best, but success can be achieved with a 21 gauge lumbar puncture needle and stylet. The resultant fat embolisation is almost always silent; osteomyelitis is the only common complication.

Administration into the lung: Surfactant is the only drug regularly given down an endotracheal tube, but drugs occasionally given this way include adrenaline, atropine, diazepam, lidocaine, midazolam, naloxone, propranolol and tolazoline. Tolazoline is the only drug where a sound case has been made for such an approach. Surfactant is best delivered using a catheter inserted just beyond the end of the endotracheal tube. Other drugs should be diluted in, or followed by, a 2 ml 'chaser' of sterile water, since using 0·9% saline for this purpose, or for regular endotracheal toilet, can impose an unpredictable sodium load on the baby.

A range of drugs, including adrenaline, betamethasone, epoprostenol, furosemide, ipratropium, nitroprusside, salbutamol and tribavirin have sometimes been administered as a fine nebulised mist. Face masks have usually been used for this in the past, but a modification of the Infant Flow® CPAP device is probably a better alternative. For a description of at least one effective way of achieving this see the article by Smedsaas-Löfvenberg et al. in Acta Paediatr 1999;**88**:89−92.

Excipients: Drugs often contain preservatives, solvents and stabilisers ('excipients'), and staff need to be aware that these can occasionally have an unpredictable effect. Such problems have occurred with particular frequency in neonatal and paediatric practice. Excessive amounts of IV benzyl alcohol can cause a 'gasping' syndrome, collapse and even death in the preterm baby (as is outlined in the web-archived monograph), so neonatal exposure needs to be minimised and very carefully monitored. Amiodarone, clindamycin, clonazepam, diazepam, heparin and lorazepam are the only drugs mentioned in the main section of this compendium where at least one commonly used UK product contains benzyl alcohol, but rather more US products still contain this excipient.

Propylene glycol is used to improve the solubility of some drugs, and the UK products that contain this solvent are noted. Guidelines say that exposure in adults should not, if possible, exceed 25 mg/kg a day − a level easily exceeded during neonatal use. While exposure to more than this does not usually cause a problem, very high levels can cause seizures, hyperosmolality and other problems (as is outlined in the web-archived monograph on enoximone). Some products for oral use in young children (including some, but not all, iron supplements) contain quite a lot of alcohol. How safe this is in the preterm baby is not entirely clear. The sulphite used in some parenteral formulations of dexamethasone is now known to be neurotoxic in mice, as is discussed in greater detail in the web commentary attached to the monograph on betamethasone (see p. 56).

It is always best to avoid any product containing fructose, glucose or sucrose when giving an older child medicine on a regular basis to minimize the risk of dental caries. These products are listed as sugar-free in this compendium (as they are in the BNF) even if they contain hydrogenated glucose syrup, maltitol, mannitol, sorbitol or xylitol.

Drugs and the body

Pharmacokinetics describes how drugs are absorbed, distributed and excreted by the body and *pharmacodynamics* how they act within it. What follows is a simple introduction to some of the (*italicised*) terms and concepts most frequently encountered.

Drugs taken by mouth are only effective if absorbed, unless, like Gaviscon® or nystatin, they act on, or in, the gut. Many antibiotics are destroyed when given by mouth, although a small alteration in structure may change a drug like benzylpenicillin (penicillin G), which is destroyed by acid, into a drug like penicillin V, which is not. Food may reduce intestinal absorption; milk, for example, reduces the absorption of tetracycline. Delayed gastric emptying, poor peristalsis or ileus will delay arrival in the upper small intestine, where most absorption occurs. Some drugs (like aciclovir) are never completely absorbed. Others, though well absorbed, also show reduced *bioavailability* because they are metabolised by the liver, before reaching the rest of the body. These are said to show extensive *first-pass* metabolism. Morphine by mouth shows about 30% bioavailability for this reason. If a drug is well absorbed, this delay can be circumvented by rectal (diazepam), buccal or nasal (midazolam) administration. Intramuscular administration is usually effective, but drug release from the intramuscular 'depot' may be slow (naloxone), or deliberately made slow (insulin), and may make IM treatment unpredictable (phenytoin). Intravenous administration is usually the most reliable strategy, but drugs (like vancomycin) may need to be given slowly because even transiently high levels cause problems (such as histamine release). Consistent *side effects* like this (and the *toxic* effects of overtreatment) are easier to anticipate than less predictable *adverse reactions*. For some drugs, tissue levels exceed plasma levels; such drugs are said to have a *volume of distribution* (V_D) in l/kg that exceeds one.

Most drugs are structurally altered by oxidation, reduction or hydrolysis in the liver, and most of the resultant products are pharmacologically inactive. However, some drugs only become active after modification. One such *prodrug*, chloral hydrate, is inert until transformed into trichloroethanol. Other drugs are 'neutralised' (and made more water soluble) by conjugation. However, N-demethylation of diazepam produces desmethyl-diazepam, which remains active in the body for longer than diazepam itself. Babies are slow to deal with many drugs because enzyme levels controlling conjugation (such as acetylation, glucuronidation, methylation and sulphation) are low after birth. Drug *interactions* can speed up (phenobarbitone) or slow down (cimetidine) the metabolism of other drugs by the liver.

Many drugs are eliminated by the kidneys. For some unmetabolised drugs, like gentamicin, glomerular filtration is the only means of elimination. The speed of elimination only changes slowly, therefore, in the weeks after birth. Other drugs, like the penicillins, are excreted with increasing rapidity after delivery as renal tubular secretion becomes more active. The dose required depends on the drug's distribution within the body, and dose frequency on its speed of elimination. This is usually proportional to the amount present, unless saturation occurs (as with phenytoin). It can be described by the time it takes for the blood level to halve (elimination *half life* or $t_{1/2}$), a relationship (Fig. 1a) that is linear when plotted on a log scale (Fig. 1b). The aim is to achieve and sustain levels in the safe therapeutic range. Response to a drug may improve as levels increase (Fig. 1c), but toxic effects may also appear, and the ratio of the toxic to the therapeutic level (*therapeutic index*) may be quite small. A drug has to be given for a time equal to 4 half lives before levels stabilise (Fig. 1d), unless a *loading dose* is given (Fig. 1e).

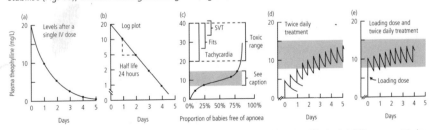

Fig. 1 Baby with a theophylline half life of 24 hours. The therapeutic range (8–15 mg/l) is shaded. SVT, supraventricular tachycardia.

Drugs and the law

Licensing

While the UK laws that control the prescribing and the supply of medicines may seem complex, they actually impose few constraints on staff working in a hospital setting. The Medicines Act of 1968, passed in the wake of the thalidomide disaster, regulates the activity of the pharmaceutical industry, making it illegal for any medicine to be marketed for human use in the UK without a product licence (marketing authorisation). These are issued by the Licensing Authority (the Ministers of Health) on the advice of the Medicines and Healthcare products Regulatory Agency (MHRA). The MHRA also oversees the manufacture, promotion and distribution of medicines, while the Committee on Safety of Medicines (CSM) advises the Agency on their efficacy, quality and safety. While these licences are not published, the relevant provisions, including indications for use, recommended precautions and dose ranges, are summarised in the manufacturer's Summary of Product Characteristics (SPC). These summaries can now be accessed via the Internet (www.medicines.org.uk), as can copies of the manufacturer's Patient Information Leaflet (PIL) drafted to make key information available in a more accessible format. Datapharm Communications also publishes the same information on a compact disc and in book format.

The 1968 Act was deliberately framed in such a way that it did not restrict 'clinical freedom', and it exempts doctors and dentists from many of the constraints placed on drug companies. It is, therefore, perfectly in order for a doctor to recommend, or administer, a drug for which no product licence exists. The Act and EC Directive 89/341/EEC also make it clear that a doctor can use an unlicensed drug in clinical trials, or give an unlicensed product that has been specially prepared or imported, for a particular ('named') patient. It is also acceptable for a doctor to use, or recommend the use of, a drug in a dose, by a route, for a condition, or for a group of patients, that differs from those mentioned in the manufacturer's product licence (so-called 'off label' or 'off licence' use). It is also legal for such a drug to be dispensed by a pharmacist, or administered by a nurse or midwife. Legislation in America and many other countries has adopted a similar approach.

This legal freedom places doctors under a heavy legal, moral and professional obligation to ensure that the recommendations they make about drug use are well founded. Such problems become acute when a manufacturer offers no advice with regard to the use of a drug for children of less than a certain age, as is, for example, currently true of almost all the drugs used to manage hypotension and hypertension in childhood. Such problems can turn children into 'therapeutic orphans'. Manufacturers are often reluctant to bear the cost of sponsoring the trials necessary to support a change to the original marketing licence, or the cost of collating all the information published in the scientific literature after a product's first commercial launch so the licence can be updated. Here it becomes particularly important for the doctor to be sure that the use to which they are putting a product is reasonable and prudent in the light of such scientific information as *is* available in print. This compendium is one aid to that end. The *BNF for children* (BNFC) offers similar guidance on how to handle some of the many situations in which older children may need to be treated in ways not covered by the manufacturer's recommendations, but it is not a referenced text. In addition it only provides limited information on how to manage drug treatment in the ill preterm baby, and it provides very little useful guidance on drug use during pregnancy and lactation.

Prescribing

The 1968 Act classifies medicines into those available for general sale (a General Sale List, or GSL drug), those only available for retail sale through a pharmacy (P) and those that can only be dispensed from a pharmacy against a prescription (a Prescription Only Medicine, or POM). Additional rules apply to Controlled Drugs (CD). All medicines, other than GSL drugs, have to be sold from a registered pharmacy *unless* they are being sold or supplied by a hospital or health centre, and are being administered in accordance with the directions of a doctor. The only POM products that could be dispensed by a community pharmacist without a doctor's prescription (except in an emergency) were, until now, the few products in the Nurse Prescribers' and Dental Practitioners' Formularies, as listed in the *British national formulary* (BNF) and the BNFC.

Non-medical prescribing: However, new legislation came into force in the UK in May 2006 that makes it possible for senior, experienced, first level nurses, midwives, specialist community public health nurses, and some pharmacists, to acquire almost exactly the same prescribing rights as doctors. Staff put forward for such training will need to be working in an area where this skill could be put to use. They will also need the background to be able to study at level 3 (degree level), to have acquired at least 3 years' post-registration clinical experience, and to have been working for at least the last year in the clinical area in which they are expecting to prescribe once trained. Their register will be annotated to record the successful completion of this training, and they will then be in a position where they can legally prescribe any licensed drug, even for 'off label' use, as long as it is not a controlled drug (where some, slightly ambiguous, restrictions still operate). Any borderline food product, dressing or appliance listed in the BNF can also be prescribed. Staff so qualified will all be at least as aware as any doctor of the need to work within the limits of their sphere of professional competence, and within any guidelines laid down by their employing authority. These developments should, once such training becomes more generally available, make it much easier for senior midwifery and nursing staff to start treatment when it is called for without first having to get a doctor to authorise this. They will also make it possible for experienced nurses and midwives to manage urgent inter-hospital transfers appropriately even when there is not a doctor on the transfer team.

There are, however, a few residual restrictions and uncertainties. It is not, for example, possible for an Independent Nurse Prescriber to initiate treatment with caffeine in a neonatal unit because this is still an unlicensed medicine in the UK. The indications for which a limited range of controlled drugs can now be prescribed are not always very precisely specified either (an area where legislation is as much a matter for the UK Home Office as for the Department of Health). Morphine can be given for suspected myocardial infarction, for 'postoperative pain relief' and for 'pain caused by trauma', but it is not clear whether this includes the pain associated with childbirth, or the trauma associated with many aspects of neonatal intensive care. Staff can also give morphine to a baby with severe necrotising enterocolitis but only, it would seem, after surgery. Diazepam, lorazepam and midazolam can be used to control 'tonic-clonic seizures' and can also be used, like morphine and diamorphine, to provide 'palliative care', but that phrase is often used to mean simply the terminal care of a patient with an untreatable condition rather than the palliation of the stress associated with the sudden urgent need to initiate artificial respiratory support. Doubtless most of these residual uncertainties will be clarified in time.

Patient Group Directions: Because legislation in the UK does not allow most nurses to prescribe, alternative, more flexible, strategies have been developed in the last 8 years to enable appropriately trained staff to assume greater personal responsibility for administering a range of POM products. An 'ad hoc' system of 'Group Protocols' was recognised as having merit by the Crown Report in 1998, and legislation was passed in 2000 making it legal for nurses to supply and administer any licensed medicine (even 'off label') to specific groups of patients under a formal agreement with a prescribing doctor. The work of pharmacists, physiotherapists and other 'paramedic' groups can be covered in a similar way. Such agreements (known as Patient Group Directions, or PGDs) need to conform to the guidance given in HSC 2000/026 (England), HDL (2001) 7 (Scotland) and WHC (200) 116 (Wales), and any Direction has to be prepared by a multidisciplinary group involving a senior doctor, pharmacist and nurse or midwife, in consultation with the local Drug and Therapeutics Committee, and then approved by the Hospital or Primary Care Trust.

While the introduction of PGDs is restricted to situations where such administration 'offers an advantage to patient care without compromising patient safety', there are many aspects of maternity care where it is clearly possible to improve the delivery of care by making better use of these, as yet very inconsistently applied, arrangements. Vaccine administration (including hepatitis B vaccine) has been the aspect of primary care most often covered by the development of PGDs. However, the administration of rhesus D immunoglobulin, the initiation of antenatal betamethasone treatment, and the provision of prophylactic antibiotic cover to any mother (and/or baby) where there has been significant prelabour rupture of membranes, are three further important aspects of maternity care that can often be improved by the development of an appropriate PGD at unit level. Unfortunately, because PGDs cannot be used to initiate treatment with a controlled drug, pethidine still remains, very inappropriately, the only controlled drug that a midwife can prescribe and administer on her own authority. There is a widespread belief that these Directions can only be used to administer a single dose of some licensed medicinal product – this is incorrect. A PGD can certainly, for example, be used in appropriate circumstances to initiate a course of antibiotic treatment.

Supplementary prescribing provides an alternative strategy for involving nurses and midwives more productively in the management of conditions where treatment needs may vary over time, allowing staff to prescribe from within the elements of a previously agreed joint management plan. Some hospitals in the UK have used this option to allow bedside intensive care staff to adjust treatment hour by hour as the patient's condition dictates, but the option has been more widely adopted in the community management of long-term medical conditions such as asthma or diabetes.

Care and use of intravascular lines

Intravascular lines serve a number of vital functions. They make it possible to give fluids, including glucose and a range of other nutrients, when oral nutrition is impossible or inappropriate. They also make it possible to monitor both arterial and central venous pressure directly and continuously, to collect blood specimens without causing pain or disturbance, and to give drugs reliably and painlessly.

These very real advantages have to be balanced against a range of very real disadvantages. Of these, infection due to localised vasculitis or insidious low-grade septicaemia is perhaps the most common. Vascular thrombosis is a hazard, and thrombi can also shed emboli. Even reactive arterial vasospasm can cause significant ischaemia. Bleeding from an arterial line can cause serious blood loss, life-threatening air embolism can occur into any central venous line, and fluid extravasation can cause severe ischaemia or chemical tissue damage with subsequent necrosis. Any baby with an intravascular line in place is at risk of sudden fluid overload if steps are not taken to make the unintentional and uncontrolled infusion of more than 30 ml/kg of fluid technically impossible (see the section on minimising hazards on p. 17). There is also a risk of reactive hypoglycaemia if any glucose infusion is stopped (or the rate changed) too abruptly.

Because complications are thought to be common and become more common with prolonged use, umbilical vein catheters have not been much used in the last 40 years, and even more rarely left in place for long when used. However, a trial involving 200 babies weighing less than 1·25 kg has recently shown that, when properly cared for, an umbilical vein catheter is no more likely to cause complications than a percutaneous central venous catheter. As long as the tip was known to be at the point where the inferior vena cava joins the right atrium, it was found to be perfectly reasonable to use this route for at least 2–3 weeks. Since the insertion of an umbilical vein catheter soon after birth requires much less skill than the insertion of a percutaneous 'long line', and also subjects the baby to less handling and less stress, it is surprising that this relatively simple approach is not more widely used.

Line care

Thrombosis: Relatively little can be done to reduce the risk of thrombosis. A small amount of heparin (q.v.) can reduce the risk of catheter occlusion, but this has little effect on the formation of mural thrombi. Whether the benefit of full heparinisation outweighs the risk remains unclear. Clinical vigilance can speed the recognition of problems when they occur, and the routine use of a lateral X-ray to identify where any central catheter has lodged can help to ensure that the tip is optimally sited (a lateral X-ray is more easily interpreted than an anteroposterior (AP) view). An attempt is usually made to site any central venous catheter in a major vein, or at the entrance to the right atrium. The larger the vessel the less the risk of occlusion (or extravasation), but the greater the hazard should this occur. Similarly, it is standard practice to site any aortic catheter either above the diaphragm (T6) or below the two renal arteries (L4) to minimise the risk of a silent renal or mesenteric artery thrombosis, and there is now good controlled trial evidence that there are fewer recognisable complications associated with high placement (although there may be a marginally increased risk of necrotising enterocolitis). Case controlled studies suggest, however, that intraventricular haemorrhage may be commoner when aortic catheters are positioned above the diaphragm, and when heparin is used to prolong catheter patency. Only a very large, properly conducted, randomised controlled trial is likely to resolve some of these uncertainties.

Limb ischaemia is usually readily recognised, but by the time it is identified much of the damage has often been done. Thrombosis of the abdominal vessels is often silent, but may be a significant cause of renal hypertension. Central venous thrombosis is also underdiagnosed, but can cause a chylous ascites by occluding the exit of the thoracic duct. Occlusion of a small vein is seldom a problem because of the nature of the anastomotic venous plexus, but occlusion of even a small artery can cause severe ischaemia if it is an 'end artery' (i.e. the only vessel supplying a particular area of the body). Even occlusion of the radial artery can sometimes cause vascular compromise if there is no significant terminal anastamosis between the radial and ulnar arteries. Every baby with an intravascular line in place should be examined regularly by the nursing staff for evidence of any of the above complications. There are good grounds for particular vigilance in the first few hours after an arterial line has been sited but, with this one exception, all lines merit equal vigilance. Treatment options are reviewed in a commentary linked to the monograph on the use of alteplase (see p. 39).

Vascular spasm: Arteries are particularly likely to go into spasm shortly after cannulation. This may make it necessary to withdraw the catheter, but a single small dose of tolazoline can sometimes correct the acute 'white leg' seen after umbilical artery catheterisation, and a continued low-dose infusion may work when a single bolus dose is only transiently effective. Papaverine has also been used experimentally in the same way.

Extravasation: Never give a drug into a drip that has started to 'tissue'. Delivery can not be guaranteed once this has happened, and some drugs (as noted in the individual drug monographs) can also cause severe tissue damage. Fluids containing calcium cause particularly severe scaring. Serious damage can also be caused by the fluids used in providing parenteral nutrition. Such problems will only be noticed promptly if every drip is so strapped that the tissue around the cannula tip can be inspected at any time. The best line of management, if extravasation is starting to cause tissue damage, involves early tissue irrigation, as outlined in the monograph on hyaluronidase on p. 130. Hot or cold compresses are of no measurable value. Neither is limb elevation.

Infection: Localised or generalised infection is probably the commonest complication of the use of intravascular lines. Indolent, usually low grade, but occasionally life threatening, blood-borne infection (septicaemia) has been reported in more than 20% of all babies with 'long lines' in some units. Infection can be devastating in the small baby, and it is a clear indictment of unit policy if the way in which a baby is cared for puts it unnecessarily at increased risk of infection. The risk of such iatrogenic infection can only be minimised by scrupulous attention to hygiene. Inadequate attention to skin sterility (see p. 237) is probably the commonest reason why cannulas and catheters later become colonised. Access should always be achieved using an aseptic approach. A gown, mask and surgical drape should also be used whenever a long line is being inserted. The risk of infection is not reduced by the use of an antiseptic or antibiotic cream. Indeed there is evidence that such use can actually increase the risk of fungal infection. Covering the insertion site with a transparent occlusive dressing helps even though increased humidity under such a dressing can speed the multiplication of skin bacteria. An impregnated chlorhexidine disc may help prevent this.

Infection most frequently enters where the catheter pierces the skin. This is why most infusion-related infections are caused by coagulase-negative staphylococci, and why Broviac lines 'tunnelled' surgically under the skin less often become infected. Complications, including infection, seem commoner in neonates if the line is inserted into an arm rather than a leg. Bacterial colonisation of the catheter hub (where the catheter connects to the giving set) can also be the precursor of overt septicaemia. Stopcocks often become contaminated, but there is no evidence that such contamination causes catheter-related infection. The risk of generalised infection is increased by the use of a long line rather than a short line. Independently of this, parenteral nutrition may, and Intralipid® certainly does, further increase the risk of systemic infection. Antibiotic treatment for this can, in turn, greatly increase the risk of life-threatening fungal septicaemia. These are strong reasons for avoiding the unnecessary use of long lines, and for only using parenteral nutrition when oral feeding is impracticable. Catheters impregnated with an antimicrobial agent have started to become available, but their use is no substitute for proper attention to other aspects of catheter hygiene. Impregnation with minocycline and rifampicin seems better than impregnation with chlorhexidine and silver sulfadiazine.

It used to be thought that the risk of infection could be reduced by resiting all infusions at regular intervals, and short cannulas are still often resited in adults once every 2–3 days to reduce the risk of phlebitis and catheter colonisation. There is, as yet, no good evidence that this approach is justified in children. It also used to be said that fluids and administration sets should to be changed daily to minimise the risk of in-use fluid contamination, but this practice is *not* now endorsed by the American Centres for Disease Control in Atlanta, Georgia. Such routines generate a lot of work, increase costs and have not been shown to reduce the risk of blood stream infection. Unnecessary interference with the infusion line could actually increase the risk. There is, however, one small controlled trial (in urgent need of confirmation) suggesting that the regular use of an in-line filter does reduce the risk septicaemia in the preterm baby, and that this remains true even if the giving set is only changed only once every 4 days. There are also good grounds for changing the administration set each time the infusion fluid is changed (although infusion with insulin may be an exception to this generalization, as explained on p. 141). This is particularly important after any blood or blood product has been given, because the presence of a thin thrombin film increases the chance of bacteria then colonising the giving set. Lipid solutions are also particularly likely to become infected, and it is probably good practice to change these once every 48 hours. In addition, some continuously infused drugs are only stable for a limited time (as outlined in the individual drug monographs) and need to be prepared afresh once every 12–24 hours. There is no evidence that other fluids (or giving sets) need to be changed more than once every 3–4 days. The catheter *must* be removed promptly once bacteraemia is documented if complications are to be minimised (a single coagulase-negative staphylococcal blood culture being the only exception to this general rule).

Air embolism: Air can kill a patient very rapidly. Air is so much more compressible than blood that once it enters the heart it tends to stay there instead of being pumped on round the body, especially if the baby is lying flat. This air then completely stops the circulation unless immediately aspirated. Umbilical vein catheters are particularly dangerous; air can easily be drawn into the heart when the baby takes a breath if there is not a tap or syringe on the end of any catheter at all times (especially during insertion). Similarly, if air gets into a giving set (through, for example, a cracked syringe) it can easily be pumped into the blood stream.

Blood loss: Babies can easily die of blood loss. Serious loss from the cord has become rare since the invention of the modern plastic umbilical clamp, but haemorrhage can still occur if no clamp has been placed on the umbilical vessels so that they can be cannulated (especially if the baby is then wrapped up for warmth with, perhaps, a 'silver swaddler', through which tell-tale blood cannot seep). Death can also occur from haemorrhage if an intravascular line becomes disconnected. To minimise this latter risk all connections in any intravascular line should always have Luer-Lok® fittings.

Use of lines

There has been a lot of confused thought as to what may, and may not, be put into what sort of intravascular line. Policy varies widely from unit to unit, and all the policies cannot possibly be right. There is equal uncertainty over who has the necessary authority to put drugs into, or take blood out of, what sort of line. True 'authority' comes with training and experience, not with the mere possession of a medical qualification.

A midwife or nurse who has been trained in the care and use of intravascular catheters will often be in a better position to give safe care than a 'qualified' but untrained and inexperienced doctor. With proper training all qualified staff working in any neonatal unit ought to be equally competent in all aspects of intravascular catheter care and use. Anyone experienced enough to give drugs into an established line should have enough experience to sample blood from such a line, and anyone who has been trained to give drugs or to sample from a venous catheter has all the knowledge necessary to use a properly inserted arterial line.

What you can safely put *into* a line depends not only on what sort of line it is, but also on what sort of fluid is already in the line (see below). This is also true of what you can reliably take *out* of a line. Any line can, in theory, be used for blood sampling, but care needs to be taken to clear the 'dead space' first. Sodium levels can only be measured from a line being infused with 0·9% sodium chloride after a volume equal to three times the dead space has been withdrawn first. Blood glucose levels cannot be measured in a blood sample taken from *any* line through which glucose is being infused, even if the catheter dead space is first cleared by temporarily withdrawing 5 ml of blood before collecting the sample for analysis. Nor can reliable blood coagulation test results be obtained from any line that has ever contained heparin. False-positive evidence of infection can also result if blood is drawn for blood culture from an already established intravascular line. Where septicaemia is suspected it is always best to collect blood direct into a culture medium from a fresh venous 'needle stab'.

Peripheral veins: These can be used for collecting blood samples and for giving almost any drug, although care should be taken when infusing a number of vasoactive drugs (as indicated in the relevant drug monographs). Drugs such as dopamine and isoprenaline are better delivered through a central venous line. Where there is no need to give a continuous infusion, a cannula can be inserted and left 'stopped off' with a rubber injection 'bung'. There is no good evidence that these benefit from heparinisation and, in any strict interpretation of the regulations, both the drug *and* the heparinised flush solution would need to be prescribed, and each administration signed for separately each time (although it has not, as yet, generally been considered necessary to record the giving of every 'flush' of saline or water).

Central veins: Drugs can be given safely into any central venous line once ultrasound, or an X-ray, has shown where the catheter tip has lodged, and this is the best route for giving any drug or infusion that tends to damage the vascular endothelium (such as solutions containing more than 10% glucose). Keep the tip away from the right atrium and mediastinal vessels since, if wall damage *does* occur, the resultant pleural or pericardial effusion will kill if not recognised promptly. Anchor the exposed end of the catheter firmly to the skin – serious complications can arise if the catheter migrates further into the body after insertion. Better still, cut the catheter to the right length before insertion. Only give drugs into an umbilical vein catheter as a last resort if the tip has lodged in a portal vein. Any midwife or nurse who has been trained to give drugs into a peripheral vein should be competent to give drugs into a central vein. However, because of the greater risk of infection when a central line is in place, such lines should not be 'broken into' either to give drugs or to sample blood unnecessarily. It will often be difficult to sample blood from a central venous line because of its length and narrow bore. Furthermore, if blood is allowed to track back up a central venous catheter there is a serious risk of a clot developing, blocking the line.

Peripheral arteries: Such lines are almost always inserted in order to monitor blood pressure, or to sample arterial blood. They should never be used for giving drugs. The right radial artery is the most frequently used vessel. It may be safe to use a continuous infusion of glucose saline into a peripheral artery, but it is probably best to limit any infusion to as small a volume of heparinised 0·18% (or 0·9%) sodium chloride as is compatible with maintaining catheter patency (see p. 127).

Central arteries: These will almost always be aortic catheters positioned through an umbilical artery. Such lines are usually sited in order to monitor blood pressure or sample post-ductal arterial blood, but they can safely be used to give glucose or total parenteral nutrition once the site of the catheter tip has been checked radiologically. Take care that this is not close to the coeliac axis, because exposing the pancreas to an infusion of concentrated glucose can cause hypoglycaemia by stimulating an excessive release of insulin. Because blood flow down the aorta is high it is also perfectly safe to give most drugs (other than some of the vasoconstrictive drugs such as adrenaline, dopamine and isoprenaline) as a slow continuous infusion into the aorta. Bolus infusions should be avoided, however, unless there is no realistic alternative (particularly if the drug is a vascular irritant) because of the risk that an excessive amount of drug will be delivered into a single vulnerable 'end artery'. Severe tissue necrosis in the area served by the internal iliac artery has been documented quite frequently when drugs such as undiluted sodium bicarbonate have been administered as a bolus into an umbilical artery during emergency resuscitation after circulatory collapse.

Compatible and incompatible fluids

All the drugs mentioned in the main section of this compendium as being suitable for intravenous use are capable of being injected into, or pickabacked onto, any existing IV infusion containing up to 0·9% sodium chloride and/or up to 10% glucose unless otherwise stated (amphotericin B, enoximone, phenytoin and erythromycin (unless buffered) being the main exceptions). Do not add drugs to any line containing blood or blood products.

Different drugs should never be mixed together, however, except as specified in the various drug monographs, without express pharmacy approval. Where a single infusion line *has* to be used to give more than one drug, and it is not practicable to delay the administration of the second drug for at least 10 minutes, different products must be separated by 1 ml of glucose saline, 0·9% sodium chloride or sterile water for injection (less will do with very narrow bore tubing). Adherence to these guidelines is particularly important where a very alkaline product such as sodium bicarbonate or THAM is being infused. Use the technique described under IV injection in the review of 'Neonatal drug administration' (see p. 6), and give the separating 1 ml bolus *slowly* over at least 2 minutes to ensure that the drug already in the IV line does not reach the patient as a sudden, dangerously rapid, surge. This is particularly important if the line contains an inotrope or vasoactive product, or a drug, such as aminophylline, cimetidine, phenytoin or ranitidine, which can cause a cardiac arrhythmia if infused too fast.

Special problems arise when it is necessary to give more than one drug continuously, and intravascular access is limited. Here terminal co-infusion (the brief mixing of two different infusates using a T tap or Y connector sited as close to the patient as possible) is sometimes known to be safe. In this situation the two drugs are only in contact for a relatively short time (although with slow infusion rates in a very small baby contact may last longer than is generally appreciated). In the most frequently encountered situations where such co-infusion is thought to be safe a statement to this effect has been added to one of the two relevant drug monographs. The documentary evidence for this practice comes (unless otherwise stated) from *Trissel's Handbook of Injectable Drugs*. Note that, even here, compatibility will have only been formally assessed for a limited range of drug concentrations.

Special considerations apply to the administration of any drug into a line containing an amino acid solution when a baby requires parenteral nutrition. Terminal co-infusion using any product that approximates fairly closely to the formulation described in this compendium is probably safe for certain drugs, as outlined in the various drug monographs. It is not, however, safe to assume that this is true for other formulations. *No* drug (other than Vitlipid®) should ever be added to any infusion containing emulsified fat (Intralipid®), nor should lipid be co-infused with any fluid containing any other drug (other than heparin, insulin, isoprenaline, noradrenaline or vancomycin). The use of a double, or triple, lumen umbilical catheter makes it possible to give drugs to a baby receiving parenteral nutrition through a single infusion site.

References

American Academy of Pediatrics. Committee on Drugs. 'Inactive' ingredients in pharmaceutical products: update (subject review). *Pediatrics* 1997;**99**:268–78.

Benjamin DK, Miller W, Garges H, *et al*. Bacteremia, central catheters, and neonates: when to pull the line. *Pediatrics* 2001;**107**:1272–6.

Burn W, Whitman V, Marks VH, *et al*. Inadvertent over administration of digoxin to low-birth-weight infants. *J Pediatr* 1978;**92**:1024–5.

Buttler-O'Hara M, Buzzard CJ, Reubens L, *et al*. A randomized trial comparing long-term and short-term use of umbilical venous catheters in premature infants with birthweights of less than 1251 grams. *Pediatrics* 2006;**118**:e25–36. [RCT]

Dann TC. Routine skin preparation before injection: unnecessary procedure. *Lancet* 1969;**ii**:96–8.

Davies MW, Mehr S, Morley CJ. The effect of draw-up volume on the accuracy of electrolyte measurements from neonatal arterial lines. *J Paediatr Child Health* 2000;**36**:122–4.

Fletcher MA, MacDonald MG. *Atlas of procedures in neonatology*, 2nd edn. Philadelphia PA: JB Lippincott, 1993.

Gillies D, Wallen MM, Morrison AL, *et al*. Optimal timing for intravenous administration set replacement. *Cochrane Database of Systematic Reviews*, 2005, issue 4, article no CD003588.

Golombek SG, Rohan AJ, Parvez B, *et al*. 'Proactive' management of percutaneously inserted central catheters results in decreased incidence of infection in the ELBW population. *J Perinatol* 2002;**22**:209–13.

Hoang V, Sills J, Chandler M, *et al*. Percutaneously inserted central catheter for total parenteral nutrition in neonates: complications rates relating to upper versus lower extremity insertion. *Pediatrics* 2008;121:e1152–9.

Hodding JH. Medication administration via the umbilical arterial catheter: a survey of standard practices and review of the literature. *Am J Perinatol* 1990;**7**:329–32.

Leff RD, Roberts RJ. Methods for intravenous drug administration in the pediatric patient. *J Pediatr* 1981;**98**:631–5.

MacDonald MG, Chou MM. Preventing complications from lines and tubes. *Sem Perinatol* 1986;**10**:224–33.

Marlow AG, Kitai I, Kirpalani H, *et al*. A randomised trial of 72- versus 24-hour intravenous tubing set changes in newborns receiving lipid therapy. *Infect Control Hosp Epidemiol* 1999;**20**:487–93. [RCT]

Moore TD, ed. *Iatrogenic problems in neonatal intensive care*. Sixty-ninth Ross Conference on Pediatric Research. Columbus, OH: Ross Laboratories, 1976.

O'Grady NP, Alexander M, Dellinger EP, *et al*. Guidelines for the prevention of intravascular catheter-related infections. *Pediatrics* 2002;**110**:e51.

Orlowski JP. Emergency alternatives to intravenous access. *Pediatr Clin North Am* 1994;**41**:1183–99.

Phillips I, Meers PD, D'Arcy PF. *Microbiological hazards of infusion therapy*. Lancaster, UK: MTP Press Ltd, 1976.

Salzman MB, Rubin LG. Intravenous catheter-related infections *Adv Pediatr Infect Dis* 1995;**10**:337–68.

Sinclair JC, Bracken MB, eds. *Effective care of the newborn infant*. Oxford: Oxford University Press, 1992. (See especially Chapter 10, pp. 188–189, Chapter 19, pp. 440–441 and Chapter 23, p. 582.)

Trissel LA. *Handbook of Injectable Drugs*, 12th edn. Bethesda, MA: American Society of Hospital Pharmacists, 2003.

van Lingen RA, Baerts W, Marquering ACM, *et al*. The use in-line intravenous filters in sick newborn infants. *Acta Paediatr* 2004;**89**:658–62. [RCT]

Minimising IV infusion and drug hazards

Occasional errors of IV fluid and drug administration are inevitable. Their reporting is important, but their occurrence should never be made the pretext for disciplinary action unless there has been obvious negligence. Medical staff sometimes share responsibility for any administrative error that does occur by prescribing in an unclear or unnecessarily complex way. Staff new in place, at all levels, frequently find themselves working under considerable pressure, and low staffing levels often impose further stress. Management shares responsibility for protecting staff from excessive pressure, for ensuring that unit policies are such as to minimise the risk of any error occurring, and (even more importantly) for seeing that the potential danger associated with any error is minimised by the use of 'fail-safe' routines like those outlined below. If senior staff over-react when mistakes occur errors may simply go unreported, increasing the risk of a recurrence.

It is, moreover, important to retain a sense of proportion in considering the issues raised by the rule that every error of drug prescribing has to be reported. While any error of *commission* is generally looked upon as a potentially serious disciplinary issue, serious errors of *omission* often go unremarked. Yet an inadvertent reduction in IV fluid administration due to tissue extravasation, failure to resite an infusion line promptly, or failure to set up the syringe pump correctly, is more likely to put a baby at hazard (from reactive hypoglycaemia) than a transient period of excess fluid administration. Note that hypoglycaemia is particularly likely to occur where a maintenance infusion of glucose saline IV is cut back or stopped abruptly so that blood can be given (for guidance on this see the monograph on blood transfusion). Similarly, failure to give a dose of medicine may sometimes be just as hazardous as the administration of too big a dose.

Drug prescribing and drug administration call for close teamwork between the medical, midwifery and nursing staff. When an error does occur it is seldom one person's sole fault, and this needs to be acknowledged if disciplinary action is called for. Where it is clear that a doctor and a midwife or nurse both share responsibility for any untoward incident, natural justice demands that any necessary disciplinary action is handled in an equable way.

Minor medication errors (i.e. any deviation from the doctor's order as written on the patient's hospital chart) are extremely common. Rates of between one per patient day and two per patient week have been reported in the United States. Prescribing errors are also common. Anonymous self-reporting schemes have been initiated in a few hospitals, as part of a more general risk management strategy, in an attempt to identify high-risk situations. Dilutional errors are particularly common in neonatal practice, and the individual drug guidelines in this compendium have been carefully framed so as to minimise these.

Ten golden rules

Attention to the following ten rules will help to minimise error and, even more importantly, ensure that when an error does occur the impact is minimised:

1 Keep the prescribing of medication to a minimum, and use once or twice daily administration where this is possible.
2 Never have more than two IV infusion lines running at the same time unless this is absolutely necessary.
3 Never put more than 30 ml of fluid at any one time into any syringe used to provide continuous IV fluid or milk for a baby weighing less than 1 kg.
4 Record the amount of fluid administered by every syringe pump by inspecting the movement of the syringe and by inspecting the infusion site once every hour. Do not rely merely on any digital electronic display.
5 In an analogous way, where the infusion of fluid from any large (0·5 l) reservoir is controlled by a peristaltic pump (or by a gravity-operated system with a gate valve and drop counter), it is always wise to interpose a burette between the main reservoir and the control unit. Limiting the amount of fluid in the burette limits the risk of accidental fluid overload, and recording the amount of fluid left in the burette every hour speeds the recognition of any administrative error.
6 Do not change the feeding or IV fluid regimen more than once, or at most twice, a day except for a very good reason. Try to arrange that such changes as do have to be made are done during the morning or evening joint management rounds.

7 Those few drugs that have to be administered over 30 minutes or more should be administered using a separate programmable syringe pump connected 'pickaback' onto an existing IV line. As an extra precaution, the syringe should never be set up containing more than twice as much of the drug as it is planned to deliver. Do not adjust the rate at which the main IV infusion fluid is administered unless there is a serious risk of hyperglycaemia, or it is necessary to place an absolute restriction on the total daily fluid intake.

8 Do not routinely flush drugs or fluids through an established IV line except in the rare situations where this is specifically recommended in this compendium. To do so can expose the baby to a dangerously abrupt 'bolus' of drug. Using fluid from the main IV line to do this can also make the baby briefly and abruptly hyperglycaemic.

9 Beware giving a small newborn baby excess sodium unintentionally. The use of flush solutions of Hep-lok®, Hepsal® or 0·9% sodium chloride can expose a baby to an unintended excess of intravenous sodium. The steady infusion of 1 ml/hour of heparinised 0·9% sodium chloride (normal saline) to maintain catheter patency is sometimes enough to double a very small baby's total daily sodium intake. So can intratracheal sodium chloride administration during tracheal 'toilet'.

10 Treat the prescribing of potentially toxic or lethal drugs (such as chloramphenicol and digoxin, etc.) with special care. There are relatively few situations where it is really necessary to use such potentially dangerous drugs.

If something *does* go wrong

Report any significant error of omission or commission promptly so that appropriate action can be taken to minimise any possible hazard to the baby. Nine times out of ten, a senior member of staff with pharmacological expertise will be able to determine that no harm has been done quite quickly and offer much needed reassurance to all concerned. If malfunction of a pump or drip regulator is suspected, switch the equipment off and replace it *without touching* the setting of the rate control switches, pass the equipment to medical electronics for checking without delay, and record the serial number of the offending piece of equipment on the incident form.

Check and double check

1 **Have you got the right drug?** *Check the strength of the formulation and the label on the ampoule as well as the box.*

2 **Has it's shelf life expired?** *Check the 'use by' date.*

3 **Has it been reconstituted and diluted properly?** *Check the advice given in the individual drug monograph in this compendium.*

4 **Have you got the right patient?** *Check the name band.*

5 **Have you got the right dose?** *Have two people independently checked steps 1–4 with the prescription chart?*

6 **Have you picked up the right syringe?** *Deal with one patient at a time.*

7 **Is the IV line patent? Have you got the right line?** *Is it correctly positioned? Could the line have tissued?*

8 **Is a separate flush solution needed?** *Have two people checked the content of the flush syringe?*

9 **Are all the 'sharps' disposed of?** *What about any glass ampoules?*

10 **Have you 'signed up' what you have done?** *Has it been countersigned?*

Writing a hospital prescription

Comprehensive guidance on how to 'write up' (or transcribe) a prescription is given for those working in the UK in the introduction to the *British national formulary*, but many of the points in this bear repetition. While the formal constraints that operate in the community do not apply in a hospital setting (see p. 10), the following guidelines still represent good practice:

Block capitals: Always use block capitals when prescribing drug names to ensure legibility. A poorly written prescription is, at best, discourteous to nurses and to pharmacists who may have to spend time checking what has been written. Illegibility can also be dangerous.

Approved names: These should always be used to ensure consistency between vials, ampoules, bottles and other labels. Proprietary names ('trade names') should only be used for compound preparations when a generic name does not exist (e.g. INFANT GAVISCON – half a dual sachet). Avoid abbreviations and contractions other than those universally used and recognised (such as THAM).

The dose: This should be given in grams (g), milligrams (mg) or micrograms. The only acceptable abbreviation for micrograms is 'microg' – never mcg, ug or μg.

Units: When the dose is in 'units' write this word out in full. Avoid the symbol 'u' because it is too easily misread, and avoid the term 'microunits'. Oxytocin (see p. 193) is the one exception to this rule. Some drug companies still use the term 'international units' (IU) but, since international agreement has now been reached as to the meaning of all such terms, this terminology is unnecessary, and best avoided.

Volumes: Volumes should always be prescribed in millilitres. This can be abbreviated to ml (but it should not be contracted to cc or cm^3).

Decimal places: Carelessness here is a major cause of potentially lethal overtreatment. Decimals should be avoided where possible and, where unavoidable, always prefaced by a zero. Write 500 mg not 0·5 g. If a decimal has to be used, write 0·5 ml not ·5 ml. Do not use a comma, use a stop (0·5 ml not 0,5 ml).

Time: This is best written using the 24 hour clock when prescribing for patients in hospital.

Route of administration: This must always be indicated. The following abbreviations are generally acceptable:

IV	Intravenous	**IM**	Intramuscular
NEB	Nebuliser	**PO**	Oral (per os)
RECT	Rectal	**SC**	Subcutaneous

All other methods of administration should be written in full (e.g. intradermal, intratracheal, etc.).

Continuous IV administration: Drugs for continuous intravenous (or, rarely, umbilical arterial) infusion can be prescribed on an IV infusion chart, and signed for on this chart in the usual way. Full details do not then need to be written up and signed for in duplicate on the main inpatient medicine chart, but the front of this chart does, as a minimum, need to be marked to show clearly what other charts are in use.

Reconstitution and dilution: Drugs often have to be reconstituted and/or diluted before they can be given to babies. It is not necessary to write down how this should be done when prescribing a drug listed in this compendium in units where all staff routinely use these guidelines because it will be assumed that reconstitution and dilution will be carried out as specified in the relevant drug monograph. Indeed, it would only cause confusion to give any instruction that was unintentionally at variance with the advice given here. Instructions *must* be given, however, where this is not the case, or if a drug is prescribed that is not in this compendium.

Limits of precision: Do not ask for impossible precision. A dose prescribed by weight will almost always have to be given to a child by volume (often after dilution, as above), and it is not generally possible to measure or administer a volume of less than 0·1 ml with any precision (as noted on p. 5).

Flexible dosage: Some drugs (such as insulin) are regularly prescribed on a 'sliding scale'. Where this is the case it may not be necessary or appropriate for a doctor to write up each individual dose given. In the same way detailed authorization for hour-by-hour dose variation within a prescribed range (such as the use of labetalol or an inotrope to control blood pressure) does not require a doctor's signature each time treatment is adjusted as long as each change in dosage is recorded and signed for on the IV chart by the relevant responsible nurse.

Management at delivery: Drugs commonly given to the baby at birth (such as vitamin K or naloxone) do not need to be written up on a medicine chart as long as their administration is fully documented in a fixed and standardised position in the maternity notes.

Emergency resuscitation: Where drugs are given in an acute emergency by a doctor or nurse during cardiorespiratory resuscitation, they do not need to be recorded in duplicate in the medicine chart as long as they are accurately recorded in the narrative record in the medical notes (along with dosage and timing) when this is subsequently written up.

Blood products and vaccines: While these are not traditionally recorded on the medicine chart, their administration must be recorded somewhere in the clinical notes along with the relevant batch number.

Dietary supplements: Vitamin and other dietary supplements for which no doctor's prescription is necessary, or once daily additions to the milk formula (such as supplemental sodium), do not need to be prescribed on the medicine chart, but administration does need to be recorded each time on the child's feed chart.

Self administration: Parents should be encouraged to give certain drugs (such as eye drops) on their own, especially where they are likely to have to continue giving such treatment after discharge from hospital. This can be done by writing 'Self-administered' in the space labelled 'Notes' on some medicine charts.

Midwife authorised prescriptions: Drugs given by a midwife on her own responsibility in the UK must be properly recorded and 'signed up' on the medicine chart. Some units ask staff to add the symbol 'M' after their signature.

Patient Group Directions: Patient safety makes it very important for all medication administered under the terms of a Patient Group Direction (PGD) to be documented on the same chart as is being used to record all the *other* drugs the patient is being given. Just transcribing such a directive onto a medicine chart is *not* an act of 'prescribing' – that occurred when the PGD was drawn up.

'As required' prescriptions: Be specific about how much may be taken, how often, and for what purpose. Specify a minimum time interval before another such dose can be given. Do not *only* write 'as required' or 'prn' (pro re nata). It will often be important to indicate a maximum cumulative daily (24 hour) dose. Patients offered analgesics 'prn' often end up undertreated. A flexible prescription (see above) can often be more appropriate.

Medication on discharge: Hospitals in the UK generally instruct staff not to issue a prescription for more of any drug then the minimum needed to continue treatment until such time as the family can get a further prescription from their general practitioner unless, as with a small minority of drugs used in the neonatal period, the drug is only obtainable from a hospital pharmacy. It should not, in other circumstances, be necessary to dispense more than 2 week's treatment. The same guidelines apply to the dispensing of drugs for outpatients. Drugs prescribed by a hospital doctor in the UK have to be dispensed by the hospital pharmacy except under circumstances clearly defined by the Principal Pharmacist (when form FP(10)HP may be used).

Telephone messages: Hospital rules vary. Most accept that under exceptional circumstances a telephone message may be accepted from a doctor by two nurses (one of whom must be a Registered Nurse and one of whom acts as a witness to the receipt of the message). It is not acceptable to prescribe controlled drugs in this way, and any other drug so prescribed should be given only once. The doctor must then confirm and sign the prescription within 12 hours. Faxed prescriptions should also be confirmed in writing within 72 hours.

Signature: Each entry must be signed for, separately, in full by a registered doctor or by a nurse with independent prescribing rights (except, in the UK, as covered by the PGD provisions outlined above). The date the entry was signed must also be recorded.

Cancellation: Drugs should not be taken for longer than necessary. Stop dates for short-course treatments (such as antibiotics) can often be recorded on the medicine chart when first prescribed. The clearest way to mark the chart is to draw a horizontal line through the name of the drug, and the date, and then date and initial the 'Date discontinued' space. Drugs often tend to be given for much longer than is necessary.

Adverse reactions and overtreatment

Adverse reactions

Any drug capable of doing good is also capable of doing harm, and unwanted reactions can be very unexpected. Some of these adverse reactions are dose related, but others are idiosyncratic. Problems may relate to the drug's main pharmacological action in the body, or to some secondary action ('side effect'). The recognition of these adverse reactions is of vital importance, but their proper documentation and reporting is frequently neglected. The Committee on Safety of Medicines (CSM) operates a simple yellow lettercard reporting system in the UK for the Medicines and Healthcare products Regulatory Agency (MHRA) that is designed to make it easier for staff to initiate such notifications. Copies of the prepaid lettercard can be found bound into the back of each new edition of the *British national formulary*. The Committee has its main base in London (telephone 0800 731 6789), but there are also five other regional reporting centres (see box below).

Doctors have a professional duty to report all serious suspected reactions even if they are already well recognised, especially if they are fatal, life-threatening, disabling or incapacitating. This is necessary so that reports can be prepared comparing the risk:benefit ratio seen with other drugs of a similar class. Doctors should also report any adverse or unexpected event, *however minor*, where this could conceivably be a response to a drug that has only been on the market for a relatively short time. Pharmacists also have a responsibility to report all important adverse reactions coming to their attention. Nurses and midwives are often the first to suspect an adverse reaction: they have a duty to see that any such reaction is brought to the attention of the appropriate doctor or pharmacist, and to initiate a report themselves if necessary. Deaths have, by law, to be reported to the coroner.

The CSM are interested in hearing about adverse reactions caused by **any** therapeutic agent (including any drug, blood product, vaccine, dental or surgical material, X-ray contrast medium, intrauterine device, etc.). Reactions observed as a result of self-medication should be reported in the same way as those seen with prescribed drugs. Drug interactions of a serious nature should also be reported. Drugs can sometimes have a delayed effect, causing problems such as later anaemia, jaundice, retroperitoneal fibrosis or even cancer. Any suspicion of such an association should always be reported. Whenever a baby miscarries, is aborted or is born with a congenital abnormality doctors should always consider whether this might have been due to an adverse drug reaction, and report all the drugs (including any self-medication) taken during the pregnancy.

Adverse reactions are particularly common when drugs are given at the extremes of life. This is, in part, because the liver and the kidneys handle drugs less efficiently, both in the first weeks of life and in old age. Nevertheless, although the CSM receives many reports relating to drug medication in the elderly, relatively few reports are received in relation to adverse events in the neonatal period. This is not because such events are uncommon, as many of the individual drug monographs in this compendium bear testimony, but because a proper tradition of reporting never seems to have become established. Yet, without such reporting, the identification of many important side effects is avoidably delayed. Because, in particular, some of the most important side effects seen in the neonatal period differ from those normally seen later in life, failure to report can also delay the recognition, and quantification, of a very real drug hazard.

Defective medicines constitute a related but different problem. Problems can occur either during manufacture, or during distribution, rendering the product either dangerous or ineffective. Whenever such a problem is suspected it should be reported *at once* to the hospital pharmacy who will, in turn, notify the national Defective Medicines Report Centre in London (telephone 020 7084 2574, or, out of office hours, 020 7210 3000) if the suspicions are confirmed.

UK MEDICINES AND HEALTHCARE PRODUCTS REGULATORY AGENCY

CHM FREEPOST, London SW8 5BR
or directly by going to the following web address: www.yellowcard.gov.uk

---

Overtreatment

Identifying the right dose of medicine to give a newborn baby is never easy, and the problem is made even more difficult if kidney or liver immaturity is compounded by illness or organ failure. Progressive drug accumulation is a very real possibility in these situations. A major error can easily arise during the drawing up of the small dose needed in a small preterm baby, particularly if prior dilution is involved. Few of these events ever get widely reported. Indeed, where the baby is already ill, the cause if death may go unrecognised. Ten-fold administration errors are not unheard of.

Luckily even after serious overtreatment most babies recover with supportive or symptomatic care (although this is not always true where drugs such as atropine, chloramphenicol, digoxin, lidocaine and potassium chloride are concerned). If the drug has been given by mouth it may be worth giving a stomach washout. A 1 g/kg oral dose of activated charcoal (repeatable every 4 hours until charcoal appears in the stool) may also be of some help, especially if it is started within 4 hours. Do not try to make the baby sick. Other forms of forced elimination such as exchange transfusion, haemoperfusion, dialysis and forced diuresis are only of limited value for a small number of drugs taken in severe excess. Whole bowel irrigation with a polyethylene glycol-electrolyte solution (such as Klean-Prep®) may occasionally be appropriate. Always seek the immediate help and advice of the nearest Poisons Centre (see below) if there are severe symptoms. For a limited number of drugs specific antidotes, antagonists or chelating agents are available; these are mentioned briefly, where appropriate, under the name of the drug for which they are of use, in the various monographs in the main section of this compendium. Specific antagonists include naloxone for opioid drugs, Digibind® for digoxin, and flumazenil for benzodiazepines. Acetylcysteine is of value after paracetamol over-dosage, methylene blue is used to control methaemoglobinaemia, and the chelating agent desferrioxamine mesylate is used in iron poisoning. The main components of supportive care are as follow.

Respiration: Airway obstruction is a real hazard in patients who go unconscious. Vomiting is not uncommon, and inhalation a real risk. Most poisons that impair consciousness also depress breathing, so artificial respiratory support may well be required. While specific opioid and benzodiazepine antagonists can be helpful, respiratory stimulants should not be used. Correct any serious metabolic acidosis (pH <7·2) with sodium bicarbonate or THAM.

Fluid and glucose intake: Reduce fluid intake to a minimum and monitor urine output while retaining normoglycaemia until it is clear that kidney function is unaffected. Stop all oral feeds if there is acidosis, hypotension and/or suspected ileus.

Blood pressure: Do not use vasopressor drugs without first getting expert advice. Cautious plasma volume expansion may help if there is serious hypotension.

Arrhythmia: Do not give drugs, especially if output is tolerably well maintained, before defining the nature of the arrhythmia and seeking advice as outlined in the monograph on adenosine. A β-blocker (such as propranolol) may help to moderate the tachyarrhythmia sometimes seen with excess theophylline, chloral hydrate, quinine, amphetamine or some of the antihistamines, and may improve cardiac output. These drugs do not seem to cause an arrhythmia in children as often as they do in adults.

Convulsions: While short-lived seizures do not require treatment, prolonged seizures should be controlled, especially if they seem to be impeding respiration. A slowly infused IV dose of diazepam (preferably the emulsified formulation) is the anticonvulsant most often used in older patients, but phenobarbitone is more usually used in the neonatal period. Either drug can, in itself, cause further respiratory depression.

Temperature control: Poisoning can cause both hypo- and hyperthermia. The rectal temperature should be measured to monitor deep body temperature, using a low reading thermometer if necessary so as not to miss hypothermia, and appropriate environmental measures taken.

INFORMATION SERVICES

UK National Poisons Centre 'hot line': 0844 892 0111

Maternal drug abuse

Drug misuse (abuse) is common, but only a small amount of misuse is associated with dependence (or addiction). Society currently displays a schizophrenic attitude to drug abuse. We seem to accept alcohol intake and smoking during pregnancy even though we know that these drugs can be addictive, and that regular use can affect the baby. There is a puritanical (and paternalistic) streak that is particularly strong amongst legislators in America, that would ban all alcohol intake in pregnancy, but there is no evidence that an intake of less than 10 units a week is harmful unless it is consumed in one go (1 'unit' of alcohol being a single pub measure of spirits, a small glass of wine or half a pint of ordinary strength beer or cider). In addition, smoking in pregnancy is now seen as one of those 'facts of life' that the medical and midwifery professions can do little to change. The attitude to other recreational drug use is more censorious, even though we know that many UK doctors occasionally take drugs themselves.

Opiate addiction presents the most serious challenge, and IV injection further increases the risk to the mother's health. Indeed the main reason for offering these mothers methadone is that it may help them to avoid the hazards associated with giving any drug intravenously. Access to oral methadone may, by limiting the woman's urge to acquire other costly drugs of doubtful purity, also help stabilise her lifestyle. Attitudes change over time. Opium and laudanum were widely used by the middle classes in Europe and North America in the 19th century. Opium was even added to many infant 'soothing syrups'. Now it has been estimated that, when no legal source is available, the average UK addict gets through £20,000 worth of heroin a year. Diet may become inadequate, and alcohol intake may rise. Judgmental attitudes can deter addicts from seeking help until problems escalate. Users may seem to have neglected their condition when the health services have actually, by their attitude, effectively excluded them from care. Despite this, many manage to lead apparently normal lives, running a family or holding down a job.

Few areas of maternity care are more in need of a collaborative, team-based approach. Little can be achieved until the woman's trust and confidence have been won. Antenatal care should identify those most in need of support. Intravenous drug users should always be tested, with their informed consent, for sexually transmitted infection, and for hepatitis B, hepatitis C and HIV infection, both to optimise the scope for treatment and to minimise the risk that the baby will also become infected. Plans for post-delivery care should also be made ahead of delivery, and the mother should know what these are.

Many heroin users also take other drugs. While recreational use of drugs such as cannabis, LSD, PCP, amphetamine, ecstasy or cocaine on their own do not usually cause neonatal withdrawal symptoms serious enough to require treatment, the same is not true for high-dose benzodiazepine use. Transferring from heroin to methadone may actually make matters worse because this does not give the immediate 'high' obtained when heroin is smoked and inhaled or taken intravenously. Cocaine may then be turned to for the 'lift' that it gives and a benzodiazepine, such as temazepam, used to reduce the 'low' that tends to follow. Fashions change, but combined addiction to heroin and temazepam is common in the UK.

Most people who misuse drugs are not drug dependent. The problem only becomes an addiction if abrupt discontinuation causes serious physical and mental symptoms to appear. This is, however, what can happen to the baby after birth. Babies exposed to opiates throughout pregnancy, or to high sustained benzodiazepine usage, often exhibit a range of symptoms (see box) 12–72 hours after birth. **None** of these, on their own, need treatment, but treatment is called for if sucking is so in-coordinate that tube feeding is required, if there is profuse vomiting or watery diarrhoea, or if the baby remains seriously unsettled after two consecutive feeds despite gentle swaddling and the use of a pacifier.

W	Wakefullness
I	Irritability
T	Tachypnoea (>60 min)
H	Hyperactivity
D	Diarrhoea
R	Rub marks
A	Autonomic dysfunction
W	Weight loss
A	Alkalosis (respiratory)
L	Lachrymatiom (tears)

Many units currently admit such babies to special care for observation and then 'score' the child's condition once every 4 hours. However, experience shows that an observer's views and their 'attitude' to drug misuse can influence the score awarded. Scores ask the observer to say how 'severe' the symptoms are. If the nurse or doctor has not cared for such a baby before, how can they decide on the severity of the symptoms? Scoring systems, though popular, can also have the perverse effect of suggesting that an increasingly sedated baby is 'improving' when the real need is to get the baby feeding and sleeping normally.

A better approach is to make the mother aware, before delivery, that the baby will need to be watched for a period, to involve the mother in this, and to care for mother and baby together. Most already feel guilty about their drug habit, and live in constant fear of having their children taken from them. A knowledge of antenatal drug intake (even if accurate) is only of limited value in predicting whether the baby will develop symptoms, and mothers need to be aware of this. If mother and baby have been cared for together both can be discharged home after 72 hours if no serious symptoms have developed.

If symptoms serious enough to make the baby unwell do develop then the logical approach is to wean the baby slowly from the drug to which the mother is habituated, rather than introducing yet another drug. Babies of mothers taking an opiate should be weaned using a slowly decreasing dose of morphine or methadone. Morphine is widely used, and the dose can be easily and rapidly adjusted up or down, but methadone may provide smoother control. Weaning should not normally take more than 7–10 days. The same approach can be used where the mother is addicted to buprenorphine, codeine or dihydrocodeine. The use of paregoric for the baby, or tincture of opium, lacks rational justification. Benzodiazepine dependency is harder to manage using this strategy, because nearly all these drugs have such a long half life. Some use chloral hydrate but this can oversedate the baby, and chlorpromazine may be a better choice. For the occasional mother with barbiturate dependency, phenobarbital should be considered but, while this may provide sedation, it does nothing to control gastrointestinal symptoms.

Although there have been 14 small controlled trials looking at strategies for managing neonatal withdrawal, the assessors have generally merely looked to see how many symptoms there were rather than how distressing and disabling the symptoms were. In addition, the assessors have usually been aware of how the babies were being treated. There is scope for some useful nursing research here.

Breastfeeding can be encouraged if the mother is on a stable dose of methadone, but it is doubtful if this should be encouraged in polydrug users since the safety of the baby cannot be assured. There is no need to place any arbitrary limit on the length of time the mother is 'permitted' to breastfeed. It should, however, be explained that weaning needs to be gradual. No baby should be left in the care of anyone taking a hallucinogen, and few would condone the possible exposure of a baby to such a drug in breast milk. The place of breastfeeding in mothers taking other drugs is summarised on pp. 284–95.

Screening urine, or meconium, for drugs serves little purpose unless serious thought is being given to care proceedings, since it is unlikely to influence management. If you tell the mother you plan to do this, you imply that you do not believe what she has told you about her drug history. If you tell her later, she will merely conclude that you are another person she can not trust. The decision of any child protection conference, or court, will be influenced purely by what is best for the child, and by the mother's ability to provide that care. Drug misuse is not in itself a sufficient reason to separate mother and child.

Babies can also become addicted to opiates and benzodiazepines *after* birth. Fentanyl and midazolam are the drugs that most often cause problems. Continuous use for even a few days can produce tolerance (the need for a progressively larger dose) and dependency (addiction). Management is the same as for addiction acquired *in utero* – a slow, tapered withdrawal of treatment. Perhaps we should do what we tell mothers to do, and avoid sustained use all together.

INSTITUTE FOR THE STUDY OF DRUG DEPENDENCE

This charitable organisation, founded in 1968, provides an information service for professionals and for researchers. It has produced a useful series of informative booklets called Drug Notes, and a series of five short leaflets called Drug Information for Women. The Institute has recently merged with the Standing Conference on Drug Abuse (SCODA) to form DrugScope. This can be contacted at:

DrugScope, 32–36 Loman Street, London SE1 0EE

Telephone 020 7928 1771

Renal failure

Since the kidney is responsible for the elimination of most drugs from the body (either before or after inactivation by the liver) an assessment of how well the kidney is functioning is an essential part of the daily care of any patient on medication. Kidney function can fluctuate rapidly in the neonatal period so it should be assessed at the time treatment is first prescribed and monitored daily.

Deterioration occurs because blood flow has decreased (*pre renal failure*), because the kidney has suffered damage (*intrinsic renal failure*) or because the urine flow has been obstructed (*post renal failure*) – although both pre and post renal failure can also cause secondary kidney damage. Clinical examination, and knowledge of the other problems involved, will often suggest where the problem lies. In babies with normal renal function sodium excretion is driven by intake, and therefore varies widely. The proportion filtered that appears in urine (fractional excretion, FE_{Na}) is equally variable:

$$FE_{Na} (\%) = \frac{Urinary\ sodium}{Plasma\ sodium} \times \frac{Plasma\ creatinine}{Urinary\ creatinine} \times 100$$

Check all concentrations are expressed in the same units. Babies with pre renal failure (who are typically oliguric and hypotensive) conserve sodium avidly under the control of aldosterone. They will have a FE_{Na} ≤3% (<5% when less than 32 weeks' gestation and less than 2 weeks old) regardless of the intake and the plasma level, except after a large dose of furosemide. Babies with established failure have a high FE_{Na} excretion because reabsorption is impaired by tubular damage.

Weigh all ill babies at least once a day because weight change is a sensitive index of fluid balance. Babies normally lose weight for 3–5 days after birth as they shed extracellular fluid (including sodium) following the loss of the placenta through which they were 'dialysed' before birth. Weight gain at this time is either a sign of excessive fluid intake or early renal failure. Even healthy growing babies only gain weight by 2% a day. Gain in excess of this is a very useful sign of kidney failure. Urine output will vary with fluid intake, but any baby putting out less than 1 ml/kg of urine per hour is almost certainly in failure. A rising plasma creatinine or a level above 88 µmol/l (>1 mg%) in a baby more than 10 days old suggests some degree of renal failure, but the plasma level should never be relied on to identify failure because it rises six times more slowly after any insult than it does in an older child or adult.

Early diagnosis is vital because the elimination of some commonly used but potentially toxic drugs, such as gentamicin, is entirely dependent on excretion in the urine. Furthermore, most acute renal failure in the neonatal period is, at least initially, pre-renal in origin – often as a result of sepsis, intrapartum stress or respiratory difficulty – and early diagnosis makes early treatment possible. Trouble can often be anticipated. The later the problem is recognised, the more difficult management becomes. The frequency with which it is necessary to rescue a baby from metabolic chaos by dialysis is inversely related to the promptness with which such a threat is recognised. A fluid balance strategy for minimising the need for dialysis is summarised on p. 276, and a strategy for the conservative management of hyperkalaemia on p. 234 (and p. 212).

Reduce all medication to the minimum as soon as there is evidence of definite renal failure to minimise the risk of toxic drug accumulation and of unpredictable interactions. Antibiotics should be given as indicated in Table 2. Flucytosine, vancomycin and cefuroxime are sometimes added to dialysis fluids to prevent peritonitis. A first dose of the appropriate antibiotic should always be given intravenously (if the baby is not already on treatment) before utilising the peritoneal dialysis fluid to sustain an appropriate blood level if there are signs of systemic infection. Sustained high aminoglycoside levels are not bactericidal (as explained on p. 120) so these drugs should not be put in peritoneal dialysis fluid. Pancuronium should be replaced by atracurium if the baby requires paralysis. Morphine may accumulate because it is renally excreted. The half life of heparin seems unaffected, but that of low molecular weight heparin is reduced. The clearance of the drugs commonly used to control arrhythmia, seizures, hypertension and hypotension are (luckily) unaffected by renal failure.

Peritoneal dialysis is the most effective strategy in most small babies, but surgical problems may make haemodialysis necessary. Commercial dialysis fluids usually contain lactate, but some ill neonates metabolise this poorly. A flexible range of fluids can be prepared containing bicarbonate by combining three different basic solutions as outlined in Table 1. Use an in-line IV burette, and adjust the glucose concentration by

Table 1 Solutions for neonatal peritoneal dialysis.

Solution	Preparation	Final concentration		
		Sodium (mmol/l)	Bicarbonate (mmol/l)	Glucose (%)
A	500 ml 5% glucose modified by removing 60 ml of fluid and adding 60 ml of 8·4% sodium bicarbonate	120	120	4·4
B	500 ml 0·9% sodium chloride	150	0	0
C	500 ml 0·9% sodium chloride modified by removing 50 ml of fluid and adding 50 ml of 50% glucose and 1·5 ml of 30% (strong) sodium chloride	150	0	5·0
Potential combinations:				
1/3 A plus 2/3 B		140	40	1·47
1/3 A plus 1/2 B plus 1/6 C		140	40	2·30
1/3 A plus 1/3 B plus 1/3 C		140	40	3·13
1/3 A plus 2/3 C		140	40	4·80

varying ingredients B and C in order to control ultrafiltration and the removal of water. Because these dialysis fluids cannot contain calcium it is necessary to give supplemental calcium intravenously. Start with 1 mmol/kg a day and adjust as necessary. Magnesium may occasionally be needed. Add heparin (1 unit/ml) if the dialysis fluid is cloudy or bloodstained to stop fibrin and clots obstructing the catheter. Watch for peritonitis by microscoping and culturing the effluent fluid daily.

Table 2 Drugs used to combat infection, and their clearance from the body in babies with severe renal failure before or during peritoneal dialysis (PD).

Drug	Dose adjustment needed	Comment
Aciclovir	Major	Quadruple the dose interval. Removal by PD is poor
Amikacin	Measure	Judge dose interval from trough serum level. Removal by PD is slow
Amoxicillin	Some	Increase the dose interval, or give one IV dose and put 125 mg/l in the PD fluid
Amphotericin	None	Give IV treatment as normal. The drug is not removed by PD
Ampicillin	Some	Increase the dose interval, or give one IV dose and put 125 mg/l in the PD fluid
Azithromycin	None	Give as normal. The drug is not removed by PD
Aztreonam	Major	Halve the dose. The drug is not removed by PD
Cefotaxime	Some	Increase the dose interval, or give one IV dose and put 125 mg/l in the PD fluid
Cefoxitin	Major	Double the dose interval, or give one IV dose and put 125 mg/l in the PD fluid
Ceftazidime	Major	Double the dose interval, or give one IV dose and put 125 mg/l in the PD fluid
Ceftriaxone	Some	Reduce the dose if there is both renal and liver failure. Removal by PD is poor
Cefuroxime	Major	Increase the dose interval, or give one IV dose and put 125 mg/l in the PD fluid
Chloramphenicol	None	Use with caution – metabolites accumulate. The drug is not removed by PD
Ciprofloxacin	Major	Halve the dose. Crystalluria may occur. The drug is not removed by PD
Clindamycin	Minimal	Give IV treatment as normal. The drug is not removed by PD
Erythromycin	None	Give IV as normal. The drug is not removed by PD
Flucloxacillin	Minimal	Give IV as normal, or give one dose IV and put 250 mg/l in the PD fluid
Fluconazole	Major	Double the dose interval or, in babies on PD, put 7 mg/l in the PD fluid
Flucytosine	Measure	Monitor the serum level or, in babies on PD, put 50 mg/l in the PD fluid
Gentamicin	Measure	Judge dose interval from trough serum level. Removal by PD is slow
Isoniazid	None	Give oral or IV treatment as normal. The drug is removed by PD
Meropenem	Major	Double the dose interval. It is not known if the drug is removed by PD
Metronidazole	Minimal	Give oral or IV treatment as normal. The drug is removed by PD
Netilmicin	Measure	Judge dose interval from trough serum level. Removal by PD is slow
Penicillin	Substantial	Use with caution – penicillin is neurotoxic. Removal by PD is poor
Rifampicin	None	Give oral or IV treatment as normal. The drug is not removed by PD
Teicoplanin	Moderate	Give if IV level can be measured, or give one IV dose and put 20 mg/l in PD fluid
Trimethoprim	Moderate	Halve the IV dose after 2 days. Removal by PD is slow
Vancomycin	Measure	Monitor serum level, or give one IV dose and put 25 mg/l in the PD fluid

Body weight and surface area

Basal metabolic rate has a fairly fixed relationship to body surface area throughout childhood and adult life. For this reason it was once common practice to use body surface area when calculating drug dosage in childhood. However, while this works reasonably well for children more than a few months old it is not really appropriate in early infancy because resting or 'basal' metabolic rate (BMR) rises rapidly in the first 2 or 3 weeks after birth even though little growth takes place, and BMR is only one of many factors influencing drug metabolism at this time.

Most paediatric reference texts have, until recently, provided nomograms that could be used to derive surface area from a knowledge of height and weight but, as this text has long argued, height (or length) is seldom measured with any real accuracy in children who cannot yet stand, and experience has shown that further errors often creep in when staff then use one of the various nomograms that have been devised without due care. What is more, as the late Edith Boyd showed in her book *The growth of the surface area of the human body*, published by the University of Minnesota Press in 1935, surface area can be predicted as accurately in very young children from a knowledge of weight alone as it can from a knowledge of height as well as weight.

In fact BMR changes so much during the first 1–2 months of life that it has *never* been sensible to use surface area to calculate how much of a drug to give during this time anyway. Changes in kidney and liver function are of much more relevance during this time, and all the treatment recommendations given in this book are based on what we know of the variable way that these two factors interact to affect how long each drug remains active in the body after administration. The table relating weight to surface area given in earlier editions of this book utilised Boyd's data but the revised figures given here (Table 3) have made use

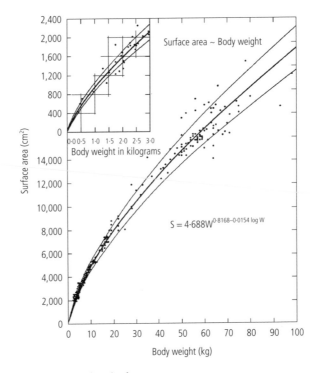

Fig. 2 Relationship between body weight and surface area.

of the additional data collected by Meban in 1983 (*J Anat* 1983;**137**:271–8). In truth, however, in young children more than 1–2 months old, it is nearly always best to simply use body weight to calculate the most appropriate dose to employ (see Johnson, *Arch Dis Child* 2008;**93**:207–11.)

Table 3 Relationship between body weight (kg) (full units down left side and part units across the top) and surface area (m²); for example, a baby weighing 2.3 kg will have a surface area of 0.17 m².

kg	·0	·1	·2	·3	·4	·5	·6	·7	·8	·9
0	–	–	0·04	0·04	0·05	0·06	0·07	0·08	0·08	0·09
1	0·10	0·10	0·11	0·11	0·12	0·12	0·13	0·14	0·14	0·15
2	0·15	0·16	0·17	0·17	0·18	0·18	0·19	0·19	0·20	0·21
3	0·21	0·22	0·22	0·23	0·23	0·24	0·24	0·25	0·25	0·26
4	0·26	0·27	0·27	0·27	0·28	0·28	0·29	0·29	0·30	0·30
5	0·31	0·31	0·32	0·32	0·32	0·33	0·33	0·34	0·34	0·35
6	0·35	0·35	0·36	0·36	0·36	0·37	0·37	0·38	0·38	0·38
7	0·39	0·39	0·39	0·40	0·40	0·40	0·41	0·41	0·41	0·42
8	0·42	0·43	0·43	0·43	0·44	0·44	0·44	0·45	0·45	0·45
9	0·46	0·46	0·46	0·47	0·47	0·48	0·48	0·48	0·49	0·49

Useful website addresses

American Academy of Pediatrics

The American Academy of Pediatrics provides a wealth of well-formulated advice available on its website. Abstracts of all the papers published in *Pediatrics* since 1948 can also be accessed. In fact, since 1997, only half the papers published by this journal have appeared in print in full. Others only appear in abstract form (and have an e-page number). Abstracts of all the articles and a full text version of all the e-published articles can be accessed and downloaded, without charge, from the journal's website.
- www.pediatrics.org

British national formulary

This formulary, sponsored jointly by the British Medical Association and the Royal Pharmaceutical Society of Great Britain, aims to provide authoritative and practical information on the selection and use of all UK licensed medicines in a clear, concise and accessible manner. It is semi-continuously updated and published afresh in book form every 6 months, but it can also be accessed online, and has grown over the years to become one of the world's most authoritative reference texts. A separate publication, *BNF for children* (or BNFC), was launched in September 2005 jointly with the Royal College of Paediatrics and Child Health, and updates of this version appear annually.
- www.bnf.org
- www.bnfc.org

Clinical Evidence

Clinical Evidence is a 'continuously updated international source of evidence on the effects of clinical interventions', based on a thorough search and appraisal of the literature. Where little good evidence exists the text says so. Relatively few perinatal issues are covered as yet (the ones in print by the time this edition went to press are mentioned in the list of references at the end of each monograph in this book), but the number covered is increasing steadily. The full text is available on the web and in PDA format, and the content is updated every 6 months. Online access to the full text is now only available to subscribers in the UK, but access remains free for those in many developing countries. The text is also currently available in German, Hungarian, Portuguese, Russian and Spanish. A summary of each monograph is also published by the BMJ Publishing Group in book form twice a year under the title *BMJ Clinical evidence handbook*.
- www.clinicalevidence.com

Cochrane Library

The Cochrane Collaboration is an international not-for-profit organisation providing up-to-date information about the effects of health care. The library contains the Cochrane Database of Systematic Reviews, the Database of Abstracts of Reviews of Effectiveness and the Cochrane Central Register of Controlled Trials. Access to the full text of all the reviews that have something useful to say about drugs mentioned in the main section of this compendium can be assessed directly from this Formulary's website, while the National Institutes of Health (NIH) website in America provides access to all existing and currently planned neonatal reviews. Access to the whole site is now available free of charge in Australia, India, Latin America, New Zealand, Scandinavia, UK and many low income countries.
- www.cochrane.org/
- www.nichd.nih.gov/cochrane/

Communicable Disease Centres

Many countries maintain a national communicable disease centre. Two that make a particularly wide range of information publicly available are the Health Protection Agency (HPA) – once the PHLS or Public Health Laboratory Service – in the UK, and the Communicable Disease Centre (CDC) in the USA.
- www.hpa.org.uk/infections/default.htm
- www.cdc.gov

Contact a Family

Families told that their child has a rare, possibly inherited, disorder often feel bereft of good-quality advice and information. Charities exist both in the UK and USA to bridge that gap. They can also offer help to those who want to contact other families facing a similar challenge.
- www.cafamily.org.uk
- www.rarediseases.org

Contraception

The website managed by the Faculty of Family Planning and Reproductive Health Care in the UK provides authoritative advice on all aspects of contraception and family planning.
- www.ffprhc.org.uk

Controlled clinical trials

Until recently it has been difficult to get information about ongoing and unpublished clinical trials. This unsatisfactory state of affairs is changing however, at least in respect of non-commercial trials. Information about these is now becoming available through the meta-Register of Controlled Trials (www.controlled-trials.com) and, for the USA, on a user-friendly site run by the National Library of Medicine. A register of trials is also available at TrialsCentral.
- www.trialscentral.org
- www.clinicaltrials.gov
- www.controlled-trials.com

Drug abuse

Drugscope is an independent registered UK charity that undertakes research, and provides authoritative advice, on all aspects of drug abuse and drug addiction.
- www.drugscope.org.uk

Drug use in children

The National Health Service (NHS) in the UK supports 'DIAL' – a medicines advisory service for pharmacists that provides information and a 'help line' on all issues relating to the use of medicine in children. It is based in Liverpool.
- www.dial.org.uk

Drug use during lactation

Thomas Hale, the pharmacist at the Tech University School of Medicine in Texas is the author of the valuable and frequently updated book *Medications and mothers' milk*, which is a mine of information on drug use during lactation. He also maintains an active and useful website. The UK Breastfeeding Network, who run an invaluable support and advice line (0844 412 4665), have issued a series of useful fact sheets about drug use during lactation that can be accessed from their website, while NHS Education for Scotland has developed a very useful eLearning programme covering that whole issue of drug use during lactation.

- http://neonatal.ama.ttuhsc.edu/lact/
- www.breastfeedingnetwork.org.uk
- www.nes.scot.nhs.uk/pharmacy/breastfeeding/index.html

Drug use during pregnancy

For a useful alphabetical list summarising how most drugs commonly used in pregnancy are classified by the American Federal Food and Drug Administration (FDA) see this well-designed Californian Perinatology Network website. One particularly useful feature of the site is the way you can, with one more click, undertake a full Medline literature search. This site also provides some information on drug use during lactation. There is a Swedish data base that assesses the link between birth defects and drug taking in pregnancy. See also the two websites giving information on teratogenicity (see below).

- www.perinatology.com/exposures/druglist.htm
- www.janusinfo.se

Genetic disease

The National Institutes of Health (NIH) in America supports a register of every known human single gene disorder (14,184 conditions at the last count). This register of 'Online Mendelian Inheritance in Man' provides a wealth of constantly updated information.

- www.ncbi.nlm.nih.gov/Omim/

History of controlled trials

For an insight into the way in which objectivity was eventually brought to bear on the many claims that doctors have always made for the drugs and treatments that they had on offer see:

- www.jameslindlibrary.org

HIV and AIDS

An authoritative website supported by the National Institutes of Health (NIH) in the USA provides extensive and very up-to-date information on the treatment of HIV and AIDS in patients of all ages, together with information on clinical trials currently in progress. The British HIV Association also has an active medical website and supports a second, more general (aidsmap), website. The University of Liverpool in the UK provides a site giving information on drug interactions.

- www.aidsinfo.nih.gov
- www.bhiva.org
- www.aidsmap.com
- www.hiv-druginteractions.org

Immunisation

The UK Department of Health has a website from which it is possible to download a range of informative leaflets suitable for parents. It also offers advice on travel issues. Another useful website is the one supported by the Institute of Child Health and Hospital for Sick Children in London.

- www.immunisation.nhs.uk
- www.gosh.nhs.uk/immunisation/

Immunisation facts

This is an independent website run by the writer who regularly writes on vaccine issues for *Hospital Pharmacy* (John Grabenstein). It focuses on US products and practices, but it provides links to a wide range of factual information from government and drug company sources.

- www.immunofacts.com

Immunisation Green Book

The 1996 edition of the UK Government's official publication *Immunisation against infectious disease* has now undergone radical revision, and these updates finally appeared in book form in December 2006. Access to the fully revised text can also

be obtained from the following website, while all the individual chapters relating to the vaccines covered in this book can also be accessed direct from this Formulary's website.

- www.immunisation.nhs.uk/article.php?id=400

Malaria

The malaria parasite is becoming progressively more resistant to many of the drugs usually used for prophylaxis and treatment. For area-specific advice on management from the World Health Organisation (WHO) and from the Communicable Disease Centre (CDC) in the USA see:

- www.who.int/ith/en/
- www.cdc.gov/travel/diseases.htm#malaria

Medicines Compendium

The information issued by the manufacturer of every product licensed for sale in the UK – the manufacturer's Summary of Product Characteristics or SPC – can be accessed electronically on the web. This information is also available in book format from Datapharm Communications. Patient Information Leaflets can also be accessed from the same website. Access is free and no longer password protected, and staff do not need to register before using this site.

- www.medicines.org.uk

Midwifery Digest

MIDIRS is a UK-based not-for-profit organisation. The website provides extensive, regularly updated information on all issues relating to childbirth. It also supports a very active inquiry service, and publishes a quarterly digest containing original articles and overviews of recent medical, midwifery and neonatal research taken from over 500 international journals. Subscribers also, for a fee, enjoy online access to over 400 regularly updated standard reading lists, and to over 100,000 articles on pregnancy, midwifery and childbirth issues.

- www.midirs.org

Motherisk Program

The Motherisk Program, backed by the expertise of the Department of Clinical Pharmacology and Toxicology at the Hospital for Sick Children in Toronto, maintains a very authoritative website dealing with the safety of drug use during pregnancy and lactation.

- www.motherisk.org

National Association of Neonatal Nurses

NANN is the main neonatal nursing organisation in the USA. Most of its benefits are only open to members, but some publications are available for purchase. Similar organisations exist in Australia and the UK. Each organisation supports its own 'in house' journal.

- www.nann.org
- www.nna.org.uk
- www.anna.org.au

National Library for Health

This UK-based facility aims to provide NHS staff, patients and the public with a comprehensive electronic information service. Look in particular at the items available by focusing on the material in the 'specialist libraries' for Women's Health and Child Health accessible direct from the Home Page. For registered users the site also provides direct access to the *British national formulary* and the Cochrane Collaboration (see above).

- www.library.nhs.uk/Default.aspx

National Institute for Clinical Excellence

This organisation provides cost–benefit advice on an as yet relatively restricted range of treatment strategies used by those working in the NHS in England and Wales.

- www.nice.org.uk

Neonatal and Paediatric Pharmacy Group

This is a UK-based website providing extensive advice for pharmacists on neonatal and paediatric pharmacy issues. It can be used to search and view abstracts of recent selected paediatric (Pharm-Line) pharmacology papers.

- www.show.scot.nhs.uk/nppg

Neonatology on the Web

This site contains an absorbing selection of classic papers and historical reports. The 'Hot Lit' links readers (perhaps a little uncritically) to a new, recently published paper each month, while the 'New Stuff' link takes you to a round up of recently updated features. There is a useful collection of bibliographies on a wide range of topics.

- www.neonatology.org

NICU-WEB

This site provides regularly updated, referenced articles on a wide range of neonatal topics written, largely from a US perspective, by staff from the University of Washington. It can also be used to gain access to NICU-NET, a web-based neonatal discussion group (see below).

- neonatal.peds.washington.edu

Nutritional Assessment Tool for Iron and Vitamins

A web-based nutritional assessment algorithm incorporating a nutritional profile of infant formulas, breast milk fortifiers and common supplements provided by the Neonatal Dietitians Interest Group, an informal network of neonatal dietitians within the British Dietetic Association.

- www.ndig.org/Nativ_whatisit.aspx

Renal failure

There are no published guidelines that relate specifically to the safe prescribing of drugs to children in renal failure, but the American College of Physicians in Philadelphia publishes an extremely useful slim book, *Dosing guidelines for adults*, and an update to the third (1999) edition is currently in preparation. An outline summary of its current advice on individual drugs can be accessed from the following university website:

- www.kdp-baptist.louisville.edu/renalbook/

Royal College of Obstetricians and Gynaecologists

This London-based college has published a small series of clinical practice guidelines (so-called 'Green Top' Guidelines) in the 'Good Practice' section of their website that cover some of the management issues mentioned in this book.

- www.rcog.org.uk

Royal College of Paediatrics and Child Health

This London-based college has a website where a number of management guidelines can be found. The British Association of Perinatal Medicine has also issued a number of important guidelines. For details see:

- www.rcpch.ac.uk
- www.bapm.org/index.php

Unicef UK Baby Friendly Initiative

The Baby Friendly Initiative is a global UNICEF (United Nations Children's Fund) programme that works to improve practice so that parents are helped and supported in making an informed choice over the way they feed and care for their babies by health professionals.

- www.babyfriendly.org.uk

Teratogens

Two large collaborative groups collate information and disseminate advice on drugs that may be teratogenic (i.e. cause fetal damage) if taken during pregnancy. The European Network of Teratology Information Services (ENTIS) covers not only Europe but also Israel and Latin America. The Organisation of Teratogen Information Specialists (OTIS) covers North America.

- www.entis-org.com
- www.otispregnancy.org

This book

BMJ Books have a website maintained by Blackwell Publishing where detailed, and regularly updated, commentaries are now being posted on an increasing number of the individual drug entries in this formulary. The site does *not* provide direct access to the main monographs themselves, but all monographs added or updated after the latest print edition went to press can be found and downloaded from this site. It also provides a cross link to all relevant Cochrane Reviews.

- www.neonatalformulary.com

Travel advice

A number of sites provide advice for members of the public thinking of travelling abroad. The following are provided by the World Health Organisation (WHO), by the Communicable Disease Centre (CDC) in America, and by the National Health Service (NHS) in the UK, respectively:

- www.who.int/ith/
- www.cdc.gov/travel
- www.fitfortravel.scot.nhs.uk

US Food and Drug Administration

The FDA (which is responsible for licensing all drug products in America) maintains a full and very informative website with good search facilities.

- www.fda.gov

Web-based discussion groups

Several web-based neonatal discussion groups now exist. Two of the most widely supported are the US-based NICU-NET (which is widely visited by doctors as well as nurses) and the UK-based neonatal-talk (which tends to focus more exclusively on nursing issues).

- www.neonatology.org/nicu-net/join.html
- www.infantgrapevine.co.uk

World Health Organisation

The WHO has long had the provision and dissemination of reliable information on a core of essential drugs 'that satisfy the priority healthcare needs of the population, selected with due regard to public health relevance, efficacy and safety, and comparative cost-effectiveness' as one of its major briefs. This website provides links to a large number of relevant documents and resources, including a model formulary (which has also now been published in book form).

- www.who.int/medicines

Part 2

Drug monographs

ACETAZOLAMIDE

Use
Acetazolamide is now rarely used in the neonatal period (except to manage glaucoma) because a trial in 1998 showed that it did more harm than good when used to treat post-haemorrhagic hydrocephalus.

Pharmacology
Acetazolamide is a specific inhibitor of the enzyme carbonic anhydrase used to decrease CSF and ocular fluid production in glaucoma and in children with idiopathic intracranial hypertension. It has also been used less widely as an anticonvulsant (particularly with petit mal and complex partial seizures in children). Its first clinical use, in 1952, was as a diuretic because it increases the renal loss of bicarbonate (and hence sodium, potassium and additional water). It is excreted unchanged in the urine with a serum half life of 4–10 hours.

The drug is not thought to cross the placenta, but high doses have been reported to cause teratogenic limb defects in animals, making its use inadvisable in the first trimester of pregnancy. Maternal treatment during lactation would only result in the baby receiving about 2% of the maternal dose on a weight-for-weight basis. Acetazolamide is a sulphonamide derivative, and complications such as agranulocytosis, thrombocytopenia, aplastic anaemia, skin toxicity and crystalluria with calculus formation have all been reported on occasion, as with many of the sulphonamide drugs.

Post-haemorrhagic hydrocephalus
Trials have shown that regular tapping, to remove CSF, has no measurable impact on long-term disability. While tapping can reduce symptomatic raised intracranial pressure, it can also cause iatrogenic meningitis. As a result, oral acetazolamide (which reduces CSF production) was used with increasing frequency over a 25-year period, in the hope that it would postpone or abolish the need for surgical intervention. However a UK-based trial (using 32 mg/kg of acetazolamide once every 8 hours, and 500 micrograms/kg of furosemide twice a day) was stopped in 1998 when it was found that that this did not change the number requiring shunt placement, and significantly increased the number (84% v 60%) who were dead or disabled at a year. Isosorbide was also used in much the same way for some years, but such use was never the subject of controlled trial evaluation. If regular tapping is necessary to keep CSF pressure below 7 cmH$_2$O, insertion of a ventricular reservoir should allow the atraumatic and safe removal of CSF until such time as growth and a reduction in the protein content of the CSF makes the insertion of a formal shunt possible. If acetazolamide has any residual role in the management of such children it is when it becomes necessary to delay definitive shunt surgery and to rely, temporarily, on the use of an external ventriculostomy drain. If a lot of CSF is removed by tapping, it may become necessary to replace the bicarbonate and potassium lost.

Electrolyte imbalance
Acetazolamide can cause hypokalaemic acidosis and gastrointestinal disturbances. Give 4 mmol/kg of sodium bicarbonate prophylactically once a day by mouth with high-dose treatment to reduce this risk, and monitor the child's electrolyte levels since a dangerous metabolic acidosis can occur if there is renal failure. It may also be necessary to give 1 mmol/kg a day of potassium chloride as an oral supplement.

Treatment
Seizures: Try 4 mg/kg by mouth (or, slowly, IV) once every 8 hours. Some infants only respond to two and a half times this dose.
Glaucoma: A dose of 4–10 mg/kg by mouth once every 8 hours has been used, but surgical goniotomy is usually the treatment of choice. Late recognition and poor treatment can cause irreversible damage to the eye.
Idiopathic intracranial hypertension: Start by offering 8 mg/kg by mouth once every 8 hours, while recognising that it may be necessary to give three times as much as this to reduce CSF production.

Supply and administration
One 500 mg vial costs £14·80. The dry powder should be reconstituted with 5 ml of sterile water. Take 1 ml of the resultant solution and dilute to 12·5 ml with glucose or glucose saline to obtain a solution for oral use containing 8 mg/ml. This solution should not be kept more than 24 hours after reconstitution even if kept at 4°C. The same preparation can be given IV where necessary as long as it is used promptly after reconstitution. A supply of vials is maintained in the hospital pharmacy. A sugar-free oral suspension with a 4-week shelf life costing a tenth as much as this can be prepared by the pharmacy on request.

References
See also the Cochrane reviews of ventriculomegaly management

Carrion E, Hertzog JH, Medlock MD, *et al.* Use of acetazolamide to decrease cerebrospinal fluid production in chronically ventilated patients with ventriculopleural shunts. *Arch Dis Child* 2001;**84**:68–71.

Kennedy CR, Ayers S, Campbell MJ, *et al.* Randomized, controlled trial of acetazolamide and furosemide in posthemorrhagic ventricular dilatation in infancy: follow-up at 1 year. *Pediatrics* 2001;**108**:597–607. [RCT]

Maertzdorf WJ, Vles JSH, Beuls E, *et al.* Intracranial pressure and cerebral blood flow velocity in preterm infants with posthaemorrhagic ventricular dilatation. *Arch Dis Child* 2002;**87**:F185–8.

Matthews YY. Drugs used in childhood idiopathic or benign intracranial hypertension. *Arch Dis Child Educ Pract Ed* 2008;**93**:19–25.

Whitelaw A. Intraventricular haemorrhage and posthaemorrhagic hydrocephalus: pathogenesis, prevention and future interventions. *Semin Perinatol* 2001;**6**:135–46.

Use

Aciclovir is used to treat herpes simplex virus (HSV) infection. It is also used, along with varicella-zoster immunoglobulin (q.v.), to treat those with varicella zoster (chickenpox) who are immuno-incompetent.

Pharmacology

Aciclovir is converted by viral thymidine kinase to an active triphosphate compound that inhibits viral DNA polymerase. It was first marketed in 1957. It has no effect on dormant viruses, and needs to be given early to influence viral replication. Oral uptake is limited and delayed and, at high doses, progressively less complete (bioavailability 10–20%). Aciclovir is preferentially taken up by infected cells (limiting toxicity) and cleared by a combination of glomerular filtration and tubular secretion. Slow IV administration is important to prevent drug crystals precipitating in the renal tubules. Always watch for signs of progressive neutropenia. Oral absorption is good but experts do not recommend oral use in the neonatal period. Signs of CNS toxicity, with lethargy, tremor and disorientation, will develop if poor renal function causes aciclovir to accumulate. The neonatal half life is about 5 hours, but 2·5 hours in adults and in children over 3 months old. Aciclovir enters the CSF and ocular fluids well. It also crosses the placenta, but there are no reports of teratogenicity. Treatment during lactation only results in the baby receiving 2% of the weight-related maternal dose.

Herpes simplex infection

Neonatal illness remains less common in the UK (1:40,000 births) than in North America, but overt infection can follow vaginal exposure to the HSV virus after a variable latent period. Lesions of the skin, eyes and mouth are usually the first signs, but an encephalitic or a generalised illness with pneumonia and hepatitis may develop without warning even, rarely, after some weeks. The virus grows readily in cell culture, and a positive diagnosis is often possible within 2–3 days. Scrapings from a skin vesicle can be used to provide rapid diagnosis by immunofluorescence. Isolates from specimens collected >36 hours after birth suggest genuine infection rather than transient colonisation. A polymerase chain reaction (PCR) test can be used to detect viral DNA in the CSF in cases of suspected encephalitis. Congenital (transplacental) infection is rare but has been documented. Babies born to women with an active genital infection at delivery are at significant risk of infection, the risk being very much lower (well below 5%) with reactivated infection. Unfortunately differentiation can be difficult, maternal infection is often silent, and routine cervical culture unhelpful. Caesarean delivery can prevent the baby becoming infected, but is of limited value if the membranes have been ruptured more than 6 hours. Only one small trial has yet assessed whether oral aciclovir (400 mg once every 8 hours from 36 weeks' gestation) can reduce the need for Caesarean delivery or risk of neonatal infection in mothers becoming infected for the first time during pregnancy. Babies who survive a generalised or encephalitic illness are often disabled. One report describing the outcome of long-term treatment has appeared to date, and two trials of sustained treatment (90 mg/kg by mouth twice a day) to limit the risk of relapse are still recruiting in America.

A mother with recurrent facial cold sores (labial herpes) will not infect her own baby because both will have the same high viral antibody titre. Ward staff with lesions need to apply topical 5% aciclovir cream every 4 hours as soon as the first symptoms develop (2 gram quantities are available without prescription), adhere to a careful handwashing routine, and wear a mask until the lesions dry. Staff with an active herpetic whitlow should not have direct hands-on responsibility for babies.

Treatment

Dose: 20 mg/kg IV once every 8 hours. The dosing interval must be at least doubled if there is renal failure.
Duration: Treat chicken pox for 1 week, and disseminated neonatal herpes simplex infection for 3 weeks (especially if there could be CNS involvement). Treat any absolute neutropenia with filgrastim (q.v.).
Eye ointment: Apply five times a day under ophthalmic supervision until 3 days after resolution is complete.

Supply and administration

Aciclovir is available in 250 mg vials of powder costing £9·10 each (Na^+ content 1·16 mmol). To prepare a solution for IV use reconstitute the 250 mg vial with 10 ml of water or 0·9% sodium chloride, and dilute to 50 ml with 5% dextrose to give an alkaline solution containing 5 mg/ml. Extravasation causes marked tissue damage (fluid pH 11). Do not refrigerate or keep for more than 12 hours after reconstitution. 100 ml of the 40 mg/ml sugar-free oral syrup costs £24; 200 mg dispersible tablets cost 20p each; 4·5 grams of 3% eye ointment costs £10.

References

See also the Cochrane reviews and the UK guideline on genital herpes in pregnancy

Caviness AC, Demmler GJ, Almendarez Y, *et al.* The prevalence of neonatal herpes simplex virus infection compared with serious bacterial illnesses in hospitalized neonates. *J Pediatr* 2008;**153**:164–9. (See also commentaries on pp. 155–8.)

Jones CA. Vertical transmission of genital herpes. Prevention and treatment options. *Drugs* 2009;**69**:421–34.

Jungmann E. Genital herpes. *BMJ clinical evidence handbook*. London: BMJ Books, 2008: pp. 517–19 (and updates). [SR]

Kimberlin DW, Lin Y-C, Jacobs RF, *et al.* Natural history of neonatal herpes simplex virus infections in the acyclovir era. *Pediatrics* 2001;**108**:223–9.

Kimberlin DW, Lin C-Y, Jacobs RF, *et al.* Safety and efficacy of high-dose intravenous acyclovir in the management of neonatal herpes simplex virus infection. *Pediatrics* 2001;**108**:230–8.

Malm G. Neonatal herpes simplex virus infection. *Semin Fetal Neonat Med* 2009;**14**:204–8.

Tiffany KF, Benjamin DK, Palasanthiran P, *et al.* Improved neurodevelopmental outcomes following long-term high-dose acyclovir therapy in infants with central nervous system and disseminated herpes simplex disease. *J Perinatol* 2005;**25**:156–61.

Tod M, Lokiec F, Bidault R, *et al.* Pharmacokinetics of oral acyclovir in neonates and in infants: a population analysis. *Antimicrob Agents Chemother* 2001;**45**:150–7.

ADENOSINE

Use
Adenosine is the drug of first recourse in the management of neonatal supraventricular tachycardia.

Physiology
Supraventricular tachycardia (usually an atrioventricular re-entry tachycardia) presents with a heart rate of 260–300 bpm. Something as simple as a strong vagal stimulus may be enough to re-establish a normal rhythm especially in the very young baby, and one very effective way of triggering this is to wrap the baby in a towel, and then submerge the baby's face in a bowl of ice-cold water for about 5 seconds. Even a cold face flannel may occasionally suffice. There is no need to obstruct the mouth or nose as submersion will cause reflex apnoea. Other approaches are, however, generally more effective in older children and a bolus dose of adenosine is now accepted as the approach of choice if IV access can be achieved.

Pharmacology
Adenosine is a short-acting purine nucleoside with a serum half life of about 10 seconds, first marketed commercially in 1992. It has the potential to slow conduction through the atrioventricular node and suppress the automaticity of atrial and Purkinje tissues. It has no negative inotropic effects and does not cause significant systemic hypotension, and can therefore be used safely in children with impaired cardiac function or early postoperative arrhythmia. Transient flushing may occur. There is no evidence that its use is dangerous in pregnancy or lactation (although respiratory side effects may occur in mothers with asthma). It has even been given to the fetus by cordocentesis. There are also some limited animal and human data to suggest that a continuous infusion into the right atrium might, by causing pulmonary vasodilatation, be of some value in babies with persistent pulmonary hypertension.

Adenosine is the drug of choice in the initial management of any supraventricular tachycardia that fails to respond to vagal stimulation. The arrival of this rapidly effective drug has greatly reduced the need for 2 joule/kg shock cardioversion, although this still occasionally remains the treatment of choice for the shocked, collapsed infant. If the problem persists or recurs, other drugs such as propranolol (q.v.), flecainide (q.v.) and amiodarone (q.v.) may be needed, but the true diagnosis needs confirmation first. Seek the advice of a paediatric cardiologist, and arrange, if necessary, to fax an ECG trace for assessment. An unsynchronised DC shock remains the only effective treatment for ventricular fibrillation, but this is very rare in infancy, even in babies with congenital heart disease.

Monitoring treatment
Try to connect the child to an electrocardiograph (and, if it is available, a multichannel recorder) before starting treatment so it is possible to look back at the trace later to establish what had been causing the tachycardia. Bradycardia with nodal escape may occur for a few seconds before a normal sinus rhythm returns.

Treatment
Arrhythmia: Give 150 micrograms/kg IV (0·15 ml/kg of a dilute solution made up as specified below) as rapidly as possible, followed by a small 'chaser' of 0·9% sodium chloride, while collecting at least a one channel ECG paper record for diagnostic purposes. A larger dose (300 micrograms/kg) is sometimes needed. Treatment can be repeated several times, where necessary, because the half life of adenosine is less than half a minute.

Lowering pulmonary vascular tone: Adenosine has very occasionally been given as a continuous IV infusion. Some have used a catheter positioned in the right atrium or (preferably) the pulmonary artery, but it is not clear how necessary this is. Start with a dose of 30 micrograms/kg per minute and double (or even treble) this if there is no response within half an hour. Treatment may be needed for 1–5 days.

Supply and administration
2 ml vials are available containing 3 mg/ml of adenosine (costing £4·40). To obtain a dilute solution for accurate 'bolus' use containing 1 mg/ml take 1 ml of this fluid and dilute to 3 ml with the 0·9% sodium chloride. To administer a continuous infusion of 30 micrograms/kg per minute give an hourly infusion of 1·8 mg of adenosine for each kg the baby weighs. Check the strength of the ampoule carefully because some hospitals stock non-proprietary ampoules of a different strength. Discard the ampoule once it has been opened. Do not refrigerate.

References

Dixon J, Foster K, Wyllie JP, et al. Guidelines and adenosine dosing in supraventricular tacvhycardia. Arch Dis Child 2005;**90**:1190–1 (See also **91**:373.)

Kothari DS, Skinner JR. Neonatal tachycardias: an update. Arch Dis Child 2006;**91**:F136–44.

Motti A, Tissot C, Rimensberger PC, et al. Intravenous adenosine for refractory pulmonary hypertension in a low-weight premature newborn: a potential new drug for rescue therapy. Pediatr Crit Care Med 2006;**7**:380–2.

Patole S, Lee J, Buettner P, et al. Improved oxygenation following adenosine infusion in persistent pulmonary hypertension of the newborn. Biol Neonat 1998;**74**:345–50.

Paul T, Bertram H, Bökenkamp R, et al. Supraventricular tachycardia in infants, children and adolescents. Paediatr Drugs 2002;**2**:171–81.

Skinner JR, Sharland G. Detection and management of life threatening arrhythmias in the perinatal period. Early Hum Dev 2008;**84**:161–72.

Sreeram N, Wren C. Supraventricular tachycardia in infants: response to initial treatment. Arch Dis Child 1990;**65**:127–9.

Wren C. Adenosine in paediatric arrhythmias. Paediatr Perinat Drug Ther 2006;**7**:114–17.

Use

'Bolus' doses of adrenaline are widely used during cardiopulmonary resuscitation in adults, but there has never been much evidence to support their use during neonatal resuscitation. Continuous infusions of adrenaline, or noradrenaline (q.v.), are increasingly used to treat cardiac dysfunction and septic shock.

Pharmacology

Adrenaline, first isolated in 1901, is the main chemical transmitter released by the adrenal gland. It has a wide range of α and β receptor effects, like noradrenaline. Metabolism is rapid, and the half life less than 5 minutes. It crosses the placenta. A *low* dose (less than 500 nanograms/kg per minute) usually causes systemic and pulmonary vasodilatation, with some increase in heart rate and stroke volume. A *high* dose causes intense systemic vasoconstriction; while blood pressure rises as a result, the effect on cardiac output depends on the heart's ability to cope with a rising afterload. Combined support with a corticosteroid may help, at least in the neonatal period. Adrenaline acts as a bronchodilator and respiratory stimulant; it also causes increased wakefulness, reduced appetite and reduced renal blood flow (partly from juxtaglomerular renin release). Excessive doses cause tachycardia, hypertension and cardiac arrhythmia. Heart block and pulmonary hypertension have more frequently been controlled using isoprenaline (q.v.).

When ventricular fibrillation causes circulatory stand still (the commonest reason for 'cardiac arrest' in an adult) intra-cardiac adrenaline should always be tried if cardiac massage on its own seems ineffective. However, when circulatory arrest due to respiratory failure (by far the commonest reason for 'cardiac arrest' in infancy) proves unresponsive to immediate artificial respiration and cardiac massage, intracardiac THAM or sodium bicarbonate (q.v.) should be tried first before giving intravenous or intracardiac adrenaline (despite much published advice to the contrary). While adrenaline can be given down an endotracheal tube, the efficacy of this route remains unclear. It is, however, pointless to give *any* drug during resuscitation until oxygen has been got into the lungs and seldom necessary to give anything once it has because, once oxygenated blood gets into the coronary artery, the heart will nearly always recover by itself. Very few of the babies found to *require* drugs during resuscitation at birth survive, and most of those who do are disabled. Most reports to the contrary come from centres that use drugs so frequently that they must have often been given unnecessarily.

Treatment

Anaphylaxis: See the monograph on immunisation. *Never* give more than a 1 microgram/kg IV bolus.

Resuscitation: The recommended dose is 10 micrograms/kg (0·1 ml/kg of 1:10,000 solution) IM or down the trachea. Only a rough estimate of weight is necessary. There is no evidence that a higher dose is better.

Croup and bronchiolitis: Giving 3 ml of a 1:1000 solution through a nebuliser does very little to reduce symptoms in babies with bronchiolitis, but reduced the number admitted in one study. It provides 1–2 hours of symptomatic relief in croup, but an oral or IM dose of dexamethasone (q.v.) provides more sustained relief.

Cardiac dysfunction: Continuous IV infusions of 30–300 nanograms/kg per minute, made up as described below, can increase output without causing vasoconstriction; higher doses should only be used if facilities exist to monitor cardiac output, especially in the first day of life.

Compatibility

It can be added (terminally) to a line containing dobutamine and/or dopamine, doxapram, fentanyl, heparin, midazolam, milrinone, morphine or standard TPN (but not lipid).

Supply and administration

Stock 1 ml ampoules containing 1 mg of L-adrenaline (1:1000) cost 56p each. To give a 100 nanogram/kg per minute infusion, place 3 mg of adrenaline for each kg the baby weighs in a syringe, dilute to 50 ml with 10% glucose saline, and infuse at 0·1 ml/hour. 0·9% saline or a less concentrated glucose, or glucose saline, solution can be used. These solutions are stable and do not need to be prepared afresh every 24 hours. Protect ampoules from light and always check their strength, because 100 micrograms/ml (1:10,000) ampoules also exist. Tissue extravasation can be dangerous and should be treated as outlined in the monograph on hyaluronidase.

References

See also the relevant Cochrane reviews and UK guideline on anaphylaxis

Barber CA, Wyckoff MH. Use and efficacy of endotracheal versus intravenous epinephrine during neonatal cardiopulmonary resuscitation in the delivery room. *Pediatrics* 2006;**118**:1028–34.

Bjornson CL, Johnson DW. Croup. *Lancet* 2008;**371**:329–39. [SR]

Germanakis I, Bender C, Hentschel R, *et al.* Hypercontractile heart failure caused by catecholamine therapy in premature neonates. *Acta Paediatr* 2003;**92**:836–8.

Heckmann M, Trotter A, Pohlandt F, *et al.* Epinephrine treatment of hypotension in very low birthweight infants. *Acta Paediatr* 2002;**91**:566–70.

McLean-Tooke APC, Bethune CA, Fay AC, *et al.* Adrenaline in the treatment of anaphylaxis: what is the evidence ? *BMJ* 2003;**327**:1332–5. [SR]

Pellicer A, Valverde E, Elorza MD, *et al.* Cardiovascular support for low birth weight infants and cerebral haemodynamics: a randomized, blinded, clinical trial. *Pediatrics* 2005;**115**:1501–12. [RCT]

Perondi MBM, Reis AG, Paiva EF, *et al.* A comparison of high-dose and standard-dose epinephrine in children with cardiac arrest. *N Eng Med J* 2004;**350**:1722–30. [RCT]

Sicherer SH, Simons FER. Self-injectable epinephrine for first-aid management of anaphylaxis. *Pediatrics* 2007;**119**:638–46.

Wyckoff MH, Wyllie J. Endotracheal delivery of medications during neonatalresuscitation. *Clin Perinatol* 2006;**33**:153–60. [SR]

Use

Albendazole is used to treat a range of parasitic diseases including hookworm, roundworm, threadworm and whipworm infection. It also has a role in the treatment of some tapeworm (cestode) infections and is the drug of choice to treat symptomatic microsporidiosis (*Enterocytozoon bieneusi* and *E. intestinalis* infection).

Pharmacology

Albendazole came into clinical use by a circuitous route. The drug bezimidazole was the first to be studied for its antiviral properties between 1947 and 1953, and it was then discovered that the related product thiabendazole was active against many roundworms. Further exploratory work with a range of related products finally led to the patenting of mebendazole by Janssen in 1971, and the development of albenazole, which was thought to have fewer side effects, 4 years later.

Parasitic infestation of the gut is so common in young children in many developing countries that it generally goes unnoticed by doctors unless it produces acute florid ill health. Indeed a quarter of all the people in the world are probably harbouring either roundworm, hookworm or whipworm infection at the present time. Forty million pregnancies are affected by hookworm infection each year. Two hundred million people in Africa have bilharziasis, and this contributes to the death annually of a quarter of a million people from complicated nephrosis and portal hypertension even though schistosomal infection is cheaply and easily treated with two 20 mg/kg oral doses of praziquantel 6 hours apart (three such doses for *S. japonicum* infection). The balance of risk supports *including* pregnant and lactating women in mass treatment programmes with praziquantel even if breastfeeding cannot be safely substituted for 48 hours after administration.

The oral absorption of albendazole is very limited in man (although improved by a simultaneous fatty meal) and what is absorbed is rapidly metabolised by the liver into the active drug, albendazole sulphoxide, which is then cleared from the body with a half life of 8–12 hours. The active metabolite slows little toxicity in animals, but is rapidly lethal to most nematode worms because of tubulin binding. High-dose treatment has been teratogenic in some animals, although fetal damage has not been identified in man, treatment should, where possible, be avoided in the first trimester of pregnancy. Use during lactation is probably safe.

Intestinal nematode parasites

Hookworm: *Ancylostoma duodenale* and *Necator americanus* are the commonest causes of this usually asymptomatic roundworm infection. Heavy infection can cause serious microcytic anaemia in young children.

Roundworm: Infection with *Ascaris lumbricoides*, the most common of all the roundworm infections, is normally asymptomatic but heavy infection can cause malnutrition. It is large enough to cause intestinal obstruction in some small children, while migration out of the bowel can cause a protean range of symptoms.

Threadworm: Threadworm, or pinworm, is a small white roundworm infection caused by *Enterobius vermicularis*.

Whipworm: Infection with *Trichuris trichiura* is commonly asymptomatic, but severe infection can affect growth and lead to bloody diarrhoea or an inflammatory colitis. Mature worms, which are 3–5 cm long, attach themselves to the wall of the large bowel, but diagnosis is usually made by identifying eggs in the stool.

Maternal treatment

Community-based studies in an area where severe anaemia from hookworm infection is extremely common have shown that a 400 mg oral dose of albendazole given in the second and third trimester of pregnancy can reduce the incidence of severe anaemia, boost birthweight and improve infant survival.

Treatment in infancy

A single 400 mg oral dose of albendazole will effectively 'deworm' children who are 2 or more years old (although 3 days' treatment is advisable for whipworm infection). Children less than a year old should only be treated if symptomatic, and WHO has tentatively suggested a 200 mg dose for such children. There is, as yet, no evidence on the safety of treatment in children less than 6 months old.

Supply

While albendazole (as a 400 mg tablet and 40 mg/ml suspension) and praziquantel (as a 150 mg pr 600 mg tablet) are both licensed for sale in the US they are, at the moment, only available on a named-patient basis in the UK from IDIS World Medicines, Surbiton, Surrey. GlaxoSmithKline (which has donated large quantities of albendazole to the WHO) is the main manufacturer in the US. Bayer makes praziquantel in Germany.

References
See also the relevant Cochrane reviews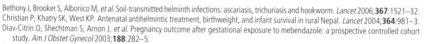

Bethony J, Brooker S, Albonico M, *et al*. Soil-transmitted helminth infections: ascariasis, trichuriasis and hookworm. *Lancet* 2006;**367**:1521–32.

Christian P, Khatry SK, West KP. Antenatal antihelmintic treatment, birthweight, and infant survival in rural Nepal. *Lancet* 2004;**364**:981–3.

Diav-Citrin O, Shechtman S, Arnon J, *et al*. Pregnancy outcome after gestational exposure to mebendazole: a prospective controlled cohort study. *Am J Obstet Gynecol* 2003;**188**:282–5.

Kalra V, Dua T, Kumar V. Efficacy of albendazole and short-course dexamethasone treatment in children with 1 or 2 ring-enhancing lesions of neurocyticercosis: a randomized controlled trial. *J Pediatr* 2003;**143**:111–4. [RCT]

Keiser J, Utzinger J. Efficacy of current drugs against soil-transmitted helminth infections: systematic review and meta-analysis. *JAMA* 2008;**299**:193748. [SR]

Montresor A, Awasthi S, Crompton DWT. Use of bezimidazoles in children younger than 24 months for the treatment of soil-transmitted helminthiasis. *Acta Tropica* 2003;**86**:223–32. (See also pp. 141–59.)

Olds GR. Administration of praziquantel to pregnant and lactating women. *Acta Trop* 2003;**86**:185–95.

Tremoulet AH, Avila-Aguero ML, Paris MM, *et al*. Albendazole therapy for *Microsporidium* diarrhea in immunocompetent Costa Rican children. *Pediatr Infect Dis J* 2004;**23**:915–18.

Use

Alteplase is a fibrinolytic drug used to dissolve intravascular thrombi. Streptokinase (q.v.) is cheaper.

Pharmacology

All fibrinolytic drugs work by activating plasminogen to plasmin, which then degrades fibrin, causing the break up of intravascular thrombi. Treatment should always be started as soon as possible after any clot has formed. Streptokinase and alteplase both have an established role in the management of myocardial infarction, but controlled trials show that benefit is limited if treatment is delayed for more than 12 hours. Alteplase, a human tissue plasminogen activator first manufactured by a recombinant DNA process in 1983, is a glycoprotein that directly activates the conversion of plasminogen to plasmin. It became commercially available in 1988. When given IV it remains relatively inactive in the circulation until it binds to fibrin, for which it has a high affinity. It is, however, rapidly destroyed by the liver, with a plasma half life of only 5 minutes. As a result, adverse effects (including excess bleeding) are uncommon in adults and usually controlled without difficulty by stopping treatment. There is little experience of use during pregnancy. The high molecular weight makes placental transfer unlikely. There is no evidence of teratogenicity, but placental bleeding is a theoretical possibility. Use during lactation seems unlikely to pose any serious problem.

There have been many reports of the use of alteplase to lyse arterial and intracardiac thrombi in the neonatal period, but it is not clear whether it is any safer or more effective than streptokinase and the drug is considerably more expensive. There is, however, probably rather less risk of an adverse effect, and less theoretical risk of an allergic reaction. Visualise the clot and take advice from a vascular surgeon before starting treatment, remembering that ultrasound review has shown that the great majority of catheter-related thrombi never give rise to symptoms. Use can certainly speed the resolution of infective endocarditis. However there is a risk of bleeding, especially if the platelet count is below 100×10^9/l, or the fibrinogen level falls below 1 g/l. Intracranial bleeding was a common complication with sustained use in one recent neonatal case series, so risk assessment is important before starting treatment. Combined use with heparin (q.v.) optimises outcome in adults with myocardial infarction, but the value of such dual treatment in babies has not been properly studied. Try and avoid venepuncture and IM injections during treatment. See the website for a commentary on the slim evidence base that currently underpins the management of clots and emboli in early infancy.

Alteplase (0·5 mg/kg) has been instilled experimentally into the cerebral ventricles of babies with severe intraventricular bleeding in an attempt to reduce post-haemorrhagic hydrocephalus, but neither of the first two trials of this strategy showed any real evidence of benefit and such treatment may provoke further bleeding.

Prophylaxis

A 1 mg/ml solution of alteplase is better (if more expensive) than heparin at keeping 'stopped-off' long lines patent. Slightly overfill the line, and aspirate before reuse to stop small emboli being shed into the lung.

Treatment

Blocked catheters: Instil a volume of alteplase (1 mg/ml) slightly greater than the catheter dead space. Other strategies, as outlined in the monograph on urokinase, may sometimes work better in lines that have been used to infuse parenteral nutrition.

Thrombi: Give 500 micrograms/kg over 30 minutes. If Doppler ultrasound shows inadequate resolution consider a second similar dose followed by a continuous infusion of 200 micrograms/kg per hour.

Monitoring

Monitor the fibrinogen level regularly during sustained treatment, and adjust the dose if the level falls below 1 g/l. Give cryoprecipitate or fresh frozen plasma (q.v.) at once if a bleeding tendency develops.

Supply and administration

10 mg (5·8 mega-units) vials of powder suitable for reconstitution using 10 ml of water for injection (as provided) cost £135. The resultant solution (containing 1 mg of alteplase per ml) must be used within 24 hours, even if stored at 4°C, but small pre-prepared syringes can be kept for 3 months at −20°C. To give 200 micrograms/kg per hour dilute the reconstituted solution with an equal volume of 0·9% sodium chloride and infuse at a rate of 0·4 ml/kg per hour. Do not dilute the reconstituted solution with anything except 0·9% sodium chloride.

References

Gittins NS, Hunter-Blair YL, Matthews J, *et al.* Comparison of alteplase and heparin in maintaining the patency of pediatric central venous haemodialysis lines: a randomised controlled trial. *Arch Dis Child* 2007;**92**:499–501. [RCT] (See also pp. 516–17.)

Gupta AA, Leaker M, Andrew M, *et al.* Safety and outcomes of thrombolysis with tissue plasminogen activator for treatment of intravascular thrombosis in children. *J Pediatr* 2001;**139**:682–8.

Hartmann J, Hussein A, Trowitzsch E, *et al.* Treatment of neonatal thrombus formation with recombinant tissue plasminogen activator: six years experience and review of the literature. *Arch Dis Child* 2001;**85**:F18–22. (See also pp. F66–72.)

Jacobs BR, Haygood M, Hingl J. Recombinant tissue plasminogen activator in the treatment of central venous catheter occlusion in children. *J Pediatr* 2001;**139**:593–6.

Monagle P, Michelson AD, Bovill E, *et al.* Antithrombotic therapy in children. [Consensus statement] *Chest* 2001;**119**:344–70S.

Whitelaw A, Evans D, Carter M, *et al.* Randomized clinical trial of prevention of hydrocephalus after intraventricular hemorrhage in preterm infants: brain-washing versus tapping fluid. *Pediatrics* 2007;**119**:e107–18. [RCT]

Use

Amikacin is commonly used to treat suspected neonatal infection in some countries, but it is usually held in 'reserve' in the UK for use against Gram-negative bacteria that are resistant to gentamicin, as well as all the other commonly used antibiotics, and should only be used on the advice of a consultant microbiologist.

Pharmacology

Amikacin is a semisynthetic aminoglycoside antibiotic first developed in 1972. It is of particular use in the treatment of Gram-negative bacteria resistant to gentamicin (such as certain *Enterobacter* species). Significant placental transfer occurs and, although the drug has not been documented as causing fetal damage, it would seem wise to monitor blood levels when amikacin is used in pregnancy to minimise the risk of fetal ototoxicity because drug accumulation has been documented in the fetal lung, kidney and placenta. Only small amounts appear in CSF or in human milk and absorption from the gut is minimal. The drug, like its parent compound, kanamycin, is largely excreted through the renal glomerulus. The half life is 7–14 hours in babies with a postmenstrual age of less than 30 weeks, and 4–7 hours at a postmenstrual age of 40 weeks (the adult half life being about 2 hours). Nephrotoxicity and cochlear or vestibular damage can occur if 'trough' blood levels in excess of those generally recommended go uncorrected, as with all aminoglycosides. The risk is increased if amikacin is prescribed for more than 10 days, follows treatment with another aminoglycoside, or is given at the same time as a diuretic such as furosemide (q.v.). Amikacin is less toxic to the neonatal kidney than gentamicin or netilmicin, however, and also probably less ototoxic. Absorption is said to be somewhat unpredictable after IM administration in very small babies. For a justification of the dose regimen recommended in this book see the monograph on gentamicin and, for a more general discussion of the prescribing of aminoglycosides in infancy, see the associated website. The dosage interval should be increased in patients with renal failure and adjusted in the light of serum antibiotic levels.

Treatment

Dose: Give 15 mg/kg IV or IM to babies less than 4 weeks old, and 20 mg/kg to babies older than this.
Timing: Give a dose once every 36 hours in babies less than 32 weeks' gestation in the first week of life. Give all other babies a dose once every 24 hours unless renal function is poor. Check the trough serum level just before the fourth dose is due and increase the dosage interval if this level is more than 8 mg/l.

Blood levels

The trough level is all that usually needs to be monitored in babies on high-dose treatment once every 24–36 hours, and this is probably only necessary as a *routine* in babies less than 10 days old or with possible renal failure. Aim for a trough level of less than 8 mg/l (1 mg/l = 1·71 μmol/l). The 1 hour peak level, when measured, should be 20–30 mg/l. Collect specimens in the same way as for gentamicin.

Supply and administration

2 ml (100 mg) vials containing 50 mg/ml cost £2·40 (Na$^+$ content 0·5 mmol). Material should not be stored after dilution. Do not mix amikacin with any other drug. IV doses do *not* need to be given slowly over 30 minutes.

References

Allegaert K, Anderson BJ, Cossey V, *et al.* Limited predictability of amikacin clearance in extreme premature neonates at birth. *Br J Clin Pharmacol* 2006;**61**:39–48.

Allegaert K, Cossey V, Langhendries JP, *et al.* Effects of co-administration of ibuprofen-lysine on the pharmacokinetics of amikacin in preterm infants during the first days of life. *Biol Neonat* 2004;**86**:207–11.

Allegaert K, Scheers I, Cossey V, *et al.* Covariates of amikacin clearance in neonates: the impact of postnatal age on predictability. *Drug Metab Lett* 2008;**2**:286–9.

Berger A, Kretzer V, Gludovatz P, *et al.* Evaluation of an amikacin loading dose for nosocomial infections in very low birthweight infants. *Acta Paediatr* 2004;**93**:356–60.

Giapros VI, Andronikou S, Cholevas VI, *et al.* Renal function in premature infants during aminoglycoside therapy. *Pediatr Nephrol* 1995;**9**:163–6.

Kenyon CF, Knoppert DC, Lee SK, *et al.* Amikacin pharmacokinetics and suggested dosage modifications for the preterm infant. *Antimicrob Agents Chemother* 1990;**34**:265–8.

Kotze A, Bartel PR, Sommers DK. Once versus twice daily amikacin in neonates: prospective study on toxicity. *J Paediatr Child Health* 1999;**35**:283–6. [RCT]

Labaune JM, Bleyzac N, Maire P, *et al.* Once-a-day individualized amikacin dosing for suspected infection at birth based on population pharmacokinetic models. *Biol Neonat* 2001;**80**:142–7.

Langhendries JP, Battisti O, Bertrand JM, *et al.* Once a day administration of amikacin in neonates: assessment of nephrotoxicity and ototoxicity. *Dev Pharmacol Ther* 1993;**20**:220–30. [RCT]

Langhendries JP, Battisti O, Bertrand JM, *et al.* Adaptation in neonatology of the once-daily concept of aminoglycoside administration: evaluation of a dosing chart for amikacin in an intensive care unit. *Biol Neonat* 1998;**74**:351–62.

Marik PE, Lipman J, Kobilski S, *et al.* A prospective randomized study comparing once- versus twice-daily amikacin in critically ill adult and paediatric patients. *J Antimicrob Chemother* 1991;**28**:753–64. [RCT]

Prober CG, Yeager AS, Arvin AM. The effect of chronologic age on the serum concentration of amikacin in the sick term and premature infant. *J Pediatr* 1981;**98**:636–40.

Vásquez-Mendoza MG, Vargas-Origel A, Ramos-Jiménez A del C, *et al.* Efficacy and renal toxicity of once daily dose of amikacin versus conventional dosage regime. *Am J Perinatol* 2007;**24**:141–6.

Use

Amiodarone is increasingly used to control persisting troublesome supraventricular, and junctional ectopic, tachycardia. It is also used to manage those fetal cardiac arrhythmias that do not respond to digitalisation or flecainide (q.v.). Use should **always** be initiated and supervised by a paediatric cardiologist because adverse reactions are not uncommon, and the manufacturers have not yet endorsed use in children. Treatment can usually be discontinued after 9–12 months.

Pharmacology

Amiodarone, a class III antiarrhythmic agent first developed in 1963, is used in the management of certain congenital or postoperative re-entry tachycardias, especially where there is impaired ventricular function. It prolongs the duration of the action potential and slows atrioventricular (AV) nodal conduction. It also increases the atrial, AV nodal and ventricular refractory periods, facilitating re-entrant rhythm suppression. Blood levels are of no value in optimising treatment or in avoiding toxicity. Combined treatment with oral propranolol (q.v.) may be needed at first, but the use of propranolol can usually be discontinued after a few months. Flecainide is probably a better first choice for automatic arrhythmias.

Tissue levels greatly exceed plasma levels (V_D ~40–80 l/kg). Amiodarone also has an extremely long half life (several weeks), and treatment usually has to be given for several days before a therapeutic response is achieved. IV treatment can be used, when necessary, to speed the achievement of a response as long as the consequent exposure to benzyl alcohol is judged acceptable. Most of the adverse effects associated with amiodarone treatment are reversible once treatment is withdrawn. Skin photosensitivity (controlled by using a sun block cream), skin discolouration, corneal microdeposits (easily seen with a slit lamp), liver disorders (with or without jaundice), pneumonitis, and peripheral neuropathy have all been reported, but such complications have not yet been seen in infancy.

Amiodarone is thought to be hazardous in pregnancy because of its iodine content, and the manufacturer has not endorsed the drug's use in children under 3 years. Such a risk may have to be accepted, however, if no other treatment can be found for maternal (or fetal) arrhythmia. For the same reason most texts recommend that patients on long-term treatment should also be monitored (with T_3, T_4 and TSH levels) for hypo- and hyperthyroidism. Such complications have not, however, been reported as yet during treatment in the first year of life. In addition, since breast milk contains a substantial amount of amiodarone there are important reasons why a mother on treatment who wishes to breastfeed should only do so under close medical supervision. While absorption is incomplete experience suggests that the baby can receive, on a weight-for-weight basis, a dose equivalent to about a third of that taken by the mother.

Drug interactions

Joint medication can prolong the half life of flecainide, digoxin, phenytoin and warfarin. Treatment with these drugs *must* be monitored, since the dose of these drugs may have to be reduced if toxicity is to be avoided. Amiodarone can prolong the QT interval and cases of torsade des pointes have been reported.

Treatment

Intravenous: Only give this drug IV in an intensive care setting, and when a rapid response is essential. Give 5 mg/kg over 30 minutes and a second similar dose if the first is ineffective. Watch for bradycardia and hypotension. Further 5 mg/kg maintenance doses can be given IV every 12 or 24 hours if necessary. Change to oral administration as soon as possible.

Oral: Give a 15 mg/kg loading dose (unless the baby has already had IV treatment) and then a maintenance dose of between 5 and 12 mg/kg once a day depending on the response achieved.

Supply and administration

3 ml ampoules containing 50 mg/ml of amiodarone hydrochloride (and 20 mg/ml of benzyl alcohol) cost £1·40. To give 5 mg/kg of amiodarone IV, place 0·5 ml (25 mg) of amiodarone for each kg the baby weighs in a syringe, dilute to 25 ml with 5% glucose (**not** sodium chloride), and give 5 ml of this dilute preparation over 30 minutes. Watch for extravasation because the excipient, Tween-80®, is very irritant and the solution quite acid (pH ~4). Try to avoid giving a continuous infusion to a child under 3 years because it can leach the plasticiser out of an IV giving set. Prepare a fresh solution each time. An oral suspension in syrup containing 20 mg/ml with a 14-day shelf life can be prepared on request. It must be protected from light.

References

Burri S, Hug MI, Bauersfeld U. Efficacy and safety of intravenous amiodarone for incessant tachycardias in infants. *Eur J Pediatr* 2003;**162**:880–4.

Etheridge SP, Craig JE, Compton SJ. Amiodarone is safe and highly effective therapy for supraventricular tachycardia in infants. *Am Heart J* 2001;**141**:105–10. (See also pp. 3–5.)

Magee LA, Downar E, Sermer M, *et al*. Pregnancy outcome after gestational exposure to amiodarone in Canada. *Am J Obstet Gynecol* 1995;**172**:1307–11.

Perry JC, Fenrich AL, Hulse JE, *et al*. Pediatric use of intravenous amiodarone: efficacy and safety in critically ill patients from a multicenter protocol. *J Am Coll Cardiol* 1996;**27**:1246–50.

Pézarda PG, Boussion F, Sentilhes L, *et al*. Fetal tachycardia: a role for amiodarone as first- or second-line therapy? *Arch Cardiovasc Dis* 2008;**101**:619–27.

Saul JP, Scott WA, Brown S, *et al*. Intravenous amiodarone for incessant tachyarrhythmias in children. A randomized, double-blind, antiarrythmic drug trial. *Circulation* 2005;**112**:3470–7. [RCT]

Ward RM, Lugo RA. Cardiovascular drugs for the new born. [Review article] *Clin Perintol* 2006;**32**:979–97.

AMODIAQUINE with ARTESUNATE

Use
Amodiaquine is generally effective against most strains of *Plasmodium falciparum* that are chloroquine sensitive (q.v.), and some that are not. Toxicity can sometimes develop with long-term use, so it is only used to treat episodes of overt infection. To stop drug resistance developing it is used together with an artemisinin such as artesunate (as outlined in the artemether monograph).

History
The search for a drug that can prevent, rather than cure, infection with the malaria parasite began in 1917 with the testing of a range of compounds on deliberately infected patients with terminal paralytic syphilis, before it was shown, in 1924, that canaries could be used instead. Knowing that the plasmodia parasite takes up methylene blue, work initially focused on quinoline/methylene blue hybrids, and clinical trials soon showed that one such drug, pamaquin, could cure naturally acquired falciparum malaria. It kills the sporozoites in the liver but not the merozoites liberated by cyclical liver cell rupture into the blood as quinine does. A number of 4- and 8-aminoquinolones were studied during the Second World War by the American Army's Malaria Research Programme before chloroquine, and then amodiaquine, came into use in the late 1940s. The artemisinin drugs artemether (q.v.) and artesunate have now emerged as the most potent drugs for combating malaria and, to prevent the emergence of drug resistance yet again, these are now routinely given together with an antimalarial such as amodiaquine or lumefantrine (as outlined in the monograph on artemether).

Pharmacology
Amodiaquine hydrochloride is a 4-aminoquinolone structurally related to chloroquine. It is well absorbed when taken by mouth and rapidly converted by the liver to the active metabolite monodesmethylamodiaquine, which is then excreted by the kidney in a relatively slow and variable way (mean plasma half life 2–3 days). Amodiaquine is no longer used to *prevent* infection but it has started to be used to *treat* infection, because there is a widespread belief that the neutropenia and liver toxicity noted in the 1980s only occurs with sustained use. This may be true but, where amodiaquine is most widely used, such toxicity could well go unrecognised. A serious overdose of amodiaquine can cause seizures and loss of consciousness but it does not appear to cause any of the life-threatening cardiovascular complications often seen after an overdose of chloroquine. However, the drug has not yet been very widely used. An attack in the last 6 months of pregnancy can seriously affect maternal health and jeopardise fetal survival. Treatment with amodiaquine, ideally with one dose of pyrimethamine (q.v.) and sulphadoxine (as Fansidar®) seems very safe, though it can briefly exacerbate tiredness, dizziness and nausea. Little is known about use during lactation, but use of the closely related drug chloroquine is extremely safe.

Treatment
During pregnancy: Give two 600 mg doses 24 hours apart and then one 300 mg dose. Co-treatment with a single 75 mg dose of pyrimethamine and 1·5 grams of sulphadoxine on the first day minimises treatment failure.
During infancy: Give two 10 mg/kg doses of amodiaquine base 24 hours apart, and then one 5 mg/kg dose after a further 24 hours. Artesunate/amodiaquine combination tablets: in infants 4·5 to <9 kg, 25 mg/67·5 mg tablets, one tablet crushed with water daily for 3 days; from 9 to <18 kg, 50 mg/135 mg tablets, one tablet daily for 3 days.
Rectal artesunate: Early rectal artesunate before transit to more distant facilities is helpful in those too ill to take oral medication. A 10 mg/kg rectal dose seems ideal, but a 100 mg suppository, given as soon as the child is ill, seems safe in 6–72-month-old children. Move to oral treatment (see above) as soon as possible

Supply
Amodiaquine with or without artesunate is not currently marketed in the UK or the US, but is available from Parke-Davis as a 200 mg tablet (Camoquine®) costing 65p. This can be crushed, suspended in water, and given by spoon. A commercial suspension has also been supplied for research purposes. It is normally described in terms of the amount of amodiaquine base (260 mg of hydrochloride = 200 mg of base).

WHO-promoted artesunate/amodiaquine combination packs are increasingly available in a variety of strengths; 25 mg/67·5 mg, 50 mg/135 mg, 100 mg/270 mg. A range of artesunate products suitable for IV, IM or rectal use are available in many countries where malaria is endemic.

References
See also the relevant Cochrane reviews

Clerk CA, Bruce J, Affipunquh PK, *et al.* A randomized, controlled trial of intermittent preventive treatment with sulfadoxine-pyremethamine, amodiaquine, or the combination in pregnant women in Ghana. *J Infect Dis* 2008;**198**:1202–11. [RCT]

Falade CO, Oqundele AO, Yusuf BO, *et al.* High efficacy of two artemisinin-based combinations (artemether-lumefantrine and artesunate plus amodiaquine) for acute uncomplicated malaria in Ibadan, Nigeria. *Trop Med Int Health* 2008.**13**:63543. [RCT]

Gomes MF, Faiz MA, Gyapong JO, *et al.* Pre-referral rectal artesunate to prevent death and disability in severe malaria: a placebo controlled trial. *Lancet* 2009;**373**:557–66. [RCT]

Massaga JJ, Kitua AY, Lemnge MM, *et al.* Effect of intermittent treatment with amodiaquine on anaemia and malarial fevers in infants in Tanzania: a randomised placebo-controlled trial. *Lancet* 2003;**361**:1853–60. [RCT]

Olliaro P, Nevill C, Le Bras J, *et al.* Systematic review of amodiaquine treatment in uncomplicated malaria. *Lancet* 1996;**348**:1196–201. [SR] (See also pp. 1184–5.)

Staedke SG, Kamya MR, Dorsey G, *et al.* Amodiaquine, sulfadoxine/pyrimethamine, and combination therapy in treatment of uncomplicated falciparum malaria in Kampala, Uganda: a randomised trial. *Lancet* 2001;**358**:368–74. [RCT]

Tagbor H, Bruce J, Browne E, *et al.* Efficacy, safety and tolerability of amodiaquine plus sulphadoxine-pyrimethamine used alone or in combination for malaria treatment in pregnancy: a randomised trial. *Lancet* 2006;**368**:1349–56. [RCT] (See also pp. 1306–7.)

Use
Amoxicillin has similar properties to ampicillin (q.v.), and there is little to choose between the two antibiotics when given IV to treat *Listeria*, β-lactamase-negative *Haemophilus* or enterococcal infection.

Pharmacology
Amoxicillin is a semisynthetic broad-spectrum, bactericidal, aminopenicillin that is active against a wide range of organisms including *Listeria*, *Haemophilus*, enterococci, streptococci, pneumococci and many coliform organisms, and is also active against *Salmonella*, *Shigella* and non-penicillinase-forming strains of *Proteus*. It still remains, 40 years after its first introduction in 1964, the drug recommended by WHO when treating bacterial respiratory tract illness in young children (along with co-trimoxazole (q.v.) if there is a risk of occult HIV infection). Analgesia alone suffices for almost 90% of cases of otitis media. The half life in the full term baby is about 4 hours (but very variable) falling to a little over 1 hour in later infancy as renal excretion improves and, because efficacy depends on keeping the blood level continuously above the minimum inhibitory dose (as with all β-lactam antibiotics), dosing frequency must reflect this. Amoxicillin readily crosses the placenta, but use during lactation exposes the baby to less than 1% of the weight-adjusted maternal dose.

The dosage policy recommended here is more than adequate, but designed to achieve high CSF levels in the face of early subclinical meningitis, and in the knowledge that the drug is very non-toxic. Potency can be enhanced by also giving clavulanic acid, which has no antibiotic properties of its own but inhibits many β-lactamase enzymes. The combination (marketed as co-amoxiclav) can cause cholestatic jaundice, and use is best reserved for treating amoxicillin-resistant organisms. Administration to women in preterm labour seems inexplicably associated with a higher risk of neonatal necrotising enterocolitis. If co-amoxiclav is used in the neonate, specify the dose to be used by the product's amoxicillin content. There is little to choose between ampicillin and amoxicillin when given parenterally, although amoxicillin is said to be more rapidly bactericidal at doses close to the minimum inhibitory concentration. Both antibiotics are well absorbed when taken by mouth, widely distributed in body tissues (including bronchial secretions), and rapidly excreted in the urine. Although amoxicillin shows better bioavailablity when taken by mouth, it can still be quite variable in young children. Adverse effects are similar to those seen with ampicillin, but rare, and diarrhoea may be slightly less common.

Prophylaxis
Mothers: While ascending infection may be an occasional cause of spontaneous preterm labour, the only antibiotic that has yet been shown to delay labour or improve outcome is clindamycin (q.v.) in women with overt bacterial vaginosis in early pregnancy. See the monograph on ampicillin for a comment on antibiotic use when labour starts before 35 weeks and the membranes ruptured before there were overt signs of labour.

Children: Give babies with structural heart disease (other than a simple ASD) 50 mg/kg of amoxicillin IV or IM half an hour before and 6 hours after any surgical procedure involving a site where infection is suspected to reduce the risk of bacterial endocarditis. Some would give gentamicin as well to those at very high risk. It may be better to give azithromycin or clindamycin rather than amoxicillin in a baby who has had more than one dose of a penicillin class antibiotic in the preceding month. Even if full surgical correction is achieved (as with a simple VSD) prophylaxis should still be offered for a further 6 months until epithelialisation is complete.

Measles: Pre-emptive antibiotic treatment may prevent complicating bacterial pneumonia, especially in countries where measles remains a dangerous illness.

Treatment
Dose: Give 100 mg/kg IV or IM if meningitis is a possibility. In all other situations a dose of 50 mg/kg is more than adequate, given (if the patient is well enough) by mouth. Otitis media only needs 25 mg/kg.

Timing: Give one dose every 12 hours in the first week of life, every 8 hours in babies 1–3 weeks old, and every 6 hours in babies 4 or more weeks old. Increase the dosage interval if there is severe renal failure. Treat otitis media for 5–7 days, septicaemia for 10–14 days, meningitis for 3 weeks and osteitis for 4 weeks. Even severe pneumonia can usually be managed by treatment three times a day for 5–7 days. Oral medication can nearly always be used to complete any sustained course of treatment.

Supply
Stock 250 mg vials cost 32p (Na⁺ content 0·8 mmol). Add 2·4 ml of water for injection to the 250 mg vial (or 4·6 ml to the 500 mg vial) to get a solution containing 100 mg/ml and always use this at once. A 100 mg/kg dose contains 0·33 mmol/kg of sodium. A sugar-free oral suspension (25 mg/ml) is available which costs £1·10 for 100 ml. It can be kept at room temperature after reconstitution, but should be used within 2 weeks.

References
See also the relevant Cochrane reviews

Addo-Yobo E, Chisaka N, Hassan M, *et al*. Oral amoxicillin versus injectable penicillin for severe pneumonia in children aged 3 to 59 months: a randomised multicentre equivalency study. *Lancet* 2004;**364**:1141–8. (See also pp. 1104–5.) [RCT]

Gras-Le Guen C, Boscher C, Godon N, *et al*. Therapeutic amoxicillin levels achieved with oral administration in term neonates. *Eur J Clin Pharmacol* 2007;**63**:657–62.

Pichichero ME, Reed MD. Variations in amoxicillin pharmacokinetic/pharmacodynamic parameters may explain treatment failure in acute otitis media. *Pediatr Drugs* 2009;**11**:243–9.

Pullen J, Driessen M, Stolk LML, *et al*. Amoxicillin pharmacokinetics in (preterm) infants aged 10 to 52 days: effect of postnatal age. *Ther Drug Monit* 2007;**29**:376–80.

Spiro DM, Tay K-Y, Arnold DH, *et al*. Wait-and-see prescription for the treatment of acute otitis media. *JAMA* 2006;**296**:1235–41. [RCT]

Use

Amphotericin B is a valuable antibiotic used in the treatment of suspected or proven systemic fungal infection. A liposomal formulation can be used if toxicity develops, but routine use is hard to justify, given the cost. The liposomal formulation is also used to treat leishmaniasis (kala-azar) as outlined in the web commentary.

Pharmacology

Amphotericin B is a polyene antifungal derived from *Streptomyces nodosum*. It has been widely used to treat aspergillosis, candidiasis, coccidioidomycosis and cryptococcosis since it was first isolated in 1953. It works by binding to a sterol moiety on the surface of the organism, causing cell death by increasing cell membrane permeability. The clinical response does not always correlate with the result of *in vitro* testing. Because amphotericin only penetrates the CSF poorly, synergistic co-treatment with flucytosine (q.v.) should be considered when treating serious systemic fungal infection. (Many now think that fluconazole (q.v.) on its own is a better choice in this situation, but no formal comparative study has yet been mounted.) Caspofungin (q.v.) is probably the drug of choice if systemic *Candida* infection fails to respond to amphotericin.

Amphotericin is a potentially toxic drug with many common adverse effects including a dose-dependent and dose-limiting impairment of renal function. Drug elimination is poorly understood, unrelated to renal function, and extremely unpredictable in the neonatal period. Significant drug accumulation is thought to occur in the liver (V_D ~4 l/kg). A low salt intake increases the risk of nephrotoxicity. Anaemia and leucopenia are not uncommon, and hypokalaemia can occur. Fever, vomiting and rigors can occur during or after IV infusion. The risk of anaphylaxis in older patients can be avoided by giving a 'test' dose of 100 micrograms/kg IV over 10 minutes, 30 minutes before the first full dose of treatment is due. Rapid infusion can cause hyperkalaemia and an arrhythmia, while an overdose has occasionally caused death. Over 80% of adults given amphotericin experience some renal impairment, but such problems seem much less common in infancy. Amphotericin crosses the placenta, but does not seem to be toxic or teratogenic to the fetus, so treatment does not need to be withheld during pregnancy. No information is available on the use of amphotericin during lactation.

Diagnosing fungal infection

Notes on the diagnosis of systemic candidiasis appear in the monograph on fluconazole.

Treatment

Standard formulation: Give 1 mg/kg IV over 4 hours once a day for 7 days, and then 1 mg/kg once every 48 hours. Incremental treatment is inappropriate, and a first 'test' dose is not necessary in a neonate. Ensure a sodium intake of at least 4 mmol/kg/day. Treatment is usually continued for 4 weeks.

Liposomal formulation: AmBisome® is the most widely studied product. Start by giving 2 mg/kg IV over 30–60 minutes once a day. Doses of up to 4 mg/kg once a day have been used in deep-seated neonatal infection involving bone or the CNS without causing recognisable toxic side effects, and doses of 5 mg/kg once a day are often used in older children with proven infection. Length of treatment has varied widely.

Supply and administration

Ready-to-use prefilled syringes (which should be stored in the dark and used within 48 hours but which do not need to be protected from light during administration) can be dispensed by the pharmacy on request.

Standard formulation: 50 mg vials of dry powder (which should be stored at 4°C) cost £4·10 (Na$^+$ content <0·5 mmol). Prepare the powder immediately before use by adding 10 ml of sterile water for injection into the vial through a wide bore needle to give a solution containing 5 mg/ml. Shake until the colloidal solution is clear. Then further dilute the drug by adding 1 ml of this colloidal solution to 49 ml of 5% glucose to give a solution containing 100 micrograms/ml. The batch used *must* have a pH above 4·2, and commercial supplies of glucose have a pH that may vary between 3·5 and 6·5. One approach is to ensure an adequate pH by always adding buffer (as described in the package insert). The alternative is to measure the pH – easily checked using Whatman pH indicator paper (cat. no. 2613991) – and only add buffer if this is shown to be necessary. Do not employ a <1 μm filter, expose to bright light or mix with any other drug.

Liposomal formulation: 50 mg vials of the liposomal preparation (AmBisome) cost £97. Add 12 ml of sterile water for injection to obtain a solution containing 4 mg/ml and shake vigorously until the powder is completely dispersed. Take 20 mg (5 ml) from the vial using the 5 μm filter provided, dilute to 20 ml with 5% glucose to give a solution containing 1 mg/ml, and infuse the prescribed amount over 30–60 minutes.

Compatibility: Do not let either product come into contact with *any* fluid other than 5% glucose.

References

Bailey JE, Meyers C, Kleigman RM, *et al*. Pharmacokinetics, outcome of treatment, and toxic effects of amphotericin B and 5-flurocytosine in neonates. *J Pediatr* 1990;**116**:791–7.

Blyth CC, Palasanthiran P, O'Brien TA. Antifungal therapy in children with invasive fungal infection: a systematic review. *Pediatrics* 2007;**119**:772–84. [SR]

Moen MD, Lyseng-Williamson KA, Scott LJ. Liposomal amphotericin B: a review of its use in empirical therapy in febrile neutropenia and in the treatment of invasive fungal infections. *Drugs* 2009;**69**:361–92. [SR]

Sobel JD. Use of antifungal drugs in pregnancy: a focus on safety. *Drug Saf* 2000;**23**:77–85.

Weitkamp TJ, Poets CF, Sievers R, *et al*. Candida infection in very low birth-weight infants: outcome and nephrotoxicity of treatment with liposomal amphotericin B (AmBisome). *Infection* 1998;**26**:11–15.

Wurthwein G, Groll AH, Hempel G, *et al*. Population pharmacokinetics of amphotericin B lipid complex in neonates. *Antimicrob Agents Chemother* 2005;**49**:5092–8.

Use

Ampicillin is a widely used antibiotic with similar properties to amoxicillin (q.v.).

Pharmacology

Ampicillin is a semisynthetic broad-spectrum aminopenicillin that crosses the placenta. A little appears in human milk but it can safely be given to a lactating mother since the baby is known to receive less than 1% of the weight-related maternal dose. Maculopapular drug rashes are *not* a sign of serious drug sensitivity, and are relatively rare in the neonatal period. The drug is actively excreted in the urine and, partly as a result of this, the plasma half life falls from about 6 hours to 2 hours during the first 10 days of life. Penetration into the CSF is moderately good, particularly when the meninges are inflamed.

Ampicillin was, for many years, the most widely used antibiotic for treating infection with *Listeria*, β-lactamase-negative *Haemophilus*, enterococci, *Shigella* and non-penicillinase-forming *Proteus* species. It is also effective against streptococci, pneumococci and many coliform organisms. Ampicillin has frequently been used prophylactically to reduce the risk of infection after abdominal surgery (including Caesarean delivery), as has cefoxitin (q.v.). Ampicillin is resistant to acids and moderately well absorbed when given by mouth, but oral medication can alter the normal flora of the bowel (causing diarrhoea), and the absorption and 'bioavailability' of ampicillin when taken by mouth does not approach that achieved by amoxicillin. The arrival of ampicillin on the market before amoxicillin, following synthesis in 1961, probably explains the former's continued common use, even though most authorities now consider amoxicillin the better product for this and a range of other reasons.

Preterm prelabour rupture of membranes (PPROM)

Prophylactic antibiotic treatment can delay delivery enough to measurably reduce the risk of neonatal problems after birth. Ampicillin is widely used but erythromycin (q.v.) may be a better option.

Care in spontaneous preterm labour

Similar prophylaxis does *not* delay delivery, or improve outcome, when labour threatens to start prematurely before the membranes rupture, but high-dose penicillin *during* delivery can reduce the risk of early-onset neonatal group B streptococcal infection. Ampicillin is sometimes given instead in the hope that this will prevent coliform sepsis as well but, as such organisms are increasingly resistant to ampicillin, all women going into unexplained spontaneous labour before 35 weeks' gestation are best given both IV penicillin and IV gentamicin. Even in pregnancies more mature than this there are grounds for giving IV penicillin (q.v.) throughout labour to reduce the risk of group B streptococcal infection if the membranes are known to have ruptured more than 6 hours before labour starts. One recent study has suggested that a combination of these two strategies would result in 80% of all the babies currently dying of *any* bacterial infection of intrapartum origin (that is babies developing symptoms within 48 hours of birth) receiving appropriate antibiotic treatment during delivery. It means giving antibiotics to between 40 and 60 women during labour to provide optimum treatment for one baby with bacterial sepsis of intrapartum origin. Many policies treat even more patients than this, and it seems possible that this could increase the risk of *late-onset* infection.

Neonatal treatment

Dose: The neonatal dose when meningitis is suspected is 100 mg/kg IV or IM. In other situations, a dose of 50 mg/kg is more than adequate, given (when the patient is well enough) by mouth.

Timing: Give every 12 hours in the first week of life, every 8 hours in babies 1–3 weeks old, and every 6 hours in babies 4 or more weeks old. Increase the dosage interval if there is severe renal failure. Sustain treatment for 10–14 days in proven septicaemia, for 3 weeks in babies with meningitis, and for 4 weeks in osteitis. Oral medication can sometimes be used to complete treatment even though absorption is limited.

Supply

500 mg vials cost £7·80. Add 4·6 ml of sterile water for injection to the dry powder to get a solution containing 100 mg/ml and always use at once after reconstitution. A 100 mg/kg dose contains 0·3 mmol/kg of sodium. The oral suspension (25 mg/ml) costs £3·40 per 100 ml. Use within 1 week if kept at room temperature (2 weeks if kept at 4°C). No sugar-free oral suspension is available.

References

See also the relevant Cochrane reviews and UK guideline on managing PPROM

Bizzarro MJ, Dembry L-M, Baltimore RS, *et al.* Changing patterns in neonatal *Escherichia coli* sepsis and ampicillin resistance in the era of intrapartum antibiotic prophylaxis. *Pediatrics* 2008;**121**:689–96.

Egarter C, Leitich H, Karas H, *et al.* Antibiotic treatment in preterm and premature rupture of membranes and neonatal morbidity: a meta-analysis. *Am J Obstet Gynecol* 1996;**174**:589–97. [SR]

Gilbert RE, Pike K, Kenyon SL, *et al.* The effect of prepartum antibiotics on the type of neonatal bacteraemia: insights from the MRC ORACLE trials. *Br J Obstet Gynaecol* 2005;**112**:830–2.

Glasgow TS, Young PC, Wallin J, *et al.* Association of intrapartum antibiotic exposure and late-onset serious bacterial infections in infants. *Pediatrics* 2005;**116**:696–702.

Kenyon SL, Taylor DJ, Tarnow-Mordi W, for the ORACLE Collaborative Group. Broad-spectrum antibiotics for preterm, prelabour rupture of fetal membranes: the ORACLE I randomised trial. *Lancet* 2001;**357**:979–88. (See also **358**:502–4.) [RCT]

Schuchat A, Zywicki SS, Dinsmoor MJ, *et al.* Risk factors and opportunities for prevention of early-onset neonatal sepsis: a multicenter case-control study. *Pediatrics* 2000;**105**:21–6.

Use

L-Arginine is an essential nutritional supplement for patients with inborn errors of metabolism affecting the urea cycle (other than arginase deficiency). In some of these conditions it can also facilitate nitrogen excretion, together with sodium phenylbutyrate and sodium benzoate (q.v.).

Biochemistry

Arginine is a naturally occurring amino acid needed for protein synthesis. Since it is synthesised in the body by the 'urea cycle' it is not, usually, an essential nutrient. Dietary supplementation becomes essential, however, in most patients with inherited urea cycle disorders because the enzyme defect limits arginine production, while dietary protein restriction limits arginine intake. Further supplementation also aids nitrogen excretion in citrullinaemia and argininosuccinic aciduria because excess arginine is metabolised to citrulline and argininosuccinic acid incorporating nitrogen derived from ammonia and aspartic acid. As citrulline and argininosuccinic acid can be excreted in the urine, treatment with arginine can lower the plasma ammonia level in both these conditions.

Treatment with arginine needs to be combined with a low protein diet and supervised by a consultant experienced in the management of metabolic disease. Treatment with oral sodium phenylbutyrate and/or sodium benzoate is also usually necessary.

Specialist advice

Specialist advice on a range of inborn errors of metabolism is available from the British Inherited Metabolic Disease Group (BIMDG), and detailed guidance on the management of hyperammonaemia is available on this group's website (www.bimdg.org,uk). Start by clicking on the red box to access a range of emergency protocols.

Treatment

Ornithine transcarbamoylase and carbamoyl phosphate synthetase deficiency: Give 25–35 mg/kg of arginine by mouth four times a day to meet the basic need for protein synthesis. Patients with acute hyperammonaemia should be given 6 mg/kg an hour as a continuous IV infusion. Some authorities recommend an initial IV loading dose of 200 mg/kg of arginine given over 90 minutes.
Citrullinaemia and argininosuccinic aciduria: Up to 175 mg/kg of arginine four times a day can be given by mouth to promote nitrogen excretion. During acute hyperammonaemia an IV loading dose of 300–600 mg/kg is given over 90 minutes followed by a continuous infusion of 12·5–25 mg/kg per hour.

Monitoring

Vomiting and hypotension have occasionally been reported as a result of treatment with IV arginine. Hyperchloraemic acidosis can occur in patients on high-dose intravenous arginine hydrochloride: pH and plasma chloride concentrations should be monitored and bicarbonate given if necessary. High arginine levels are thought to contribute to the neurological damage seen in arginase deficiency, and it is therefore recommended that plasma arginine levels should be monitored during long-term use and kept between 50 and 200 µmol/l.

Supply and administration

L-Arginine can be made available (as a free base) in powder form for oral use from SHS International; 100 grams costs £8·40. This is a chemical, not a pharmaceutical, product. Regular supplies can be made available on prescription to patients with urea cycle disorders in the UK, as long as these are marked ACBS (Advisory Committee on Borderline Substances). L-Arginine is also available from Special Products Ltd as a sugar-free medicine in 200 ml bottles costing £20 each. Add 185 ml of purified water to the contents of the bottle to obtain 200 ml of a 100 mg/ml liquid which remains stable for 2 months. This can, if necessary, be mixed with milk, fruit juice or food.

A 100 ml IV infusion pack containing 10 grams of L-arginine (as the hydrochloride) is available from Special Products Ltd for £12. So are 10 ml (500 mg/ml) ampoules costing £3.

References

Brusilow SW. Arginine, an indispensable amino acid for patients with inborn errors of urea synthesis. *J Clin Invest* 1984;**74**:2144–8.
Brusilow SW, Horwich AL. Urea cycle enzymes. In: Scriver CR, Beaudet AL, Sly WS, *et al.*, eds. *The metabolic and molecular bases of inherited disease*, 8th edn. New York: McGraw-Hill, 2001: pp. 1909–64.
Leonard JV. Disorders of the urea cycle and related enzymes. In: Fernandes J, Saudubray J-M, van den Berghe G, *et al.*, eds. *Inborn metabolic diseases. Diagnosis and treatment*, 4th edn. Berlin: Springer-Verlag, 2006: pp. 263–72.
Wraith JE. Ornithine carbamoyltransferase deficiency. *Arch Dis Child* 2001;**84**:84–8.

Use

Artemether is a relatively new antimalarial now widely used in countries where many *Plasmodium falciparum* and some *Plasmodium vivax* parasites have become resistant to most other drugs.

Pharmacology

Extracts of the herb *Artemesia annua* (sweet wormwood) have been used to treat fever in China for many centuries. The key ingredient seems to be the sesquiterpene lactone called qinghaosu (or artemisinin), which was first isolated by Chinese chemists in 1971. Artemisinin, and its derivatives, artemether and artesunate, have since been shown to clear malarial parasites from the blood more rapidly than other drugs, although parasitic recrudescence is common unless a second antimalarial is taken at the same time, or the drug is taken for at least 7 days. They also reduce gametocyte carriage (the sexual form of the parasite capable of infecting any blood-sucking mosquito), but they have no sporontocidal activity. Artemisinin and its derivatives are all hydrolysed quite rapidly in the body to the active metabolite dihydroartemisinin which then accumulates within the cytoplasm of the parasite, disrupting calcium homeostasis. A cure cannot be relied on without multidose treatment because the half life is much shorter than that of most other antimalarial drugs. Combined treatment with a second antimalarial is generally considered essential to stop the parasite becoming as resistant to this new drug as it has already become to most of the other drugs used in the past, and a product containing 20 mg of artemether and 120 mg of lumefantrine (Coartem®) the most widely studied combination. Artesunate with amiodarone (q.v.) is a second widely used combination.

Published reports of the use of artemisinin in over 700 pregnancies have not identified any adverse treatment-related pregnancy outcomes, but animal experiments suggest that use can cause the early embryo to die and be resorbed. Nothing is yet been published the use of these drugs during lactation.

Managing severe malaria

Additional supportive care is necessary in any seriously ill child, as outlined in the monograph on quinine.

Oral treatment

Dose: Give children weighing 5–15 kg one tablet of Coartem crushed, if necessary, in a little water. Quinine (q.v.) is still, at the moment, the only well-studied treatment for any child weighing less than 5 kg.

Timing: Give six doses over 3 days (at 0, 8, 24, 36, 48 and 60 hours). Repeat if it is vomited within an hour.

Children too ill to take a drug by mouth

Early treatment is critically important and, in rural settings where it may take more than 6 hours to get definite care started, a strategy for giving a rectal suppository before the child reaches medical care can halve the risk of death or long-term disability.

Artemether: Rectal artemether seems at least as effective as IV quinine in infants with cerebral malaria. Give babies under 9 kg one 40 mg suppository daily until oral treatment can be started. Babies over 9 kg should have a loading dose of 80 mg (two suppositories) on the first day and 40 mg/day thereafter.

Supply

Tablets of Coartem containing 20 mg of artemether and 120 mg of lumefantrine are now widely available from WHO and are also available in North America. A dispersible tablet has also been developed to aid administration to young children. Similar tablets (costing €1) are available in Europe under the trade name Riamet®. Counterfeit products are currently known to be circulating in South East Asia. Suppositories containing 40 mg of artemether are available from Dafra Pharma in Belgium.

References

See also the relevant Cochrane reviews

Abdulla S, Sagara I, Borrmann S, *et al.* Efficacy and safety of artemether-lumefantrine dispersible tablets compared with crushed commercial tablets in African infants and children with uncomplicated malaria: a randomised, single-blind, multicentre trial. *Lancet* 2008;**372**:1819–27. [RCT] (See also pp. 1786–7.)

Aceng JR, Byarugaba JS, Tumwine JK. Rectal artemether versus intravenous quinine for the treatment of cerebral malaria in children in Uganda: randomised controlled trial. *BMJ* 2005;**330**:334–6. [RCT] (See also pp. 317–18.)

Barnes KI, Mwenechanya J, Tembo M, *et al.* Efficacy of rectal artesunate compared with parenteral quinine in initial treatment of moderately severe malaria in African children and adults: a randomised study. *Lancet* 2004;**363**:1598–605. [RCT]

Dorsey G, Staedke S, Clark TD, *et al.* Combination therapy for uncomplicated falciparum malaria in Ugandan children. *JAMA* 2007;**297**:2210–19. [RCT]

Fanello CI, Karema C, van Doren W, *et al.* A randomised trial to assess the safety and efficacy of artemether-lumefantrine (Coartem Rm) for the treatment of uncomplicated Plasmodium falciparum malaria in Rwanda. *Trans R Soc Trop Med Hyg* 2007;**101**:344–50. [RCT]

Gomes MF, Faiz MA, Gyapong JO, *et al.* Pre-referral rectal artesunate to prevent death and disability in severe malaria: a placebo-controlled trial. *Lancet* 2009;**373**:557–66. [RCT] (See also pp. 522–3.)

Karunajeewa HA, Mueller I, Senn M, *et al.* A trial of combination antimalarial therapies in children from Papua New Guinea. *N Engl J Med* 2008;**359**:2545–57. [RCT] (See also pp. 1601–3.)

McGready R, Tan SO, Ashley EA, *et al.* A randomised controlled trial of artemether-lumefantrine versus artesunate for uncomplicated *Plasmodium falciparum* treatment in pregnancy. *PLoS Med* 2008;**5**:e253. [RCT]

Ratcliff A, Siswantoro H, Kenangalem E, *et al.* Two fixed-dose artemisinin combinations for drug-resistant falciparum and vivax malaria in Papua, Indonesia: an open-label randomised comparison. *Lancet* 2007;**369**:75765. [RCT]

SEAQUAMAT Trial Group. Artesunate versus quinine for treatment of severe falciparum malaria: a randomised trial. *Lancet* 2005;**366**:717–25. [RCT] (See also **367**:110–12.)

ASPIRIN (Acetylsalicylic acid)

Use
Aspirin is now seldom given to children under 16 because it is thought that use during a viral illness can trigger Reye syndrome (an acute life-threatening encephalopathy with fatty liver degeneration), but it is still used in Kawasaki disease, in children with severe rheumatoid arthritis, and to limit clot formation after cardiac surgery. The web commentary reviews aspects of safe use during pregnancy and lactation.

Pharmacology
Aspirin has been better studied in pregnancy than almost any other drug. Self-treatment to relieve headache around the time of conception seems (as with all non-steroidal anti-inflammatory drugs other than paracetamol (q.v.)) to increase the risk of miscarriage, but a 75 mg daily dose started shortly after conception *reduces* the risk of repeated miscarriage in women with phospholipid antibodies. Early low dose use also produces a 10% reduction in the risk of pre-eclampsia and of perinatal death. Low dose use for 3 days before and on the day of any long haul flight also probably reduces the risk of deep vein thrombosis. Even high-dose use does not seem to be teratogenic, but sustained high-dose use may increase the risk of bleeding and has been associated with premature duct closure and a rise in perinatal mortality. Episodic use during lactation seems harmless because the baby only ingests ~3% of the weight-related maternal dose, but little is known about continuous high-dose treatment, and the elimination pathways are saturable, making ibuprofen (q.v.) a much safer alternative.

Kawasaki disease
Kawasaki is an acute febrile illness, first described by clinicians in Japan in 1967, that has now been recognised in many parts of the world, sometimes in epidemic form (making an unrecognised infection its likely cause). Most children are under 5 and, typically, under 2 years old. Features include high fever for at least 5 days with a variable rash, conjunctivitis, inflammation of the oral mucosa, swollen neck glands, and redness and swelling of the hands and feet with later desquamation. Other common features include abdominal pain, vomiting, diarrhoea, aseptic meningitis, arthritis and mild liver dysfunction. Mild cases may go unrecognised, but nearly a third of children with overt disease develop serious inflammation of the coronary arteries, sometimes leading to dangerous aneurysm formation, if treatment is not started early. A high platelet count during convalescence further increases the risk of coronary thrombosis and myocardial infarction. However 90% respond to a single 2 g/kg dose of human immunoglobulin (q.v.) given IV over 12 hours, if this is given within a week of the onset of symptoms, and this greatly reduces the risk of secondary complications. Aspirin is also given (see below), both to reduce fever and because of the drug's known antithrombotic (platelet-inhibiting) properties. Patients with severe or progressive vasculitis should be referred promptly to a paediatric cardiologist.

Treatment
Early Kawasaki disease: Give 8 mg/kg by mouth four times a day for 2 weeks to control acute symptoms. (A 30 mg/kg dose four times a day is often recommended, but there is no evidence that this higher dose further reduces the risk of cardiac complications.)
Later prophylaxis: Low-dose treatment (5 mg/kg once a day by mouth) is usually given for 2 months during convalescence, and such treatment is usually maintained indefinitely where echocardiography shows continued coronary artery involvement. A similar prophylactic dose is used after Fontan and Blalock–Taussig shunt surgery, and is also often given for 3 months after certain other forms of cardiac surgery to minimise the risk of clot formation until endothelial lining cells finally cover all postoperative scar tissue.

Monitoring
Oral absorption can be variable during the acute inflammatory phase of Kawasaki disease. It is wise, therefore, to monitor the serum salicylate level in children given high-dose treatment, aiming for a serum level of 250 mg/l (1 g/l = 7·2 mmol/l). Levels in excess of 450 mg/l are often toxic, causing nausea, vomiting, sweating and hyperventilation. Young children may become acidotic; IV sodium bicarbonate will correct this and aid drug elimination by helping to keep urine pH above 7·5.

Supply
To obtain a 5 mg/ml sugar-free solution for oral use add one 75 mg tablet of dispersible aspirin to 15 ml of water, and use immediately. Tablets cost less than 1p each.

References
See also the relevant Cochrane reviews

Askie LM, Duley L, Henderson-Smart DJ, *et al.* Antiplatelet agents for prevention of pre-eclampsia: a meta-analysis of individual patient data. *Lancet* 2007;**369**:1791–8. [SR] (See also pp. 1791–2 and **370**:1685–6.)

Council on Cardiovascular Disease in the Young, American Heart Association. Diagnosis, treatment and long-term management of Kawasaki disease. *Pediatrics* 2004;**114**:1708–33. www.pediatrics.org/cgi/content/full/114/6/1708.

Farquharson RG, Quenby S, Greaves M. Antiphospholipid syndrome in pregnancy: a randomised, controlled trial of treatment. *Obstet Gynecol* 2002;**100**:408–13. [RCT]

Kozer E, Nikfar S, Costei A, *et al.* Aspirin consumption during the first trimester of pregnancy and congenital anomalies: a meta-analysis. *Am J Obstet Gynecol* 2002;**187**:1623–30. [SR]

Li D-K, Liu L, Odouli R. Exposure to non-steroidal anti-inflammatory drugs during pregnancy and risk of miscarriage: population based cohort study. *BMJ* 2003;**327**:368–71. (See also 2004;**328**:108–9.)

Li JS, Yow E, Berezny KY, *et al.* Clinical outcomes of palliative surgery including a systematic-to-pulmonary artery shunt in infants with cyanotic congenital heart disease. Does aspirin make a difference. *Circulation* 2007;**116**:293–7. (See also pp. 236–7.)

Use

Atosiban seems at least as good at briefly arresting early preterm labour as most of the other IV strategies tried to date, and causes fewer side effects than the use of a β-sympathomimetic such as ritodrine or salbutamol (q.v.). Nifedipine (q.v.) is a rather cheaper alternative that can be given by mouth.

Pharmacology

Oxytocin and vasopressin (q.v.) are two closely related nonapeptides secreted by the posterior part of the pituitary gland. Oxytocin, which the pituitary secretes in a pulsatile manner, and which is also produced by the ovaries, the placenta, the fetal membranes and the myometrium, has long been recognised as having an important role in the initiation of term and preterm labour. Contractions are stimulated when oxytocin binds to receptors on uterine muscle, and oxytocin also stimulates decidual prostaglandin secretion. Because of this, much time has recently been spent synthesising compounds with a structure that mimics that of oxytocin well enough for these molecules to attach themselves to the oxytocin receptors, blocking the action of oxytocin itself (having what is often termed a 'tocolytic' effect). Atosiban was first introduced into clinical use in 1998 and shown to inhibit labour at least as effectively as any betamimetic. It can sometimes cause nausea and headache, but seldom causes the tachycardia or the other unpleasant maternal side effects associated with betamimetic use. It has a large volume of distribution (V_D ~18 l/kg) and is cleared from the body in a biphasic manner – the effective half life being about 18 minutes. Despite its low molecular weight, relatively little seems to cross the placenta, and there is no reason to think that its appearance in breast milk is of any clinical significance. The European manufacturers have only been authorised, as yet, to recommend use when labour looks likely to cause delivery at 24–33 weeks' gestation, but a single 6·75 mg dose IV may be useful in controlling the fetal distress that can be caused by uterine hyperstimulation. No trial has yet been undertaken to look at the relative merits of atosiban and the calcium channel antagonist nifedipine. The only *indirect* analysis available suggests that babies born after nifedipine tocolysis may be marginally less likely to develop respiratory distress, but in all other respects the outcomes were very similar. For a further comment on the various drugs that have been used to at least briefly arrest labour see the monograph on nifedipine.

Sustained drug use to prevent preterm labour

Although a number of drugs are capable of delaying delivery in mothers in early preterm labour for long enough to give betamethasone (q.v.) and, if necessary, arrange hospital transfer, there is no evidence that *sustained* treatment with any of these drugs is capable of delaying delivery for more than a few days. Atosiban shows marginally more promise than most in this regard. In the only important trial reported to date (limited to women in whom uterine quiescence was successfully achieved with atosiban), pregnancy lasted another 33 days in the 261 women who were given 30 micrograms a minute of this drug as a continuous subcutaneous infusion, but only 27 days in the 251 given a placebo infusion. Treatment with progesterone (q.v.) is another strategy currently undergoing controlled trial assessment. A recent (2010) Cochrane review found that no benefit of atosiban was shown in delaying or preventing preterm birth compared to placebo or betamimetics and suggests that further well-designed controlled trials, including a placebo arm, are needed.

Treatment

Initial loading dose: Give an initial 6·75 mg IV dose of atosiban base over 1 minute.
Maintenance infusion: Give 12 ml per hour of a solution made up as described below for 3 hours, and then continue the infusion at a rate of 4 ml an hour for no more than 2 days.

Supply and administration

0·9 ml vials of atosiban acetate (which contain 6·75 mg of atosiban base) cost £19 and are used to initiate treatment. 5 ml vials containing 37·5 mg of atosiban base cost £53; draw the contents from two such vials into a syringe and dilute to 50 ml with 0·9% sodium chloride or 5% glucose to give a solution containing 1·5 mg/ml, and infuse this as described above. Store vials at 4°C, and use promptly once opened.

References

See also the relevant Cochrane reviews and UK guideline on tocolytic use

Afschar P, Schöll W, Bader A, *et al.* Prospective randomised trial of atosiban *versus* hexoprenaline for acute tocolysis and intrauterine resuscitation. *Br J Obstet Gynaecol* 2004;**111**:316–18. [RCT]

Coomarasamy A, Knox EM, Gee H, *et al.* Effectiveness of nifedipine *versus* atosiban for tocolysis in preterm labour: a meta-analysis with an indirect comparison of randomised trials. *Br J Obstet Gynaecol* 2003;**110**:1045–9. [SR]

European Atosiban Study Group. The oxytocin antagonist atosiban versus the beta-agonist terbutaline in the treatment of preterm labour. A randomized, double blind, controlled trial. *Acta Obstet Gynaecol Scand* 2001;**80**:413–22. [RCT]

Husslein P, Roura L, Duden Hausen J, *et al.* Clinical practice evaluation of atosiban in preterm labour management in six European countries. TREASURE study group. *Br J Obstet Gynaecol* 2006;**113**(suppl 3);105–10. [RCT] (See also **114**:1043–4.)

Sanchez-Ramos L, Huddleston JF. The therapeutic value of maintenance tocolysis: an overview of the evidence. *Clin Perinatol* 2003;**30**:841–54.

Shim J-Y, Park YW, Yoon BH, *et al.* Multicentre, parallel-group, randomised, single-blind study of the safety and efficacy of atosiban versus ritodrine in the treatment of acute preterm labour in Korean women. *Br J Obstet Gynaecol* 2006;**113**:1228–34. [RCT]

Simhan HN, Caritis SN. Prevention of preterm delivery. [Review] *N Engl J Med* 2007;**357**:477–87.

Tsatsaris V, Carbonne B, Cabrol D. Atosiban for preterm labour. *Drugs* 2004;**64**:375–82.

Valenzuela GJ, Sanchez-Ramos L, Romero R, *et al.* The Atosiban PTL-089 Study Group. Maintenance treatment of preterm labour with the oxytocin antagonist atosiban. *Am J Obstet Gynecol* 2000;**182**:1184–90. [RCT]

Worldwide Atosiban versus Beta-agonists Study Group. Effectiveness and safety of the oxytocin antagonist atosiban versus beta-adrenergic agonists in the treatment of preterm labour. *Br J Obstet Gynaecol* 2001;**108**:133–42. [RCT]

Use

Atracurium besylate is a relatively short-acting alternative to pancuronium (q.v.). Suxamethonium and mivacurium (q.v.) are also commonly use when only brief paralysis is necessary.

Pharmacology

Atracurium, like pancuronium, is a non-depolarising muscle relaxant that works by competing with acetylcholine at the neuromuscular junction's receptor site – an effect that can be reversed with anticholinesterases such as neostigmine (q.v.). It was first developed as an analogue of suxamethonium and patented in 1977. Atracurium is particularly popular in anaesthetic practice because it has no vagolytic or sympatholytic properties, and is eliminated by non-enzymatic Hofmann degradation at body temperature independently of liver or kidney function. It is non-cumulative, and only effective for about 20 minutes (30 minutes in older children). Weight-for-weight young children do not need as high a dose as adults. Little seems to cross the placenta, and no concerns have been identified as a result of use during pregnancy, delivery or lactation. Atracurium (400 micrograms/kg injected into the umbilical vein, or 1 mg/kg injected into the fetal buttock) has been shown to reliably abolish all fetal movement for about half an hour.

The manufacturer has not yet endorsed the use of atracurium in children less than 1 month old, and one UK neonatal centre reported four serious adverse reactions in late 2000 after staff gave atracurium while preparing babies for tracheal intrubation. Three babies became so hypoxic, bradycardic and unventilatable that they died. While this still remains, after 9 years, an isolated report, the occurrence does underline the importance of reminding staff that they should never use any muscle relaxant, except under supervision, until they are confident they can always sustain an airway and deliver mask ventilation if intubation proves difficult.

Cicatracurium is a more potent single-isomer refinement of atracurium. It takes rather longer (23 minutes) to cause muscle paralysis, but it is less likely to trigger histamine release. The usual bolus dose is 200 micrograms/kg IV, but there is, as yet, only limited experience of use in very young children.

Treatment

Pre-intubation paralysis: A 300 microgram/kg IV dose of atracurium causes almost complete paralysis after 2 minutes. A 500 microgram/kg dose will almost always provide sustained muscle relaxation for 15–35 minutes in babies less than a year old. Always flush the bolus through into the vein.
Continuous infusion: IV infusions of 400 micrograms/kg of atracurium per hour can provide sustained neuromuscular blockade in babies less than 1 month old. Older patients need 500 micrograms/kg per hour. Babies requiring paralysis should always be sedated as well, and provided with pain relief where necessary.

Compatibility

A continuous infusion of atracurium can, if necessary, be given (terminally) into a line containing adrenaline, dobutamine, dopamine, fentanyl, heparin, isoprenaline, midazolam, milrinone or morphine.

Antidote

Most of the effects of atracurium can be reversed by giving a combination of 10 micrograms/kg of glycopyrronium (or 20 micrograms/kg of atropine) and 50 micrograms/kg of neostigmine as outlined in the glycopyrronium monograph, although reversal is seldom called for given atracurium's short half life.

Supply and administration

Atracurium: 2·5 ml ampoules containing 25 mg cost £1·80; larger ampoules are also available. Multidose vials are available in North America, but are best avoided in young children because they contain benzyl alcohol. Store at 2–8°C. To give a bolus injection of atracurium take 0·5 ml from a 10 mg/ml ampoule and dilute to 5 ml with 5% glucose or glucose saline to obtain a preparation containing 1 mg/ml (1000 micrograms/ml) for accurate administration. To give a continuous infusion of 500 micrograms/kg per hour, draw 2·5 ml of atracurium besylate for each kg the baby weighs from the ampoule into a syringe, dilute to 50 ml with 0·9% sodium chloride or 10% glucose in 0·18% sodium chloride, and infuse at 1 ml per hour. A less concentrated solution of glucose or glucose saline can be used if appropriate. Make up a fresh solution daily.
Cisatracurium: 10 ml ampoules containing 20 mg of cisatracurium cost £7·50. Both the single dose and the multidose ampoules available in North America contain benzyl alcohol. Store at 2–8°C.

References

Bryson HM, Faulds D. Cisatracurium besilate: a review of its pharmacology and clinical potential in anaesthetic practice. *Drugs* 1997;**53**:848–68.
Clarkson A, Choonara I, Martin P. Suspected toxicity of atracurium in the neonate. *Paediatr Anaesth* 2001;**11**:631–2.
Flynn PJ, Frank M, Hughes R. Use of atracurium in caesarean section. *Br J Anaesth* 1984;**56**:599–604.
Martin LD, Bratton SL, O'Rourke PP. Clinical uses and controversies of neuromuscular blocking agents in infants and children. *Crit Care Med* 1999;**27**:1358–68.
Piotrowski A. Comparison of atracurium and pancuronium in mechanically ventilated neonates. *Intensive Care Med* 1993;**19**:401–5.
Sparr HJ, Beuafort TM, Fuchs-Buder T. Newer neuromuscular blocking agents. How do they compare with established agents? *Drugs* 2001;**61**:919–42.

Use
Atropine is now less routinely used prior to surgery, but is still used during and after surgery to the eye. Ipratropium is a related compound occasionally used, by inhalation, as a bronchodilator.

Pharmacology
The medicinal properties of the Solanaceae have been known for many centuries, and pure atropine was first isolated from deadly nightshade root in 1833. The Venetians had called this plant 'herba bella donna' because the ladies used water distilled from the plant as a cosmetic to beautify the eye (by dilating the pupil). Linnaeus later gave the plant the Latin botanical name *Atropa belladonna* in recognition of its toxicity and use as a poison (Atropos being the name of one of the Greek fates who could 'cut the slender thread of life'). Atropine blocks the muscarinic effects of acetylcholine on the postganglionic autonomic nerve fibres, producing a vagal block that can abolish the sudden bradycardia caused by operative vagal stimulation. The half life in adults is 4 hours, but is longer in infancy. Use prior to anaesthesia reduces oropharyngeal secretions, but it also reduces lower oesophageal sphincter tone and does nothing, directly, to reduce the risk of laryngospasm. Bronchial secretions become more viscid and less copious; gastrointestinal secretions and motility are reduced.

Atropine is moderately well absorbed by the small intestine (V_D ~3 l/kg). It crosses the placenta with ease, and has been known to affect the fetal heart rate. Small amounts are thought to appear in breast milk but no neonatal symptoms have ever been reported. It has a role in heart block due to digoxin poisoning, and in patients with serious reflex (vagal) bradycardia. Atropine eye drops are used to achieve sustained dilatation of the pupil after ocular surgery (as described in the monograph on eye drops) but excess usage can lead to ileus and other problems, especially when the standard 1% drops are used. Its use to make surgery unnecessary in babies with pyloric stenosis merits further evaluation.

Treatment with atropine
Oral premedication: Some doubt the need to use *any* drug prior to the induction of anaesthesia in most neonates as long as there is IV access. When a 'premed' is judged appropriate an intramuscular injection can usually be avoided by giving 40 micrograms/kg of atropine by mouth 2 hours before induction so long as gut motility is normal. Glycopyrronium (q.v.) is now a commonly used alternative.

Parenteral premedication: A 10 microgram/kg IV bolus produces an effect within half a minute that lasts at least 6 hours. A subcutaneous or IM dose will be maximally effective after 30–60 minutes.

Pyloric stenosis: A 10 microgram/kg dose IV once every 4 hours before feeds can often check the contractile spasm of the pyloric muscle. Treatment should be continued for 3 weeks, but can be undertaken at home after a few days, once vomiting has stopped, using twice this dose by mouth once every 4 hours.

Reversing neuromuscular blockade: See the monograph on glycopyrronium.

Digoxin toxicity: Give 25 micrograms/kg IV for AV block. Ten times as much is occasionally given.

Eye drops: 0·5% drops given twice a day for 5–7 days maintains dilatation of the pupil after surgery.

Treatment with ipratropium
Giving inhaled ipratropium with, or instead of, salbutamol (q.v.) counteracts the bronchoconstrictor effect of acetylcholine. The usual dose in babies with bronchopulmonary dysplasia is 25 micrograms/kg, every 8 hours, but larger doses have been used. Protect the eye from direct exposure to avoid glaucoma. Little is absorbed systemically, making inhalational use safe during pregnancy and lactation.

Toxicity
Check the dose of atropine carefully – even a moderate overdose will cause tachycardia, flushing and dilatation of the pupils. A severe overdose will cause respiratory depression, convulsions and coma requiring barbiturate sedation, ventilatory support for respiratory depression, and steps to control hyperpyrexia. Neostigmine (q.v.) will counteract some of the effects of a severe overdose.

Supply and administration
Atropine: 1 ml 600 microgram ampoules cost 60p each. Dilute 0·1 ml of the ampoule with 0·9 ml of 0·9% saline in a 1 ml syringe to obtain a solution containing 60 micrograms/ml.

Ipratropium: 1 ml preservative-free, isotonic, 250 microgram nebules cost 25p each. Take 0·1 ml for each kg the baby weighs and dilute to 2 ml with normal saline for use in a nebuliser.

References
See also the Cochrane review of anticholinergic drug use

Bonthala S, Sparks JW, Musgrove KH, *et al*. Mydriatics slow gastric emptying in preterm infants. *J Pediatr* 2000;**127**:327–30.

Kawahara H, Imura K, Yagi M, *et al*. Motor abnormality in the gastroduodenal junction in patients with infantile hypertrophic pyloric stenosis. *J Pediatr Surg* 2001;**36**:1641–5.

Shorten GD, Bissonnette B, Hartley E, *et al*. It is not necessary to administer more than 10 µg.kg^{-1} of atropine to older children before succinylcholine. *Can J Anaesth* 1995;**42**:8–11. (See also pp. 1–7.)

Singh UK, Kumar R, Prasad R. Oral atropine for infantile hypertrophic pyloric stenosis. *Indian Pediatr* 2005;**42**:473–6.

Singh UK, Kumar R, Suman S. Successful management of infantile hypertrophic pyloric stenosis with atropine sulfate. *Indian Pediatr* 2001;**38**:1099–105.

AZITHROMYCIN

Use
Azithromycin is a macrolide antibiotic related to erythromycin (q.v.) that is now increasingly used to treat neonatal *Chlamydia*, *Mycoplasma* and *Ureaplasma* infections, and to reduce whooping cough cross infection. A single dose can also speed recover in children with severe cholera (*Vibrio cholerae* infection).

Pharmacology
Azithromycin is an azalide developed in 1988 by structurally modifying the erythromycin molecule that works, like erythromycin, by interfering with bacterial protein synthesis. Although it is slightly less potent against Gram-positive organisms it demonstrates superior *in vitro* activity against a wide variety of Gram-negative bacilli, including *Haemophilus influenzae*. A single dose is a more effective way of treating childhood cholera than a 3-day course of erythromycin, and probably as effective as a single dose of ciprofloxacin (c.v.). Azithromycin is moderately well absorbed when taken by mouth (40% bioavailability) and better tolerated than erythromycin because it triggers fewer gastrointestinal side effects. It has a very low peak serum level and a very high volume of distribution (V_D ~23 l/kg) consistent with data showing extensive tissue distribution and intracellular accumulation, and this makes it particularly effective against intracellular microorganisms such a *Chlamydia* and *Legionella*. CSF levels are low but there is substantial penetration into brain tissue. Much of the drug undergoes biliary excretion (terminal half life ~5 days), and the rest is inactivated in the liver – properties that make once a day treatment more than adequate, but can also make it important to give a first loading dose. The interactions with other drugs sometimes seen with erythromycin do not seem to occur with azithromycin. The manufacturers have not yet recommended use in children less than 6 months old.

There is little published information relating to use in pregnancy, but the macrolide antibiotics are not, as a class, considered teratogenic. Drug transfer across the placenta is limited, and a breastfed baby only ingests ~5% of the weight-adjusted maternal dose. Systemic use in infancy may increase the risk of pyloric stenosis.

Prophylaxis
Bacterial endocarditis: Give a single 10 mg/kg dose to any baby with congenital heart disease if they have had a penicillin class antibiotic in the past month before surgery involving any site where infection is suspected.
Trachoma: Endemic disease can be much reduced in the whole community by giving all children under 11 years a single 20 mg/kg dose, once every 3 months.
Whooping cough: Children with this are much less likely to infect others if given 5 days' treatment.

Maternal treatment
A single 1 gram dose by mouth eliminates maternal genital infection due to *Chlamydia trachomatis*. A 2 gram dose has been used as an alternative to IM benzathine or procaine benzylpenicillin (q.v.) in adults with early syphilis, but the efficacy of such an approach has not yet been assessed in women who are pregnant.

Treatment in infancy
Systemic infection: Give a single 10 mg/kg oral loading dose, and then 5 mg/kg once a day. Authorities in the UK suggest that treatment should not be continued for more than 3 days, but those in North America favour a 5-day course. There is almost no information on use in the first month of life.
Conjunctivitis: A single oral 20 mg/kg dose is an effective treatment for *Chlamydia* conjunctivitis, including chronic follicular trachoma. Giving 1·5% eye drops twice a day for 3 days is also very effective.

Supply and administration
Small 600 mg packs of powder costing £5 are normally reconstituted with 9 ml of water to give 15 ml of a fruit-flavoured sucrose-sweetened oral suspension containing 40 mg/ml of azithromycin, which is stable for 5 days after reconstitution. Further dilution in order to give a very low dose accurately should only be done just before use. Eye drops and an American IV formulation have not yet been licensed in the UK, but could be imported.

References
See also the relevant Cochrane reviews

Atik B, Thanh T, Luong VQ, *et al*. Impact of annual targeted treatment of infectious trachoma and susceptibility to infection. *JAMA* 2006;**296**:1488–97. [RCT]

Cochereau I, Meddeb-Ouertanu A, Khairallah M, *et al*. 2-day treatment with azithromycin 1·5% eye drops versus 7-day treatment with tobramycin 0·3% for purulent bacterial conjunctivitis: multicentre, randomised and controlled trial in adults and children. *Br J Ophthalmol* 2007;**91**:465–9. [RCT]

House JI, Ayele B, Porco TC, *et al*. Assessment of herd protection against trachoma due to repeated mass antibiotic distributions: a cluster-randomised trial. *Lancet* 2009;**373**:1111–18. [RCT] (See also **373**:1061–3 and **374**:449–50.)

Khan WA, Saha A, Rahman A, *et al*. Comparison of single-dose azithromycin and 12-dose 3-day erythromycin for childhood cholera: a randomised, double-blind trial. *Lancet* 2002;**360**:1722–7. [RCT]

Rieder G, Rusizoka M, Todd J, *et al*. Single-dose azithromycin versus penicillin G benzathine for the treatment of early syphilis. *N Engl J Med* 2005;**353**:1236–44. [RCT] (See also pp. 1291–3.)

Solomon AW, Mabey DCW. Trachoma. *BMJ clinical evidence handbook*. London: BMJ Books, 2009: pp. 227–8 (and updates). [SR]

Srinivasan R, Yeo TH. Are newer macrolides effective in eradicating pertussis? *Arch Dis Child* 2005;**90**:322–4. [SR]

West SK, Muroz B, Mkocha H, *et al*. Infection with Chlamydia trachomatis after mass treatment of a trachoma hyperendemic community in Tanzania: a longitudinal study. *Lancet* 2005;**366**:1296–300.

Wright HR, Turner A, Taylor HR. Trachoma. [Review] *Lancet* 2008;**371**:1945–54. [SR]

Zar HJ. Neonatal chlamydial infections. Prevention and treatment. *Pediatr Drugs* 2005;**7**:103–10.

Use

BCG vaccine is used to reduce the risk of tuberculosis (TB) in children without evidence of cell-mediated immunity to *Mycobacterium tuberculosis* or *M. bovis*. Tuberculosis is a notifiable illness.

Product

BCG vaccine contains a live attenuated strain of *M. bovis* (bacillus Calmette–Guérin). The product was developed after 13 years of research involving 200 serial subcultures. It was first used in France in 1921 and has been widely used in the international control of tuberculosis since 1950. Tuberculosis is still a severe illness, especially in the first year of life, and there is clear evidence that correctly administered neonatal BCG vaccination greatly reduces the risk of serious infection in early childhood without obscuring the diagnosis of active infection by intradermal testing. Immunity probably wanes after 10–15 years, but re-vaccination is not considered appropriate. The protection conferred is not absolute, but a review of prospective studies shows a mean protective efficacy of 75% against serious early infection. BCG vaccination forms part of WHO's global immunisation programme, but it is not routinely offered at present to children living in countries where the community prevalence is low. Recent studies have also suggested that use in resource-poor countries may improve all-cause infant mortality in some non-specific (as yet unexplained) way. The newly developed interferon-γ (T.SPOT-TB and QuantiFERON-TB) tests have greater specificity and their use may reduce the number of children judged to need treatment, but reliance on these tests still needs further study.

Indications

Babies being cared for in a family or household where there is a patient with active respiratory tuberculosis under treatment should be given prophylactic isoniazid (q.v.) for 6 months from birth, and then vaccinated at 6 months if the Mantoux test remains negative. Current policy in the UK is that BCG should also be offered to all children born in (or likely to spend a considerable time in) an area where prevalence currently exceeds 40:100,000, and to any child whose parents or grandparents were born in a country where prevalence is that high. There are many parts of Asia, India, South America and sub-Saharan Africa where TB is currently much commoner than this (see website commentary). Prior tuberculin testing is *not* necessary before giving BCG in this way to children less than 6 years old. Tuberculin-negative children of any age should be offered BCG if there is a clear history of contact exposure, or a case in the family in the last 6 years, and vaccination should also be offered, as opportunity permits, to those who were born in, or lived for several months in, a country where the prevalence of TB is high. Vaccination is probably best delayed in the very preterm baby until shortly before discharge, because this may improve conversion. However, postponing it longer than this runs the risk that vaccination will never get offered until the period of greatest vulnerability is past.

Drug interactions

BCG can be given at the same time (but not into the same arm) as another vaccine. Leave a 4-week interval after giving any live vaccine (other than the oral polio vaccine) before giving BCG. Do not give any other vaccine into the arm into which BCG was given for 3 months to minimise the risk of lymphadenitis.

Contraindications

Live BCG vaccine should not be given to anyone who is immunodeficient, immunosuppressed or on high-dose corticosteroid treatment (any dose equivalent to more than 1 mg/kg of prednisolone per day, as summarised in the monograph on hydrocortisone). In countries like the UK, where the prevalence of TB is low, BCG (unlike other live vaccines) should not be given to babies who are HIV positive, or to babies born to mothers who are HIV positive, until the child's HIV status has become clear. In high prevalence countries the balance of risk is very different. Avoid administration in any area of skin actively affected by eczema.

Administration

Babies less than 12 months old should receive 0·05 ml intradermally; older children receive 0·1 ml. Strict attention *must* be paid to the technique used if 'conversion' is to be achieved and complications avoided. Injections are normally given into the left upper arm over the point where the deltoid muscle is attached to the humerus to minimise the risk of scarring. This point is only a little above the middle of the upper arm: vaccination is often inappropriately administered higher than this (over the bulk of the deltoid muscle). The skin only needs to be cleaned first if it is overtly dirty. If spirit is used it must be allowed to dry. Soap and water is better. Do not use an antiseptic. Use a 1 ml (Mantoux) syringe and a 10 mm long 26 gauge short-bevel needle (with the bevel facing upwards). A separate syringe and needle must be used for each child to avoid transmitting infection. Stretch the skin between thumb and finger and insert the needle parallel with the surface about 3 mm into the superficial layers of the dermis. The tip should remain visible through the skin and a raised, blanched 3 mm bleb will appear if the injection has been given correctly. If no resistance is encountered the tip is almost certainly too deep and needs to be repositioned. Give the injection slowly and leave the injection site uncovered to facilitate healing. Successful administration will usually, but not invariably, cause a papule to appear at the injection site after 2–4 weeks which may ulcerate before healing to leave a small flat scar after 1–3 months. Babies should become tuberculin positive within 6 weeks if vaccination was effective (but routine testing to confirm this is not generally thought necessary).

Adverse reactions

Early reactivity: A very early response to BCG administration that progresses to pustule formation within 3–5 days (Koch phenomenon) strongly suggests that the subject has active TB.

Continued on p. 54

Other problems: If the slow local reaction generally expected eventually turns into a discharging ulcer this should be covered with a simple, dry, non-occlusive dressing (occlusive dressings can delay healing). The lesion will still heal over 1–2 months and should only leave a small scar if the injection technique was sound. Lymphadenitis may occur. More serious local reactions should be referred to the doctor responsible for the local TB contact clinic. If disseminated infection does occur antitubercular treatment may need to be given (the Danish strain of BCG [1331] being sensitive *in vitro* to isoniazid and rifampicin). For the management of anaphylaxis (an extremely rare occurrence) see the monograph on immunisation.

Documentation
The identification of high-risk babies remains poorly organised in many UK maternity units at present. Parents need to be approached in the antenatal period so that babies likely to benefit can be identified before birth and agreement reached regarding the need for early vaccination. Early post-delivery discharge and the fragmentation of postnatal care have further damaged the systems that used to exist for delivering and documenting such prophylaxis reliably in many Health Districts. Vaccination *must* be documented in the child's personal health record (red book) and in the computerised community child health record – failure to do this can render later interpretation of the child's tuberculin status very difficult. Make a note of the batch number and the expiry date, as well as the date of administration. In some UK maternity units it has also long been standard practice to tell the local TB contact clinic about all babies offered BCG at birth.

Mantoux testing
Tuberculin (tuberculin PPD) is a purified protein made from sterile, heat-treated products of the growth and lysis of *M. tuberculosis* that produces induration of the skin after intradermal injection. The peak extent of any induration induced (ignoring any associated erythema or redness) is documented to the nearest millimetre.

Testing for active tuberculosis: Inject 0·1 ml of tuberculin PPD containing 20 units/ml intradermally into the middle third of the flexor surface of the previously cleaned forearm producing a 'bleb' about 7 mm in diameter (using the same technique as described above for giving BCG). Induration on review 48–72 hours later that extends more than 5 mm indicates a positive response, and induration extending 15 mm or more at this time is a strong reaction probably indicative of active infection. Interpretation is unreliable after 96 hours.

Tests for cellular immunity: A more concentrated (100 units/ml) preparation of PPD can be used, in the same way, to document the existence of cellular immunity if the response to the low-dose test is negative.

Supply
BCG: 1 ml amber vials of lyophilised material (containing enough material to vaccinate 7–8 children) are manufactured by the Danish Statens Serum Institut (SSI). Supplies are distributed within the UK by Farillon for the Department of Health. Vials should be stored at 2–8°C, protected from light and used within 18 months. Do not allow the associated diluent (in vials labelled 'diluted Sauton SSI') to freeze. Reconstitute the vials using this diluent. Do *not* use water for injection. Draw up 1 ml of the diluent using a long needle and transfer this to the BCG vial without attempting to clean the rubber stopper with any antiseptic, detergent or alcohol-impregnated swab. Invert the vial a few times but do not shake it. Swirl the vial round gently to resuspend the material before drawing up each dose. Discard any material not used within 4 hours.

Tuberculin: 1·5 ml vials of tuberculin PPD (in vials of 20 units/ml and 100 units/ml) are available from SSI in Denmark. Store at 2–8°C, and protect from light. Do not freeze. A Patient Group Direction can not currently be used to authorise use because the product's European marketing authorisation does not cover the UK.

References

See also the full UK website guidelines

Abubakar I, Laundry MT, French CE, *et al*. Epidemiology and treatment outcome of childhood tuberculosis in England and Wales 1999–2006. *Arch Dis Child* 2008;**93**:1017–21.

Bergamini BM, Losi M, Valenti F, *et al*. Performance of commercial blood tests for the diagnosis of latent tuberculosis infection in children and adolescents. *Pediatrics* 2009;**123**:e419–24.

Bothamley GH, Cooper E, Shingadia D, *et al*. Tuberculin testing before BCG vaccination. *BMJ* 2003;**327**:243–4. (See also p. 932.)

Hawkridge A, Hatherill M, Little F, *et al*. Efficacy of percutaneous versus intradermal BCG in the prevention of tuberculosis in South African infants: randomised trial. *BMJ* 2008;**337**:a2052 and a2086. [RCT] (See also pp. 1246–7.)

Joint Tuberculosis Committee of the British Thoracic Society. Control and prevention of tuberculosis in the United Kingdom: code of practice 2000. *Thorax* 2000;**55**:887–901.

Roth A, Jensen H, Garly M-L, *et al*. Low birth weight infants and Calmette–Guérin bacillus vaccination at birth. *Pediatr Infect Dis J* 2004;**23**:544–50.

Shingadia D. Diagnosis of tuberculosis. In: David TJ, ed. *Recent advances in paediatrics 24*. London: RSM Press, 2007: pp. 237–53.

Shingadia D, Novelli V. The tuberculin skin test: a hundred, not out? *Arch Dis Child* 2008;**93**:189–90. (See also pp. 200–3.)

Soysal A, Millington KA, Bakir M, *et al*. Effect of BCG vaccination on risk of *Mycobacterium tuberculosis* infection in children with household tuberculosis contact: a prospective community-based study. *Lancet* 2005;**366**:1443–51. (See also pp. 1414–6 and **337**:391–4.)

Thayyil-Sudhan S, Kumar A, Singh M, *et al*. Safety and effectiveness of BCG vaccination in preterm babies. *Arch Dis Child* 1999;**81**:F64–6.

Trunz BB, Fine PEM, Dye C. Effect of BCG vaccination on childhood tuberculosis and miliary tuberculosis worldwide: a meta-analysis and assessment of cost-effectiveness. *Lancet* 2006;**367**:1173–80. [SR] (See also pp. 1122–4.)

Use
Betaine is used in the management of inherited metabolic diseases associated with homocystinuria.

Biochemistry
Homocysteine is an intermediate in the breakdown of the amino acid methionine. Homocysteine has toxic effects on the brain and predisposes to lens dislocation, thromboembolism, osteoporosis and Marfanoid habitus. Betaine (*N,N,N*-trimethylglycine) acts as a methyl group donor, allowing hepatic methyltransferases to convert homocysteine to methionine. Since methionine is less toxic than homocysteine, this can be beneficial in homocysteinuria.

Causes of homcystinuria
Classical homocystinuria: This results from cystathionine β-synthase deficiency. A few patients are detected by neonatal screening programmes but most patients present with developmental delay, dislocated lenses, skeletal abnormalities or thromboembolic disease. Betaine is used in patients who do not respond to pyridoxine (q.v.) and who either can not comply with, or are inadequately controlled by, a low methionine and low protein diet. Betaine lowers plasma and urine homocysteine concentrations, and usually improves symptoms such as behaviour and seizures. Women with homocystinuria should continue with treatment during pregnancy to minimise the risk of thromboembolic disease and, possibly, the risk of fetal loss.

Other causes: Homocystinuria can also be caused by deficiency of methylenetetrahydrofolate reductase (MTHFR) or disorders of cobalamin metabolism (which may be accompanied by methylmalonic aciduria or megaloblastic anaemia). Patients with these rare disorders can present in many different ways, including acute neonatal encephalopathy and developmental delay. Betaine is the best available treatment for MTHFR deficiency; such patients should also be given 5 mg/day of folic acid. Betaine is also used in defects of cobalamin metabolism if homocystinuria persists despite pharmacological doses of vitamin B_{12} (q.v.).

Treatment
Start by giving 100 mg/kg/day by mouth, divided into 2–3 doses. The dose is then adjusted by monitoring the plasma homocysteine level, but doses in excess of 150 mg/kg/day seldom confer additional benefit.

Monitoring
Plasma methionine concentrations rise during treatment in classical homocystinuria, and monitoring is recommended to ensure that potentially toxic levels (>1000 μmol/l) do not develop. Clinicians need to be aware that acute cerebral oedema has (very rarely) been reported a few weeks after starting treatment.

Supply
Most patients in the UK were, until about 5 years ago, treated with betaine hydrochloride provided by Fluka Chemicals. This company traditionally charged £12 for 100 grams of the crystalline powder, supplied on the understanding that it is a chemical, and not a pharmaceutical, product. A palatable strawberry-flavoured medicine is now available as a 'special' from Special Products Ltd; 100 ml costs £40. Reconstitute the dry powder with 55 ml of purified water to obtain a liquid containing 50 mg/ml, and use within 28 days. A pharmaceutical product is also now available from Orphan Europe, who import it from an FDA approved supplier in the US. It comes with a 1 gram (1·7 cc) measuring scoop. The cost of 100 grams from this supplier is £140. The powder is usually administered mixed in a drink.

References
Devlin AM, Hajipour L, Gholkar A, *et al*. Cerebral edema associated with betaine treatment in classical homocystinuria. *J Pediatr* 2004;**144**:545–8.
Mudd SH, Levy HL, Kraus JP. Disorders of transsulfuration. In: Scriver CR, Beaudet AL, Sly WS, *et al*., eds. *The metabolic and molecular bases of inherited disease*, 8th edn. New York: McGraw-Hill, 2001: pp. 2007–56.
Ogier de Baulny H, Gérard M, Saudubray J-M, *et al*. Remethylation defects: guidelines for clinical diagnosis and treatment. *Eur J Pediatr* 1998;**157**(suppl 2):S77–83.
Ronge E, Kjellman B. Long term treatment with betaine in methylenetetrahydrofolate reductase deficiency. *Arch Dis Child* 1996;**74**:239–41.
Rosenblatt DS, Fenton WA. Inherited disorders of folate and cobalamin transport and metabolism. In: Scriver CR, Beaudet AL, Sly WS, *et al*., eds. *The metabolic and molecular bases of inherited disease*, 8th edn. New York: McGraw-Hill, 2001: pp. 3897–934.
Rosenblatt DS, Fowler B. Disorders of cobalamin and folate transport and metabolism. In: Fernandes J, Saudubray J-M, van den Berghe G, *et al*., eds. *Inborn metabolic diseases. Diagnosis and treatment*, 4th edn. Berlin: Springer-Verlag, 2006: pp. 341–56.
Wilken DEL, Wilken B, Dudman NPB, *et al*. Homocystinuria – the effects of betaine in the treatment of patients not responsive to pyrodixine. *N Engl J Med* 1983;**309**:448–53.

Use

Maternal treatment with betamethasone accelerates surfactant production by the fetal lung reducing the incidence of neonatal respiratory distress, a property it shares with dexamethasone (q.v.).

Pharmacology

The pharmacology of betamethasone and dexamethasone are very similar. See the website commentary for observational evidence that, antenatally, betamethasone seems to be safer than dexamethasone.

Indications for antenatal use

The seminal paper that first identified a strategy for preventing, rather than curing, surfactant deficiency was published more than 30 years ago. The first clue came from the observation that experimental lambs delivered prematurely failed to develop the respiratory problems seen in control animals if exposed to corticosteroids before delivery. A randomised placebo-controlled trial that eventually recruited more than a thousand mothers from New Zealand soon confirmed that two 12 mg IM doses of betamethasone caused a significant reduction in the incidence of respiratory distress in babies born more than 8 weeks early, and a fall in neonatal mortality in all babies born more than 3 weeks early. Doubling this dose brought about no further improvement in outcome. No study has ever looked to see if a smaller dose might be equally effective.

It took 20 years for this strategy to gain general acceptance and, in the interim, a further 11 trials were mounted to replicate the original findings. The most recent Cochrane review of all the 21 trials ever done shows that antenatal treatment with 24 mg of betamethasone *or* dexamethasone is associated with a 40–60% reduction in the risk of neonatal respiratory distress, and with a similar reduction in cerebroventricular haemorrhage, in necrotising enterocolitis and in early systemic infection, and that this, in turn, results in fewer deaths, and in a reduction in the cost and duration of neonatal care. Benefit 'appears to apply to babies born at *all* gestational ages at which respiratory distress syndrome may occur' and one recent trial showed that it also reduced problems for babies electively delivered at 37–38 weeks' gestation. Babies delivered less than 24 hours after prophylaxis is started derive only limited benefit, and it is now clear that benefit wanes after a week. Twins seem to benefit just as much as singleton babies but, because they were not separately identified in many trials, the available sample size is currently too small to establish this. Giving one more dose once a week to women not delivered within 7 days further reduced the number of babies troubled by respiratory problems after birth in the Australasian (ACTORDS) trial and there were no detectable adverse effects in the 2-year survivors. Only long-term follow up will show if there are any late consequences. Giving more than this delivers no additional benefit and may further retard fetal growth, while fortnightly repetition (as in the MACS trial) delivered no benefit. Delaying further prophylaxis until delivery again seems imminent can also work well (as long as delivery can then be delayed for at least 36 hours) as the Obstetrix trial showed in March 2009.

No adverse late consequence of exposure to a single course of betamethasone could be detected when the children of the mothers recruited into the first trial in New Zealand were recontacted after 30 years. Women with hypertension and fetal growth retardation were excluded from many early trials, but we now know that these babies benefit too. Use (under prophylactic antibiotic cover) was also beneficial where there has been prelabour rupture of membranes, but use in mothers with diabetes remains less well established, since treatment could affect diabetic control. Repetitive antenatal treatment slows fetal growth but the effect was too small to be detectable at discharge in most trials, and non-existent in the most recent trial (Garite *et al.*, 2009).

Maternal prophylaxis

First course of treatment: Give 12 mg of betamethasone base as a deep IM injection, and a second dose after 24 hours while trying to delay delivery for 48 hours. Oral treatment cannot be recommended on the basis of the only small trials conducted to date. While prophylaxis is of no proven benefit when delivery threatens before 24 weeks' gestation, it should not be denied to those at risk of delivery at 23 weeks if requested.

Repeat treatment: If delivery does not occur for 7 days and then again becomes likely in the next 7 days, consider giving another 12 mg dose and try to delay delivery for 24 hours, since respiratory problems and their complications can be serious after delivery before 30 weeks' gestation (and a reducible risk before 33 weeks).

Supply

Celastone®, a product that contains both betamethasone sodium phosphate and the more long-acting ester bet amethasone acetate, was used in all the more important perinatal trials, but this product is still not on sale in the UK. Indeed, the only formulation routinely available in the UK is a 1 ml ampoule containing 5·3 mg of betamethasone sodium phosphate (4 mg of betamethasone base) costing £1·20, and the ampoules provided by some manufacturers contain sodium metabisulphite. 500 microgram (5p) tablets are also available.

References

See also the relevant Cochrane reviews and UK guideline **DHUK**

Crowther CA, Doyle LW, Haslam RR, *et al*. Outcomes at 2 years of age after repeat doses of antenatal corticosteroids. *N Engl J Med* 2007;**357**:1179–89. [RCT] (See also pp. 1191–8 and editorial on pp. 1248–50.)

Garite TJ, Kurtzman J, Maurel K, *et al*. Impact of a 'rescue course' of antenatal corticosteroids: a multicenter randomized placebo-controlled trial. *Am J Obstet Gynecol* 2009;**200**:248:e1–9. [RCT] (See also pp. 217–18.)

Joseph KS, Netta F, Scott H, *et al*. Prenatal corticosteroid prophylaxis for women delivering at late preterm gestation. *Pediatrics* 2009;**124**:e835–43.

Lee BH, Stoll BJ, McDonald SA, *et al*. Adverse neonatal outcomes with antenatal dexamethasone versus antenatal betamethasone. *Pediatrics* 2006;**117**:1503–10.

Murphy KE, Hannah ME, Willan AR, *et al*. Multiple courses of antenatal corticosteroids for preterm birth (MACS): a randomised controlled trial. *Lancet* 2008;**372**:2143–51. [RCT] (See also pp. 2094–5.)

Use
Two rare, recessively inherited, metabolic diseases respond to biotin treatment.

Biochemistry
Biotin is one of the water-soluble group B vitamins. It is found in a wide range of foods including eggs, liver, kidneys and some vegetables. Nutritional deficiency is extremely rare. Biotin is a cofactor for four carboxylases: propionyl-CoA carboxylase, pyruvate carboxylase, 3-methyl-crotonyl-CoA carboxylase and acetyl-CoA carboxylase. Holocarboxylase synthetase catalyses the covalent attachment of biotin to these proteins. When carboxylases are degraded, biotin is liberated by the action of biotinidase and recycled.

Pathology
Deficiency of either holocarboxylase synthetase or biotinidase leads to 'multiple carboxylase deficiency'.

Holocarboxylase synthetase deficiency: These children present as neonates or infants with feeding problems, encephalopathy, metabolic acidosis and urinary organic acids compatible with the four carboxylase deficiencies. Lymphocytes and fibroblasts can be used to confirm the enzyme deficiency. Mothers of patients are sometimes given 10 mg of biotin a day during any subsequent pregnancy, although it is not clear whether such prenatal treatment is actually necessary.

Biotinidase deficiency: Children with this rare condition present in the first 2 years of life, usually with seizures or developmental delay. Rashes and alopecia are common. Biotinidase can be measured in blood.

In both conditions, there is a good response to pharmacological doses of biotin but, if treatment is delayed, irreversible brain damage will often have occurred. Although screening at birth has not yet been initiated in the UK (as it has in some countries) it does have the potential to prevent most of these problems. Screening also brings to light cases of *partial* biotinidase deficiency. It is not yet clear whether these children benefit from routine supplementation, but supplementation seems harmless enough in itself. There have been no convincing reports of benefit from biotin in patients with an isolated carboxylase deficiency.

Treatment
Patients with either holocarboxylase synthetase or biotinidase deficiency usually respond to 5–10 mg of biotin a day (irrespective of weight or age) but doses of up to 100 mg a day may be needed in a few patients. Treatment can usually be given by mouth, but a parenteral preparation is available.

Supply
The need for high-dose biotin treatment is so uncommon that there is no regular pharmaceutical preparation on the market. It is possible for hospital pharmacies to get 5 mg tablets in packs of 20 and ampoules containing 5 mg/ml intended for IM use through John Bell and Croydon, 54 Wigmore Street, London W1H 0AU (telephone 020 7935 5555) by special request on a 'named patient' basis from Roche Products Ltd. A suspension could be prepared on request.

References
Baumgartner ER, Suormala T. Biotin-responsive disorders. In: Fernandes J, Saudubray J-M, van den Berghe G, *et al.*, eds. *Inborn metabolic diseases. Diagnosis and treatment*, 4th edn. Berlin: Springer-Verlag, 2006: pp. 332–9.
McVoy JR, Levy HL, Lawler M, *et al.* Partial biotinidase deficiency: clinical and biochemical features. *J Pediatr* 1990;**116**:78–83.
Moslinger D, Stockler-Ipsiroglu S, Scheibenreiter S, *et al.* Clinical and neuropsychological outcome in 33 patients with biotinidase deficiency ascertained by nationwide newborn screening and family studies in Austria. *Eur J Pediatr* 2001;**160**:277–82. (See also **161**:167–9.)
Packman S, Cowan MS, Golbus MS, *et al.* Prenatal treatment of biotin-responsive multiple carboxylase deficiency. *Lancet* 1982;**i**:1435.
Salbert BA, Pellock JM, Wolf B. Characterization of seizures associated with biotinidase deficiency. *Neurology* 1993;**43**:1351–5.
Suormala T, Fowler B, Duran M, *et al.* Five patients with biotin-responsive defect in holocarboxylase formation. *Pediatr Res* 1997;**41**:667–73.
Thuy LP, Jurecki E, Nemzer L, *et al.* Prenatal diagnosis of holocarboxylase syntherase deficiency by assay of the enzyme in chorionic villus material followed by prenatal treatment. *Clin Chim Acta* 1999;**284**:59–68.
Wastell HJ, Bartlett K, Dale D, *et al.* Biotinidase deficiency: a survey of 10 cases. *Arch Dis Child* 1988;**63**:1244–9.
Weber P, Scholl S, Baumgartner ER. Outcome in patients with profound biotinidase deficiency: relevance of newborn screening. *Devel Med Child Neurol* 2004;**46**:481–4.
Wolf B. Disorders of biotin metabolism. In: Scriver CR, Beaudet AL, Sly WS, *et al.*, eds. *The metabolic and molecular bases of inherited disease*, 8th edn. New York: McGraw-Hill, 2001: pp. 3935–64.

Use

Red cell concentrates, or 'plasma reduced cells' (previously called 'packed cells'), and red cell suspensions, are used to correct serious symptomatic anaemia.

Products

Blood is not sterile, and viruses can be transmitted during transfusion, although the risk of cell-associated virus transmission is now routinely minimised by prior leucodepletion (i.e. the removal of virtually all white cells). Vigorous action has also been taken to minimise the risk from variant Creutzfeldt–Jakob disease. Donors are screened for the presence of hepatitis B, hepatitis C and HIV-1 antibodies, but these take some time to develop after the onset of infection. Ill and preterm babies born to mothers lacking cytomegalovirus (CMV) antibodies also face a significant risk of neonatal CMV infection if given CMV seropositive blood. Malaria, and other blood-borne parasites, pose a significant risk in areas where these are endemic.

A unit of 'whole blood' (haematocrit 35–45%) is prepared by adding 450 ml of donor blood to 63 ml of anticoagulant (usually citrate phosphate dextrose with added adenine – CPD-A), but the main product now provided for clinical use is a 230 ml concentrate with a haematocrit of 55–75% made from this by removing most of the plasma. Such packs are not only leucodepleted, but also contain virtually no functional platelets. They can be stored for 5 weeks, but blood less than 7 days old should be supplied for neonatal use where possible because the potassium and acid load are less, there will be fewer microaggregates, and the oxygen carrying capacity will be greater (the concentration of 2,3-diphosphoglycerate in the red cells falls with time). Most clotting factors remain relatively stable when so stored, but factor V and factor VIII levels fall by 75% within 10 days. Blood for intrauterine and exchange transfusion is plasma reduced to a haematocrit of ~70% and prepared from CMV-negative CPD-A blood. It is also irradiated if the baby is having, or has had, an intrauterine transfusion. However when a 'top up' transfusion proves necessary in early infancy, a red cell suspension in optimal added solution (usually CPD or SAG-M) is now usually issued. Such suspensions, which contain no clotting factors, increasingly come in 40–45 ml 'minipacks' (1 unit of donor blood usually being used to prepare 4–6 such packs). Such products can be used for up to 5 weeks after preparation. Such suspensions should ***never*** be used for an exchange transfusion.

Matching

The laboratory needs to check the recipient's ABO and Rh D blood group, and to test for the existence of any irregular antibodies before donor blood is released. Maternal blood is still used for detailed matching in some districts, as long as the mother's and baby's ABO groups are compatible, because infants less than 4 months old rarely make antibodies to red cells, and any neonatal IgG antibody will usually be derived from the mother. If unmatched group 0 Rh D-negative blood ever needs to be used in an emergency, an attempt should be made to discuss this with a consultant haematologist first.

Adverse reactions

Allergic reactions with urticaria are rare in the neonatal period. Symptomatic treatment with 1 mg of chlorphenamine maleate IM (previously known as chlorpheniramine maleate) may be appropriate. Intravascular haemolysis due to ABO incompatibility is rare but potentially fatal. Immediate signs include flushing, dyspnoea, fever, hypotension and oliguria, with haemoglobinaemia and haemoglobinuria. Stop the transfusion at once, take specimens for laboratory analysis and watch for renal failure, hyperkalaemia and a coagulopathy. Rhesus, Kell, Kidd (Jk^a) and Duffy (Fy^a) antibodies may cause late reticuloendothelial haemolysis with jaundice and anaemia.

Clinical factors

Intravascular blood volume almost always falls significantly during the first few hours of life as plasma leaves the intravascular compartment, but soon stabilises at 80–90 ml/kg with a haematocrit that reflects the extent and direction of any placental transfusion at delivery. Umbilical vein obstruction (as from a tight nuchal cord) can leave a baby hypovolaemic at birth. Capillary haemoglobin and haematocrit values for term babies in the first 3 months of life are shown in Fig. 1 and Fig. 2 (opposite). Replicate laboratory haemoglobin estimates from capillary samples can vary by 6 g/l, so apparent changes of 10 g/l may merely reflect sampling error. A capillary haemoglobin may also exceed the venous haemoglobin by 10 g/l. Packed cell volume (PCV) measurements using a centrifuge provide a more rapid and satisfactory way of screening for anaemia in the neonatal period. They are more reproducible, require less blood and provide an immediate side-ward answer.

Venous PCV or 'haematocrit' values for term babies are shown in Fig. 2. Babies born more than 8 weeks early have values that are about 5% lower than these at birth, and the lower limit of the normal range 4–12 weeks after birth is also lower than in term babies (giving a minimum PCV of 20% instead of 25%). Capillary values exceed venous values by at least 2% (and often by 4–8% in the first few days of life). Such differences can be minimised if free flowing blood is collected from a warm, well-perfused heel. Microcentrifuge measurement methods always exceed particle counting estimates by 1–2%.

Indications for transfusion

Symptomatic babies with a venous haematocrit of less than 40% at birth merit transfusion once a sample of blood has been collected from both the baby and the mother for diagnostic purposes. Watch for the hypovolaemic baby with a normal haematocrit immediately after birth; haematocrit values normally rise in the first 12 hours of life, but in such babies there will be a fall. Such babies may have lost a quarter to a half of all their blood (20–40 ml/kg). Acute loss is best managed by a prompt rapid transfusion, but chronic anaemia at birth is better managed by exchange transfusion. Since it is the fall in plasma volume rather than the fall in haemoglobin that poses the immediate threat after acute blood loss, 0·9% sodium chloride or pentastarch (q.v.) can be given while waiting for blood to arrive if the patient's condition is critical.

Continued

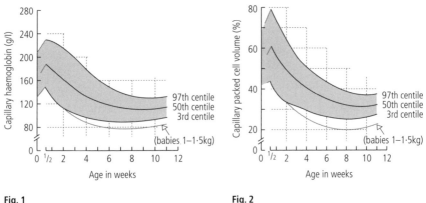

Fig. 1   **Fig. 2**

Most healthy preterm babies do not need transfusion until their haematocrit falls below 20%, but very oxygen-dependent babies and babies with other cardiorespiratory problems are seldom allowed to develop an untreated haematocrit below 30%. Mortality actually *rose* in critically ill adults in a trial designed to keep the haemoglobin above 100 g/l, and morbidity was unaffected in a paediatric trial where a level of 70 g/l rather than 95 g/l provided the threshold for transfusion. Babies who have had a lot of blood samples taken run a risk of becoming iron deficient, because four-fifths of all the body's iron stores are present as molecular haemoglobin at birth. However, it is not difficult, with a little thought, to keep loss from sampling below 0·6 ml/kg a day (as several trials into neonatal erythropoietin (q.v.) have shown), and these babies seldom needed to be transfused more than once or twice, or exposed to more than one donor, even if they weighed less than 1 kg at birth. Early cord clamping (before 2 minutes) only makes such anaemia worse. Such babies are more often iron deficient 6 months later, and infants with iron-deficiency anaemia make slower neurodevelopmental progress.

Administration

Treat anaemia with 25 ml/kg of blood over 1–2 hours. Multiple small transfusions from different donors are wasteful, and put the patient at increased risk. It is ***not*** usually necessary to calculate a specific replacement volume, or give a 'covering' diuretic. Give blood through a fresh giving set with a 170–200 μm filter into a line previously set up and primed with 0·9% sodium chloride. Terminal co-infusion into a line containing glucose is also safe, and does not cause measurable haemolysis, so it is better to do this than terminate the glucose infusion and precipitate reactive hypoglycaemia when it is not practicable to erect a separate intravenous line. Check the cross-match particulars and the patient's name, and record all the details in the case notes.

Supply

Cross-matched blood stored at 4°C is available from the local blood bank. Group O Rhesus-negative, CMV-negative, plasma-reduced blood is available for emergency use. Use within 4 hours of removal from the fridge. Use a minipack containing about 40–45 ml of red cell concentrate where possible, particularly if more than one transfusion is likely to be needed within the next 7 days, to conserve stocks and minimise the risk of exposure to several donors. A unit of blood costs £55, and a minipack £15 to dispense.

References

See also the relevant Cochrane reviews and UK guideline

Alverson DC. The physiologic impact of anemia in the neonate. *Clin Perinatol* 1995;**22**:609–25. (See also pp. 657–69.)

Brotanek JM, Fosz J, Weitzman M, *et al*. Secular trends in the prevalence of iron deficiency among US toddlers, 1976–2002. *Arch Pediatr Adolesc Med* 2008;**162**:374–81.

Hosono S, Mugishima H, Fujita H, *et al*. Umbilical cord milking reduces the need for red cell transfusions and improves neonatal adaptation in infants born less than 29 weeks' gestation: a randomised controlled trial. *Arch Dis Child* 2008;**93**:F14–9. [RCT] (See also pp. F2–3.)

Jankov RP, Roy RND. Minimal haemolysis in blood co-infused with amino acid and dextrose solutions *in vitro*. *J Paediatr Child Health* 1997;**33**:250–2.

Lacroix J, Hébert PC, Hutchison JS, *et al*. Transfusion strategies for patients in pediatric intensive care units. *N Engl J Med* 2007;**356**:1609–19. [RCT]

Murray NA, Roberts IAG. Neonatal transfusion practice. [Review] *Arch Dis Child* 2004;**89**:F101–7.

van Rheenen PF, Brabin BJ. A practical approach to timing cord clamping in resource poor settings. *BMJ* 2006;**333**:954–8. [SR]

von Lindern JS, Brand A. The use of blood products in perinatal medicine. [Review] *Semin Fetal Neonat Med* 2008;**13**:271–81.

Use

Powdered products are now commercially available for modifying the nutritional content of human breast milk when this is used to feed the very preterm baby. However, the benefits have been modest to date, and the variability of expressed breast milk does not make 'tailored' supplementation any easier.

Immunological factors

Human milk is the ideal food for almost every baby. Although the various artificial products available seem to meet all the key nutritional needs of the term and preterm baby (as outlined in the monograph on milk formulas) feeding with unpasteurised human milk still confers a number of unique, if poorly understood, immunological advantages. While it is now recommended that all 'donor' milk should be pasteurised before use, mother's own milk is best used without pasteurisation. Milk collected in the home is safe for 8 days if kept at 4°C, and is best *not* frozen. Cells are damaged by storage and by freezing, but the immunoprotective constituents remain stable when stored at 0–4°C for 3 days, when frozen at –20°C for 12 months, or when pasteurised at 56°C for 30 minutes. Use thawed milk at once.

Nutritional factors

All these products are designed to enhance the nutritional value of human milk. Do not insist on an arbitrary upper limit to oral intake – some preterm babies do very well on a daily intake of 220 ml/kg when 2 or 3 weeks old. The milk of a mother delivering a preterm baby usually has a relatively high protein content in the first couple of weeks of life, and too high a protein intake could, theoretically, be hazardous. Fortification is probably best not started, therefore, until about 2 weeks after delivery. It seldom needs to be continued once breastfeeding is established, or the baby weighs 2 kg.

All the products listed in Table 1 enhance the protein and calorie content of the milk. They also provide minerals to improve bone growth (an important requirement for very preterm babies – as discussed in the monograph on phosphate). For details of four other products quite widely used in Europe, Australia and North America see the web commentary.

Table 1 Composition per 100 ml of human milk after fortification.

	Protein (g)	Fat (g)	Carbohydrate (g)	Energy (kcal)	Na (mmol)	Ca (mmol)	P (mmol)	Fe (mg)	Zn (mg)	Vit D (µg)	Vit K (µg)
Mature human breast milk (Widdowson 1977)	1·3	4·2	7·4	70	0·7	0·9	0·5	0·1	0·4	<0·1	0·2
Cow & Gate: Nutriprem fortifier® 2 sachets (4·1 g) per 100 ml	2·1	4·2	10·4	86	1·1	2·5	1·9	0·1	0·8	≥5	6·4
Mead Johnson: Enfamil® 4 sachets (2·8 g) per 100 ml	2·4	5·2	7·8	84	1·4	3·2	2·1	1·5	1·1	3·9	4·6
Milupa: Eoprotin® 4 scoops (4·2 g) per 100 ml	2·1	4·2	10·4	85	1·1	2·5	2·0	0·1	0·8	5	6·5
SMA: Breast milk fortifier® 2 sachets (4 g) per 100 ml	2·3	4·4	9·8	85	1·4	3·1	2·0	0·1	0·6	7·6	11·2

Supplementation

Human milk contains relatively little protein, and a plasma urea of less than 1·6 mmol/l may be a sign of suboptimal protein intake. Very preterm babies fed on fortified breast milk will benefit from additional sodium (either as sodium chloride (q.v.) or as some other salt) in the first few weeks of life, until their obligatory renal sodium loss decreases. Babies on Nestle FM85® will also need, and babies on Enfamil® and Similac® may well benefit from, further vitamin D (q.v.). Breastfed babies also almost certainly need additional vitamin K (q.v.) to prevent late vitamin K deficiency bleeding once fortification ceases, unless they have been given a total 'depot' supply of 1 mg IM at birth, irrespective of their weight at delivery, and it is probably easier to start such supplementation early. From about a month of age all preterm breastfed babies benefit from sustained supplementation with oral iron (q.v.), and a few need zinc (q.v.). The commercially available breast milk fortifiers do not address these needs. Whether it helps to give further vitamin A (q.v.) by mouth is still unclear.

Supply

Enfamil has been widely used in the USA, but it is not commercially available in the UK. While the SMA product is not on general release, it is available in boxes containing 50 × 2 gram sachets to units stocking and using SMA low birthweight formula milk. Eoprotin® is supplied in 200 gram tins costing £15 each and Nutriprem fortifier® in boxes containing 50 × 1·5 gram sachets costing £10. The powder is best added just before the baby is fed. Do not use any of these products to further fortify artificial formula milks.

References

See also the relevant Cochrane reviews

Breast Feeding Network 2009. Expressing and storing breast milk. www.breastfeedingnetwork.org.uk/pdfs/BFNExpressing&Storing.pdf.
Cowett RM, ed. Nutrition and metabolism of the micropremie. [A series of 13 review articles] *Clin Perinatol* 2000;**27**:1–254.
Hands A. Safe storage of expressed breast milk in the home. *MIDIRS Midwifery Digest* 2003;**13**:278–85. [SR]
Jones E, King C, eds. *Feeding and nutrition in the preterm infant*. Edinburgh: Elsevier Churchill Livingstone, 2005.
Royal College of Midwives. *Successful breastfeeding*, 3rd edn. Edinburgh: Churchill Livingstone, 2002.

Use

Inhaled steroids (like budesonide) are central to the management of asthma and useful in the management of croup. Prophylactic use has done little to reduce the incidence of ventilator-induced chronic lung disease, but one small study suggests that direct liquid intratracheal co-instillation with surfactant may be more effective.

Pharmacology

Budesonide (patented in 1975) and beclometasone dipropionate (called beclomethasone dipropionate in the USA) are steroids of almost equivalent potency with strong glucocorticoid and negligible mineralocorticoid activity. Fluticasone propionate is a related compound which is about twice as potent on a weight-for-weight basis. They are widely used topically on the skin or by inhalation into the lung (as in asthma) and have little systemic effect unless high-dose treatment is employed. There is no contraindication to their use during pregnancy and lactation: indeed it is particularly important to keep asthma under stable control during pregnancy. Administration is generally from an aerosol or dry powder inhaler. Suspensions of budesonide and fluticasone can also be nebulised, but there seems to be no comparable preparation of beclometasone.

Intratracheal steroid use in the preterm baby

Early prophylactic use: The OSECT trial compared inhaled budesonide versus systemic dexamethasone, and early versus delayed, treatment in 570 ventilated babies of less than 30 weeks' gestation using a factorial design. Inhalation seemed almost as effective as systemic treatment when started early, and less likely to cause hyperglycaemia or a rise in blood pressure. Fewer babies treated early (systemically or by inhalation) died, or were still oxygen dependent at 36 weeks (55% v 59%), but the difference was not statistically significant. Outcome at 7 years was similar in the four trial groups. Because of concern for the long-term consequences of early postnatal steroid use (as outlined in the monograph on dexamethasone), there is now a consensus that systemic steroid treatment should only be given to babies displaying clear signs of serious lung damage (bronchopulmonary dysplasia) more than a week after birth. There is, however, one small study suggesting that, in the very oxygen-dependent baby, early treatment may reduce this risk if budesonide is co-administered with surfactant to help optimise distribution within the lung as a *liquid*. There were few early side effects, but the long-term outcome is not yet known.
Treatment of established disease: A recent overview of trial information suggests that while aerosolised or nebulised budesonide or beclometasone can be of some help in weaning babies from ventilator support, they are not as effective as systemic steroids. Use may, however, help to reduce or abolish the need for systemic treatment with dexamethasone in a few babies with chronic lung disease.

Inhaled steroid use in croup

Croup (the sudden onset of hoarseness, a barking cough and distressing inspiratory stridor) is common in young children. It is mainly viral in origin, though atopy plays a part in some children. Symptoms often settle almost as fast as they arise. Brief steroid use can reduce admission, and only 1% of those admitted require intubation (once cases of bacterial epiglottitis are recognised for what they are).

Treatment

Early prophylactic use: One small study has suggested that instilling 250 micrograms/kg of budesonide premixed with 100 mg/kg of the surfactant beractant directly into the trachea (see below) may reduce the risk of chronic lung disease in the very preterm baby. This should *only* be attempted as part of a clinical trial.
Managing ventilator-induced chronic lung disease: 200 (or 500) micrograms of budesonide inhaled twice a day may occasionally aid extubation but is of no other demonstrable long-term benefit. The drug has usually been given from a metered dose aerosol inhaler into a rigid 'aerochamber' during hand ventilation. Mask administration using a jet nebuliser after extubation can reduce the child's 'symptom score' but trials have failed to show any more general clinical benefit. It may be wise to protect the eyes during mask administration. Only a tenth of the administered dose reaches the baby.
Use in croup: Two 1 mg doses of nebulised budesonide 30 minutes apart can reduce the need for hospital admission as effectively as a single 0·6 mg/kg oral (or IM) dose of dexamethasone (q.v.).

Supply and administration

500 microgram (2 ml) Respules® of budesonide, designed for face mask nebulisation, cost £1·60 each. For direct intratracheal instillation mix 8 ml (200 mg) of beractant with 2 ml (500 micrograms) of budesonide in a syringe and give 5 ml/kg of this in 3–4 aliquots into the trachea at 2–5-minute intervals. The effect of using any *other* surfactant is, as yet, unknown, and could involve putting twice as much fluid into the lung. Fluticasone proprionate is available in 2 ml 500 microgram Nebules® (costing 90p) for jet nebuliser use.

References

See also relevant Cochrane reviews

Berger WE, Qaqundah PY, Blake K, *et al*. Safety of budesonide inhalation suspension in infants aged six to twelve months with mild to moderate persistent asthma or recurrent wheeze. *J Pediatr* 2005;**146**:91–5. [RCT]

Wilson TT, Waters L, Patterson CC, *et al*. Neurodevelopmental and respiratory follow-up results at 7 years for children from the United Kingdom and Ireland enrolled into a randomized trial of early and late postnatal corticosteroid treatment, systematic and inhaled (the Open Study of Early Corticosteroid Treatment). *Pediatrics* 2006;**117**:2196–205. [RCT]

Yeh TF, Lin HC, Chang CH, *et al*. Early intratracheal installation of budesonide using surfactant as a vehicle to prevent chronic lung disease in preterm infants: a pilot study. *Pediatrics* 2008;**121**:e1310–18. [RCT]

BUPIVACAINE

Use

Bupivacaine is a widely used local anaesthetic. It takes rather longer than lidocaine (q.v.) to become effective, and is much more toxic, but the pain relief it provides lasts four times as long.

Pharmacology

Bupivacaine is an amide local anaesthetic, like lidocaine, that blocks the conduction of nerve impulses by decreasing the nerve membrane's permeability to sodium ions. It was first developed in 1957. Sensory nerves are more readily affected than motor nerves. A small amount (~6%) is excreted unchanged in the urine, but most is metabolised by the liver, the neonatal half life being about 8 hours (at least twice as long as in adults). Tissue levels exceed plasma levels (neonatal steady state V_D ~4 l/kg). All local anaesthetic drugs are potentially toxic. Most are more toxic to the brain than the heart, causing tremor, restlessness, apnoea and fits before they cause an arrhythmia, but the reverse is true of bupivacaine. Check the maximum dose for the baby and do not put more than this in the syringe. Have an IV line in place. Accidental injection into a blood vessel can be particularly dangerous, so aspirate before injecting. Epidural bupivacaine (with or without an opioid) provides lumbar block before surgery and during childbirth. Tissue infiltration can provide local sensory block.

Lidocaine becomes fully effective in adults within 2−4 minutes, and blocks all local sensation for about an hour. Bupivacaine, in contrast, takes up to half an hour to become fully effective after infiltration but then blocks all sensation for 2−8 hours (and probably longer than this in the neonate). Anaesthetists have used intraoperative bupivacaine nerve blocks and wound infiltration (in a dose not exceeding 2 mg/kg) to reduce postoperative pain. Epidural bupivacaine has been used during abdominal surgery to avoid the need for morphine in young children, with its attendant risk of respiratory depression. Low epidural blocks have been used, in the same way, during the surgical treatment of inguinal hernia in the preterm baby, obviating the need for a general anaesthetic. The subcutaneous infusion of up to 400 micrograms/kg of bupivacaine an hour postoperatively for up to 3 days into the region of any major incision can also deliver significant pain relief.

Ropivacaine, a related aminoamide anaesthetic first introduced in 1997, has now started to be used to provide caudal and lumbar epidural block in children. Early experience suggests that it is less toxic and produces less motor block for a given degree of sensory block. The dose used in infancy is 1 ml/kg of a 0·2% solution, followed by a continuous infusion of 200 micrograms/kg per hour (or 400 micrograms/kg per hour in infants more than 6 months old) continued for not more than 72 hours.

Maternal bupivacaine is systemically absorbed after epidural administration, crosses the placenta readily, and is detectable in the cord blood in a dose that is high enough to interfere transiently with auditory brainstem evoked responses, but not high enough to induce any significant neurobehavioural changes. The same probably goes for ropivacaine. The amount excreted in human milk is negligible.

Pain relief

Infiltrative local anaesthesia: Do not exceed a dose of 2 mg/kg (0·8 ml/kg of 0·25% bupivacaine), and do not repeat this dose for 8 hours. Use a pulse oximeter (and/or ECG monitor) to detect any early adverse cardiorespiratory effect. *It is essential to avoid accidental injection into a blood vessel.*
Epidural block: Give up to 0·8 ml/kg of 0·25% bupivacaine slowly into the caudal epidural space over 1−2 minutes, aspirating intermittently to check for the presence of blood or CSF. This should produce adequate anaesthesia for inguinal or perineal surgery after about 15 minutes.

Toxicity

Apnoea or a change in heart rate is usually the first sign that too much drug has entered the circulation. Immediate ventilatory support can minimise acidosis (which further augments the drug's toxicity). Hypotension may respond to dobutamine (q.v.). Thiopental sodium (q.v.) may be needed if fits interfere with ventilation. Complete recovery can be anticipated unless an arrhythmia develops that is resistant to these measures and to a 10 microgram/kg bolus of clonidine.

Supply

10 ml ampoules containing 25 mg of plain bupivacaine hydrochloride (i.e. 0·25% bupivacaine) cost 98p. Note that more concentrated ampoules (0·5% and 0·75%), and ampoules containing adrenaline, are also marketed. 10 ml ampoules containing 20 mg of ropivacaine hydrochloride cost £1·40.

References

Bösenberg AT, Thomas J, Cronje L, *et al*. Pharmacokinetics and efficacy of ropivacaine for continuous epidural infusion in neonates and infants. *Pediatr Anaesth* 2005;**15**:739−49.
de La Coiussaye JE, Bassoul B, Brugada J, *et al*. Reversal of electrophysiological and haemodynamic effects induced by high dose bupivacaine by the combination of clonidine and dobutamine in anesthetised dogs. *Anesth Analg* 1992;**74**:703−11.
Gallagher TM. Regional anaesthesia for surgical treatment of inguinal hernia in preterm babies. *Arch Dis Child* 1993; **69**:623−4.
Rapp HJ, Molnar V, Austin S, *et al*. Ropivacaine in neonates and infants − a population pharmacokinetic evaluation following single caudal block. *Paediatr Anaesth* 2004;**14**:724−32.
Tirotta CF, Munro HM, Salvaggio J, *et al*. Continuous incisional infusion of local anesthetic in pediatric patients following open heart surgery. *Pediatr Anesth* 2009;**19**:571−6. [RCT]
Wolf AR, Hughes D. Pain relief for infants undergoing abdominal surgery: comparison of infusions of IV morphine and extra-dural bupivacaine. *Br J Anaesth* 1993;**70**:10−16.

Use

Cabergoline is used to treat hyperprolactinaemic amenorrhoea and galactorrhoea. Use can also, occasionally, be justified to suppress lactation after childbirth.

Pharmacology

Bromocriptine is a derivative of ergot that functions as a dopamine D_2 agonist. It was first used to treat patients with Parkinson disease in 1974 (but is now only used for this purpose in patients who suffer a fluctuant response when treated by levodopa alone). It was once widely used to suppress lactation (see web archive) but side effects resulted in a general switch to the use of cabergoline in the late 1980s.

Carbergoline is a closely related drug that is well absorbed when given by mouth, is metabolised in the liver with a half life of 2–4 days, and is excreted largely in the bile. It is a potent, long-lasting inhibitor of prolactin secretion that has now become the most widely used drug in the management of hyperprolactinaemia. Indeed a single dose twice a week will restore ovulation in most women with hyperprolactinaemic amenorrhoea. The manufacturers have recommended that treatment should be stopped before women try to conceive, but there is no evidence of teratogenicity in man and a real possibility that withdrawal could prevent ovulation or result in vision-threatening increase in size if the tumour is already large. While high-dose treatment can cause fibrotic heart valve changes, and this should be watched for, such changes seem rare with low-dose treatment. Nor does low-dose treatment seem to cause a problem during lactation in patients with a prolactinoma, and the baby ingests, on a weight-related basis, less than 1% of the maternal dose. It is, however, often possible to stop treatment during pregnancy and during lactation because prolactinomas usually only grow slowly at this time.

Effect on lactation

Milk formation during late pregnancy occurs under the combined stimulus of oestrogens, prolactin (placental lactogen) and progesterone. Insulin and cortisol may also have a role. Oestrogens antagonise the effects of prolactin, and lactation is stimulated when oestrogen levels fall after delivery.

Oestrogens were once used widely to suppress lactation in the puerperium, but they were found to be relatively ineffective, and to increase the risk of potentially life-threatening thromboembolism. Trials undertaken between 1972 and 1984 showed 2·5 mg of bromocriptine given twice a week for 2 weeks to be a more effective alternative. However, most drug trials only looked at the immediate effect of drug treatment and there is some evidence that although bromocriptine reduces pain, engorgement and milk production 1 week after delivery more than a breast binder, the situation is reversed 2 weeks later.

Over the next 10 years reports started to appear of mothers having seizures, strokes, heart attacks and sudden severe hypertension while taking bromocriptine to suppress lactation. While it is difficult to know whether these symptoms were caused by the use of bromocriptine, problems were, however, reported with sufficient frequency for the manufacturers to stop recommending the use of bromocriptine to suppress lactation in 1994. Since discomfort is only a transient problem there can seldom be a case for using *any* drug to suppress lactation in most mothers, but drug use can still be justified in certain situations. Continued milk production can certainly cause acute anguish to some mothers coping with a stillbirth or early neonatal death. Here cabergoline is probably the drug of choice (even though it gets little mention in the recent Cochrane review). It seems to be relatively free from the problems associated with the use of bromocriptine to suppress lactation, although that could be because it has not, as yet, been as widely used. However, post-treatment rebound certainly seems less marked. If either drug is used for this purpose, treatment should certainly be stopped at once if the mother experiences any severe headache or visual disturbance.

Use to suppress lactation

A single 1 mg dose of cabergoline by mouth is usually enough to suppress lactation immediately after delivery. If lactation has already been established, give four 250 mg doses at 12-hour intervals.

Supply

500 microgram scored tablets of cabergoline are available (costing £3·70 each), as are 2·5 mg tablets of bromocriptine (costing 18p each).

References
See also the relevant Cochrane reviews

Bhattacharyya S, Shapira A, Mikhailidis DP, *et al*. Drug-induced fibrotic valvular heart disease. *Lancet* 2009;**374**:577–85. [SR]

Caballero GA, Caballero DJL. Caberbolina: Nuevo dopaminérgico a dosis única en la inhibición de la lactación. *Acta Ginecológica* 1996;**53**:172–9. [RCT]

Caballero-Gordo A, Lopez-Nazareno N, Calderay M, *et al*. Single-dose inhibition of puerperal lactation. *J Reprod Med* 1991:**36**:717–21.

Colao A, Abs R, Barcena DG, *et al*. Pregnancy outcomes following carbergoline treatment: extended results from a 12 year observational study. *Clin Endocrinol (Oxf)* 2008;**68**:66–71.

Dutt S, Wong F, Spurway JH. Fatal myocardial infarction associated with bromocriptine for postpartum lactation suppression. *Aust NZ J Obstet Gynaecol* 1998;**38**:116–19.

European Multicentre Study Group for Cabergoline in Lactation Inhibition. Single dose cabergoline versus bromocriptine in inhibition of puerperal lactation: randomised, double-blind, multicentre study. *BMJ* 1991;**302**:1367–71. [RCT]

Martin NM, Tan T, Meeran K. Dopamine agonists and hyperprolactinaemia. [Editorial] *BMJ* 2009;**338**:554–5. [*BMJ* 2009;**338**:b381.]

Rains CP, Bryson HM, Fitton A. Cabergoline. *Drugs* 1995;**49**:255–79. [SR]

Webster J. A comparative review of the tolerability profiles of dopamine agonists in the treatment of hyperprolactinaemia and inhibition of lactation. *Drug Safety* 1996;**14**:228–38.

Use

Caffeine reduces apnoea and speeds extubation, so decreasing the time very preterm babies spend ventilated and in supplemental oxygen. Use also seems to decrease the number of survivors with disability.

Pharmacology

Caffeine citrate is a general stimulant that increases metabolic rate, central chemoreceptor sensitivity to CO_2 and inspiratory drive. It crosses the placenta easily, and an intake of more than 300 mg a day (equivalent to 8 cups of tea or 3 cups of strong coffee) probably increases in the risk of miscarriage and stillbirth (see web commentary). The amount in the breast milk of mothers on a normal diet is of no clinical significance, even though the neonatal half life (60–140 hours) is 16 times as long as it is in adults. Caffeine is well absorbed by mouth, and IV treatment is seldom necessary. It is mostly excreted, unchanged, in the urine in the first month of life, but clearance rises and approaches the rate found in adults in infants over 4 months old. Use marginally reduces weight gain for a few weeks, but it can reduce the number needing surgery for retinopathy of prematurity (ROP), and use does not increase the risk of necrotising enterocolitis. Benefit is most marked in the ventilator-dependent baby started on treatment within 3 days of birth. Tachycardia and agitation are the first signs of toxicity, while a 10-fold overdose can cause hyperglycaemia, hypertonia and heart failure.

Managing neonatal apnoea

Caffeine is now preferred to theophylline (q.v.) when managing apnoea, once sepsis, hypoglycaemia, subtle seizures and respiratory exhaustion have been excluded, but medication is no substitute for a sensible nursing strategy. While simple bradycardia can be detected with an ECG monitor and central apnoea with a transthoracic impedance or other movement monitor, a pulse oximeter picks up what really matters – clinically significant spells of hypoxaemia. A prone (face-down) posture, or a left lateral position, may help but there is very little evidence for the long-held view that it is reflux of milk back into the lower oesophagus that commonly triggers apnoea, and all babies are best nursed supine (on their backs) after discharge even if this leaves them marginally more oxygen dependent. Neither does bolus feeding cause more apnoea than continuous feeding. Constant positive airway pressure (CPAP) may help (and a similar nasal devise can also be used to provide ventilatory support). So too may doxapram (q.v.), but stimulants seldom help when obstructive apnoea is due to reflex glottic closure, or sleep-associated pharyngeal hypotonia, and caffeine can make reflux worse. Serious apnoea is commonest in the very preterm baby, becomes more troublesome a few days after birth and is uncommon in babies with a postmenstrual age of more than 33 weeks, so treatment can usually be stopped 2 weeks before discharge and any monitor removed a week after treatment ceases. Developmental delay is commoner when serious apnoea persists longer than this.

Drug equivalence

There is only 1 mg of caffeine in 2 mg of caffeine citrate. Most neonatologists worldwide have, for the last 25 years, quoted the amount of caffeine citrate used when prescribing or writing about this drug, but the UK drug regulator has now said that prescribers should state the amount of caffeine base to be given. This advice now makes it essential to always specify either the amount of caffeine **citrate** to be given (as has been traditional and recommended by this book for the last 15 years) or, to avoid confusion, the amount of caffeine **base** required.

Treatment

Neonatal apnoea: Give a loading dose of 20 mg/kg of caffeine *citrate* IV or by mouth, followed by a maintenance dose of 5 mg/kg (or *very* occasionally 10 mg/kg) IV or by mouth once every 24 hours.
Later apnoea: In the few babies who merit treatment at a postmenstrual age of more than 52 weeks it is sometimes necessary to give a maintenance dose of 5 mg/kg of caffeine *citrate* four times a day.
Facilitating extubation: The dose used to control neonatal apnoea (see above) will usually suffice. A higher loading dose of 80 mg/kg IV followed by 20 mg/kg once a day may further speed tracheal extubation in a few babies of less than 30 weeks' gestation, but it often causes quite significant tachycardia (170–190 bpm).

Blood levels

Measurement seldom influences management. While the usual target plasma level is 10–20 mg/l, a few babies respond better to a level of 25–35 mg/l. Signs of toxicity only occur when the level exceeds 50 mg/l (1 mg/l = 5·14 µmol/l). Samples do not need to be collected at any set time.

Supply

IV products: Two commercial products designed mainly for IV use, but also marketed for oral use, are available. Each 3 ml (20 mg/ml) vial in America costs $15, and each 1 ml (10 mg/ml) ampoule in the UK costs £5. Do not give IM, and do not freeze. The UK product label highlights the amount of caffeine **base** present.
Oral products: Many centres in America, and some in the UK, continue to make a more easily used (and cheaper) sugar-free preparation 'in house' with a 1-year shelf life that is useable for a month once opened.

References

See also the relevant Cochrane reviews

Pillekamp F, Hermann C, Keller T, *et al*. Factors influencing apnea and bradycardia of prematurity – implications for neurodevelopment. *Neonatology* 2007;**91**:155–61.
Schmidt B, Roberts RS, Davis P, *et al*. Caffeine therapy for apnea of prematurity. *N Engl J Med* 2006;**354**:2112–21. [RCT]
Schmidt B, Roberts RS, Davis P, *et al*. The long-term effects of caffeine therapy for apnea of prematurity. *N Engl J Med* 2007;**357**:1893–1902. [RCT] (See also pp. 1967–8.)
Steer P, Flenady V, Shearman A, *et al*. High dose caffeine citrate for extubation of preterm infants: a randomised controlled trial. *Arch Dis Child* 2004;**89**:F499–503. [RCT]

Use

Calcium gluconate can be given orally or IV to control symptomatic neonatal hypocalcaemia, but IM magnesium sulphate (q.v.) may be preferable in babies presenting 4–10 days after birth.

Pharmacology

Calcium increases myocardial contractility and ventricular excitability and is occasionally useful in adults with profound cardiovascular collapse. It can also be used to control cardiac hyperexcitability in severe neonatal hyperkalaemia (as outlined in the monograph on polystyrene sulphonate resins). Dietary supplementation during pregnancy has been shown to reduce the risk of maternal hypertension and pre-eclampsia in high-risk women. Calcium should not be used during cardiopulmonary resuscitation, and is not required for the mild transient hypocalcaemia caused by citrate administration during exchange transfusion.

Some degree of hypocalcaemia is common in the first 2 days of life with apathy and hypotonia, especially if there is intrapartum asphyxia or respiratory distress. Late hypocalcaemia on the other hand is usually associated with increased tone, jitteriness and multifocal seizures 4–10 days after birth in an otherwise well child. Seizures are usually associated with a serum calcium of less than 1·7 mmol/l and more specifically an ionised calcium of less than 0·64 mmol/l. Hypomagnesaemia is also often present (<0·68 mmol/l). Most such babies have a QTc of >0·2 seconds on their ECG.

There is no evidence that hypocalcaemia causes permanent neurological damage, and little evidence that an asymptomatic baby with transient hypocalcaemia requires any treatment. Calcium gluconate is probably the treatment of choice for early symptomatic hypocalcaemia, but extravasation can cause severe permanent tissue damage with IV administration, and has even made partial limb amputation necessary on occasion. Intramuscular magnesium sulphate may be preferable in the first line management of transient late neonatal hypocalcaemia. Calcium gluconate can also be given orally, but calcium glubionate and lactobionate (Calcium-Sandoz®) is a cheaper and more convenient formulation for sustained oral use. Phenobarbital (q.v.) is effective in controlling seizures but should not be allowed to mask symptoms in the rare baby in whom hypocalcaemia does not resolve within 48 hours. Look for evidence of parathyroid disturbance in mother and/or baby, or maternal vitamin D deficiency, if problems persist.

Correcting hypocalcaemia

Urgent IV correction: Correct serious hypocalcaemia by giving 2 ml/kg (0·46 mmol/kg) of 10% calcium gluconate slowly IV over 5–10 minutes if oral correction does not seem appropriate. This is more than the dose recommended in most British texts, but conforms to practice in North America. Watch for arrhythmia and extravasation, and avoid all intra-arterial and IM administration. A further 2·5 ml/kg can be given IV each day for the next 2–3 days, either as a continuous infusion or as four slow bolus doses, while investigations continue into the cause of any persisting abnormality if oral administration is not possible.

Rapid oral correction: Give 4 ml/kg of Calcium-Sandoz syrup (~2 mmol/kg of calcium) a day in divided doses. This more than doubles the calcium intake provided by most artificial infant milks.

Routine supplementation: Give 0·5 ml/kg of the Calcium-Sandoz syrup (~250 micromol/kg of calcium) four times a day.

Compatability

Do not add calcium to any solution containing bicarbonate, sulphate or phosphate, and do not let any IV fluid containing calcium come into even brief contact with any other IV administered drug. An insoluble salt precipitates out on contact with ceftriaxone, and the same may be true of some other drugs.

Tissue extravasation

A strategy for the early treatment of tissue extravasation due to IV administration is described in the monograph on hyaluronidase.

Supply

One 10 ml ampoule of 10% calcium gluconate contains 1 gram of calcium gluconate (or 89 mg of calcium) and costs 60p. 1 ml of this stock preparation, designed primarily for IV use, contains 0·22 mmol (0·46 mEq) of calcium. The product should not be used to supplement the calcium content of parenteral nutrition because of its high aluminium content. An oral syrup (Calcium-Sandoz) containing calcium glubionate and calcium lactobionate in sucrose (containing 22 mg (0·54 mmol) of calcium per ml) is available from the pharmacy on request (cost £1·10 for 100 ml). It is said that this product should be avoided in patients with galactosaemia, because the glubionate is metabolised to galactose.

References

See also relevant Cochrane reviews

Hofmeyr GJ, Duley L, Atallah A. Dietary calcium supplementation for prevention of pre-eclampsia and related problems: a systematic review. *Br J Obstet Gynecol* 2007;**114**:933–43. [SR]

Hsu SC, Levine MA. Perinatal calcium metabolism: physiology and pathophysiology. *Sem Neonatol* 2004;**9**:23–36.

Mimouni F, Tsang RC. Neonatal hypocalcaemia: to treat or not to treat ? [Review] *J Am Coll Nutr* 1994;**13**:408–15.

Porcelli PJ, Oh W. Effects of single dose calcium gluconate infusion in hypocalcaemic preterm infants. *J Perinatol* 1995;**12**:18–21.

Srinivasan V, Morris MC, Helfaer MA, *et al.* Calcium use during in-hospital pediatric cardiopulmonary resuscitation: a report from the national registry of cardiopulmonary resuscitation. *Pediatrics* 2008;**121**:e1144–51.

Use

Captopril is of value in the management of babies with congestive cardiac failure. It is also used to control hypertension in older children, but IV labetalol followed by oral nifedipine (q.v.) offers a more secure and reliable strategy for controlling serious hypertension in infancy. Captopril is also used to reduce proteinuria in nephrotic syndrome.

Blood pressure

The way systolic pressure normally varies with postmenstrual age in the first year of life is summarised in the monograph on hydralazine.

Pharmacology

A range of drugs used to treat heart failure and hypertension work by inhibiting the angiotensin-converting enzyme (ACE) responsible for converting angiotensin I to the potent vasoconstrictor angiotensin II. These drugs are contraindicated in renovascular disease, and are feto-toxic in pregnancy, but breastfeeding is not contraindicated since the baby only gets about 0·1% of the maternal dose (on a weight-for-weight basis). Hyperkalaemia is a hazard in patients on potassium-sparing diuretics (like spironolactone) or on potassium supplements. The half life of captopril is only 1–2 hours, but the clinical effect persists much longer than this, possibly because of reconversion of inactive metabolites back to active drug. The half life of enalaprilat is 1–2 days. Because the neonatal response to treatment with an ACE inhibitor is very variable, and some babies become profoundly hypotensive with even a small dose, it is essential first to give a small test dose and then increase the dose cautiously. This seems particularly true in babies under a month old. Reversible adverse effects (including apnoea, seizures and renal failure as well as severe unpredictable hypotension) have been unacceptably common when these drugs were used to control hypertension in the first few months of life. What is more worrying, such episodes have sometimes occurred unpredictably in small babies on maintenance treatment. ACE inhibitors can, however, be of help in infants with chronic congestive failure by decreasing the afterload on the heart, although babies with a left-to-right shunt seldom seem to benefit.

Treatment

Neonatal use: Start by giving 10 micrograms/kg of captopril by mouth once every 8 hours and monitor blood pressure carefully. The dose can then be increased progressively, as necessary, to no more than 100 micrograms/kg once every 8 hours.

Older children: Start by giving a 100 microgram/kg test dose and monitor blood pressure every 15 minutes for at least 2 hours. Start treatment by giving this dose once every 8 hours, and increase the dose cautiously to no more than 2 mg/kg per dose.

Use of enalapril

Enalapril maleate is an alternative oral prodrug which is hydrolysed in the liver to the even more potent ACE inhibitor enalaprilat (enalaprilat itself being available as an IV preparation in North America but not in the UK). The oral bioavailability of enalapril is ~60% in adults, but variably less than this in neonates. The neonatal response is *very* variable, as is the duration of action. As a result the starting dose in neonates should be 10 micrograms/kg once a day. A starting dose of 100 micrograms/kg is probably safe in older children, and oral doses as high as 1 mg/kg once a day are occasionally used later in the first year of life. The dose should be titrated up slowly as required, watching for possible signs of early renal failure. The drug's main advantage over captopril is the longer half life and the availability of an IV formulation. The manufacturers have not endorsed the use of this drug in children. Liver failure is a rare hazard.

Supply and administration

Captopril and enalapril both come in tablet form (and are only stable when so formulated). Various strengths are available, some costing as little as 5p each. The tablets dissolve easily in water, so a 25 mg tablet dissolved in 25 ml of tap water gives a 1 mg/ml sugar-free solution that is stable for 24 hours. A solution of captopril in fractionated coconut oil for oral use with a 3-month shelf life can also be obtained by the pharmacy from Cardinal Health Martindale Products in the UK on request. The North American IV preparation of enalaprilat contains benzyl alcohol.

References

Bult Y, van den Anker J. Hypertension in a preterm infant treated with enalapril. *J Pediatr Pharm Pract* 1997;**2**:229–31.

Gantenbein MH, Bauersfeld U, Baenziger O, *et al*. Side effects of angiotensin converting enzyme inhibitor (captopril) in newborns and young infants. *J Perinat Med* 2008;**36**:448–52.

Hanssens M, Keirse MJ, Vankelecom F, *et al*. Fetal and neonatal effects of treatment with angiotensin-converting enzyme inhibitors in pregnancy. *Obstet Gynecol* 1991;**78**:128–35. [SR]

Leversha AM, Wilson NJ, Clarkson PM, *et al*. Efficacy and dosage of enalapril in congenital and acquired heart disease. *Arch Dis Child* 1994;**70**:35–9.

Mulla H, Tofeig M, Bu'Lock F, *et al*. Variations in captopril formulations used to treat children with heart failure: a survey in the United Kingdom. *Arch Dis Child* 2007;**92**:409–11.

O'Dea RF, Mirkin BL, Alward CT, *et al*. Treatment of neonatal hypertension with captopril. *J Pediatr* 1988;**113**:403–6.

Perlman JM, Volpe JJ. Neurologic complications of captopril treatment of neonatal hypertension. *Pediatrics* 1989;**83**:47–52.

Tack ED, Perlman JM. Renal failure in sick hypertensive premature infants receiving captopril therapy. *J Pediatr* 1988;**112**:805–10.

Use

Carbamazepine has been in use for generalised tonic-clonic (grand mal) and partial (focal) epilepsy since 1963. It is a valuable first line drug in the sustained, long-term control of epilepsy in infancy and later childhood and has been used for benign infantile convulsions. It can only be given by mouth or per rectum.

Pharmacology

Carbamazepine is well but slowly absorbed from the digestive tract, and extensively metabolised in the liver before being excreted in the urine along with carbamazepine-10,11-epoxide (one of its primary active metabolites). Peak absorption is delayed when the drug is given as a tablet rather than as a liquid or chew-tab. The amount offered should also be increased 25% when the drug is given into the rectum because of incomplete absorption. Drug clearance is low at birth (half life 24 hours), but higher in infancy (3–15 hours) than in adult life. The volume of distribution in neonates is 1·5 l/kg.

Start by giving a low dose and increase this gradually. Use should probably be avoided in children with cardiac conduction defects, and caution is appropriate in children with a history of cardiac, hepatic or renal disease. Use frequently exacerbates myoclonic and absence seizures. Side effects are rare but include leucopenia, dystonia and hyponatraemia, and an overdose can cause drowsiness, respiratory depression and convulsions. Babies may also manifest vomiting, urinary retention, tachycardia and dilated pupils. One small study found carbamazepine useful in controlling the convulsions that occur in neonatal encephalopathy as long as a first introductory 10 mg/kg oral loading dose was given, and this regimen probably deserves further study.

Maternal use during pregnancy is associated with a slightly increased risk of microcephaly, and also spina bifida, and women are therefore advised to take a folic acid supplement (5 mg daily) prior to, and for 12 weeks after, conception. Serious malformation is otherwise uncommon and, although some mild dysmorphic features are often detectable, there is no evidence that exposure before birth has any impact on the child's later cognitive development. The baby may be hypoprothombopenic at birth, but this bleeding tendency is corrected by giving the baby at least 100 micrograms/kg (usually 1 mg) of IM vitamin K (q.v.) at birth. Small amounts of the drug appear in breast milk but maternal treatment is not a contraindication to breastfeeding because the baby will only receive 5% of the maternal dose when intake is calculated on a mg/kg basis.

Drug interactions

Concurrent treatment with erythromycin, isoniazid, lamotrigine or valproate (q.v.) causes a rise in the serum level of carbamazepine. The use of two anticonvulsants always increases the risk of drug toxicity.

Treatment

Experience is limited. Give 5 mg/kg every 12 hours. A larger dose may be necessary in babies over 2 weeks old (maximum intake 15 mg/kg every 12 hours), but larger doses should be introduced slowly. Where oral treatment is not possible a slightly larger dose of the oral suspension can be given into the rectum after dilution with an equal volume of water to minimise the laxative effect of the standard suspension's high osmolarity (a dose that can probably be repeated if the baby passes a stool within 2 hours of administration).

Blood levels

The optimum anticonvulsant plasma concentration is 4–12 mg/l (1 mg/l = 4·23 μmol/l). Levels can be measured in 50 μl of plasma (or about 150 μl of heparinised whole blood) from a sample taken shortly before treatment was due. It is, however, important to realise that the drug level in a young baby can take a week to stabilise. Levels above 30 mg/l cause severe toxicity.

Supply

A caramel-flavoured, sugar-free suspension containing 20 mg/ml of carbamazepine (and 25 mg/ml of propylene glycol) is available at a cost of £2·30 per 100 ml. 125 mg suppositories cost £2 each.

References

Gaily E, Kantola-Sorsa E, Hiilesmaa V, et al. Normal intelligence in children with prenatal exposure to carbamazepine. Neurology 2004;**62**:28–32.

Kini U, Adab N, Vinten J, et al. Dysmorphic features: an important clue to the diagnosis and severity of fetal anticonvulsant syndromes. Arch Dis Child 2006;**91**:F80–5.

Korinthenberg R, Haug C, Hannak D. The metabolism of carbamazepine to CBZ-10,11-epoxide in children from the newborn age to adolescence. Neuropediatrics 1994;**25**:214–16.

MacKintosh DA, Baird-Lampert J, Buchanan N. Is carbamazepine an alternative maintenance therapy for neonatal seizures? Dev Pharmacol Ther 1987;**10**:100–6.

Matsufuji H, Ichiyama T, Isumi H, et al. Low-dose carbamazepine therapy for benign infantile convulsions. Brain Dev 2005;**27**:554–7.

Miles ME, Lawless ST, Tennison MB, et al. Rapid loading of critically ill patients with carbamazepine suspension. Pediatrics 1990;**86**:263–6.

Morrow J, Russell A, Guthrie E, et al. Malformation risks of antiepileptic drugs in pregnancy: a prospective study from the UK Epilepsy and Pregnancy Register. J Neurol Neurosurg Psychiat 2006;**77**:193–8.

Morselli PL, Franco-Morselli R, Bossi L. Clinical pharmacokinetics in newborns and infants: age related differences and therapeutic implications. Clin Pharmacokinet 1980;**5**:485–527 (See particularly p. 507.)

Orney A, Cohen E. Outcome of children born to epileptic mothers treated with carbamazepine during pregnancy. Arch Dis Child 1996;**75**:517–20.

Singh B, Singh P, al Hifze I, et al. Treatment of neonatal seizures with carbamazepine. J Child Neurol 1996;**11**:378–82.

Veuvonen PJ, Tokola O. Bioavailability of rectally administered carbamazepine mixture. Br J Pharmacol 1987;**24**:839–40.

Use

Carglumic acid is primarily used to treat *N*-acetylglutamate synthase deficiency, a rare urea cycle disorder. It may also reduce ammonia concentrations in some neonates with branched chain organic acidaemias.

Biochemistry

N-acetylglutamate is the natural activator of carbamoyl phosphate synthetase (CPS I), which is the first step in the urea cycle. Patients with *N*-acetylglutamate synthase (NAGS) deficiency present with hyperammonaemia in the neonatal period or later in life. Carglumic acid (*N*-carbamoyl-ʟ-glutamic acid or *N*-carbamylglutamate), currently marketed under the trade name Carbaglu®, is a synthetic analogue of *N*-acetylglutamate, and it has been used since the early 1980s to control hyperammonaemia in patients with NAGS deficiency. After starting carglumic acid most patients with this disorder tolerate a normal protein intake when they are well, although other measures may be needed, particularly when they are ill. A few patients with partial CPS-I deficiency may also respond to carglumic acid.

In the branched-chain organic acidaemias (methylmalonic, propionic and isovaleric acidaemias) hyperammonaemia is thought to result, at least partly, from inhibition of NAGS, and carglumic acid does appear to reduce the ammonia concentration in some, but not all, children with one of these disorders.

Investigating neonatal hyperammonaemia

Plasma ammonia levels do not normally exceed 150 μmol/l and levels above 200 μmol/l strongly suggest the presence of an inborn error of metabolism. Further investigations should include analysis of plasma amino acids, urine organic acids and urine orotic acid. NAGS is a rare cause of hyperammonaemia; and is hard to distinguish from carbamoyl phosphate synthetase deficiency. A rapid response to carglumic acid strongly suggests the diagnosis: if the drug is available, it can be given whilst other forms of treatment are being set up.

Treatment

Trial of responsiveness: A trial dose of 200 mg/kg (oral or nasogastric) has been recommended in patients with hyperammonaemia, followed by monitoring of the plasma ammonia concentration every 2 hours; further doses may be given if there is a partial response. It is, however, important not to delay other treatment of hyperammonaemia, including haemodialysis and prompt treatment with sodium benzoate, sodium phenylbutyrate and arginine (q.v.).
Long-term management of NAGS deficiency: The total daily dose is usually between 10 and 100 mg/kg a day. It should be given in divided doses 2–4 times a day before food. During illness it may be helpful to double the dose; no intravenous preparation is available.

Monitoring

Plasma ammonia and amino acids should be monitored, as in other urea cycle disorders, aiming to keep the plasma ammonia concentration below 60 μmol/l and the plasma glutamine level below 800 μmol/l while maintaining a normal essential amino acid profile.

Supply and administration

Supplies of carglumic acid (Carbaglu) are available from Orphan Europe. This product was awarded EU marketing authorisation in 2003, and was also identified by the FDA in America for 'fast track' approval as an orphan drug in 2007. It is only licensed for use in NAGS deficiency. The product is currently only available in 200 mg tablet form and in packs of 5 or 60 tablets. The tablets currently cost £45 each.

References

Bachmann C, Colombo JP, Jaggi K. *N*-acetylglutamate synthetase (NAGS) deficiency: diagnosis, clinical observations and treatment. *Adv Exp Med Biol* 1982;**153**:39–45.
Guffon N, Schiff M, Cheillan D, *et al*. Neonatal hyperammonaemia: the *N*-carbamoyl-ʟ-glutamic acid test. *J Pediatr* 2005;**147**:260–2.
Kuchler G, Raboier D, Poggi-Travert F, *et al*. Therapeutic use of carbamylglutamate in the case of carbamoyl-phosphate synthetase deficiency. *J Inherit Metab Dis* 1996;**19**:220–2.
Leonard JV. Disorders of the urea cycle and related enzymes. In: Fernandes J, Saudubray J-M, van den Berghe G, *et al*., eds. *Inborn metabolic diseases. Diagnosis and treatment*, 4th edn. Berlin: Springer-Verlag, 2006: pp. 263–72.

Use
L-Carnitine is used in the management of a range of rare genetic conditions associated with carnitine deficiency.

Nutritional factors
Carnitine (3-hydroxy-4-*N*-trimethylaminobutyric acid) is a small, water-soluble molecule. It is essential for the entry of long-chain fatty acids into the mitochondria, where they are oxidised. Most of the body's carnitine is found in skeletal and cardiac muscle. Carnitine can be synthesised in the body from lysine and methionine, although synthetic pathways are relatively immature at birth, but most is usually provided by dietary red meat and dairy produce. Human milk and whey-based formula milks all contain L-carnitine, but soya-based preparations seldom do, making primary nutritional deficiency a possibility. Dialysis and defects of renal tubular reabsorption (Fanconi syndrome) can cause secondary dietary deficiency.

Pharmacology
Primary systemic carnitine transporter deficiency is an extremely rare condition resulting from a defect in the uptake of carnitine across cell membranes. It usually presents with hypoglycaemia, cardiomyopathy or myopathy, and is generally associated with a total plasma carnitine level of less than 10 μmol/l. It is diagnosed on the basis of carnitine uptake by fibroblasts *in vitro*.

Secondary systemic carnitine deficiency occurs in organic acidaemias and fatty oxidation defects. In these conditions carnitine binds to accumulating intermediate metabolites and is excreted with them in the urine. Organic acidaemias usually present with encephalopathy, often within a few days of birth. Fatty acid oxidation defects present in the neonatal period or later with hypoglycaemic encephalopathy, or with a cardiac or skeletal myopathy. All these conditions are recessively inherited and their management should, wherever possible, be guided by a consultant experienced in the management of metabolic disease.

Carnitine is of proven value in primary carnitine deficiency. Use also forms part of the standard strategy for managing organic acidaemias (such as isovaleric, methylmalonic and propionic acidaemias and glutaric aciduria type I). Its use in fatty acid oxidation defects is more controversial. Reports of supplementation in patients on dialysis, on valproate (q.v.) or with Fanconi syndrome have suggested only variable or equivocal benefit. Treatment should always be with the naturally occurring L isomer and not the racemic (DL) mixture. The main dose-related adverse effects of oral treatment are nausea, vomiting, abdominal cramp, diarrhoea and a fish-like smell. Treatment with carnitine may possibly increase the risk of arrythmias in fatty acid oxidation disorders. A number of controlled trials have failed to show that routine supplementation reduces apnoea, makes episodic hypoglycaemia less common, or improves growth, either in orally or in parenterally fed preterm babies. Women requiring carnitine supplementation should not stop treatment during pregnancy or lactation.

Treatment
Urgent IV treatment: Give 4 mg/kg per hour (0·2 ml per hour of the solution made up as described below) as a continuous IV infusion during acute metabolic decompensation. An initial loading dose is no longer generally considered necessary.
Oral treatment: The usual dose is 25 mg/kg four times a day by mouth.

Compatibility
While formal tests of compatibility do not seem to have been done, problems have not been encountered when carinitine is terminally co-infused with arginine, sodium benzoate and sodium phenylbutyrate.

Supply and administration
An oral preparation in sucrose, dispensed as a 30% paediatric solution (containing 300 mg/ml of L-carnitine), is available commercially costing £1·10 per ml. It can be mixed with a flavoured drink to make it more palatable. It contains sorbitol and sucrose. For IV use, 5 ml ampoules containing 1 gram of L-carnitine, costing £12 each, are obtainable on request; to give 100 mg/kg take 1 ml of this preparation for each kg that the baby weighs, dilute to 10 ml with 0·9% sodium chloride, and infuse 5 ml as described above. The product is stable at room temperature for 24 hours after reconstitution in this way.

References
See also the relevant Cochrane reviews

O'Donnell J, Finer NN, Rich W, *et al*. Role of L-carnitine in apnea of prematurity: a randomized controlled trial. *Pediatrics* 2002;**109**:622–6. [RCT]
Roe CR, Ding J. Mitochondrial fatty acid oxidation disorders. In: Scriver CR, Beaudet AL, Sly WS, *et al*., eds. *The metabolic and molecular bases of inherited disease*, 8th edn. New York: McGraw-Hill, 2001: pp. 2297–326.
Scaglia F, Longo N. Primary and secondary alterations of neonatal carnitine metabolism. *Sem Perinatol* 1999;**23**:152–61.
Stanley CA, Bennett MJ, Mayatepek E. Disorders of mitochondrial fatty acid oxidation and related metabolic pathways. In: Fernandes J, Saudubray J-M, van den Berghe G, *et al*., eds. *Inborn metabolic diseases. Diagnosis and treatment*, 4th edn. Berlin: Springer-Verlag, 2006: pp. 175–90.
Whitfield J, Smith T, Solluhub H, *et al*. Clinical effects of L-carnitine supplementation on apnea and growth in very low birth weight infants. *Pediatrics* 2003;**111**:477–82. [RCT]
Zelnik N, Isler N, Goez H, *et al*. Vigabatrin, lamotrigine, topiramate and serum carnitine levels. *Pediatr Neurol* 2008;**39**:18–21.

Use

Carob seed flour is being used to thicken the feed of term babies with troublesome gastroesophageal reflux. There is no good evidence, as yet, that this approach is of any value in the preterm baby.

Pharmacology

Carob seed flour is a galactomanan refined from the seed of the carob (or locust) bean tree, *Ceratonia siliqua*. The gum is widely used as a thickening agent and stabiliser in the food industry. The commercial products Carobel® and Nestargel® both contain calcium lactate, and Carobel also contains maltodextrin (giving the product a marginally higher energy content). It is probably wise to monitor the red cell galactose-1-phosphate level in babies with known galactosaemia when using these products. A minority of babies develop loose stools, but this is seldom a serious problem.

Rice- and maize-based products are also often used to thicken feeds. While there are theoretical grounds for thinking that the thickening quality of these starches may not be sustained quite as long once food enters the stomach because amylase enzymes in the saliva probably initiate partial digestion, no comparative studies have yet been attempted to test this possibility.

Possetting and reflux

One in two full-term babies 'posset' or spits up milk once or twice a day in the first few weeks of life, and nearly a fifth have been shown to bring material back up out of their stomach. Such symptoms seldom merit treatment unless the regurgitated acid is causing oesophagitis or the problem is interfering with growth although, in the preterm baby and the child with developmental delay, there is also a risk of aspiration pneumonia. Leaving a nasogastric tube in place between feeds doubles the incidence of reflux in the preterm baby. Many babies also bring up small amounts of milk when they 'burp' and bring air back that they swallowed while feeding, but any true vomiting that comes on for the first time in a child more than a few weeks old usually has a different explanation. Problems nearly always diminish spontaneously within a few weeks or months of birth, and mothers usually only bring term babies for review when problems persist several months. Active treatment is seldom called for, and may simply serve to initiate a chain of progressively more aggressive, but unnecessary, investigation and treatment. While a systematic review shows that feed thickening can sometimes help, there are no grounds for preferring one commercial product over any other. Some clinicians think that cow's milk allergy is commoner in such children – although which causes which is, as yet, unclear. A few children call for additional treatment as outlined in the monograph on Gaviscon®.

Treatment in the term baby

Bottle feeding: Thicken each 100 ml (~3 fluid ounces) of formula milk with approximately 1 gram of carob seed flour as outlined below depending on which product is used.

Breast feeding: Mix a thin paste using half a scoop of Nestargel or one scoop of Carobel and 25 ml of water or expressed milk, and give a small quantity to the baby before and during each feed; 3–6 teaspoons will generally suffice.

Supply and administration

Instant Carobel, marketed by Nutricia Clinical, comes in 135 gram boxes costing £2·60. The powder also contains maltodextrin (giving the product a calorie content of 2·5 kcal/g). Add 2 level (0·6 grams) scoops of powder to each 100 ml of hand-warm milk; shake well and leave to thicken for 3–4 minutes. Such a feed contains just under 1·2 grams per 100 ml of carob seed flour.

Nestargel, marketed by Nestlé, comes in 125 gram tins costing £2·60. It contains no metabolisable carbohydrate and a calorie content of only 0·4 kcal/g, but it does contain rather more calcium lactate than Carobel. To make a 1% thickened feed, add one scoop (1 gram) of powder to 100 ml of water, bring gently to the boil, and simmer gently for 1 minute. Cool and then mix in the powdered formula milk as usual.

Both these products can be prescribed on the NHS in the UK when treating troublesome reflux vomiting, as long as the prescription is marked with the initials 'ACBS' (meaning that the prescription complies with the advice issued by the Advisory Committee on Borderline Substances).

References

See also the relevant Cochrane reviews

Corvaglia L, Ferlini M, Rotatori R, *et al*. Starch thickening of human milk is ineffective in reducing the gastroesophageal reflux in preterm infants: a crossover study using intraluminal impedience. *J Pediatr* 2006;**148**:265–8. [RCT]

Horvath A, Dziechciarz P, Szajewska H. The effect of thickened-feed intervention on gastroesophageal reflux in infants: systematic review and meta-analysis of randomiized, controlled trials. *Pediatrics* 2008;**122**:e1268–77. [SR]

Khoshoo V, Edell D, Thompson A, *et al*. Are we overprescribing antireflux medications for infants with regurgitation? *Pediatrics* 2007;**120**:947–9.

Peter CS, Wiechers C, Bohnhorst B, *et al*. Influence of nasogastric tubes on gastroesophageal reflux in preterm infants: a multiple intraluminal impedence study. *J Pediatr* 2002;**141**:277–9.

Vandenplas Y, Salvatore S, Hauser B. The diagnosis and management of gastro-oesophageal reflux in infants. *Early Hum Dev* 2005;**81**:1011–24.

Wenzl TG, Schneider S, Scheels F, *et al*. Effects of thickened feeding on gastroesophageal reflux in infants: a placebo-controlled crossover study using intraluminal impedance. *Pediatrics* 2003;**111**:e355–9. [RCT]

Xinias L, Mouane N, Le Luyer B, *et al*. Cornstarch thickened formula reduces oesophageal acid exposure time in infants. *Dig Liver Dis* 2005;**37**:23–7. [RCT]

Use

Caspofungin is very expensive but it is often the antifungal drug of choice when systemic infection with a *Candida* organism proves resistant to treatment with fluconazole (q.v.), and when *Aspergillus* infection proves resistant to conventional management with high-dose amphotericin B (q.v.).

Pharmacology

Caspofungin is the first of a new class of antifungals (the echinocandins), first licensed for clinical use in 2001, that works by inhibiting the synthesis of β-(1,3)-D-glucan, an integral component of fungal cell walls. Caspofungin demonstrates good *in vitro* and *in vivo* activity against *Aspergillus* and a range of *Candida* species, including *C. albicans*, *C. prapsilosis*, *C. tropicalis* and *C. glabrata*, and in a controlled trial published in 2002 adults with invasive candidiasis responded to caspofungin better than they did to amphotericin. There were also fewer side effects. It is not effective in cryptococcal infection. There are, however, very few published reports as yet of this drug's use in very young children, and the manufacturer is not yet ready to recommend use in children less than 12 years old. The drug was found to be embryo-toxic and to interfere with fetal bone formation when given, in a standard dose, to pregnant rats and rabbits but nothing, understandably, is yet known about the effect of its use in women during pregnancy or lactation.

Caspofungin blood levels decline in a polyphasic manner, the brief α phase in adults being followed by a 9–11-hour β phase and a 40–50-hour γ phase as widespread tissue redistribution is followed by slow hydrolysis, acetylation and chemical degradation before the resultant metabolites are finally excreted in the urine and faeces. Little pharmacokinetic data in neonates has yet been published, but the volume of distribution in infancy would seem to be even higher than it is in adult life while the β phase half life is shorter, making a rather higher dose necessary.

Drug interactions

Patients taking any of the hepatic enzyme-inducing drugs, such as carbamazepine, dexamethasone, nelfinavir, nevirapine, phenytoin and rifampicin, probably need to be given a rather higher daily dose because of enhanced drug elimination.

Treatment

Relatively little is known about treatment in the first year of life. The most appropriate IV dose is probably 2 mg/kg once a day, given as a 1-hour infusion. Treatment was continued for 2–3 weeks in most reports published to date. The dose given does not normally need to be reduced in patients in renal failure, but it is probably not wise to continue giving high-dose treatment to patients showing signs of liver failure.

Supply and administration

Caspofungin comes as a powder ready for reconstitution in 50 mg vials that cost £330 each. Vials should be stored at 4°C, but brought to room temperature before the powder is dissolved using 10·5 ml of sterile 0·9% sodium chloride. For accurate low-dose administration further dilute the resultant solution to 25 ml with more 0·9% sodium chloride to obtain a solution containing 2 mg/ml of caspofungin, and use this within 24 hours. Caspofungin is incompatible with glucose, and has to be given into a line that only contains 0·9% sodium chloride or compound sodium lactate.

References

Belet N, Ciftçi E, Ince E, *et al*. Caspofungin treatment of two infants with persistent fungaemia due to *Candida lipolytica*, *Scand J Infect Dis* 2006;**38**:559–62.

Dodds AES, Lewis ES, Lewis LJS. Pharmacology of systematic antifungal agents. *Clin Infect Dis* 2006;**43**:S29–39.

Fisher BT, Zaoutis T. Caspofungin for the treatment of pediatric fungal infections. *Pediatr Infect Dis J* 2008;**27**:1099–101.

Franklin JA, McCormick J, Flynn PM. Retrospective study of the safety of caspofungin in immunocompromised pediatric patients. *Pediatr Infect Dis J* 2003;**22**:747–9.

Gamock-Jones KP, Keam SJ. Caspofungin: in pediatric patients with fungal infections. *Pediatr Drugs* 2009;**11**:259–69.

Manzar S, Kamat M, Pyati S. Caspofungin for refractory candidemia in neonates. *Pediatr Infect Dis J* 2006;**25**:282–3.

McCormack PL, Perry CM. Caspofungin: a review of its use in the treatment of fungal infection. *Drugs* 2005;**65**:2049–68.

Mora-Duarte J, Betts R, Rotstein C, *et al*. Comparison of caspofungin and amphotericin B for invasive candidiasis. *N Engl J Med* 2002;**247**:202–09. [RCT]

Natarajan G, Lulic BM, Rongkavilit C, *et al*. Experience with caspofungin in the treatment of persistent fungemia in neonates. *J Perinatol* 2005;**25**:770–7.

Odio CM, Araya R, Pinto LE, *et al*. Caspofungin therapy in neonates with invasive candidiasis. *Pediatr Infect Dis J* 2004;**23**:1093–7.

Rüping MJGT, Vehreschild JJ, Cornely OA. Patients at high risk of invasive fungal infections. When and how to treat. *Drugs* 2008;**68**:1941–61. [SR, in adult patients only]

Saez-Lorens X, Macias M, Maiya P, *et al*. Pharmacokinetics and safety of caspofungin in neonates and infants less than 3 months of age. *Antiomicrob Agents Chemother* 2009;**53**:869–75.

Smith PB, Steinbach WJ, Cotton CM, *et al*. Caspofungin for the treatment of azole resistant candidemia in a premature infant. *J Perinatol* 2007;**27**:127–9.

Steinbach WJ. Antifungal agents and children. *Pediatr Clin North Am* 2005;**52**:895–915.

Walsh TJ, Adamson PC, Seibel NL, *et al*. Pharmacokinetics, safety, and tolerability of caspofungin in children and adolescents. *Antimicrob Agents Chemother* 2005;**45**:4636–45.

Yalaz M, Akisu M, Hilmioglu S, *et al*. Successful caspofungin treatment of multi-drug resistant Candida parapsilosis septicaemia in an extremely low birth weight neonate. *Mycoses* 2006;**49**:242–5.

Zaoutis TE, Jafri HS, Huang L-M, *et al*. A prospective, multicenter study of caspofungin for the treatment of documented *Candida* or *Aspergillus* infections in pediatric patients. *Pediatrics* 2009;**123**:877–84.

CEFALEXIN = Cephalexin (USAN and former BAN)

Use

Cefalexin is one of the few cephalosporin antibiotics that can be given by mouth. It should only be used in the neonatal period when the sensitivity of the organism under treatment is known. Cefuroxime (q.v.) is a closely related antibiotic with slightly different sensitivities suitable for IV or IM use.

History

Stimulated by the discovery of penicillin, many other moulds were soon studied to see if they had antimicrobial properties. This soon led Brotzu to discover *Cephalosporium acremonium* in 1948 in a sewage outlet in Sardinia, extracts of which were soon shown to be active against a range of Gram-negative, as well as Gram-positive, bacteria. However it took 12 years of hard work before the team working with Florey in Oxford had a product (called cephalosporin C, because it had been isolated as a pure crystalline sodium salt) ready for clinical use. Its structure was similar to that of penicillin, but it was *not* destroyed by β-lactamase-producing bacteria. Plans to market cephalosporin C were thwarted when Beechams brought methicillin onto the market in 1960, but a wide range of semisynthetic analogues were developed over the next 20 years. Cefalexin was one of the first in 1967. Various 'second generation' products, including cefoxitin and cefuroxime with a wider spectrum of antibiotic activity, arrived 5 years later, and a third generation of very broad-spectrum cephalosporins, including cefotaxime, ceftazidime and ceftriaxone (q.v.), followed between 1976 and 1979.

Pharmacology

Cefalexin is a first generation cephalosporin which is reasonably active against nearly all Gram-positive cocci (including group B streptococci) and most Gram-negative cocci other than enterococci. Gram-positive rods are relatively resistant. While the drug is relatively resistant to staphylococcal β-lactamase, it has no useful activity against meticillin-resistant strains. It should not be used for infections in which *Haemophilus influenzae* is, or is likely to be, implicated, or used as an alternative to penicillin for syphilis. Although most *Bacteroides* species are susceptible to cefalexin, this is not true of *Bacteroides fragilis*. Cefalexin has no useful activity against *Listeria*, *Citrobacter* and *Enterobacter* or against *Serratia* and *Pseudomonas* species, and it only penetrates CSF poorly.

Cefalexin, unlike most cephalosporins, is acid resistant, and well absorbed when taken by mouth, although absorption is delayed and incomplete when the drug is taken on a full stomach. The dose recommended here takes this into account. Oral treatment usually only has a modest effect on the balance of other bacteria in the gut. Cefalexin is actively excreted by the kidney, the plasma half life falling from 5 hours at birth to about 2·5 hours at 4 weeks. Babies more than a year old clear cefuroxime from their plasma almost as fast as adults ($t^{1}/_{2}$ = 0·9 hours). Dosage intervals should be extended in babies with severe renal failure. Problems associated with treatment are uncommon but the same as for all cephalosporins, as discussed in the monograph on ceftazidime. Only modest amounts cross the placenta, and there is no evidence of teratogenicity. The baby ingests less than 1% of the weight-related maternal dose when the mother takes this drug while breastfeeding.

Treatment

Give 25 mg/kg by mouth once every 12 hours in the first week of life, every 8 hours in babies 1–3 weeks old, and every 6 hours in babies older than this. The dosage interval should be increased in babies with renal failure.

Supply

Cefalexin is available as a 25 mg/ml oral suspension. Reconstitute the granules or powder with water and use the resultant suspension within 10 days. 100 ml of the sugar-free, non-proprietary product costs £1·30. There are no parenteral formulations available.

References

Boothman R, Kerr MM, Marshall MJ, *et al*. Absorption and excretion of cephalexin in the newborn infant. *Arch Dis Child* 1973;**48**:147–50.

Creatsas G, Pavlatos M, Lolis D, *et al*. A study of the kinetics of cephalosporin and cephalexin in pregnancy. *Curr Med Res Opin* 1980;**7**:43–7.

Disney FA, Dillon H, Blumer JL, *et al*. Cephalexin and penicillin in the treatment of group A beta-haemolytic streptococcal sore throat. *Am J Dis Child* 1992;**146**:1324–9. [RCT]

Kefetzis D, Siafas C, Georgakopoulos P, *et al*. Passage of cephalosporins and amoxicillin into the breast milk. *Acta Paediatr Scand* 1981;**70**:285–8.

McCracken GH Jr, Ginsburg CM, Clahsen JC, *et al*. Pharmacologic evaluation of orally administered antibiotics in infants and children: effect of feeding on bioavailability. *Pediatrics* 1978;**62**:738–43.

Tetzlaff TR, McCracken GH Jr, Thomas, ML. Bioavailability of cephalexin in children: relationship to drug formulations and meals. *J Pediatr* 1978;**92**:292–4.

Use

Cefotaxime is a broad-spectrum cephalosporin largely reserved for use in the management of neonatal meningitis. It should not be used on its own if *Listeria* or *Psudomonas* infection is a possibility.

Pharmacology

Cefotaxime is a bactericidal antibiotic introduced into clinical use in 1976 with the same range of activity against Gram-positive organisms as most other third generation cephalosporins (cf. the monograph on cefoxitin), and exceptional activity against most Gram-negative organisms. Unfortunately it is not active against *Listeria monocytogenes*, enterococci or *Pseudomonas*. Tissue penetration is good and CSF penetration is usually more than adequate when there is meningeal inflammation. Maternal use presents no problem during pregnancy, and during lactation exposes the baby to considerably less than 1% of the weight-adjusted maternal dose. The neonatal half life (2–6 hours) varies with gestation and with postnatal age. The drug's primary metabolite, desacetylcefotaxime, which also displays antibiotic activity, has a neonatal half life twice as long as this. Most of the drug is renally excreted.

Cefotaxime is widely considered to be the antibiotic of choice in the management of most cases of Gram-negative neonatal meningitis at present although, for most infections, there is probably little to choose between cefotaxime and ceftazidime (q.v.). Ceftriaxone (q.v.) is sometimes used in this situation when there is no risk of jaundice because it only has to be given once a day. There is some limited evidence to suggest that the outcome in proven bacterial meningitis *may* be improved by the simultaneous early administration of dexamethasone (q.v.), although controlled trial evidence for this form of treatment is currently only available in respect of treatment for *Haemophilus influenza* meningitis in patients over 6 weeks old.

The neonatal use of the third generation cephalosporins such as cefotaxime and ceftazidime should probably be limited to the management of proven Gram-negative septicaemia and meningitis because several units have reported the emergence of resistant strains of *Enterobacter cloacae* when cefotaxime is used regularly in the first line management of possible neonatal sepsis (including coagulase-negative staphylococcal infection). The same potential exists with other organisms (such as *Serratia* and *Pseudomonas* species) where inducable β-lactamase production is a possibility.

Diagnosing meningitis

The signs of meningitis are seldom as clear cut in the neonatal period as they are in later childhood and (since babies with meningitis do not always have a positive blood culture) the organism may be missed if a lumbar puncture (LP) is not done when blood is obtained for culture. Even if it is delayed until the baby has been stabilised, an LP should still be done (and done within 2 hours of initiating antibiotic treatment to be sure of isolating the organism), since diagnosis will often influence decisions regarding treatment. Flex the hips and knees, but do not bend the neck to limit respiratory embarrassment. A Gram stain will usually reveal meningitis, but the cell count seen in normal babies overlaps with that seen in babies with early meningitis. The same is true of CSF protein and glucose levels. A combination of ampicillin and an aminoglycoside is widely used in early-onset meningitis of uncertain origin, but cefotaxime should replace ampicillin if Gram-negative organisms are seen (ceftazidime being more appropriate if pseudomonas infection is suspected). Meropenem should be held in reserve for use when a β-lactamase-resistent organism is suspected. Penicillin can replace ampicillin in group B streptococcal infection. Vancomycin should be reserved for proven staphylococcal infection. Viral culture should always be undertaken if no bacteria are seen. Confirm sterility with a second LP after 24–48 hours if the response is uncertain. Meningitis (whatever its cause) is a notifiable condition in the UK.

Treatment

Severe neonatal infection calls for treatment with 50 mg/kg slowly IV (or IM) once every 12 hours in the first week of life, every 8 hours in babies 1–3 weeks old, and once every 6 hours in babies older than this. The dosage interval should be increased in babies with severe renal failure. A single 100 mg/kg IV or IM dose can be used (instead of ceftriaxone) to treat neonatal gonococcal eye infection.

Supply

Stock 500 mg vials, which should be protected from light, cost £2·10. The dry powder should be reconstituted with 2·3 ml of water for injection to give a solution containing 200 mg/ml.

References

Clark RH, Bloom BT, Spitzer AR, *et al*. Empiric use of ampicillin and cafotaxime, compared to ampicillin and gentamicin, for neonates at risk for sepsis is associated with an increased risk of neonatal death. *Pediatrics* 2006;**117**:67–74.
de Man P, Verhoeven BAN, Verbrugh HA, *et al*. An antibiotic policy to prevent emergence of resistant bacilli. *Lancet* 2000;**355**:973–8.
Heath PT, Nik Yusoff NK, Baker CJ. Neonatal meningitis. [Review] *Arch Dis Child* 2003;**88**:F173–8. (See also pp. F179–84.)
Kafetzis DA, Brater DC, Kapiki AN, *et al*. Treatment of severe neonatal infections with cefotaxime: efficacy and pharmacokinetics. *J Pediatr* 1982;**100**:438–9.
Kearns GL, Jacobs RF, Thomas BR, *et al*. Cefotaxime and desacetylcefotaxime pharmacokinetics in very low birth weight neonates. *J Pediatr* 1989;**114**:461–7.

CEFOXITIN

Use
Cefoxitin sodium is a broad-spectrum second generation cephalosporin with enhanced activity against anaerobic bacteria, which is used prophylactically, like ampicillin (q.v.), in patients undergoing abdominal surgery and increasingly, on its own, in the routine postoperative care of children with a ruptured appendix.

Pharmacology
Cephalosporins are all *N*-acylated derivatives of 7-β-aminocephalosporanic acid with a β-lactam ring fused to a six-membered dihydrothiazine ring, first found amongst the fermentation products of *Cephalosporin acremonium*. A wide range of semisynthetic products have been produced since 1948. First generation products rapidly gave way to products with greater resistance to the β-lactamase enzymes that could be given parenterally. Most of these have now given way to third generation products with enhanced antibacterial activity, but some are still used for specialised purposes. Cefoxitin has retained its utility because of its ability to control anaerobic infection and its better than average activity against *Bacteroides fragilis*. Most Gram-positive cocci are moderately susceptible, but *Pseudomonas* species and *Listeria monocytogenes* are resistant, as are enterococci and *Enterobacter*. CSF penetration is poor and elimination rapid in urine, the neonatal half life (3–4 hours) being nearly four times as long as in adults. Problems associated with treatment are uncommon but largely the same as for all cephalosporins, as discussed in the monograph on ceftazidime. Use can be considered safe during pregnancy and lactation. There is no evidence of teratogenicity, and the baby ingests less than 1% of the weight-related dose if the mother takes the drug while breastfeeding (little of which would be absorbed anyway).

Caesarean delivery
Antibiotic prophylaxis can never be a substitute for good surgical technique and meticulous asepsis. Despite this, controlled trials have shown, quite unequivocally, that a policy of routine antibiotic prophylaxis is associated with a three-fold reduction in the risk of serious postoperative infection, localised wound infection and endometritis, as well as the much commoner risk of postoperative fever, in women undergoing Caesarean delivery. Furthermore the magnitude of the benefit seems as great for elective section as it is for section after the onset of labour. Analyses also show that, except in units with a quite exceptionally low postoperative infection rate, such a policy cuts costs. Yet despite the combined evidence provided by more than 90 controlled trials, and the parallel evidence from other trials of prophylaxis during abdominal surgery, the adoption of routine prophylaxis remains uncommon outside North America. The cephalosporins and broad-spectrum penicillins (usually ampicillin) seem to be equally effective. The use of an aminoglycoside or metronidazole as well as a broad-spectrum penicillin and the duration of prophylaxis both deserve further study. One day of prophylaxis (starting, if necessary, after the umbilical cord has been cut) provides substantial protection. Continued treatment for several days, or the routine use of two antibiotics, have been shown to further reduce the risk of perioperative infection, but this could have a detrimental effect on the bacterial ecology of the unit and increase the risk of infection from multiresistant organisms (an issue that has received far too little attention in studies to date).

Maternal prophylaxis
Mothers offered prophylaxis at Caesarean delivery usually receive four doses of 2 grams either IV or deep IM at 6-hour intervals. It is not unreasonable to delay the first dose until the umbilical cord has been clamped.

Neonatal treatment
Babies should be given 40 mg/kg IV once every 12 hours in the first week of life, once every 8 hours when 1–3 weeks old, and once every 6 hours in babies older than this. The dose interval should be doubled when renal function is seriously impaired.

Supply and administration
1 and 2 gram vials are on sale in Europe and North America (costing approximately £5 and £10 each), but no company is currently marketing this antibiotic in the UK. For IV administration dissolve the powder from a 1 gram vial with 9·5 ml of water for injection and shake well to give a solution containing 100 mg/ml. For IM administration the contents of the 1 gram vial should be dissolved with 2 ml of *plain* 1% lignocaine hydrochloride (noting that IM treatment is not recommended in small babies). When giving 2 grams IM to an adult it is best to give two separate 1 gram injections.

References
See also the Cochrane reviews of antibiotic prophylaxis for surgical delivery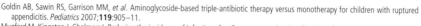

Goldin AB, Sawin RS, Garrison MM, *et al*. Aminoglycoside-based triple-antibiotic therapy versus monotherapy for children with ruptured appendicitis. *Pediatrics* 2007;**119**:905–11.

Mugford M, Kingston J, Chalmers I. Reducing the incidence of infection after Caesarean section: implications of prophylaxis with antibiotics for hospital resources. *BMJ* 1989;**299**:1003–6.

Regazzi MBG, Chirico G, Cristiani D, *et al*. Cefoxitin in newborn infants. *Eur J Clin Pharmacol* 1983;**25**:507–9.

Roos R, von Hattingberg HM, Belohradsky BH, *et al*. Pharmacokinetics of cefoxitin in premature und newborn infants studied by continuous serum level monitoring during combination therapy with penicillin and amikacin. *Infection* 1980;**8**:301–6.

Use

Ceftazidime is widely used in the management of Gram-negative (including *Pseudomonas aeruginosa*) infection, although cefotaxime (q.v.) is more often used for Gram-negative meningitis. However the frequent use of any third generation cephalosporin can rapidly lead to many babies becoming colonised by resistant organisms. It also increases the risk of invasive candidiasis in babies weighing less than 1 kg at birth.

Pharmacology

Ceftazidime is a valuable third generation bactericidal cephalosporin (cf. the monograph on cefoxitin) first patented in 1979. It is resistant to most β-lactamase enzymes and has good *in vitro* activity against a wide range of Gram-negative bacteria, including *P. aeruginosa*. It is reasonably active against group A and group B streptococci and against *Streptococcus pneumoniae*, but only has limited efficacy with most other Gram-positive organisms. Ceftazidime is not effective against enterococci, *Listeria, Helicobacter* or *Bacteroides fragilis*, and the widespread regular use of this (or any other) cephalosporin can result in an increasing proportion of babies becoming colonised with enterococci and with other potentially dangerous organisms. Generalised fungal infection is also a potential hazard. Ceftazidime should not, therefore, be used on its own in the management of neonatal infection due to an unidentified organism. Ceftazidime is widely distributed in most body tissues including respiratory secretions, ascitic fluid and cerebrospinal fluid (CSF), although CSF penetration is rather variable unless the meninges are inflamed. There is no clear evidence that aminoglycosides are synergistic.

Ceftazidime crosses the placenta freely, but there is no evidence of teratogenicity. Treatment during lactation is equally acceptable since this exposes the baby to less than 1% of the maternal dose on a weight-adjusted basis. The drug is not absorbed when taken by mouth and is excreted unchanged in the urine. The half life is 4–10 hours at birth, but half this in babies more than a week old. Adverse effects are not common with *any* of the cephalosporin antibiotics in the neonatal period, but hypersensitivity reactions are occasionally seen in older patients (sometimes overlapping with hypersensitivity to penicillin). Rashes, phlebitis and leucopenia have all been reported. Diarrhoea can progress to pseudomembranous colitis, due to an overgrowth of antibiotic-resistant bowel organisms, such as *Clostridium difficile* and, if this is not recognised and treated with metronidazole (q.v.), this could prove fatal. A very high blood level, usually because of a failure to reduce dose frequency when the patient is in renal failure, can cause CNS toxicity and fits (as is true of all the β-lactam antibiotics). Bleeding due to hypoproteinaemia (easily reversed by giving vitamin K) has been associated with the prolonged use of cephalosporins in malnourished patients. Ceftriaxone is, on theoretical grounds, the cephalosporin most likely to cause such a problem of all the products listed in this compendium.

Some 5% of patients given a cephalosporin develop a transient positive Coombs' test (and this can interfere with the cross-matching of blood), but frank haemolytic anaemia is extremely uncommon. Tests may wrongly suggest that there is glucose in the urine because of interference with the alkaline copper reduction test, and interference with the Jaffé reaction may affect the measurement of creatinine (giving a false high reading that can be particularly misleading when renal failure is a concern).

Treatment

Give 25 mg/kg of ceftazidime IV or deep IM once a day in the first week of life, once every 12 hours in babies 1–3 weeks old, and once every 8 hours in babies older than this. Doses of 50 mg/kg should be used in the treatment of suspected or proven meningitis. The dosage interval should be increased in babies with renal failure.

Supply and administration

Ceftazidime is supplied as a powder in 500 mg vials under reduced pressure costing £4·40 each. For IM administration add 1·6 ml of water to provide a solution containing 250 mg/ml. The bubbles of carbon dioxide will disappear after 1–2 minutes. Reconstitute for intravenous use with 4·6 ml of water for injection to produce a solution containing 100 mg/ml. Ceftazidime should not be put in the same syringe, or administered in a giving set at the same time, as vancomycin or an aminoglycoside.

References

Bégué P, Michel B, Chasalette JP, *et al*. Etude clinique multicentrique et pharmacocinétique de la ceftazidime chez l'enfant et le nouveau-né. *Pathol Biol* 1996;**34**:525–9.

Cotton CM, McDobald S, Stoll B, *et al*. The association of third-generation cephalosporin use and invasive candidiasis in extremely low birth-weight infants. *Pediatrics* 2006;**118**:717–22.

de Louvois J, Dagan R, Tessin I. A comparison of ceftazidime and aminoglycoside based regimens as empirical treatment of 1316 cases of suspected sepsis in the newborn. *Eur J Pediatr* 1991;**151**:876–84.

Tessin I, Trollfors B, Thringer K, *et al*. Concentrations of ceftazidime, tobaramycin and ampicillin in the cerbospinal fluid of newborn infants. *Eur J Pediatr* 1989;**148**:678–81.

van den Anker JN, Hop WCJ, Schoemaker RC, *et al*. Ceftazidime pharmacokinetics in preterm infants: effect of postnatal age and postnatal exposure to indomethacin. *Br J Clin Pharmacol* 1995;**40**:439–43.

van den Anker JN, Schoemaker RC, Hop WCJ, *et al*. Ceftazidime pharmacokinetics in preterm infants: effects of renal function and gestational age. *Clin Pharmacol Ther* 1995;**58**:650–9.

CEFTRIAXONE

Use

Ceftriaxone is a versatile and useful cephalosporin antibiotic that only needs to be given once a day. It should only be given with great caution to any child with a high unconjugated bilirubin level.

Pharmacology

Ceftriaxone is a β-lactamase-resistant 'third generation' cephalosporin first patented in 1979 that is active, like cefotaxime and ceftazidime (q.v.), against some important Gram-positive and most Gram-negative bacteria. Because of good CSF penetration, even when the meninges are not inflamed, it is now often used as a simpler alternative to cefotaxime in the treatment of early meningitis due to organisms other than *Listeria monocytogenes* and faecal streptococci (enterococci). It is also used to treat *Salmonella typhi* infection in countries where this organism is becoming resistant to chloramphenicol (q.v.), and to treat gonorrhoea (*Neisseria gonorrhoea* infection). The drug is excreted unaltered almost equally in bile and urine, so treatment does not normally require adjustment unless there is both renal and hepatic failure. It has a longer half life than other cephalosporins, the plasma half life falling from 15 hours at birth to a value only a little in excess of that found in adults (7 hours) over some 2–4 weeks. It crosses the placenta and also appears in amniotic fluid. There is no evidence of teratogenicity in animals, but only limited information regarding its safety during human pregnancy. Very little appears in breast milk: the baby of any mother treated during lactation would be exposed to less than 1% of the maternal dose on a weight-adjusted basis, and little of this would be absorbed.

Ceftriaxone displaces bilirubin from its plasma albumin-binding sites, thereby increasing the amount of free, unconjugated bilirubin. This initially made many clinicians reluctant to recommend its use in babies less than 6 weeks old, and the drug should only be used in babies at risk of developing unconjugated hyperbilirubinaemia if a lower than usual threshold is adopted for starting phototherapy (q.v.). High doses often cause a transient precipitate to form in the biliary tract, and small asymptomatic renal stones occasionally form with sustained use. Ceftriaxone has very occasionally caused severe neonatal erythroderma ('red baby' syndrome). Severe, potentially lethal, haemolysis is another very rare complication. Other problems are very uncommon but the same as for all cephalosporins, as discussed in the monograph on ceftazidime.

Gonorrhoea

The incidence of this sexually transmitted disease, which can cause vaginal discharge, dysuria and heavy or intermenstrual bleeding, varies greatly in different parts of the world, and a single 250 mg IM dose of ceftriaxone is now widely used to treat maternal infection. If it is not possible to test for possible co-infection with *Chlamydia* it may be appropriate to give a single 1 gram dose of azithromycin (q.v.) as well by mouth. There is also a high risk of reinfection unless sexual partners are also seen and treated. Babies run a 30–50% risk of becoming infected at birth, and a 4% chance of developing serious eye infection in the absence of prompt prophylaxis (as outlined in the monograph on eye drops). The presence of intracellular Gram-negative diplococci on a conjunctival Gram stain is virtually diagnostic. The eyes become increasingly purulent and inflamed, and sight can be put at risk if treatment is not started promptly. Untreated discharge from the eye can also cause cross infection. Generalised septicaemia can occur, and this can cause a destructive septic arthritis if early signs are not sought with diligence. Neonatal ophthalmia is a notifiable disease in the UK.

Drug interactions

Never give ceftriaxone IV to any child who is being or has recently been given any IV fluid (such as TPN or Ringer lactate) that contains calcium – precipitation could be potentially lethal. Use cefotaxime instead.

Treatment

Neonatal gonococcal eye infection: A single 125 mg IM dose was shown to be a simple and very effective treatment strategy in one African trial (use 40 mg/kg in any low birthweight baby). Consider giving oral azithromycin or erythromycin (q.v.) as well if there is a possibility of chlamydial co-infection.

Other sepsis: Give 50 mg/kg IM or, preferably, IV once a day for 7 days. Use with great caution in young babies with unconjugated jaundice. Use a 75 mg/kg dose for meningitis in babies over 4 weeks old.

Supply and administration

250 mg vials cost £2·70. They contain 0·9 mmol of sodium. Dissolve the powder in this vial in 4·8 ml of water for injection to obtain a 50 mg/ml solution for IV administration. It is only necessary to give this slowly over an hour if the baby has a relatively high unconjugated bilirubin level. To make IM (but *not* IV) injection less painful dissolve the 250 mg of powder with 0·9 ml of plain 1% lidocaine hydrochloride to make a 250 mg/ml solution.

References

See also the Cochrane review of gonococcal infection in pregnancy

Duke T, Michael A, Mokela D, *et al*. Chloramphenicol or ceftriaxone, or both, as treatment for meningitis in developing countries? *Arch Dis Child* 2003;**88**:536–9.

Laga M, Naamara W, Brunham RC, *et al*. Single-dose therapy of gonococcal ophthalmia neonatorum with ceftriaxone. *N Engl J Med* 1986;**315**:1382–5. [RCT]

Lamb HM, Ormrod D, Scott LJ, *et al*. Ceftriaxone. *Drugs* 2002;**62**:1041–89. [SR]

Moran J. Gonorrhoea. *BMJ clinical evidence handbook*. London: BMJ Books, 2009: pp. 519–20 (and updates). [SR]

Nathan N, Borel T, Djibo A, *et al*. Ceftriaxone as effective as long-acting chloramphenicol in short-course treatment of meningococcal meningitis during epidemics: a randomised non-inferiority study. *Lancet* 2005;**366**:308–13. [RCT]

Use

This non-toxic, broad-spectrum antibiotic was quite widely used for some years in the prophylactic management of babies considered to be at increased risk of intrapartum infection.

Pharmacology

Cefuroxime is a β-lactamase-resistant second generation cephalosporin first patented in 1973, which is active against most Gram-positive organisms (including group B streptococci and penicillin-resistant staphylococci) and a wide range of Gram-negative organisms. It is reasonably active against *Haemophilus influenzae* and *Neisseria gonorrheae*, but inactive against *Listeria*, enterococci and *Bacteroides* and *Pseudomonas* species. It only penetrates the CSF poorly, but has sometimes been used prophylactically, like cefoxitin (q.v.), in neonates undergoing abdominal surgery. Coagulase-negative staphylococci are increasingly resistant to this antibiotic. It was once advocated for use (on its own) in asymptomatic babies at birth who were thought to be at risk as a result of prolonged rupture of membranes, maternal pyrexia or meconium aspiration because of its broad spectrum and low potential toxicity for some years. However, controlled trial evidence to support this strategy does not yet exist, and such use has declined in recent years. While prophylactic treatment is certainly simplified by using a single broad-spectrum antibiotic administered once or twice a day, there are very few situations in which prophylactic treatment has ever been shown to be of clinical value in the neonatal period.

Cefuroxime itself is ineffective when given by mouth (less than 1% is recovered in the urine), but about a third of the administered dose is absorbed when the drug is given as the lipophilic acetoxyethyl ester, cefuroxime axetil. There are no published reports of the use of this formulation in children less than 3 months old, but it has been widely used to treat otitis media and other respiratory infections in children older than this. It is just as effective as treatment with co-amoxiclav, and less likely to cause troublesome loose stools. Alternative oral cephalosporins include cefalexin (q.v.), and cefixime.

Cefuroxime is largely excreted by the kidney. Little crosses the placenta and only negligible amounts are found in breast milk. On a weight-for-weight basis the baby will be exposed to less than 1% of the maternal dose. The plasma half life falls from 6 hours at birth to about 3 hours at 2 weeks. Babies more than a month old clear cefuroxime from their plasma almost as fast as adults (half life 1 hour), but dosage intervals should be extended in babies with severe renal failure. Toxic adverse effects are rare but oral treatment does sometimes cause nausea and vomiting and a change in stool frequency, and pseudomembranous colitis has occasionally been reported. Other problems are uncommon but much the same as for all cephalosporins (as discussed in the monograph on ceftazidime).

Lyme disease

Lyme disease, like syphilis, is caused by a spirochete (*Borrelia burgdorferi*) – human infection being caused by the bite of an infected animal tick. Illness is rare in the UK, but not uncommon in much of Europe and North America. While a migrating annular skin lesion (erythema migrans) is the classic presentation, symptoms are very variable. Fetal infection was first recognised in 1985, and it is now realised that the risk to the fetus is comparable to that from congenital syphilis. While tetracycline (or doxycline) is generally considered the treatment of choice, sustained high-dose treatment with cefotaxime is generally preferred in pregnancy and childhood. Mothers should be given 2 grams of cefotaxime IV three times a day for 2–4 weeks, and babies treated as indicated below for 2–4 weeks.

Treatment

Systemic: Give 25 mg/kg IM or IV once every 12 hours in the first week of life, every 8 hours in babies 1–3 weeks old, and every 6 hours in babies older than this. Double this dose when treating Lyme disease in a baby less than 4 weeks old. The dosage interval needs to be increased if there is serious renal failure.

Oral: Give 15 mg/kg of cefuroxime axetil by mouth once every 12 hours for severe infection. There is no experience of use in babies under 3 months old.

Supply

250 mg vials of the dry powder (costing 94p) should be reconstituted by adding 2·4 ml of sterile water to the vial to get a solution containing 100 mg/ml. A 25 mg/ml suspension of cefuroxime axetil containing sucrose is available as a powder for oral use after reconstitution with water; 100 ml costs £7·70.

References

Donn KH, James NC, Powell JR. Bioavailablity of cefuroxime axetil formulations. *J Pharm Sci* 1994;**83**:842–4.

Eppes SC, Childs JA. Comparative study of cefuroxime axetil versus amoxicillin in children with early Lyme disease. *Pediatrics* 2002;**109**:1173–9. [RCT]

Gardner T. Lyme disease. In: Remington JS, Klein JO, eds. *Infectious diseases of the fetus and newborn infant*, 5th edn. Philadelphia: WB Saunders, 2001: pp. 519–641.

Gooch WM, Blair E, Puopolo A, *et al*. Effectiveness of five days of therapy with cefuroxime axetil suspension for treatment of acute otitis media. *Pediatr Infect Dis J* 1996;**15**:157–64. [RCT]

Smith J, Finn A. Antimicrobial prophylaxis. [Commentary] *Arch Dis Child* 1999;**80**:388–92.

Stanek G, Strle F. Lyme borreliosis. [Seminar] *Lancet* 2003;**362**:1639–47. (See also 2004;**363**:901.)

CHLORAL HYDRATE

Use

Chloral hydrate has been widely used as a short-term sedative and hypnotic drug for more than a century. It is of no use in controlling pain. The web commentary reviews strategies for safe use in the first year of life.

Pharmacology

Chloral hydrate was synthesised in 1832 and first used as a hypnotic in 1869. Its chemical resemblance to chloroform led early workers to believe that it might work by liberating chloroform in the blood stream. It is rapidly and effectively absorbed from the stomach and then metabolised by liver enzymes to trichloroacetic acid and the active hypnotic meta-bolite trichloroethanol (TCE). Further conjugation results in the drug's eventual excretion in the urine as a glucuronide. The half life of TCE shows troubling variability, and is at least three times as long in early infancy (10–50 hours) as it is in toddlers and in adult life. It is even longer in the preterm baby, and in babies with hepatic or renal disease, making drug accumulation a potential hazard with repeated administration. Hypotension and respiratory depression have been described, and even a low dose may increase the frequency of brief, self-correcting bradycardia. Long-term use has also, on occasion, been thought to cause jaundice and an increased metabolic acidosis in the neonate. The main adverse effects of oral administration (nausea, vomiting and gastric irritation) can be minimised by giving the drug with a small amount of milk or fruit juice, and this also serves to disguise the drug's unpleasant taste. An overdose can cause coma and a potentially dangerous arrhythmia, probably best controlled using propranolol (q.v.).

Triclofos sodium, which causes less gastric irritation, has the same hypnotic and sedative action as chloral hydrate. Like chloral hydrate it is also rapidly hydrolysed to TCE; 75 mg of triclofos is therapeutically equivalent to 45 mg of chloral hydrate. Neither drug has been recommended by the manufacturers for use in children under 2 years.

Adult insomnia

Chloral hydrate is a good short-term nocturnal sedative for adult patients who find it difficult to sleep while in hospital, and it seems less potentially addictive than the widely used short-acting benzodiazepine temazepam. The usual adult dose of chloral hydrate is 1 gram given well diluted with water, and the usual dose of temazepam is 20 mg. Long-term use is strongly discouraged. Both drugs appear in human milk but published studies show that the breastfed baby only ingests about 5% of the weight-related maternal dose. Chloral hydrate does not seem to be teratogenic, but there is some concern that sustained benzodiazepine use could be.

Infant sedation

Single-dose treatment: A 45 mg/kg oral dose of chloral hydrate usually produces about 1 hour's deep sleep after about 45 minutes. In term babies a 75 mg/kg dose is occasionally used prior to CT scanning, etc., but such babies should be monitored because this dose can produce mild hypoxaemia. Rectal administration is sometimes used. A single 100 mg/kg dose is probably safe in infants more than a month old, but only if a pulse oximeter is employed and the child is kept under close surveillance. Staff must also be aware that it can take a **very** variable time for the sedative effect to wear off.

Sustained sedation: A 30 mg/kg oral dose of chloral hydrate given once every 6 hours for 1–2 days has been used as an alternative to 400 micrograms/kg of diazepam once every 6 hours in the management of babies with cerebral irritation. It has also been used in some centres to sedate babies requiring respiratory support, but drug accumulation is known to occur variably with repeated use in ill and preterm babies.

Antidote

Flumazenil (as described in the monograph on midazolam) may be of some value in the management of an overdose, but propranolol may be needed to control any arrhythmia.

Supply

An oral elixir of chloral hydrate in glucose (Welldorm®) containing just under 30 mg/ml (143 mg per 5 ml) is available costing less than 5p/ml. Stocks may be stored at room temperature (5–25°C). 25, 50, 100 and 200 mg suppositories of chloral hydrate can be obtained from Novo on request.

A solution of triclofos in syrup (costing £9·40 for 100 ml) is available containing 100 mg/ml. It should be used within 7 days if further diluted. Midwives in the UK have the little known right to supply chloral hydrate and triclofos to women on their own authority in the course of their professional practise.

References

See also the UK guideline on the safe care of any sedated child

Allegaert K, Daniels H, Naulaers G, et al. Pharmacodynamics of chloral hydrate in former preterm infants. Eur J Pediatr 2005;**164**:403–7.

American Academy of Pediatrics Committee on Drugs and Committee on Environmental Health. Use of chloral hydrate for sedation in children. Pediatrics 1993;**92**:471–3.

Donovan KL, Fisher DJ. Reversal of chloral hydrate overdose with flumazenil. BMJ 1989;**298**:1253.

Jacqz-Aigrain E, Burtin P. Clinical pharmacokinetics of sedatives in neonates. Clin Pharmacokinet 1996;**31**:423–43.

Mason KP, Sanborn P, Zurakowski D, et al. Superiority of pentobarbital versus chloral hydrate for sedation in infants during imaging. Radiology 2004;**230**:537–42.

Napoli KL, Ingrall CG, Martin GR. Safety and efficacy of chloral hydrate sedation in children undergoing echocardiography. J Pediatr 1996;**129**:287–91.

Pershad J, Palmisano P, Nichols M. Chloral hydrate: the good and the bad. Pediatr Emerg Care. 1999;**15**:432–5.

Sury MRJ, Hatch DJ, Deeley T, et al. Development of a nurse-led sedation service for paediatric magnetic resonance imaging. Lancet 1999;**353**:1667–71.

Use

Chloramphenicol is used for *Salmonella* infection (the cause of notifiable typhoid and paratyphoid fever) and occasionally used to control meningitis and ventriculitis (because of good CSF penetration). It is also used for sepsis and pneumonia in countries because oral absorption is good and most alternatives remain expensive.

History

Chloramphenicol came into widespread neonatal use soon after it first became available in 1949. Then, early in 1959, came a report describing three babies who suffered a 'fatal cardiovascular collapse' (so-called gray baby syndrome). It was not, however, until the result of a prospective controlled trial was published in December of that year that the potential toxicity of treatment with 100–150 mg/kg per day (the dose then normally recommended) was generally accepted. Coming only 4 years after it was realised that sulphonamides could cause kernicterus and death in the jaundiced preterm baby (as described in the monograph on sulfadiazine), neonatologists had to accept that two widely used drugs had both killed many hundreds of babies over a 10-year period. That most had only been given antibiotics to *prevent* infection only added to the anguish. The drug's potential toxicity seems to be a lesson that each new generation of clinicians has to learn afresh, because more deaths from dosing errors were reported in 1983.

Pharmacology

Chloramphenicol kills *Haemophilus influenzae*, and *Neisseria* spp., and stops the growth of rickettsiae and most bacteria. It penetrates all body tissues well: the CSF concentration averages 60% of the serum level, while brain levels are said to be nine times higher because of high lipid solubility. Despite this, cefotaxime (q.v.) has now become the drug of choice in the management of suspected or proven Gram-negative meningitis (partly because 2–5% of all strains of *H. influenzae* are now resistant to chloramphenicol). The parenteral drug (chloramphenicol succinate) only becomes biologically active after hydrolysis and, because this can be delayed in the neonate, levels of the active antibiotic can be *very* unpredictable. The oral drug (chloramphenicol palmitate) also requires prior hydrolysis by pancreatic enzymes, which makes it unwise to give the drug by mouth when first starting treatment in early infancy. Much of the inactive ester is excreted by the renal tubules (especially in children), and most of the active drug is first metabolised to the inactive glucuronide, so the dose does not usually need to be modified when there is renal failure. Excretion and metabolic inactivation are, however, influenced by postnatal age. The half life decreases from a mean of 27 hours in the first week of life to 8 hours by 2–4 weeks, and 4 hours in children over 4 months old. Maternal treatment does not seem to pose a hazard to the baby at any stage of pregnancy as some texts claim, and it only exposes the baby to about 5% of the weight-related maternal dose during lactation, so the only reason to discourage breastfeeding is the small (~1:40,000) risk that this could trigger aplastic anaemia – a consideration that applies to the mother at least as much as it does to the baby. There are a few reports of haemolysis in patients with G6PD deficiency.

Drug interactions

Co-treatment with phenobarbital or rifampicin tends to lower the plasma chloramphenicol level. The effect of phenytoin is more variable, but chloramphenicol can slow the elimination of phenytoin.

Treatment

Neonatal treatment: Give a loading dose of 20 mg/kg IV and then 12 mg/kg orally or IV once every 12 hours in babies less than a week old. Babies 1–4 weeks old should have further doses every 8 hours in the absence of renal failure or liver damage. *Check the dose given carefully: an overdose can be fatal*.
Older children: Children over 4 weeks old can usually be started on 25 mg/kg every 8 hours. The first doses should be given IV or IM in any child who is ill, but further treatment can then be given by mouth.
Eye drops: See the eye drop monograph.

Blood levels

Levels should be monitored where facilities exist when this drug is used in babies less than 4 weeks old. Aim for a peak serum concentration of 15–25 mg/l (1 mg/l = 3·1 μmol/l). Levels over 35 mg/l may cause transient marrow suppression. Levels over 50 mg/l can cause cardiovascular collapse.

Supply

1 gram vials of chloramphenicol succinate cost £1·40. Add 9·2 ml of water to give a solution containing 10 mg in 0·1 ml. No oral suspension of the palmitate salt is now commercially available in the UK, but a sugar-free suspension with a 4-week shelf life can be provided on request.

References

Duke T, Poka H, Dale F, *et al*. Chloramphenicol versus benzylpenicillin and gentamicin for the treatment of severe pneumonia in children in Papua New Guinea: a randomized trial. *Lancet* 2002;**359**:474–80. [RCT]
Mulhall A, de Louvois J, Hurley R. Chloramphenicol toxicity in neonates: its incidence and prevention. *BMJ* 1983;**2**:1424–7.
Rojchgot P, Prober CG, Soldin S, *et al*. Initiation of chloramphenicol therapy in the newborn infant. *J Pediatr* 1982;**101**:1018–21.
Smith AL, Weber A. Pharmacology of chloramphenicol. *Pediatr Clin North Am* 1983;**30**:209–36.
Weber MW, Gatchalian SR, Ogunlesi O, *et al*. Chloramphenicol pharmacokinetics in infants less than three months of age in the Philippines and The Gambia. *Pediatr Infect Dis J* 1999;**18**:896–901.

CHLOROQUINE

Use
Chloroquine was, for a long time, the world's most widely used antimalarial drug, but the most common and virulent parasite, *Plasmodium falciparum*, is now becoming very resistant to this drug. Chloroquine can still be used, however, when *P. ovale,* and *P. malariae* infection needs treatment, and *P. vivax* is also usually still sensitive.

Pharmacology
Chloroquine (a 4-aminoquinoline developed during World War II) is well absorbed, widely distributed in body tissues, slowly metabolised by the liver, and only very slowly cleared from the body. There is no evidence that standard dose treatment during pregnancy is hazardous and good evidence that weekly prophylaxis is not just safe, but also advisable where disease is endemic. Use during lactation exposes the baby to less than 5% of the weight-adjusted maternal dose, which is probably not enough to protect the baby from infection.

Malaria
Malaria, caused by four closely related parasites spread by the bite of the night-feeding female *Anopheles* mosquito, currently kills 2 million people in the tropics each year – most of them children. Residents develop considerable immunity over time, but pregnancy makes women more vulnerable, and infection during pregnancy increases the risk of anaemia, miscarriage, stillbirth and prematurity. Transplacental spread is uncommon but infection sometimes occurs during delivery, although florid symptoms (including fever, jaundice, an enlarged liver and spleen and low platelet count) usually only manifest themselves 2–8 weeks later. Diagnosis of infection, however acquired, depends on recognising the intracellular parasite in a thick smear of stained blood on a microscope slide. Infection is considered severe if there is shock, acidosis, hypoglycaemia or cerebral symptoms, or more than 5% of red cells are involved. In *P. vivax* and *P. ovale* infections, treatment with chloroquine can leave some organisms dormant in the liver unless primaquine is given as well (see below). There are a few areas where even *P. vivax* has now become resistant to chloroquine, and here it can still be appropriate to treat overt infection with mefloquine (15 mg/kg by mouth followed, after 12 hours, by a second 10 mg/kg dose) or artemether (q.v.) where this is available.

Drug resistance
Chloroquine prophylaxis is still appropriate in the Middle East and Central America. WHO advice on travel, and the prevalence of drug-resistant organisms across the world, can be found on www.who.int/ith. Similar advice can also be found in the *British national formulary* and the related children's formulary (BNFC). Go to http://www.cdc.gov/malaria/ for up-to-date advice from the CDC in America.

Prophylaxis
See the monograph on proguanil with atovaquone for a discussion of prevention and prophylaxis.

Treatment
Prevention in visitors: Offer children 5 mg/kg of chloroquine *base* by mouth once a week in areas where sensitive parasites are endemic. Start 1 week before entering the area and stop 4 weeks after leaving. Consider giving proguanil (q.v.) as well.
Cure: Give a 10 mg/kg loading dose of chloroquine *base* IV or by mouth, and then three 5 mg/kg doses (given at 24-hour intervals) starting 6 hours after the loading dose was given. In *P. vivax* or *P. ovale* infections there may be a case for giving primaquine after this to eliminate any dormant liver parasites.

Eradicating liver organisms
Giving 300 micrograms/kg of primaquine once a day by mouth for 2 weeks will usually kill residual organisms. A higher dose may occasionally be necessary but increases the risk of haemolysis in those with the Mediterranean and Asian variants of G6PD deficiency. Use in young children has not been well studied.

Toxicity
Excess chloroquine is toxic to the heart and the CNS. Prompt high-dose diazepam (2 mg/kg daily) and ventilation seem beneficial. Gastric lavage may be appropriate once the airway has been protected, and activated charcoal may reduce gut absorption. IV adrenaline helps control hypotension. Correct any acidosis. Phenytoin or a β blocker can be used to treat arrhythmia. Dialysis is not helpful.

Supply
Chloroquine base: A 10 mg/ml syrup is available; 75 ml costs £3·40.
Primaquine base: 7·5 and 15 mg tablets cost about 70p each. A 3 mg/ml suspension can be prepared that retains its potency for at least a week if stored at 4°C.

References
See also the relevant Cochrane reviews

Hill DR, Baird JK, Parise ME, *et al*. Primaquine: report from the CDC expert meeting on malaria chemoprophylaxis I. *Am J Trop Med Hyg* 2006;**75**:402–15.
Laufer MK, Thesing PC, Eddington ND, *et al*. Return of chloroquine efficacy in Malawi. *N Engl J Med* 2006;**355**:1959–66. [RCT] (See also pp. 1956–7.)
Leslie T, Mayan MI, Hasan MA, *et al*. Sulfadoxine-pyrimethamine, chlorproguanil-dapsone, or chloroquine for the treatment of *Plasmodium vivax* malaria in Afghanistan and Pakistan: a randomized controlled trial *JAMA* 2007;**297**:2201–19. [RCT]
Obua C, Hellgren U, Ntale M, *et al*. Population pharmacokinetics of chloroquine and sulfadoxine and treatment response in children with malaria: suggestions for an improved dose regimen. *Br J Clin Pharmacol* 2008;**65**:493–501.
Wolfe MS, Cordero JF. Safety of chloroquine in chemosuppression of malaria during pregnancy. *BMJ* 1985;**290**:1466–7.

Use

Chlorothiazide is a thiazide diuretic used to control the pulmonary oedema seen in preterm babies with chronic ventilator-induced lung disease. It is also used in the control of fluid retention in congestive heart failure, preferably in combination with spironolactone (q.v.). Furosemide (q.v.) is a useful short-term alternative in both conditions where oral treatment is not possible or a rapid response is required.

Pharmacology

Chlorothiazide is a diuretic that was first developed commercially in 1957. It crosses the placenta but shows no definite evidence of teratogenicity, although there is one study suggesting some increased risk associated with use in the first trimester of pregnancy. Diuretic use is, nevertheless, generally considered unwise in pregnancy, except in women with heart disease, because it alters the course of pre-eclampsia and may decrease placental perfusion. Chlorothiazide is moderately well absorbed when taken by mouth and is excreted unchanged into the lumen of the proximal straight tubule where it acts by inhibiting the absorption of sodium and chloride from the urine in the distal tubule, doubling the excretion of potassium, and causing a five-fold increase in sodium excretion. The plasma half life (about 5 hours in the preterm baby) is much shorter than the functional half life. It increases when there is renal failure, making drug accumulation possible. Kernicterus is a theoretical possibility in the very jaundiced baby because the drug competes with bilirubin for the available plasma albumin-binding sites.

Hydrochlorothiazide is an alternative, closely related, thiazide with very similar properties. Since the usual dose of hydrochlorothiazide is only 1·5 mg/kg twice a day by mouth it is important not to confuse the two products. Chlorothiazide and hydrochlorothiazide are both excreted in breast milk, but the baby receives less than 2% of the maternal dose on a weight-for-weight basis. Reports that use during lactation can cause thrombocytopenia are unsubstantiated, as are suggestions that thiazide diuretics suppress lactation.

Diuretics are routinely used in patients with heart failure. They can also improve lung compliance in babies with chronic lung damage and pulmonary oedema, but further studies are needed to confirm whether sustained thiazide treatment really reduces the need for supplemental oxygen (as suggested by one small trial). Diuretics often stimulate increased aldosterone secretion, and the addition of spironolactone, which counteracts the sodium retaining and potassium excreting effect of aldosterone on the distal tubule, is thought to enhance the response to thiazide use. Combined treatment with spironolactone does, however, cause urinary calcium loss of a magnitude similar to that incurred by furosemide use, and this can cause serious bone demineralisation in the preterm baby. It can also cause nephrocalcinosis detectable on ultrasound (but not, usually, on X-ray), although this appears to resolve in later infancy when treatment is stopped. While there are good grounds for giving spironolactone to babies with heart failure (as outlined in the monograph on that drug), it is not yet clear whether such treatment does more good than harm in the preterm baby with chronic lung damage.

Treatment

Heart failure: Give 10 mg/kg of chlorothiazide and 1 mg/kg of spironolactone twice a day by mouth. Babies that fail to respond to a standard dose sometimes respond to twice this dose. Potassium supplements are not usually necessary with such combined treatment.

Chronic lung disease: Babies with chronic ventilator-induced lung damage may benefit from a similar dose of chlorothiazide. Whether they should also receive spironolactone requires further study.

Supply

Chlorothiazide is available commercially, to special order, as a suspension containing 50 mg/ml (costing about £12 for 100 ml), but this formulation has to be imported from America at present. This formulation contains sucrose and saccharin. A sugar-free suspension could also be prepared from powder on request, but this suspension is known to have a reduced shelf life. A similar oral suspension of hydrochlorothiazide could be prepared if required.

References

See also the relevant Cochrane reviews

Albersheim SG, Solimano AJ, Sharma EK, *et al*. Randomised double blind trial of long term diuretic therapy for bronchopulmonary dysplasia. *J Pediatr* 1989;**115**:615–29. [RCT]

Atkinson SA, Shah JK, McGee G, *et al*. Mineral excretion in premature infants receiving various diuretic therapies. *J Pediatr* 1988;**113**:540–5.

Engelhardt B, Blalock A, DanLevy S, *et al*. Effect of spironolactone-hydrochlorothiazide on lung function in infants with chronic bronchopulmonary dysplasia. *J Pediatr* 1989;**114**:619–24. [RCT]

Kao LC, Durand DJ, McCrea RC, *et al*. Randomised trial of long-term diuretic therapy for infants with oxygen-dependent bronchopulmonary dysplasia. *J Pediatr* 1994;**124**:772–81. [RCT]

Wells TG. The pharmacology and therapeutics of diuretics in the pediatric patient. *Pediatr Clin North Am* 1990;**37**:463–504.

CHLORPROMAZINE

Use
Chlorpromazine hydrochloride is a widely used antipsychotic or 'neuroleptic' drug. It was first used in 1952 in the treatment of schizophrenia, but has also been widely used in the short-term management of severe anxiety. It is still used as a short-term tranquilliser in patients of all ages.

Pharmacology
Chlorpromazine hydrochloride is a phenothiazine used to reduce agitation without causing respiratory depression. The phenothiazines have an antihistaminic effect and are sometimes used to combat nausea. They have also been used to reduce peripheral and pulmonary vascular resistance, and were so used for a few years in the 1980s in the management of neonatal respiratory distress. While chlorpromazine was initially most widely offered to psychiatric patients, the drug soon became even more widely used in the 1950s as an adjunct in preoperative medication, and as a joint agent in sedation anaesthesia because of the way it potentiates the hypnotic, narcotic and analgesic effects of other drugs. Such use has now diminished.

Chlorpromazine is well absorbed by mouth, although absorption is said to be occasionally unpredictable. Deep IM injection is generally considered preferable to IV administration though this is occasionally painful. It is metabolised by the liver into a wide number of different breakdown products with a half life of about 30 hours in adults and a half life twice as long as this at birth. Attempts to correlate plasma levels with the clinical effects of treatment have been largely unsuccessful, probably because tissue drug levels greatly exceed those in plasma (V_D >8 l/kg). The drug crosses the placenta and unpredictable maternal hypotension has been reported following use during labour, but there is no evidence of teratogenicity. The baby only receives about 3% of the weight-related maternal dose during lactation, and there is only a single, unevaluatable report of this making the baby drowsy. Extrapyramidal signs have occasionally been suspected for a few days after delivery in babies born to mothers on long-term high-dose antenatal medication. Use in babies less than 1 year old has not yet been endorsed by the manufacturer, and very few reports have been published relating to use in the neonatal period. It is, however, sometimes used in the management of babies born to non-opioid drug-abusing mothers. It is also very good at sedating babies with chronic respiratory problems who become seriously agitated and distressed after weeks of care on a ventilator. There is one unconfirmed report of naloxone (q.v.) being an effective antidote after an overdose.

Neonatal abstinence syndrome
Many different drugs provoke similar withdrawal symptoms in the baby after birth. Restlessness, irritability and excessive wakefulness are the commonest problems seen. Autonomic dysfunction can include sneezing, yawning, sweating and temperature instability. Feeding can prove difficult. Symptoms can be very unpleasant and occasionally, if particularly severe, dangerous. Those that persist after feeding, swaddling and the use of a dummy or pacifier should be managed with a tapering dose of methadone or morphine (q.v.) if the mother has been taking a narcotic (opioid) drug, but chlorpromazine is an understudied alternative that may achieve weaning faster than a tapering dose of morphine. Using phenobarbital (q.v.) as well may sometimes help where there is a mixed dependency. With amphetamine and most opiate abuse, serious symptoms usually present within 1–2 days, peak early and subside fairly rapidly, because these drugs have a fairly short half life. Symptoms present more insidiously with other drugs, such as diazepam and the barbiturates, with a longer half life. Some illicit drugs, such as marijuana (cannabis), seldom cause symptoms. For a fuller discussion see the methadone website commentary.

Treatment
Start by offering 1 mg/kg by mouth every 8 hours. Most authorities suggest that the *total* daily dose should not exceed 6 mg/kg.

Supply
An oral syrup containing 5 mg/ml of chlorpromazine hydrochloride (costing 90p for 100 ml) is available. It can be diluted 10-fold for accurate administration by the pharmacy on request, but the diluted preparation only has a 2-week shelf life. A 1 ml ampoule containing 25 mg of chlorpromazine hydrochloride (costing 60p) is available for intramuscular use.

References
See also relevant Cochrane reviews

Chasnoff IA, ed. Chemical dependency in pregnancy. *Clin Neonatol* 1991;**18**:1–191.
Johnson K. Withdrawal from drugs of addiction in newborn infants. In: David TJ, ed. *Recent advances in paediatrics 22*. London: RSM Press, 2005: pp. 73–83.
Mazurier E, Gambonie G, Barbotte E, Grare A, *et al*. Comparison of chlorpromazine versus morphine hydrochloride for treatment of neonatal abstinence syndrome. *Acta Paediatr* 2008;**97**:1358–61. (See also pp. 1321–3.)
McElhatton PR. The use of phenothiazines during pregnancy and lactation. *Reprod Toxicol* 1992;**6**:475–90.
Nielsen HC, Wiriyathian S, Rosenfeld CR, *et al*. Chlorpromazine excretion by the neonate following chronic in utero exposure. *Pediatr Pharmacol* 1983;**3**:1–5.
Theis JGW, Selby P, Ikizler Y, *et al*. Current management of neonatal abstinence syndrome: a critical analysis of the evidence. *Biol Neonat* 1997;**71**:345–66.
Yoshida K, Smith B, Craggs M, *et al*. Neuroleptic drugs in breast-milk: a study of pharmacokinetics and of possible adverse effects in breast-fed infants. *Psychol Med* 1998;**28**:81–91.

CIPROFLOXACIN

Use

Ciprofloxacin is a quinolone antibiotic with broad-spectrum activity against a wide range of infectious organisms that can be given by mouth. A single 20 mg/kg dose can be used to treat cholera, and also offers protection to those who have been in contact with a case of meningococcal infection.

Pharmacology

Ciprofloxacin is a fluoroquinolone, first patented in 1982, with broad-spectrum activity against many Gram-positive and Gram-negative bacteria, and against other organisms such as *Chlamydia* and rickettsiae (although gonococci are becoming progressively more resistant). It is particularly useful in the management of enterobacter and other infections resistant to all cephalosporins and all the widely used aminoglycosides. Because it can be given by mouth (oral bioavailability 70%), it is particularly useful in the treatment of pulmonary infection with *Pseudomonas aeruginosa* and systemic infection with *Salmonella*. Intravenous administration can be painful, and cause local erythema and phlebitis unless a slow rate of infusion is used. Ciprofloxacin crosses the placenta and diffuses into most body fluids well. Very adequate levels have also been documented in the CSF (>1·0 milligram/l) in infants with ventriculitis. It is partly metabolised in the liver but largely excreted unchanged in the urine (where crystalluria may occur if fluid intake is not maintained). The steady-state half life does not seem to have been studied in babies less than a month old, but the half life in children and adults is not dissimilar (3−4 hours). Dosage only requires review where there is serious renal or liver dysfunction.

Although the use of this drug was initially discouraged in children because studies had shown lasting damage to the cartilage of weight-bearing joints during growth in animals, no reports of any such complication have appeared following its use in childhood, although transient arthralgia may occur. Nalidixic acid (the first widely used quinolone antibiotic) caused similar cartilage damage to growing animals, but was never shown to cause a comparable problem in children. There is one isolated report that has suggested that the drug may stain the primary dentition green. Nevertheless, while the drug should not be used in the neonatal period where other alternative treatment strategies are available, use has sometimes proved extremely effective in the treatment of severe septicaemia or meningitis, and *P. aeruginosa* infection, even though the manufacturers have never formally recommend its use children less than 6 years old. The dose quoted here is in line with most published reports of the drug's use in children (see website commentary), and in line with American advice, but is twice as high as is recommended in most UK texts. There is some suggestion that the drug can cause seizures in patients with an underlying epileptic tendency, and some risk of haemolytic anaemia in babies with G6PD deficiency. Maternal treatment only exposes the breastfed baby to about 3% of the maternal weight-related dose.

Drug interactions

Ciprofloxacin treatment increases the half life of theophylline and (to a lesser extent) caffeine. The dose of theophylline may need to be halved if toxic side effects are to be avoided. Ciprofloxacin can cause prolongation of the QT interval and should be avoided in those with congenital long QT syndrome.

Treatment

Dose: Give 10 mg/kg IV over 30−60 minutes when treating severe infection. Oral treatment with a marginally higher dose (12 mg/kg) may well suffice when treating pulmonary infection.
Timing: Give one dose every 12 hours in the first 3 months of life, and every 8 hours in babies older than this (unless the plasma creatinine is over twice that of normal). Treatment is usually continued for 10−14 days.

Supply

Ciprofloxacin lactate for IV use is available in 50 ml bottles containing 100 mg of ciprofloxacin (costing £8·60) from the pharmacy. A 10 mg/kg dose contains 0·76 mmol/kg of sodium. Bottles must be discarded promptly after they have been opened; capped syringes can be prepared for IV use by the pharmacy on request to minimise drug wastage. A sugar-free oral suspension of ciprofloxacin hydrochloride containing 50 mg/ml is available (100 ml costs £15).

References

American Academy of Pediatrics, Committee on Infectious Diseases. The use of systemic fluoroquinolones. *Pediatrics* 2006;**118**:1287−92.

Chalumeau M, Tonnelier S, d'Athis P, *et al*. Fluoroquinone safety in pediatric patients: a prospective, multicenter, comparative cohort study in France. *Pediatrics* 2003;**111**:e714−19.

Gendrel D, Chalumeau M, Moulin F, *et al*. Fluoroquinolones in paediatrics: a risk for the patient or for the community? [Review] *Lancet Infect Dis* 2003;**3**:537−46.

Lipman J, Gous AGS, Mathivha LR, *et al*. Ciprofloxacin pharmacokinetic profiles in paediatric sepsis: how much ciprofloxacin is enough? *Intensive Care Med* 2002;**28**:493−500.

Saha D, Khan WA, Karim MM, *et al*. Single-dose ciprofloxacin versus 12-dose erythromycin for childhood cholera: a randomized controlled trial. *Lancet* 2005;**366**:1085−93. [RCT] (See also pp. 1054−5.)

Singh UK, Sinha RK, Prassad B, *et al*. Ciprofloxacin in children: is arthropathy a limitation ? *Indian J Pediatr* 2000;**67**:386−7.

van den Oever HLA, Verteegh FGA, Theweesen EAPM, *et al*. Ciprofloxacin in preterm neonates: case report and review of the literature. *Eur J Pediatr* 1998;**157**:843−5.

CLINDAMYCIN

Use

Clindamycin is used in the prophylaxis and treatment of anaerobic infections, and to protect against bacterial endocarditis and intrapartum group B streptococcal infection in subjects allergic to penicillin. Prompt early use may also reduce the risk of very preterm birth in some women with overt bacterial vaginosis.

Pharmacology

Clindamycin hydrochloride is an antibiotic related to lincomycin that has a mainly bacteriostatic effect on Gram-positive aerobes and a wide range of anaerobic bacteria. It acts by inhibiting protein synthesis in much the same way as erythromycin. It was originally isolated from the soil fungus *Streptomyces lincolnensis*, and first synthesised in 1967. It is rapidly absorbed when given by mouth, and penetrates most tissues well, although CSF penetration is poor. The drug is metabolised by the liver with an adult half life of 2–3 hours. The dose given does not normally need to be changed when there is renal failure because only a little is excreted unmetabolised in the urine. The half life is long, and troublesomely variable (3–15 hours) in the preterm baby, falling to adult values by 2 months, and the manufacturers do not recommend IV use in babies less than 4 weeks old. The risk of diarrhoea, and of occasionally fatal antibiotic-related pseudomembranous colitis (characterised by bloody diarrhoea and abdominal pain), has limited the neonatal use of this antibiotic. Treatment must be stopped at once if this adverse reaction is suspected. Oral vancomycin (15 mg/kg every 8 hours) and parenteral nutrition are often used to treat this colitis, which seems to be due to *Clostridium difficile* toxin. Other adverse effects include skin rashes and other hypersensitivity reactions, blood dyscrasias and disturbances of hepatic function. The drug is still sometimes used as an alternative to sodium fusidate (q.v.) in the management of resistant staphylococcal osteomyelitis, and to control the anaerobic sepsis associated with necrotising enterocolitis (although the only controlled trial raised the possibility that clindamycin might increase the risk of late stricture formation). Clindamycin is occasionally used in the management of protozoal infection (including malaria and toxoplasmosis). It is now increasingly used to treat overt bacterial vaginosis, and some also advocate screening for asymptomatic vaginosis in early pregnancy if vaginal pH exceeds 4·5. There is no evidence of teratogenicity, and treatment during lactation only exposes the baby to about 3% of the maternal dose on a weight-for-weight basis. There is just one anecdotal report of a baby who passed two bloody stools while being breastfed by such a mother.

Prophylaxis

Bacterial vaginosis: Clindamycin (5 grams of the 2% vaginal cream once a day for 7 days, or 300 mg twice daily by mouth for 5 days) reduced the risk of very preterm birth in two recent trials when given to women with a clearly abnormal vaginal flora or frank bacterial vaginosis in *early* pregnancy (≤19 weeks).

Maternal group B streptococcal carriage: Clindamycin (900 mg IV once every 8 hours) can be used, like penicillin (q.v.) or erythromycin, to reduce the risk of the baby becoming infected during delivery.

In children with heart defects: Short courses of clindamycin are sometimes given during surgery involving a site where infection is suspected to reduce the risk of endocarditis in patients who are allergic to penicillin, or who have received more than a single dose of penicillin in the past 4 weeks. Give 20 mg/kg of clindamycin by mouth 1 hour before the procedure is due. Azithromycin (q.v.) is a useful oral alternative.

Treatment

Neonates: Give 5 mg/kg by mouth or (slowly) IV once every 8 hours for 7–10 days to manage severe staphylococcal infection, or the anaerobic septicaemia sometimes associated with neonatal necrotising enterocolitis. Very immature babies may be at risk from benzyl alcohol, which is an excipient of the IV product. Babies more than 2 weeks old with normal liver function may benefit from one dose every 6 hours.

Older children: Give infants with severe infection over 2 months old 10 mg/kg IV once every 6 hours.

Supply and administration

300 mg (2 ml) ampoules of clindamycin phosphate (containing 0·9% w/v benzyl alcohol) cost £6·20. To obtain a solution containing 5 mg/ml for accurate administration, first dilute the contents of the 300 mg ampoule to 15 ml with 5% glucose, and then take 0·25 ml (5 mg) of this solution for each kg that the baby weighs, dilute this with 0·75 ml/kg of 5% glucose, and infuse over at least 10 minutes. Clindamycin palmitate could also be made available as an oral suspension. This is stable for 2 weeks at room temperature after reconstitution. A 40 gram pack of the 2% vaginal cream costs £11·80.

References

See also the relevant Cochrane reviews

Bell MJ, Shackelford P, Smith R, *et al*. Pharmacokinetics of clindamycin phosphate in the first year of life. *J Pediatr* 1984;**105**:482–6.

Deajani AS, Taubert KA, Wilson W, *et al*. Prevention of bacterial endocarditis: recommendations by the American Heart Association. *JAMA* 1997;**277**:1794–801.

Faix RG, Polley TZ, Grasela TH. A randomised, controlled trial of parenteral clindamycin in neonatal necrotising enterocolitis. *J Pediatr* 1988;**112**:271–9. [RCT]

Hall CM, Milligan DWA, Berrington J. Probable adverse reaction to a pharmaceutical excipient. *Arch Dis Child* 2004;**89**:F184.

Koren G, Zarfin Y, Maresky D, *et al*. Pharmacokinetics of intravenous clindamycin in newborn infants. *Pediatr Pharmacol* 1986;**5**:187–92.

Larsson P-G, Fåhraeus L, Carlsson B, *et al*. Late miscarriage and preterm birth after treatment with clindamycin: a randomised consent design study according to Zelen. *Br J Obstet Gynecol* 2006;**113**:629–37. [RCT] (See also pp. 1483–4.)

Ugwamadu A, Manyonda I, Reid F, *et al*. Effect of early oral clindamycin on late miscarriage and preterm delivery in asymptomatic women with abnormal vaginal flora and bacterial vaginosis: a randomised controlled trial. *Lancet* 2003;**361**:983–8. [RCT]

Use

Clonazepam, like lorazepam (q.v.), is sometimes used in the neonatal period to control severe, continuous seizure activity resistant to routine anticonvulsant treatment, despite increasing concern that its sedative effect may sometimes mask the fact that cortical seizure activity has not been suppressed.

Pharmacology

Clonazepam is a benzodiazepine that is completely and readily absorbed from the gastrointestinal tract, peak plasma levels occurring after 60–90 minutes. Steady state tissue levels exceed plasma levels (V_D ~3 l/kg). Clonazepam is extensively metabolised to inactive compounds but the neonatal half life is 24–48 hours. It may be given IV if rapid onset of action is required. Clonazepam has been used since the mid-1970s as an anticonvulsant in various types of epilepsy, but is now mostly used in the management of panic attacks and some movement disorders, including hyperekplexia, and in the treatment of myoclonic and absence seizures. It crosses the placenta but no adverse fetal effects have been noted. It has also been used in late pregnancy without causing any obvious sedation of the infant after birth, but appears in breast milk in the same way as other benzodiazepines. Babies so exposed need to be monitored for signs of drowsiness, and apnoea is a theoretical possibility.

Clonazepam has often been given as a slow, continuous, IV infusion in the neonatal period, but this approach is of no particular benefit since clonazepam is only slowly cleared from the brain (unlike diazepam). In addition, its onset of action will be seriously delayed if an initial loading dose is not given. There are no good controlled trial data on the use of clonazepam in the control of neonatal seizures. Drug tolerance becomes a problem if treatment is continued for any extended period, and increasing seizure activity may occur if the serum level exceeds 125 µg/l. See the phenobarbital website for a discussion of how best to control seizures resistant to phenobarbital and phenytoin.

Major adverse effects are drowsiness, ataxia and behavioural changes. Bronchial hypersecretion and salivation are said to be a problem in infancy, particularly if there is neurological dysfunction with impaired swallowing. As with all benzodiazepine anticonvulsants, withdrawal of clonazepam should be gradual – over at least 6 weeks if medication has been used for any length of time – in order to reduce the risk of withdrawal (rebound) seizures.

Drug interactions

Concurrent treatment with phenytoin or carbamazepine reduces the half life of clonazepam.

Treatment

Try 100 micrograms/kg IV as a slow bolus injection once every 24 hours for 2–3 days in babies resistant to routine anticonvulsant medication.

Antidote

Flumazenil is a specific antidote (as described in the monograph on midazolam).

Blood levels

Plasma levels are usually 30–100 µg/l (1 µg/l = 3·16 nmol/l), but levels do not always correlate with clinical efficacy.

Supply and administration

Stock ampoules containing 1 mg in 1 ml of solvent, costing 63p each, come supplied with a further 1 ml ampoule of water for injection. The content of *both* ampoules should be drawn into a syringe *immediately* before use, and then diluted to 10 ml with 10% glucose saline to give a solution that contains 100 micrograms/ml, suitable for slow bolus IV administration. Such a solution should **not** be used to give a continuous IV infusion. Each 1 ml ampoule contains 30 mg of benzyl alcohol and a significant (but unspecified) amount of propylene glycol. Clonazepam is a schedule 4 controlled drug in the UK.

References

André M, Boutroy MJ, Bianchetti G, *et al*. Clonazepam in neonatal seizures: dose regimes and therapeutic efficiency. *Eur J Clin Pharmacol* 1991;**40**:193–5.
André M, Boutroy MJ, Dubrruc C, *et al*. Clonazepam pharmacokinetics and therapeutic efficacy in neonatal seizures. *Eur J Clin Pharmacol* 1986;**30**:585–9.
Boylan GB, Rennie JM, Chorley G, *et al*. Second-line anticonvulsant treatment of neonatal seizures: a video-EEG study. *Neurology* 2004;**62**:486–8. [RCT]
Dhahar E, Raviv R. Sporadic major hyperekplexia in neonates and infants: clinical manifestations and outcome. *Pediatr Neurol* 2004;**31**:30–4.
Rivera S, Villeha F, do Saint Martin A, *et al*. Congenital hyperekplexia: five sporadic cases. *Eur J Pediatr* 2006;**165**:104–7.

CODEINE PHOSPHATE

Use

Codeine is an opioid analgesic frequently given by mouth to adults together with aspirin or paracetamol. Use is now being discouraged because of evidence that it is becoming a drug of addiction. An overdose can also be dangerous. Paracetamol (q.v.) on its own is more often used to provide oral analgesia in young children.

Pharmacology

Codeine was first isolated from the opioid juices left over after morphine had been extracted from poppy juice in 1832. The name chosen came from the Greek word *codeia* meaning a poppy capsule. Codeine is only a mild narcotic but it is probably as effective an antitussive (cough suppressant) as morphine. When given by mouth its analgesic effect starts to become apparent after 30 minutes and peaks at 2 hours. Absorption is as rapid but less complete after rectal administration, making a larger dose necessary. Few pharmacokinetic studies have yet been done in early infancy. Tissue levels exceed plasma levels (V_D ~3 l/kg). The drug is partly metabolised by the liver (morphine being one of the metabolites), and it is increasingly thought that metabolism to morphine probably explains much of the drug's analgesic effect. The extent to which this occurs seems to depend on which genetic variant of the CYP2D6 cytochrome P450 enzyme the child has inherited, making the exact analgesic effect of any given dose hard to predict except in a child who has taken the drug before. Contrary to general belief it certainly seems to cause as much nausea, vomiting, constipation and ileus as a dose of morphine of similar analgesic potency. It also causes as much respiratory depression and hypotension (due to histamine release). Much is finally excreted after conjugation with glucuronic acid in the urine, making repeated, or high-dose, administration hazardous where there is renal or liver failure. Little has been published relating to the use of codeine in babies less than 3 months old.

Excess medication can cause somnolence and respiratory depression, and death has been reported as a result of accidental ingestion. Some cough medicines contain quite a lot of codeine. Even 5-year-old children have died after taking more than 5 mg/kg of codeine a day in this way. For this reason the *British National Formulary* strongly discourages the use of any cough mixture containing codeine in children less than 1 year old. Codeine is also an ingredient of many of the compound analgesic preparations routinely available in the UK (including a range of preparations that are available 'over the counter') even though it is a schedule 2 controlled drug – a fact that those travelling abroad need to bear in mind.

Codeine crosses the placenta but there is no evidence of teratogenicity. Tolerance develops with repeated usage and withdrawal symptoms have been documented, even in infancy. Heavy maternal usage in the period immediately before delivery can even, occasionally, cause neonatal symptoms of opiate withdrawal 1–2 days after delivery. Codeine, and its active metabolite morphine, are also excreted into breast milk. While the highest blood level usually achieved is less than a third of the lowest therapeutic blood level, a minority of babies inherit a gene that results in their metabolising very much more of the codeine into morphine, and there is one recent report where this may have caused death from opiate toxicity. The baby of any breastfeeding mother taking codeine for more than 1–2 days **must**, therefore, be monitored for lethargy and somnolence.

Treatment

Dose: Give 1 mg/kg by mouth, or IM, or 1·5 mg/kg rectally. Never give the drug IV because of the risk of anaphylactoid hypotension.

Timing: Never give a dose more than once every 6–8 hours in the first 3 months of life, or every 4–6 hours in children older than that, and never give repeat medication without looking for signs of respiratory depression.

Antidote

An overdose causes drowsiness, pinpoint pupils and hypotension and can cause dangerous respiratory depression. Naloxone (q.v.) is a specific antidote for all the opiate drugs.

Supply

A sugar-free linctus containing 5 mg/ml of codeine phosphate is available on request (100 ml costs 90p). It can be further diluted if requested. The linctus can also be given rectally if oral treatment is not possible. An IM preparation is available, but it would probably be more appropriate, in this situation, to give IV or IM morphine (q.v.). Staff need to be aware that some tablets of co-codamol, which is widely used as an analgesic after childbirth, contain as much as 30 mg of codeine as well as 500 mg of paracetamol.

References

Koren G, Cairns J, Chitayat D, *et al*. Pharmacogenetics of morphine poisoning in a breastfed neonate of a codeine-prescribed mother. *Lancet* 2006;**368**:704. (See also 2008;**372**;606 – 7 and 625 – 6.)

Magnani B, Evans R. Codeine intoxication in the neonate. *Pediatrics* 1999;**104**:e75.

McEwan A, Sigston PE, Andrews KA, *et al*. A comparison of rectal and intramuscular codeine phosphate in children following neurosurgery. *Paediatr Anaesth* 2000;**10**:189 – 93. [RCT]

Meny RG, Naumburg EG, Alger LS, *et al*. Codeine and the breastfed neonate. *J Hum Lactation* 1993;**9**:237 – 40.

Williams DG, Hatch CJ, Howard RF. Codeine phosphate in paediatric medicine. *Br J Anaesth* 2001;**86**:413 – 21.

Williams DG, Patel A, Howard RF. Pharmacogenetics of codeine metabolism in an urban population of children and its implications for analgesic reliability. *Br J Anaesth* 2002;**89**:839 – 45.

Zhang WY, Li Wan Po A. Analgesic efficacy of paracetamol and its combination with codeine and caffeine in surgical pain – a meta-analysis. *J Clin Pharmacol Ther* 1996;**21**:261 – 82. [SR]

Use

Co-trimoxazole is used to treat cholera (*Vibrio cholerae* infection) and to prevent and treat *Pneumocystis carinii* infection. It is an effective treatment for two important protozoan intestinal infections (isosporiasis and cyclosporiasis). It has also been used to treat uncomplicated falciparum malaria, and is sometimes used in the management of neonatal meningitis because of good tissue and CSF penetration. Trimethoprim (q.v.) is now quite often used on its own for most respiratory and urinary tract infections.

Pharmacology

Co-trimoxazole is a 5:1 mixture of two different antibiotics that inhibit folic acid synthesis in protozoa and bacteria (and, to a lesser degree, in man). It was first marketed in 1969. The bacteriostatic effect of the long-acting sulphonamide (sulfamethoxazole) is augmented by the synergistic effect of trimethoprim. The two drugs in combination are active against most common pathogens except *Pseudomonas* and *Mycobacterium tuberculosis*. Both drugs are well absorbed by mouth, and actively excreted by the kidney with half lives of about 12 hours. They also cross the placenta with ease. CSF levels approach half those in the plasma, while levels in urine and in bronchial and vaginal secretions exceed those in plasma. Use during lactation only exposes the baby to about 3% of the weight-adjusted maternal dose.

Because both drugs are folate antagonists, the manufacturers still caution against their use during pregnancy, but teratogenicity has only been encountered in folate-deficient animals and the drug has now been in widespread clinical use for more than 30 years. The manufacturers have also declined to recommend use in babies less than 6 weeks old, but there is no specific reason for this caution other than the risk of haemolytic anaemia in babies with G6PD deficiency, and the risk of kernicterus (although sulfamethoxazole competes for the protein-binding sites usually available to bilirubin in babies with jaundice less than most of the other sulphonamide antibiotics). Caution is understandable, however, given the unnecessary deaths caused by the prophylactic use of sulphonamide drugs in the early 1950s (as outlined in the monograph on sulfadiazine). Rapid IV administration can cause an allergic reaction or anaphylaxis. Other adverse effects, which can be fatal, are usually only seen in elderly patients, or following high-dose treatment in patients with AIDS. Nevertheless, since the problems (including rashes, erythema multiforme and marrow depression) are almost certainly due to the sulphonamide component, trimethoprim is now increasingly prescribed on its own.

Drug interactions

Treatment with co-trimoxazole increases the plasma half life of phenytoin.

Prescribing

Specify the *total* amount of active drug in milligrams. Thus 20 mg/kg of sulfamethoxazole and 4 mg/kg of trimethoprim is prescribed as 24 mg/kg of active drug.

Prophylaxis

Immunodeficiency: Give 24 mg/kg by mouth once a day to babies with possible combined immune deficiency, or overt HIV, to reduce the risk of bacterial infection, and of fungal *Pneumocystis carinii* pneumonia. This is probably worth continuing indefinitely. There are no data in children under 1 year that help to determine when to discontinue prophylaxis. In adults CD4 percentage is a better indicator of immune competence and prophylaxis is often stopped after 12–18 months unless the CD4 count is below 200 cells/μl.

Measles: Complications in a resource-poor country can be reduced by giving co-trimoxazole for 7 days.

Treatment

Dose: Treat severe systemic infection with 24 mg/kg of active drug by mouth (or IV, if oral treatment is impracticable). Avoid in babies with limited renal function, unless the plasma sulfamethoxazole trough level is kept below 120 mg/l (1 mg/l = 3·95 mmol/l), and in babies with serious unconjugated jaundice.

Timing: Give once a day in the first week of life, and once every 12 hours after that. Treat *Pneumocystis* once every 6 hours in babies over 4 weeks old, even if the blood level exceeds 120 mg/l.

Supply and administration

The sugar-free paediatric oral suspension with 48 mg of active drug per ml costs £1·10 per 100 ml. 5 ml ampoules for IV use containing 96 mg/ml (costing £1·60 per ampoule) are also available: to give the standard neonatal dose (24 mg/kg) dilute 0·25 ml/kg of the contents of the ampoule into at least 15 times the same volume of 10% glucose in 0·18% sodium chloride and then infuse this over 2 hours. The IV preparation contains 45% w/v propylene glycol. Avoid IM use in small children. More concentrated solutions have been given using a central line.

References

See also the relevant Cochrane reviews

Chintu C, Bhat GJ, Walker AS, *et al*. Co-trimoxazole as prophylaxis against opportunistic infections in HIV-infected Zambian children (CHAP): a double-blind randomised placebo-controlled trial. *Lancet* 2004;**364**:1865–71.[RCT] (See also 2005;**365**:749–50.)

Escobedo AA, Almirall P, Alfonso M, *et al*. Treatment of intestinal protozoan infections in children. *Arch Dis Child* 2009;**94**:478–82.

Fehintola FA, Adedeji AA, Tambo E, *et al*. Cotrimoxazole in the treatment of acute uncomplicated falciparum malaria in Nigerian children: a controlled clinical trial. *Clin Drug Invest* 2004;**24**:149–55. [RCT]

Garly M-L, Balé C, Martins CL, *et al*. Prophylactic antibiotics to prevent pneumonia and other complications after measles: community based randomised double blind placebo controlled trial in Guinea-Bissau. *BMJ* 2006;**333**:1245–7 [RCT] (See also p. 1234.)

Graham SM. Prophylaxis against *Pneumocystis carinii* pneumonia for HIV-exposed infants in Africa. *Lancet* 2002;**360**:1966–8.

Use

The use of a single 2-day course of dexamethasone or, preferably, betamethasone (q.v.) to accelerate surfactant production in the fetal lung *before* birth is known to be safe, but the safety of sustained high-dose use in the weeks *after* birth remains extremely uncertain.

Pharmacology in pregnancy

Dexamethasone, a potent glucocorticoid steroid that is well absorbed by mouth, was developed in 1958. It crosses the placenta, and has a half life of about 3 hours. It appears as effective as betamethasone, the drug first used for this purpose, in accelerating surfactant production by the preterm fetal lung, reducing the risk of death from respiratory distress. Maternal treatment alters fetal heart rate and its variability, and marginally enhances renal maturation. Treatment can control virilisation in fetuses with congenital adrenal hyperplasia, and 4 mg a day may improve the outcome if maternal lupus erythematosus causes fetal heart block (with salbutamol if the heart rate is <55 bpm). It is not known if treatment during lactation affects the baby, but treatment with prednisolone (q.v.) *is* known to be safe.

Pharmacology in the neonate

Dexamethasone can speed extubation in a minority of babies with laryngeal oedema. It can also reduce the amount of time that preterm babies with acute lung injury due to some combination of mechanical ventilation, low-grade infection and oxidative stress (so-called bronchopulmonary dysplasia or BPD) need to spend in oxygen before discharge home. Steroids should not be given lightly, however, because their use is associated with a 50% increase in the risk of secondary infection, while protein catabolism also affects growth. The associated rise in blood pressure and blood glucose rarely calls for intervention, and the marked hypertrophy of the ventricular myocardium seen in a minority is reversible, but steroid use increases the risk of nephrocalcinosis in babies on diuretics. Gastrointestinal haemorrhage and perforation can occur, while continuous treatment for over 10 days can also cause adrenal suppression for 2–4 weeks. If steroids are going to be beneficial, some improvement will almost always be seen within 48 hours.

Increased survival, rather than time in oxygen is, however, what matters. Improved survival free from evidence of chronic lung disease at 36 weeks postmenstrual age has only been seen when treatment is limited to babies who are still ventilator dependent and in substantial oxygen 7–14 days after birth. Intervention outside this 'time window' seems to have no measurable impact on survival. Even more worryingly, the combined results from 11 trials involving 1388 children followed after discharge show more disability among the steroid-treated children (although frequent steroid treatment in control children in some studies complicates any analysis). Perhaps, as with all drugs, dexamethasone can do good and do harm. Used early the harm may predominate because many of those treated never stood to benefit anyway.

Unfortunately, despite 15 years of widespread use, we still know little about the best dose to use, or the optimum length of treatment. Inhaled steroids have not proved as effective as was hoped, as the monograph on budesonide makes clear. Neither have short, 3-day 'pulses' of treatment proved an advance. However, Durand's low-dose regimen (see below) has been shown to improve pulmonary function in the first week of treatment as effectively as the regimen used in the past while reducing corticosteroid exposure by two-thirds, and the short-term outcome of the Australian DART trial, which had to close early for lack of support (see web commentary), has now confirmed this. In the end, however, any *short*-term benefit seen may only be worth having if the *long*-term outcome is equally reassuring – an issue still unaddressed by any large study. In so far as use reduces BPD it may achieve this largely be facilitating earlier extubation.

One study has suggested that treating established BPD with a tapering 3-week course of hydrocortisone (75 mg/kg in total) may be as effective as standard high-dose dexamethasone treatment (6 mg/kg in total) and generate fewer adverse effects. Many will take this as evidence that the use of a different corticosteroid is worth more study; others that this just shows that the early studies used too high a dose of dexamethasone, even though one recent meta-analysis has suggested that a high dose might be better.

Drug equivalence

4 mg of dexamethasone base is equivalent to 4·8 mg of dexamethasone phosphate or 5 mg of dexamethasone sodium phosphate. Minimise confusion by prescribing the amount of **base** to be given.

Prophylaxis

Congenital adrenal hyperplasia: Giving the mother 7 micrograms/kg of dexamethasone *base* once every 8 hours, preferably before the 8th week of pregnancy, reduces virilisation in the affected female fetus, but may have some impact on working memory in children treated unnecessarily. Reduce the dose in the third trimester to minimise side effects. Hydrocortisone (q.v.) is used once diagnosis is confirmed after birth.

Fetal lung maturation: Give 12 mg of dexamethasone *base* IM to the mother and repeat once after 24 hours if there is a risk of preterm delivery. Oral treatment (four 6 mg doses once every 12 hours) is sometimes preferred, although one small trial has suggested that the outcome is marginally less satisfactory. One important observational study suggests that betamethasone may be better.

Early BPD: Early postnatal steroid use can no longer be justified except as part of a formal controlled trial.

Meningitis: 300 micrograms/kg of dexamethasone *base* twice a day IV, IM or by mouth for 2 days started *early* can reduce the risk of subsequent deafness in young children with early *Haemophilus* or pneumococcal meningitis (possibly by moderating the toxic effect of the rapid bacterial lysis caused by treatment with cefotaxime). It did not improve outcome when used in a recent large trial in Africa.

Continued

Treating chronic lung disease

Ventilated preterm babies who are still seriously oxygen dependent 7–10 days after birth are at serious risk of developing chronic lung disease. While parents may understandably want treatment with dexamethasone tried if it is starting to look as though progressive lung disease may jeopardise survival, it remains uncertain which – if any – of the following treatment strategies is best. Low-dose strategies are now favoured.

DART trial regimen: 60 micrograms/kg of dexamethasone *base* twice a day IV (or orally), on days 1–3, 40 micrograms/kg twice a day on days 4–6, 20 micrograms/kg twice a day on days 7–8, and 8 micrograms/kg twice a day on days 9–10 (a total of 712 micrograms/kg over 10 days). Repeat once if necessary.

Durand trial regimen: 100 micrograms/kg of dexamethasone *base* IV twice a day for 3 days, and then 50 micrograms/kg twice a day for 4 days (a total of 1 mg/kg over 7 days).

Traditional regimen: 250 micrograms/kg of dexamethasone *base* orally or IV twice a day for 7 days was, until about 10 years ago, the most widely used regimen. Some babies were also offered a second course.

Treating other conditions

Hypotension: One 100 micrograms/kg dose followed, if necessary, by 50 micrograms/kg IV twice a day for 1–2 days often 'cures' inotrope-resistant neonatal hypotension. Low-dose hydrocortisone is also effective.

Facilitating extubation in the preterm baby: Even if the DART regimen (see above) does not reduce chronic lung damage, it *does* facilitate extubation and less than half this dose seemed to help in one small study.

Treatment for post-intubation laryngeal oedema: Three 200 micrograms/kg doses of dexamethasone *base* orally or IV at 8-hourly intervals (started at least 4 hours and preferably 12 hours before the endotracheal tube is removed) may aid extubation in babies and in older children with an oedematous or traumatised larynx .

Croup: Viral croup responds to a single 600 micrograms/kg dose of oral dexamethasone *base* as well as it does to an IM dose. Inhaled budesonide (q.v.) is another alternative of comparable efficacy.

Surgical stress: To cover possible adrenal suppression, babies on dexamethasone or who last completed a course of dexamethasone lasting more than 1 week less than 4 weeks ago should receive 1 mg/kg of hydrocortisone IV prior to surgery and then every 6 hours IV or IM for 24–48 hours.

Supply and administration

Several products exist. Stock 1 ml vials containing 4 mg of dexamethasone phosphate (costing £1) contain 3·3 mg of dexamethasone base. *Avoid products with a sulphite preservative* (for reasons outlined in the website commentary). Draw 0·3 ml of fluid from the vial into a syringe and dilute to 10 ml with 5% glucose to get a solution containing 100 micrograms/ml of base for IV or oral use. Scored 500 microgram tablets are available (costing 3p each). So is a cheap sugar-free 0·4 mg/ml oral solution (Dexsol®) with a 3-month shelf life, which can be further diluted if necessary just before use (although this contains propylene glycol).

References

See also the relevant Cochrane reviews

Ausejo M, Saenz A, Pham B, *et al*. The effectiveness of glucocorticoids in treating croup: meta-analysis. *BMJ* 1999;**319**:595–600. [SR]

Bjornson CL, Klassen TP, Williamson J, *et al*. A randomized trial of a single dose of oral dexamethasone for mild croup. *N Engl J Med* 2004;**351**:1306–13. [RCT] (See also pp. 1283–4.)

Brook CGD. Antenatal treatment of a mother bearing a fetus with congenital adrenal hyperplasia. *Arch Dis Child* 2000;**82**:F176–8. (See also associated commentaries pp. 178–81.)

Doyle LW, Davis PG, Morley CJ, *et al*. Low-dose dexamethasone facilitates extubation among chronically ventilator-dependent infants: a multicenter, international, randomized, controlled trial. *Pediatrics* 2006;**117**:75–83. [RCT] (See also 2007;**119**:716–21.)

Doyle LW, Halliday HL, Ehrenkranz RA, *et al*. Impact of postnatal systematic corticosteroids on mortality and cerebral palsy in preterm infants: effect modification by risk for chronic lung disease. *Pediatrics* 2005;**115**:655–61. [SR] (See also p. 794.)

Gaissmaier RE, Pohlandt F. Single-dose dexamethasone treatment of hypotension in preterm infants. *J Pediatr* 1999;**134**:701–5. [RCT]

Hirvikoski T, Nordenström A, Lindholm T, *et al*. Cognitive function in children at risk for congenital adrenal hyperplasia treated prenatally with dexamethasone. *J Clin Endocrinol Metab* 2007;**92**:542–8.

Jaeggi ET, Fouron J-C, Silverman ED, *et al*. Transplacental fetal treatment improves the outcome of prenatally diagnosed complete atrioventricular heart block without structural heart disease. *Circulation* 2004;**110**:1542–8.

Johnson D. Croup. *BMJ Clinical evidence handbook*. London: BMJ Books, 2009: pp. 76–9 (and updates). [SR]

Lukkassen IMA, Hassing MBF, Markhirst DG. Dexamethasone reduces reintubation rate due to postextubation stridor in a high-risk paediatric population. *Acta Paediatr* 2006;**95**:74–6.

Noori S, Siassi B, Durand M, *et al*. Cardiovascular effects of low-dose dexamethasone in very low birth weight neonates with refractory hypotension. *Biol Neonat* 2006;**89**:82–7.

Onland W, Offringa M, De Jaegere AP, *et al*. Finding the optimal postnatal dexamethasone regimen for preterm infants at risk of bronchopulmonary dysplasia: a systematic review of placebo-controlled trials. *Pediatrics* 2009;**123**:367–77. [SR]

Tanney K, Davis JW, Hegarty J, *et al*. Is a low dose dexamethasone regimen effective in extremely low birth weight babies with evolving bronchopulmonary dysplasia? [Abstract] *Neonatology* 2009;**95**:380.

van der Heide-Jalving M, Kamphuis PJGH, van der Laan MJ, *et al*. Short- and long-term effects of neonatal glucocorticoid therapy: is hydrocortisone an alternative to dexamethasone? *Acta Paediatr* 2003;**92**:827–35.

Yeh TF, Lin YJ, Lin HC, *et al*. Outcomes at school age after postnatal dexamethasone for lung disease of prematurity. *N Engl J Med* 2004;**350**:1304–13. [RCT] (See also pp. 1349–51.)

Use

Diamorphine has been used to control neonatal pain, but morphine (q.v.), which has been more fully evaluated, is equally effective. The monograph on methadone has a discussion of maternal addiction.

Pharmacology

Diamorphine hydrochloride is a potent semisynthetic opioid analgesic. Because it is all converted, within minutes, to morphine and 6-monoacetylmorphine in the body, almost all the drug's properties and adverse effects, including reduced peristalsis, urinary retention and respiratory depression are essentially the same as for morphine. It is well absorbed by mouth, but bioavailability is reduced by rapid first pass liver metabolism. Some enters the CNS after bolus IV administration causing intense euphoria, and it is this that probably makes the drug so addictive. Clearance is very variable, inversely related to gestational age, and essentially the same as for morphine. High solubility is the drug's only clinical advantage, because this makes it possible to give a large intramuscular dose in a small-volume injection, but this is of no relevance to its use in infancy. Indeed there are *no* good reasons for using diamorphine rather than morphine in young children, and parents can be very disconcerted to discover, possibly by chance, that their child is on heroin. It was first manufactured on a commercial basis in 1898, but eventually banned in America in 1924 after its full addictive potential became apparent. Many other countries have since introduced similar bans. Placental transfer is rapid, but there is no reason why a mother given diamorphine in labour should not breastfeed, although the baby may be too drowsy to suckle vigorously for several hours, unless offered naloxone (q.v.).

Maternal addiction

While there have been suggestions that diamorphine could be teratogenic, the malformations reported conform to no discernible pattern, and all the mothers in the studies reported had been taking heroin of uncertain purity as well as other drugs during pregnancy. Fetal growth is often reduced, and there may be an increased risk of fetal death. Most mothers in the UK admitting to opiate addiction are now placed on methadone (q.v.) during pregnancy to minimise these problems. Even so, babies exposed to *any* opiate drug in pregnancy, including methadone, show slight (but significant) developmental delay when 2–3 years old.

While morphine is still used in a few centres to control any symptoms of withdrawal that appear in the baby after delivery, methadone is now the drug more widely used. Some babies seem to benefit from being given phenobarbital (q.v.) as well, and there is a belief that chlorpromazine (q.v.) can be helpful if an opiate is not the only illicit drug that the mother is taking. The use of paregoric (a variable cocktail of opium, glycerin, alcohol and benzoic acid) lacks rational justification. Some assessment scales have the perverse effect of suggesting that an increasingly sedated baby is improving, but the main aim of treatment must be to improve the baby's ability to feed normally as well as sleep normally, and an unnecessarily complex weaning strategy merely serves to delay discharge. Mothers are sometimes discouraged from breastfeeding, but lactation can be used as part of a controlled weaning strategy as long as the mother is not also taking other serious drugs of abuse, since the baby only receives, on a weight-for-weight basis, about 5–10% of the maternal dose.

Pain relief

Give ventilated babies in serious pain a loading dose of 180 micrograms/kg IV followed by a maintenance infusion of 15 micrograms/kg an hour (or 6 ml/hour *for 1 hour* followed by 0·5 ml/hour of a solution made up as described below) accepting that this can depress respiration in a 'trigger' ventilated baby. Sedation only requires 9 micrograms/kg an hour IV (0·3 ml/hour). Intranasal administration gives good relief after ~20 minutes.

Antidote

Naloxone is a specific antidote for all the opioid drugs.

Supply and administration

10 mg ampoules of diamorphine (costing £1·40) can be provided on request. The ampoule should be reconstituted with 1 ml of water to give a solution containing 10 mg/ml. To set up a continuous infusion, dilute this reconstituted liquid to 10 ml with 0·9% sodium chloride; place 1·5 ml of this diluted preparation for each kg the baby weighs in a syringe, dilute to 50 ml with 10% glucose saline, and infuse at a rate of 0·5 ml/hour in order to provide a continuous infusion of 15 micrograms/kg per hour. The drug is stable in solution so it is not necessary to change the infusate daily.

Storage and administration of diamorphine is controlled under Schedule 2 of the UK Misuse of Drugs Regulations 1985 (Misuse of Drugs Act 1971).

References

See also the relevant Cochrane reviews

Barker DP, Simpson J, Barrett DA, *et al*. Randomised double blind trial of two loading dose regimens of diamorphine in ventilated newborn infants. *Arch Dis Child* 1995; **73**:F22–6. [RCT]

Barrett DA, Barker DP, Rutter N, *et al*. Morphine, morphine 6 glucuronide and morphine 3 glucuronide pharmacokinetics in newborn infants receiving diamorphine infusions. *Br J Clin Pharmacol* 1996;**41**:531–7.

Drugscope. *Substance misuse in pregnancy*. London: Drugscope, 2005.

Hunt RW, Tzioumi D, Collins E, *et al*. Adverse neurodevelopmental outcome of infants exposed to opiate in-utero. *Early Hum Dev* 2008;**84**:29–35. [SR]

Kidd S, Brennan S, Stephen R, *et al*. Comparison of morphine concentration-time profiles following intravenous and intranasal diamorphine in children. *Arch Dis Child* 2009;**94**:974–8.

Use
Diazepam is a sedative and anxiolytic. Its effect as a muscle relaxant is used in the management of neonatal tetanus. Seizures are better controlled using other benzodiazepines such as lorazepam or midazolam (q.v.).

Pharmacology
Diazepam is an anxiolytic, first marketed in 1963, that has also been used to control status epilepticus. It has a long half life (20–60 hours), and the drug and its pharmacologically active metabolite N-desmethyl diazepam both accumulate in maternal and fetal tissues ($V_D \sim 1.3$ l/kg). The neonatal half life is even longer, and a maternal dose of 30 mg or more in the 15 hours before delivery (once commonly used to manage toxaemia) can cause severe hypotonia, respiratory depression, temperature instability and feeding difficulty, particularly in babies of short gestation. Some (but not all) reports suggest that high-dose exposure in early pregnancy could be teratogenic. Withdrawal symptoms with jitteriness and hypertonia are common in babies born to women using this drug in an addictive way during pregnancy. Use during lactation only exposes the baby to a tenth of the maternal dose (on a weight-for-weight basis), but there are reports of sedation and poor weight gain, particularly in babies who had also been exposed to diazepam before delivery.

Neonatal tetanus
Tetanus (lock-jaw), due to infection with *Clostridium tetani*, was recently estimated by WHO to be causing the death of up to 6% of all newborn babies in some parts of the world. This anaerobic, spore-forming, Gram-positive bacillus typically gains access to the body through a wound or area of damaged tissue contaminated by dirt or faecal material, giving off a neurotoxin with an effect similar to strychnine that last several weeks. Ear drops, if contaminated, can cause tetanus in young children with chronic otitis media. Umbilical infection must be suspected *immediately* in any baby starting to develop increasingly frequent, stimulus triggered muscle spasms and sympathetic overactivity 4–14 days after birth. Start high-dose metronidazole (q.v.) or, if that is unavailable, IV or IM penicillin, and debride any gangrenous tissue. Give a 150 mg/kg IM dose of human (or equine) tetanus immunoglobulin at once to neutralise systemic toxins, and consider one intrathecal dose (1000 units of the preservative-free IV product diluted to 2 ml with sterile water) in patients presenting early. Give 0.5 ml of tetanus toxoid into a different limb. Minimal handling, care in a quiet dark room, tube feeding and sedation with IM paraldehyde (q.v.), followed by regular oral (or IV) diazepam, can minimise the painful spasms. A continuous IV infusion of magnesium sulphate (q.v.) reduced the need for other medication in one recent trial in adult patients. Some babies need respiratory support. Prior maternal immunisation (two 0.5 ml doses of vaccine a month apart) and appropriate cord care could completely eliminate this painful, costly illness.

Treatment
Tetanic muscle spasm: A titration of 0.5 mg/kg per hour IV will usually control spasm, but a few need double this dose. Switch to oral (or rectal) treatment and then reduce the dose used over 2–4 weeks. Depression of the swallowing reflex can render oral secretions hazardous. Monitor respiration.
Seizures: A 300 microgram/kg dose IV will stop most seizures for several hours. A 500 microgram/kg rectal dose is usually, but not always, equally effective. Other anticonvulsants, such as lorazepam or midazolam, provide more sustained control.

Antidote
Flumazenil is a specific antidote (as described in the monograph on midazolam).

Supply and administration
Diazepam: Use the emulsified IV preparation (Diazemuls®) in the neonate; 2 ml (10 mg) ampoules cost 32p. Dilute any continuous infusion in 10% glucose, and use within 6 hours. Other IV formulations contain potentially toxic benzyl alcohol (15–55% w/v), and some also contain 40% w/v propylene glycol. A 1 mg/ml oral solution is available in some countries. A rapidly absorbed rectal preparation (Stesolid®) is also available in 2.5 ml tubes containing 2.5, 5 or 10 mg of diazepam per tube (costing 90p to £1.60 each). Avoid the IM route – it is painful, and absorption is slow and incomplete. Diazepam is a UK schedule 4 controlled drug.
Tetanus immunoglobulin: Human antitetanus immunoglobulin (HTIG) is available for IM use in 250 unit ampoules, and in £15 prefilled syringes. A lyophilised IV product is also available; it is distributed in the UK by the Blood Transfusion Service. Store at 4°C.
Tetanus vaccine: 0.5 ml vials of an adsorbed tetanus toxoid suspension cost 74p. For details of the combined vaccine used in infancy see the monograph on the whooping cough vaccine. Store at 4°C.

References
See also the relevant Cochrane reviews and UK guideline on tetanus immunisation

Ahmadsyah I, Salim A. Treatment of tetanus: an open study to compare the efficacy of procaine penicillin and metronidazole. *BMJ* 1985;**291**:648–50.

Khoo BH, Less EL, Lam KL. Neonatal tetanus treated with high dose diazepam. *Arch Dis Child* 1978;**53**:737–9.

Miranda-Filho D de B, Ximenes R A de A, Barone AA, *et al*. Randomised controlled trial of tetanus treatment with antitetanus immunoglobulin by the intrathecal or intramuscular route. *BMJ* 2004;**328**:615–17. [RCT]

Ogatu BR, Newton CRJC, Crawley J, *et al*. Pharmacokinetics and anticonvulsant effects of diazepam in children with severe falciparum malaria and convulsions. *Br J Clin Pharmacol* 2002;**53**:49–75.

Tullu MS, Deshmukh CT, Kamat JR. Experience of pediatric tetanus. Cases from Mumbai. *Indian Pediatr* 2000;**37**:765–71.

Use

Diazoxide is used to treat intractable hypoglycaemia in the neonate when this is being caused by persisting excessive insulin production (hyperinsulinism).

Pharmacology

Diazoxide was once quite widely used to control hypertension in pregnancy, but high-dose (75 mg) bolus use can cause dangerous hypotension, while use during labour can affect uterine tone and delay labour unless oxytocin is prescribed as well. Use in labour can also have a transient impact on neonatal glucose homeostasis. Use during lactation has not been studied but, because of the drug's low molecular weight, it probably appears in breast milk. Diazoxide is now most commonly used to control the hypoglycaemia caused by hyperinsulinism. Insulin secretion by pancreatic β cells is controlled by ATP-sensitive potassium (K_{ATP}) channels. In the presence of glucose the channels close, leading to depolarisation of the cell membrane, an influx of calcium ions and insulin secretion. Diazoxide inhibits insulin secretion by opening these channels.

Neonatal hyperinsulinism sometimes resolves within 1–2 days of birth (as it does in infants of diabetic mothers) making drug treatment quite unnecessary. In other babies, hyperinsulinism can persist for some weeks (usually following intrauterine growth retardation or perinatal asphyxia) and diazoxide can be helpful in these patients. More persistent hyperinsulinaemic hypoglycaemia ('nesidioblastosis') is a heterogeneous condition, but most cases appear to result from genetic defects and many cases respond to treatment with diazoxide. However, an IV line for giving glucose **must** remain in place until a management regimen has been established that eliminates all risk of damaging symptomatic hypoglycaemia. If this proves difficult there must be no delay in arranging prompt tertiary referral. Some severe cases require partial pancreatectomy (for focal adenomatous islet cell hyperplasia) or subtotal pancreatectomy (for diffuse β cell hyperfunction).

Diazoxide is well absorbed by mouth and has a long half life (10–20 hours), so it can usually be given by mouth. In patients only thought to have transient hyperinsulinism, fasting tolerance should be monitored for about 5 days after diazoxide is withdrawn to ensure that there is no longer a risk of hypoglycaemia. Complete resolution is less likely in cases of hyperinsulinism persisting beyond the neonatal period, but the severity of the problem decreases with time and in most children it is possible to withdraw treatment after 5–6 years. Excessive hair growth is almost inevitable if treatment is continued for more than a few months, and leucopenia and eosinophilia are also seen on occasion. Although diazoxide is a thiazide derivative, it has an *anti*diuretic effect: giving chlorothiazide (q.v.) prevents fluid and salt retention and helps to raise glucose concentrations. A few patients who do not have the K_{ATP} channel defect benefit (for reasons that are not very clear) from being given 100–800 micrograms/kg of oral nifedipine (q.v.) once every 8 hours. The management of children who can not be stabilised with diazoxide is outlined in the monograph on octreotide.

Diagnosis

Any baby who is persistently found to need more than 9 mg/kg of IV glucose a minute to maintain a normal blood glucose level is almost certainly displaying at least transient evidence of hyperinsulinism.

Treatment

Diazoxide: Start by giving 5 mg/kg once every 8 hours (orally rather than IV where possible) as soon as it is clear that there is hyperinsulinaemia. Doses higher than this are seldom necessary, but a few babies derive optimum benefit when given 20 mg/kg a day. If the baby is going to respond, some benefit will be seen within 48 hours. The dose can then be reduced gradually once normoglycaemia has been achieved, but care *must* be taken not to let the blood glucose level fall below 3·5 mmol/l. Treatment can usually be stopped once a child only seems to need a 1·5 mg/kg dose, but 'weaning' should only be attempted in a hospital setting.

Chlorothiazide: Give all babies less than a few months old 4 mg/kg of chorothiazide by mouth as well two or three times a day to minimise the risk of excessive fluid retention.

Managing episodes of hypoglycaemia

Hypoglycaemia is particularly dangerous when caused by a high insulin level because, in this situation, fatty acid and ketone body formation is reduced. Give 0·5–1 mg of glucagon (q.v.) IM if IV access is not immediately available, but get IV glucose started after this to counteract the rebound in insulin this will cause.

Supply

Ampoules of diazoxide (300 mg in 20 ml) cost £30 each. Protect from light. A sugar-free oral suspension that is stable for a week can be made from a powder provided by Idis World Medicine, and a 50 mg/ml oral suspension (Proglycem®) containing 7·25% alcohol is available in America.

References

Hoe FM, Thornton PS, Wanner LA, *et al*. Clinical features and insulin regulation in infants with a syndrome of prolonged neonatal hyperinsulinism. *J Pediatr* 2006;**148**:207–12.

Kapoor RR, Flanagan SE, James C, *et al*. Hyperinsulinaemic hypoglycaemia. [Review] *Arch Dis Child* 2009;**94**:450–7.

Lindley KJ, Dunne MJ. Contemporary strategies in the diagnosis and management of neonatal;hyperinsulinaemic hypoglycaemia. [Review] *Early Hum Dev* 2005;**81**:61–72.

Michael CA. Intravenous labetalol and intravenous diazoxide in severe hypertension compromising pregnancy. *Aust N J Obstet Gynaecol* 1986;**26**:26–9. [RCT]

Mohnike K, Blankenstein O, Pfluetzner A, *et al*. Long-term non-surgical therapy of severe persistent congenital hyperinsulinism with glucagon. *Horm Res* 2008;**70**:59–64.

Use
Didanosine is always used in combination with other drugs and is not first line treatment for the control of human immunodeficiency virus (HIV) infection.

Pharmacology
Didanosine (DDI or ddI) is a nucleoside reverse transcriptase inhibitor (NRTI), developed in 1986, with many of the same properties as lamivudine (q.v.), though lamivudine is better tolerated. Didanosine is quite rapidly hydrolysed and inactivated by stomach acid and, as a result, the drug usually comes co-formulated with an antacid. The drug's bioavailability is also further reduced if it is taken with, or shortly after, food. Clearance is related to postnatal age, rising rapidly in the first week of life and then more slowly over the next 3–4 months. Serious adverse effects include retinal depigmentation, optic neuritis, peripheral neuropathy and pancreatitis – most of which are dose related and all of which can be difficult to detect in a young child. All the NRTI drugs occasionally cause liver damage with hepatomegaly, hepatic steatosis and potentially life-threatening lactic acidosis. Sustained use in combination with protease inhibitors such as nelfinavir or ritonavir (see the monograph on lopinavir with ritonavir) can also cause a marked loss of subcutaneous facial and limb fat and an increase in truncal and abdominal fat. Didanosine crosses the placenta, but there is no evidence as yet to suggest that it is toxic to the embryo or fetus. Nothing is known about excretion into breast milk.

Managing overt HIV infection in infancy
No strategy has yet been found for eliminating HIV from the body once it has taken hold, making the prevention of mother-to-child transmission the over-riding priority (as outlined in the monograph on zidovudine), but a wide, and some-what confusing, range of drugs are now available that can slow or halt disease progression.

The drugs currently available are all potentially toxic, and expensive, and they need to be taken, consistently and in the right dose, for life. New information on optimum management becomes available so frequently that anyone treating this condition *must* first familiarise themselves with the latest information posted on the NIH website (www.AIDSinfo.nih.gov) or CHIVA (the children's section of the British HIV Association) website (www.bhiva.org/chiva). Diagnosis and manage-ment must also be discussed with, and supervised by, someone with extensive experience of this condition. Treatment in infancy will be influenced by any prior treatment that the mother has received, but will optimally include zidovudine and lamivudine plus either nevirapine or a protease inhibitor such as lopinavir, nelfinavir or ritonavir in countries where this is affordable. Any clinical deterioration, virological change, or CD4 cell count change, may well call for a complete change of treatment.

Early postnatal prophylaxis
Monotherapy: The usual neonatal dose is 60 mg/m^2 by mouth twice a day, increasing to 100 mg/m^2 twice a day by 3 months old. This is equivalent to a dose of about 3 mg/kg by mouth twice a day in any baby less than 3 months old, and a dose of 4·5 mg/kg at 3 months. Use a lower dose when there is renal impairment.
Combination treatment: Give babies also taking another antiviral drug 100 mg/m^2 once a day.

Monitoring
Pancreatitis is an uncommon but dangerous complication that may be hard to diagnose in a young child. Even an asymptomatic rise in serum amylase or lipase levels merits at least the prompt suspension, if not a complete change, of treatment. Many authorities recommend retinal examination once every 6 months after prior dilatation of the pupils, especially in young children.

Supply
25 mg tablets of didanosine (and an antacid) cost 44p each. These need to be chewed before being swallowed, but they can also be crushed and dispersed in water or apple juice. Didanosine is also usually available as a 10 mg/ml suspension, buffered in an antacid, on a 'named patient' basis which is stable for a month if kept at 4°C. It can not be given IV or IM.

References
American Academy of Pediatrics. Human immunodeficiency virus infection. In: Pickering LK, ed. *Red book: 2003 report of the Committee on Infectious Diseases*, 26th edn. Elk Grove Village, IL: American Academy of Pediatrics, 2003: pp. 360–82.

Kovacs A, Cowles MK, Britto P, *et al*. Pharmacokinetics of didanosine and drug resistance mutations in infants exposed to zidovudine during gestation and postnatally and treated with didanosine or zidovudine in the first three months of life. *Pediatr Infect Dis J* 2005;**24**:503–9.

Mueller BU, Butler KM, Stocker VL, *et al*. Clinical and pharmacokinetic evaluation of long term therapy with didanosine in children with HIV infection. *Pediatrics* 1994;**94**:724–31.

Perry CM, Noble S. Didanosine. An updated review of its use in HIV infection. *Drugs* 1999;**58**:1099–135. [SR]

Rongkavilit C, van Heeswijk RP, Limpongsanurak S, *et al*. Pharmacokinetics of stavudine and didanosine coadministered with nelfinavir in human immunodeficiency virus-exposed neonates. *Antimicrob Agents Chemother* 2001;**45**:3583–90.

Use

Digoxin is still sometimes used, along with a second antiarrhythmic drug, to manage supraventricular tachycardia. It is of little real value in the management of other cardiac problems in the newborn period.

Pharmacology

William Withering's description in 1785 of the value of foxglove leaf as a herbal remedy for 'dropsy' (or cardiac failure) is well known. The active ingredient, digoxin, is still sometimes given to women (250 micrograms, three times a day) to control supraventricular tachycardia *in utero*, because placental transfer is relatively brisk after maternal digitalisation. Aim for a level at the top of the therapeutic range. It is by no means universally effective, however, especially in the hydropic fetus, and flecainide (q.v.) is generally considered a better first option. Quinidine sulphate (starting with 200 mg every 6–8 hours) has occasionally been of benefit in fetuses with atrial flutter after prior digitalisation. Adenosine (q.v.) is the most appropriate first line treatment for this arrhythmia after birth. Digoxin is present in breast milk but this excretion can be ignored when considering clinical management. Digoxin is largely eliminated by the kidney without prior degradation (clearance exceeding GFR). Marked tissue binding occurs, the myocardial levels being linearly related to (and some 20 times) the serum concentration, and twice as high in infancy as in adults, while the neonatal serum half life (55–90 hours) is nearly three times as long as in adults (V_D ~9 l/kg). Clearance is not affected by the serum level, so doubling the dose will double the serum concentration.

Drug interactions

Patients on amiodarone will need – and patients on indometacin may need – a lower dose. The same is occasionally true with erythromycin. Arrhythmias have been reported when digitalised patients are given pancuronium or suxamethonium.

Treatment

The conventional starting dose in micrograms/kg is:

Weight	Total slow IV loading dose	Total oral loading dose	Daily oral maintenance dose
<1·5 kg	20	25	5·0
1·5–2·5 kg	30	35	7·5
>2·5 kg	35	45	10·0

Seek consultant advice. Give half the total loading dose immediately, and a quarter of the total dose after 8 and 16 hours. Digoxin is rather erratically absorbed IM and bioavailability when given by mouth is only 80% of that achieved by IV administration (as reflected above). Use a reduced dose in babies with renal failure and monitor the blood level. ***Check each dose carefully***. An overdose can cause serious arrhythmia and a life-threatening reduction in cardiac output without warning.

Toxicity

While ECG signs may appear when the neonatal serum level exceeds 2 micrograms/l, *clinical* symptoms (with partial AV block or a PR interval of >0·16 seconds) only appear when the level exceeds 3 micrograms/l. Serum levels are not the best way to define toxicity. Control hyperkalaemia with salbutamol (q.v.). Give atropine for AV block, and lignocaine or (if this fails) phenytoin (q.v.) for tachyarrhythmia. Severe bradycardia or block may require transvenous pacing. Ventricular fibrillation will only respond to a DC shock. Control severe toxicity with IV digoxin-specific antibody fragments (Digibind®) in a dose of 0·4 mg for each kg the child weighs multiplied by the measured (or assumed) serum level in micrograms per litre.

Blood levels

Levels can take 10 days to stabilise because of the 2–4-day half life. Collect at least 0·2 ml of serum or plasma 6 or more hours after the last dose was administered (1 microgram/l = 1·28 nanomol/l).

Supply

1 ml (100 microgram) ampoules cost £5·20. The oral syrup (Lanoxin PG®) containing 50 micrograms/ml costs 9p per ml. Both products contain 10% v/v ethanol; the ampoules contain 43% and the syrup 5% v/v propylene glycol. Do not give digoxin IM. Digibind is available in 38 mg vials costing £94 each.

References

See also the relevant Cochrane reviews

Balaguer GM, Jordán GI, Caritg BJ, *et al*. Taquicardia paroxistica supraventricular en el niòo y el lactante. *Ann Pediatr* 2007;**67**:133–8.
Hastreiter AR, John EG, van der Horst RL. Digitalis, digitalis antibodies, digitalis-like immunoreactive substances, and sodium homeostasis: a review. *Clin Perinatol* 1988;**15**:491–522.
Husby P, Farstad M, Brock-Utne JG, *et al*. Immediate control of life-threatening digoxin intoxication in a child by use of digoxin-specific antibody fragments (Fab). *Paediatr Anaesth* 2003;**13**:541–6.
Skinner JR, Sharland G. Detection and management of life threatening arrhythmias in the perinatal period. *Early Hum Dev* 2008;**84**:161–72.
Yukawa E, Akiyama K, Suematsu F, *et al*. Population pharmacokinetic investigation of digoxin in Japanese neonates. *J Clin Pharmacol Ther* 2007;**32**:381–6.

Use

Dobutamine seems to be better than dopamine (q.v.) at improving systemic blood flow, and there is a growing consensus that – although they are harder to measure – cardiac output and systemic tissue perfusion usually matter more than blood pressure. Milrinone (q.v.) should be tried if dobutamine proves ineffective.

Physiology

The normal relationship between systolic blood pressure and gestation at birth is shown in Fig. 1. Pressures rise significantly during the first week of life and then more slowly after that; 95% of babies will have a systolic value within ±35% of the relevant mean shown in Fig. 2 during the first 10 days of life. Thus the most likely value for a 6-day-old baby of 25 weeks' gestation is 50 mmHg, and most will have a systolic pressure of between 33 and 67 mmHg (95% confidence intervals).

Pharmacology

Dobutamine hydrochloride is a synthetic inotropic catecholamine developed in 1973 by the systemic alteration of isoprenaline with a view to reducing some of the latter's unwanted adrenergic effects (i.e. chronotropism, arrhythmias, vascular constriction). It has to be given IV because of rapid first pass metabolism. Dobutamine is a β_1 agonist like dopamine, but in high doses its β_2 effects can decrease rather than increase peripheral resistance. For a brief summary of how drug receptors act see the monograph on noradrenaline. It is about four times as potent as dopamine in stimulating myocardial contractility in low concentration, and of proven value in increasing left ventricular output in the hypotensive preterm neonate, but has less effect than dopamine on blood pressure because it has little effect on systemic vascular resistance. The right dose to use needs to be *individually assessed* because clearance is very variable in children (something that can be done after 10–15 minutes because of the drug's short half life). Tachycardia may occur, and increased pulmonary blood pressure leading to pulmonary oedema has been reported. In general, however, side effects are rare as long as the dose does not exceed 15 micrograms/kg per minute. Extravasation seldom causes the sort of tissue damage seen with dopamine. Note that manufacturers have still not formally endorsed the use of dobutamine in children.

Treatment

Start with 10 micrograms/kg per minute (1 ml/hour of a solution made up as described below). Adjust this dose if necessary after ~20 minutes because of the drug's variable half life (see above), accepting that a few babies need twice as much as this. Prepare a fresh solution every 24 hours.

Compatibility

It is compatible with noradrenaline and the same drugs as for dopamine (q.v.). Do not mix with sodium bicarbonate.

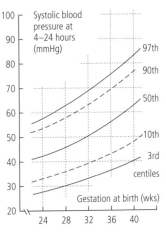

Fig. 1

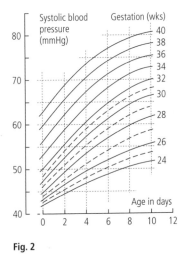

Fig. 2

Supply and administration

20 ml vials of dobutamine hydrochloride costing £5·20 each contain 12·5 mg/ml of dobutamine. To give 10 micrograms/kg of dobutamine per minute place 2·4 ml (30 mg) of this solution for each kg that the baby weighs in a syringe, dilute to 50 ml with 10% glucose or glucose saline, and infuse at a rate of 1 ml/hour. Less concentrated solutions of glucose or glucose saline can be employed.

References

See also relevant Cochrane reviews

Evans N. Which inotrope for which baby? *Arch Dis Child* 2006;**91**:F213–20.
Martinez AM, Padbury JF, Thio S. Dobutamine pharmacokinetics and cardiovascular responses in critically ill neonates. *Pediatrics* 1992;**89**:47–51.
Northern Neonatal Nursing Initiative. Systolic blood pressure in babies of less than 32 weeks gestation in the first year of life. *Arch Dis Child* 1999;**80**:F38–42.
Osborn D, Evans N, Kluckow M. Randomised trial of dobutamine versus dopamine in preterm infants with low systemic blood flow. *J Pediatr* 2002;**140**:183–91. [RCT]
Steinberg C, Notterman DA. Pharmacokinetics of cardiovascular drugs in children: inotropes and vasopressors. *Clin Pharmacokinet* 1994;**27**:345–67.

DOMPERIDONE

Use
This drug is, at present, quite widely used across Europe to treat children with gastro-oesophageal reflux, although there is little evidence of efficacy, and some evidence that it could increase the risk of arrhythmia. It has sometimes been used to manage postoperative gastrointestinal stasis although, in infancy, erythromycin (q.v.) is a better studied alternative. Severe nausea and vomiting is best treated with ondansetron (q.v.).

Pharmacology
Domperidone is a dopamine D_2-receptor antagonist used to relieve nausea and vomiting. It stimulates gastric and upper intestinal motility, and also acts on the chemoreceptor trigger zone. Like metoclopramide (q.v.) it seems to *increase* gastro-oesophageal, and *decrease* pyloric, sphincter tone. It first came into clinical use in 1978 largely as a potent antiemetic. Because of its effect on prolactin excretion it has, like metoclopramide, sometimes been given to women in order to stimulate lactation but the manufacturers have never endorsed the drug's use for this purpose even though several papers, and one recent small controlled trial, have suggested that use can augment the milk supply of some mothers who were having to express their milk following the birth of a preterm baby. For a review of all the drugs that have been used to stimulate lactation see the website linked to the metoclopramide monograph.

Dystonic and extrapyramidal reactions can occur, but are much rarer than with metoclopramide, probably because only a little of the drug crosses the blood:brain barrier. Domperidone is rapidly metabolised by the liver after absorption into the portal vein following oral administration and, because of this 'first pass' metabolism, systemic bioavailability is quite low (15%). Rectal bioavailability is much the same, but the blood level only peaks after an hour (rather than 30 minutes) when the drug is given rectally. The volume of distribution in adults is high (V_D ~5·5 l/kg) and the elimination half life about 7 hours, most of the drug being excreted in the bile and the urine, mainly as inactive metabolites. The only intravenous formulation was withdrawn after high-dose use was occasionally found to cause arrhythmia and even sudden death, and a serious oral overdose could, conceivably, be equally dangerous. Very few pharmacokinetic studies seem to have been undertaken into the drug's use in infancy or childhood. Sustained use for more than 12 weeks is not recommended even in adults, and the manufacturers have not, as yet, made any recommendation as to use in children, except to control the nausea and vomiting caused by cytotoxic drugs and by radiotherapy. Although the drug has a license for use in Canada, it has not been approved for use in the United States, and the US authorities have recently taken steps to try and stop its illegal importation and unapproved use.

Very few formal studies have been undertaken into the use of domperidone in children, and the only trials done to date suggest that domperidone does little for babies with gastro-oesophageal reflux. Since it has now been shown to interfere with cardiac conduction, causing QT prolongation, this risk should be assessed in any infant so treated because cisapride was eventually withdrawn from sale in Europe and North America after it was found to cause similar problems. Little is known about use during pregnancy, but the drug is not teratogenic in animals. Maternal use during breastfeeding is not contraindicated because the baby will receive less than 1% of the maternal dose when intake is calculated on a weight-for-weight basis.

Treatment
Mother: A 10 mg (or 20 mg) dose three times a day for 1–2 weeks may help initiate lactation in the mothers of babies too premature to be put to the breast. Use for longer than this has not yet been studied.
Baby: The usual dose is 300 micrograms/kg by mouth, repeatable every 4–8 hours as necessary. There is relatively little experience of sustained use, and no published data on the drug's use in babies less than 1 month old. It is probably wise to do a paired ECG test to see if treatment significantly prolongs the QT time.

Supply
Domperidone is available as a 1 mg/ml sugar-free suspension (100 ml costs 90p). Small quantities (packs containing not more than twenty 10 mg doses) are available 'over the counter' in the UK to treat flatulence, epigastric discomfort and heart burn in adults, but it has never been licensed for use in the United States.

References

Bines JE, Quinlan J-E, Treves S, *et al*. Efficacy of domperidone in infants and children with gastroesophageal reflux. *J Pediatr Gastroenterol Nutr* 1992;**14**:400–5. [RCT]

da Silva OP, Knoppert DC, Angelini MM, *et al*. Effect of domperidone on milk production in mothers of premature newborns: a randomized, double-blind, placebo-controlled trial. *Can Med Assoc J* 2001;**164**:17–21. [RCT]

Djeddi D, Kongolo G, Lefiax C, *et al*. Effect of domperidone on QT interval in neonates. *J Pediatr* 2008;**153**:663–6. (See also pp. 596–8.)

Grill BB, Hillemeier AC, Semeraro LA, *et al*. Effects of domperidone therapy on symptoms and upper gastrointestinal motility in infants with gastroesophageal reflux. *J Pediatr* 1985;**106**:311–16.

Hegar B, Alatas S, Advani N, *et al*. Domperidone versus cisapride in the treatment of infant regurgitation and increased acid gastro-oesophageal reflux: a pilot study. *Acta Paediatr* 2009;**98**:750–5. [RCT]

O'Meara A, Mott M. Domperidone as an antiemetic in pediatric oncology. *Cancer Chemother Pharmacol* 1981;**6**:147–9.

Pritchard DS, Baber N, Stephenson T. Should domperidone be used for the treatment of gastro-oesophageal reflux in children? Systematic review of randomised controlled trials in children aged 1 month to 11 years old. *Br J Clin Pharmacol* 2005;**59**:725–9. [SR]

Wan E W-X, Davey K, Page-Sharp M, *et al*. Dose–effect study of domperidone as a galactogogue in preterm mothers with insufficient milk supply, and its transfer into milk. *Br J Clin Pharmacol* 2008;**62**:283–9. [RCT]

Use

Dopamine is widely used to treat neonatal hypotension, but it has a variable, unpredictable, dose-dependent impact on vascular tone, and use too often fails to recognise that adequate tissue perfusion, rather than supply pressure *per se*, must be the main aim of treatment. Hydrocortisone (q.v.) may work better, and a dobutamine or adrenaline (q.v.) infusion is a more logical strategy if low cardiac output is the primary problem.

Physiology

Hypotension is currently overdiagnosed (see web commentary), and the 'rule of thumb' that so classifies any baby with a mean arterial pressure, in mmHg, that is less than gestation, in weeks, can often result in a quarter of all day-old babies being classed as hypotensive (Fig. 1). In addition an apparent response to treatment may simply reflect the rise in pressure that normally occurs anyway during the first 2 days of life.

Pharmacology

Dopamine hydrochloride is a naturally occurring catecholamine precursor of noradrenaline (q.v.) that was first synthesised in 1910 and shown to be a neurohormone in 1959. *Low*-dose infusion (2 micrograms/kg per minute) normally causes dopaminergic coronary, renal and mesenteric vasodilatation, but there is little evidence that this is clinically beneficial, and good controlled trial evidence that such treatment does *not* protect renal function, although it does cause some increase in urine output. *High* doses cause vasoconstriction, increase systemic vascular resistance and eventually decrease renal blood flow. While a moderate dose increases myocardial contractility and cardiac output in adults and older children, a dose of more than 10 micrograms/kg per minute can cause an increase in systemic resistance, a fall in gut blood flow and a *reduction* in cardiac output in the neonate especially in the first few days of life. The use of this drug in children has not yet been endorsed by the manufacturer.

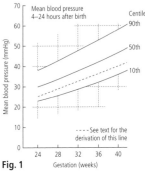

Fig. 1

Correct any acidosis first, and look to see if there is a reason for the hypotension before just treating the symptom itself. Use high-dose treatment with caution after cardiac surgery, or where there is coexisting neonatal pulmonary hypertension, because the drug can cause a detrimental change in the balance between pulmonary and systemic vascular resistance. High doses can also cause tachycardia and arrhythmia in adults. Lack of response may suggest vasopressin (q.v.) exhaustion. Side effects are easily controlled by stopping the infusion because the half life is only 5–10 minutes. There are no known teratogenic effects.

Drug interactions

There are reports of phenytoin and tolazoline causing severe hypotension in patients on dopamine.

Treatment

Start by giving 3 micrograms/kg per minute (or 0·3 ml/hour of a solution made up as described below), and increase this every half an hour as necessary because the response (like the drug's blood level) is known to vary greatly. Always use ultrasound to check the haemodynamic response when using a dose of more than 10 micrograms/kg per minute. Prepare a fresh infusion daily, and stop high-dose treatment slowly.

Compatibility

Dopamine is inactivated by alkali but can be added (terminally) to a line containing fentanyl, lignocaine, midazolam, milrinone, morphine or standard TPN (with or without lipid). See also the monograph on heparin.

Supply and administration

Supply: One stock 5 ml (200 mg) ampoule (pH 2·5–4·5) costs £4·50. To give an infusion of 1 microgram/kg per minute of dopamine, place 0·75 ml (30 mg) of the concentrate for each kg the baby weighs in a syringe, dilute to 50 ml immediately before use with 10% glucose or glucose saline and infuse at a rate of 0·1 ml/hour. (A less concentrated solution of glucose or glucose saline can be used where necessary.)

Administration: Extravasation can cause serious tissue damage, and the management of this is discussed in the monograph on hyaluronidase. Indeed serious blanching along the line of the vein can, in itself, be enough to cause tissue ischaemia, and any infusion is always best given through a 'long line'.

References

See also relevant Cochrane reviews

Batton B, Zhu X, Fanaroff J, *et al*. Blood pressure, anti-hypotensive therapy, and neurodevelopment in extremely preterm infants. *J Pediatr* 2009;**154**:351–7.

Dempsey EM, Al Kazzani F, Barrington KJ. Permissive hypotension in the extremely low birthweight infants with signs of good perfusion. *Arch Dis Child* 2009;**94**:F241–4.

Dempsey EM, Barrington KJ. Evaluation and treatment of hypotension in the preterm infant. *Clin Perinatol* 2009;**36**:75–85.

Laughon M, Bose C, Allred E, *et al*. Factors associated with treatment for hypotension in extremely low gestational age newborns during the first postnatal week. *Pediatrics* 2007;**119**:273–80.

Limperopoulos C, Bassan H, Kalish LA, *et al*. Current definitions of hypotension do not predict abnormal cranial ultrasound findings in preterm infants. *Pediatrics* 2007;**120**:966–77.

DOXAPRAM

Use
Oral or IV doxapram can be useful in preterm babies who continue to have troublesome apnoea despite treatment with caffeine citrate (q.v.). The effects of caffeine and doxapram appear to be additive.

Pharmacology
Doxapram (first developed commercially in 1964) stimulates all levels of the cerebrospinal axis, and respiration appears to be stimulated at doses that cause little general excitation. A plasma concentration of 2 mg/l doubles minute volume in healthy adults, but there is no evidence of any additive benefit from raising the plasma level above 1 mg/l in babies. High doses cause convulsions, and subconvulsive doses can still cause tachycardia, hypertension, hyperpyrexia, jitteriness, laryngospasm and vomiting.

Oral caffeine is usually considered the drug of choice in the management of idiopathic neonatal apnoea but adding doxapram can sometimes bring additional benefit. The drug is usually given as a continuous infusion, but oral treatment is often very effective as long as the dose is doubled to compensate for poor absorption. Developmental delay is not uncommon in survivors and, while severe apnoea may merely be the first sign of some existing cerebral dysfunction that later manifests as developmental delay, a drug-related effect cannot be ruled out until an appropriately designed trial is done. Nasal continuous positive airway pressure (CPAP) may make tracheal intubation and ventilation unnecessary.

Doxapram is metabolised by the liver, the half life in babies (about 7 hours) being double that seen in adults. It is longer still in the first week of life. Significant tissue accumulation occurs (V_D ~6 l/kg), and some of the metabolic breakdown products are also potentially metabolically active. The optimum respiratory response is usually seen with a plasma level of 2–4 ng/ml, but the dose needed to achieve this plasma level varies. Adverse effects are increasingly common when the level exceeds 5 ng/ml. The dose recommended in certain neonatal texts (2·5 mg/kg per hour) is almost certainly potentially toxic in some babies (especially if there is evidence of an intraparenchymal cerebral bleed or an existing seizure disorder). Watch for adverse effects (including hyperexcitability, AV heart block and a rise in blood pressure if more than 1 mg/kg per hour has to be infused for more than 36–48 hours), remembering that doxapram's use in children has not yet been endorsed by the manufacturers.

Treatment
IV administration: Start with 2·5 mg/kg as a loading dose over at least 5–10 minutes followed by a maintenance infusion of 300 micrograms/kg per hour (0·3 ml/hour of a solution made up as described below) and increase the dose cautiously as required. Babies over a week old sometimes only respond to a continuous infusion of 1 or even 1·5 mg/kg per hour. Tissue extravasation can cause skin damage.

Oral administration: Babies who respond to IV doxapram can usually be transferred onto oral maintenance treatment. Take half the total daily dose found effective intravenously and give this once every 6 hours by mouth diluted in a little 5% glucose. High-dose oral treatment sometimes slows gastric emptying. Such problems can usually be resolved by reverting to IV treatment.

Post-anaesthetic use: A single 1 mg/kg IV bolus will sometimes rouse the postoperative preterm baby.

Compatibility
Doxapram can probably be added (terminally) into a line containing standard TPN (but not lipid) when absolutely necessary.

Supply and administration
5 ml (100 mg) ampoules cost £2·10. To give an infusion of 1 mg/kg per hour of doxapram, place 2·5 ml of the concentrate for each kg the baby weighs in a syringe, dilute to 50 ml with 10% glucose or glucose saline, and infuse at 1 ml/hour. (A less concentrated solution of glucose or glucose saline can be used where necessary.) Doxapram is stable in solution, so IV lines do not require changing daily; nor does IV material made available for oral use. The US formulation contains 0·9% benzyl alcohol.

References
See also the relevant Cochrane reviews

Barbé F, Hansen C, Badonnel Y, *et al.* Severe side effects and drug plasma concentrations in preterm infants treated with doxapram. *Ther Drug Monit* 1999;**21**:547–52.

Dani C, Bertini G, Pezzati M, *et al.* Brain hemodynamic effects of doxapram in preterm infants. *Biol Neonat* 2006;**89**:69–74.

De Villiers GS, Walele A, Van der Merwe P-L, *et al.* Second-degree atrioventricular heart block after doxapram administration. *J Pediatr* 1998;**133**:149–50.

Huon C, Rey E, Mussat P, *et al.* Low-dose doxapram for treatment of apnoea following early weaning in very low birthweight infants: a randomised double-blind study. *Acta Paediatr* 1998;**87**:1180–4. [RCT]

Malliard C, Boutroy M, Fresson J, *et al.* QT interval lengthening in premature infants treated with doxapram. *Clin Pharmacol Ther* 2001;**70**:540–5.

Miyata M, Hata T, Kato N, *et al.* Dynamic QT/RR relationship of cardiac conduction in premature infants treated with low-dose doxapram hydrochloride. *J Perinat Med* 2007;**35**:330–3.

Poets CF, Darraj S, Bohnhorst B. Effect of doxapram on episodes of apnoea, bradycardia and hypoxaemia in preterm infants. *Biol Neonat* 1999;**76**:207–13.

Sreenan C, Etches PC, Demianczuk N, *et al.* Isolated developmental delay in very low birth weight infants: association with prolonged doxapram therapy of apnea. *J Pediatr* 2001;**139**:832–7. (See also 2002;**141**:296–7.)

Use

A Gastrografin® enema can be both diagnostic and therapeutic in a young baby with low intestinal obstruction. Macrogols (which act by enhancing the water content of stool in the colon) are the best way to relieve and to control constipation in later infancy.

Pathophophysiology

Once X-rays and clinical examination have rendered a diagnosis of atresia, volvulus or an obstructing hernia unlikely, and the possibility that the failure to pass stool is an iatrogenic complication of opiate sedation has been ruled out, a range of other diagnostic possibilities require consideration.

Meconium plug syndrome: All that may be required to relieve a 'plug' of hard dried gelatinous meconium in the distal colon in the term baby after birth is a 1 mg glycerin suppository plus, on occasion, a rectal washout. Similar problems in the absence of an obvious 'plug' are not uncommon in the preterm baby.

Meconium ileus: Obstruction in the terminal ileum makes meconium ileus a more likely possibility. A disimpacting enema may be all that is needed to deal with the sticky viscid meconium, but a minority require the resection of 20–40 cm of small bowel and a primary re-anastomosis. Most of these children will be found to have cystic fibrosis, requiring treatment with pancreatin (q.v.) and access to long-term, high-quality care to try and minimise the inevitable pulmonary complications of this recessively inherit condition.

Milk curd obstruction: Early milk feeding can sometimes result in undigested milk curds reaching the far end of the small bowel and impacting there. A Gastrografin enema carried out skilfully can be both diagnostic and therapeutic but some cases come to surgery, especially if there has been a focal perforation. The problem, if recognised promptly, should have no long-term consequences and can be distinguished from necrotising enterocolitis (NEC) because there is no intramural gas on X-ray and histology fails to reveal any bacterial invasion of the gut wall.

Faecal constipation: Serious constipation is rare in the first year of life. When it does occur it is probably best treated (once Hirschsprung disease has been excluded), as in older children, by using an osmotic agent to increase the water content of the stool. Here there is good evidence that the best approach is to use a macrogol (polyethylene glycol) first to disimpact the rectum and then, in a lower dose, for a sustained period until bowel tone returns to normal. Delay can cause behavioural problems to develop, and the longer the problem is left unaddressed the longer it will take for function to recover. Chronic idiopathic pseudo-obstruction (Heneyke *et al.* 1999) is one extremely rare cause of very severe intestinal dysmotility due to an, as yet, poorly understood disorder of the enteric neuromusculature that can present with intractable constipation from a very early age.

Treatment

Bowel impaction in the neonate: A Gastrografin enema, administered under fluoroscopic control, has been widely used to disimpact the lower bowel in babies without resort to surgery ever since Helen Noblett first described this approach in 1969. A rectal biopsy to exclude Hirschsprung disease is called for if the stool pattern does not become normal after this.

Constipation in later infancy: Give 600 mg/kg of macrogol once a day by mouth. More may sometimes be needed, especially at first. Manufacturers have not recommended use in children less than 1 year old.

Supply and administration

Macrogols: Non-absorbed polymers of high molecular weight (such as polyethylene glycol 3350) are usually used. Movicol Paediatric Plain® (which contains supplementary electrolytes) is the commercial product most often used in Europe. Dissolve one 6·5 gram sachet of powder (costing 15p) in 65 ml of water immediately before use to obtain a 100 mg/ml solution. An identical generic product is available in America, but here an electrolyte-free product (Miralax®) in 17 gram packs is most commonly used to treat constipation.

Gastrografin: 100 ml of this iodinated monomeric contrast medium (sodium and meglumine amidotrizoate) costs £14. Dilute 15–30 ml with five times as much 0·9% sodium chloride and then give slowly into the rectum through a plain 8 French gauge catheter while screening the enema's progress into the colon.

Glycerol: Pre-moistened l gram suppositories (costing 7p each) are often given to preterm babies.

References

Abhayabkar A, Carcani I, Clayden G. Constipation in children. *BMJ Clinical evidence handbook*. London: BMJ Books, 2008: pp. 80–1 (and updates). [SR]

Burke MS, Ragi JM, Karamanoukian HL, *et al*. New strategies for nonoperative management of meconium ileus. *J Pediatr Surg* 2002;**37**:760–4.

Candy D, Belsey J. Macrogol (polyethylene glycol) laxatives in children with functional constipation and faecal impaction: a systematic review. *Arch Dis Child* 2009;**94**:156–60. [SR]

Hajivassiliou CA. Intestinal obstruction in neonatal pediatric surgery. *Semin Pediatr Surg* 2003;**12**:241–53.

Heneyke S, Smith VV, Spitz L, *et al*. Chronic intestinal pseudo-obstruction: treatment and long term follow up of 44 patients. *Arch Dis Child* 1999;**81**:21–7.

Keckler SJ, St Peter SD, Spilde TL, *et al*. Current significance of meconium plug syndrome. *J Pediatr Surg* 2008;**43**:896–8.

Noblett HR. Treatment of uncomplicated mecomium ileus by gastrografin enema: a preliminary report. *J Pediatr Surg* 1969;**4**:190–7.

Pijpers MAM, Tabbers MM, Benninga MA, *et al*. Currently recommended treatments of childhood constipation are not evidence based: a systematic literature review on the effect of laxative treatment and dietary measures. *Arch Dis Child* 2009;**94**:117–31. [SR]

ENOXAPARIN

Use
Enoxaparin is a fractionated, low molecular weight, derivative of heparin (q.v.) with most of the same properties as the parent compound, but a longer duration of action, given subcutaneously rather than IV.

Pharmacology
Enoxaparin was first prepared by the depolymerisation of porcine heparin in 1981. A range of other low molecular weight heparins are now available, including certoparin, dalteparin sodium, reviparin sodium and tinzaparin sodium. All have very similar properties, although the recommended dose of the various products is not always identical. This monograph will concentrate on the use of enoxaparin because this is the product that has been most widely studied in pregnancy and the neonatal period. The pharmacology of this fractionated peptide is as outlined in the monograph on heparin. Manufacturers have not yet recommended use in children in the UK or USA. Danaparoid sodium is often used in adults allergic to heparin or developing thrombocytopenia while taking low molecular weight heparin.

Low molecular weight products have a longer half life, cause less osteoporosis and thrombocytopenia, and have a more predictable pharmacodynamic (anticoagulant) effect. Despite this the effective dose varies widely, and needs to be individually titrated. Neonates also generally need a high dose (as with heparin). Administration by subcutaneous rather than IV injection makes treatment much easier, but also makes an overdose less easily treatable. There is no evidence of teratogenicity. Lactation during treatment is also safe: the high molecular weight makes significant transfer into breast milk very unlikely, and any drug entering the milk would be inactivated in the gut before absorption. In 12 babies who did breastfeed while the mothers took 40 mg a day the anti-Xa level did not change.

Maternal thromboembolism
Prophylaxis: Give 40 mg subcutaneously once a day from early pregnancy until 6 weeks after delivery (20 mg in women weighing under 50 kg). High-risk patients with thrombophilia, immobility, obesity, pre-eclampsia or a past history of deep vein thrombosis should have 40 mg twice a day. Delay use on the day operative (or epidural) delivery is planned until 4 hours after the procedure is over.
Treatment: Give a 1 mg/kg subcutaneous injection once every 12 hours. Start treatment promptly, as soon as a clot or embolus is seriously suspected, after first taking blood for a full thrombophilia screen (see below) and confirm that renal and liver function are normal. Then adjust treatment for maintenance purposes to optimise the peak anti-Xa level. *Always* revert to heparin from the day before until 6 hours after delivery while continuing to give just 40 mg of enxaparin once a day. Anticoagulant use makes epidural anaesthesia potentially dangerous.

Neonatal treatment
Prophylaxis: Experience is extremely limited. Try 750 micrograms/kg once every 12 hours (or 500 micrograms/kg in babies over 2 months old).
Treatment: A subcutaneous dose of 1·7 mg/kg once every 12 hours normally produces an anti-Xa level of 0·5–1·0 units/ml, but all treatment needs to be individualised. Preterm babies sometimes need over 2 mg/kg, while babies over 2 months old usually only need about 1 mg/kg every 12 hours.

Dose monitoring
Take blood 3–4 hours after the subcutaneous injection to assess the peak anti-Xa level, and adjust the dose to achieve a level of 0·6–1·0 units/ml during treatment, and 0·35–0·7 units/ml during prophylaxis.

Antidote
Protamine sulphate will usually stop overt haemorrhage as summarised in the monograph on heparin.

Supply and administration
The drug is available in a range of prefilled syringes containing 100 mg/ml (10,000 units/ml) of enoxaparin; 0·2, 0·4, 0·6, 0·8 and 1·0 ml syringes cost from £3·20 to £6·70 each. 300 mg (0·3 ml) ampoules containing 0·9% benzyl alcohol exist in America. To make a more dilute 10 mg/ml preparation for accurate neonatal use, draw 0·1 ml into a 1 ml syringe and make up to 1 ml with water for injection just before use.

References
See also the UK guideline on thromboprophylaxis in pregnancy

Ho SH, Wu JK, Hamilton DP, *et al*. An assessment of published pediatric dosage guidelines for enoxaparin: a retrospective review. *J Pediatr Hematol Oncol* 2004;**26**:561–5.

Lim W, Eikelboom JW, Ginsberg JS. Inherited thrombophilia and pregnancy associated venous thromboembolism. [Review] *BMJ* 2007;**334**:1318–21.

Malowany JI, Managle P, Knoppert DC, *et al*. Enoxaparin for neonatal thrombosis: a call for a higher dose in neonates. *Thromb Res* 2008;**122**:826–30.

McLintock C, McCowan LME, North RA. Maternal complications and pregnancy outcomes in women with mechanical prosthetic heart valves treated with enoxaparin. *B J Obstet Gynaecol* 2009;**116**:1585–92.

Michaels LA, Gurian M, Hegyi T, *et al*. Low molecular weight heparin in the treatment of venous and arterial thromboses in the premature infant. *Pediatrics* 2004;**114**:703–7.

Paidas MJ, Ku D-HW, Arkel YS. Screening and management of inherited thrombophilias in the setting of adverse pregnancy outcome. *Clin Perinatol* 2004;**31**:783–805.

Streif W, Goebel G, Chan AKC, *et al*. Use of low molecular mass heparin (enoxaparin) in newborn infants: a prospective cohort study of 62 patients. *Arch Dis Child* 2003;**88**:F365–70.

Use

Replacement therapy using recombinant DNA technology is starting to make it possible to treat a few conditions caused by a specific congenital enzyme deficiency. While this treatment, which may need to be continued for life where stem cell transplantation is not an option, is both burdensome and expensive, its use can be justified for some seriously disabling conditions – especially if started early.

Pharmacology

Animal cell lines are genetically engineered to secrete the missing human enzyme which is then given intravenously once every 1–2 weeks after careful purification. Premedication may come to be needed for transfusion reactions.

Congenital enzyme deficiencies

Gaucher disease: This is a recessively inherited lysosomal storage disorder (LSD) in which sphingolipid accumulation occurs because of acid β-glucosidase deficiency. Manifestations are very variable, and the diagnosis is seldom obvious at birth. It presents with anaemia, thrombocytopenia and a bleeding tendency, noticeable enlargement of the liver and spleen, and progressive skeletal problems. Several thousand patients with type I disease (in which there is no neurological involvement) have now received *imiglucerace* enzyme replacement therapy which, if sustained, can render patients almost symptom free. However, because the enzyme does not cross the blood:brain barrier, this is of little help to the minority with early progressive neurological involvement (type II disease). Treatment should not be stopped during pregnancy or lactation.

Hurler syndrome: In this LSD, mucopolysaccharides accumulate because of a recessively inherited deficiency of α-L-iduronidase. Patients with severe symptoms are classed as having Hurler syndrome, and those with only minor symptoms as having Scheie disease. *Laronidase* enzyme replacement therapy can contain symptoms but, because it does not cross the blood:brain barrier, stem cell transplantation is usually offered, despite the risk involved, once a match is found.

Pompe disease: In this LSD, a recessively inherited α-glucosidase enzyme deficiency causes excess glycogen to accumulate in muscle. Expression is variable. In the infantile form hypertrophic cardiomyopathy and profound myopathy used to cause death within 18 months. *Myozyme* enzyme replacement therapy has been a spectacular success for these children if started early, although some skeletal myopathy may remain – especially if it is already present when treatment is started.

Treatment

Never initiate treatment with any of these products except in consultation with a specialist advisory centre.

Imiglucerase: Give 60 units/kg IV slowly over 1–2 hours once every 2 weeks.

Laronidase: Give 100 units/kg (0·58 mg/kg) as a slow IV infusion through a 0·2 μm line filter once a week.

Myozyme: Give 20 mg/kg as a slow IV infusion through a 0·2 μm line filter once every 2 weeks.

Supply and administration

Keep all vials at 2–8°C, but let these come to room temperature for 20 minutes before reconstitution. Give all early doses of laronidase and myozyme over 4 hours (later doses can often be given a little quicker).

Imiglucerase: 200 unit vials cost £550. Reconstitute the powder with 5·1 ml of water to obtain a 40 units/ml solution. Take a syringe containing 5 ml/kg of 0·9% sodium chloride, add the appropriate amount of reconstituted imiglucerase, and then give this IV over not less than 60 minutes within 3 hours of reconstitution.

Laronidase: 500 unit (5 ml) vials cost £460. Dilute the required dose in enough 0·9% sodium chloride to end up with 100 ml of infusate and then give this IV. Do not agitate the solution and do not use a filter needle.

Myozyme: 50 mg (10 ml) vials cost £385. Reconstitute the powder by allowing 10·3 ml of water to run slowly down the side of the vial. Check that the solution is colourless and clear (a few colourless strands may persist). Draw into a large syringe, and add enough 0·9% sodium chloride to achieve a concentration of 0·5–4 mg/ml.

References

Anderson H, Kaplan P, Kacena K, *et al*. Eight-year clinical outcomes of long-term replacement therapy for 884 children with Gaucher disease type I. *Pediatrics* 2008;**122**:1182–90.

Chien Y-H, Lee N-C, Thurberg BL, *et al*. Pompe disease in infants: improving the prognosis by newborn screening and early treatment. *Pediatrics* 2009;**124**:e1116–25.

Clarke LA, Wraith JE, Beck M, *et al*. Long-term efficacy and safety of laronidase in the treatment of mucopolysaccadidosis I. *Pediatrics* 2009;**123**:229–40.

Coman DJ, Hayes IM, Collins V, *et al*. Enzyme replacement therapy for mucopolysacchiridoses: opinions of patients and families. *J Pediatr* 2008;**152**:723–7.

Elstein Y, Eisenberg V, Granbovsky-Grisaru S, *et al*. Pregnancies in Gaucher disease: a 5-year study. *Am J Obstet Gynecol* 2004;**190**:435–41.

Grabowski GA, Kacena K, Cole JA, *et al*. Dose–response relationships for enzyme replacement therapy with imiglucerase/alglucerase in patients with Gaucher disease type I. *Genet Med* 2009;**11**:90–100.

Vanier M-T. Disorders of sphingolipid metabolism. In: Fernandes J, Saudubray J-M, van den Berghe G, *et al*., eds. *Inborn metabolic diseases. Diagnosis and treatment*, 4th edn. Berlin: Springer-Verlag, 2006: pp. 479–94.

Vellodi A, Tylski SA, Davies EH, *et al*. Management of neuropathic Gaucher disease: revised recommendations. *J Inherit Metab Dis* 2009;**32**:660–4.

Wraith JE. Mucopolysaccharidoses and oligosaccharidoses. In: Fernandes J, Saudubray J-M, van den Berghe G, *et al*., eds. *Inborn metabolic diseases. Diagnosis and treatment*, 4th edn. Berlin: Springer-Verlag, 2006: pp. 495–507.

Wynn RF, Mercer J, Page J, *et al*. Use of enzyme replacement therapy (laronidase) before hematopoietic stem cell transplantation for mucopolysaccharidosis I: experience in 18 patients. *J Pediatr* 2009;**154**:135–9. (See also pp. 609–11.)

EPOPROSTENOL (Prostacyclin)

Use
Epoprostenol has not lived up to its early promise as a treatment for babies with persistent transitional circulation, but there have been a few reports of IV (or nebulised) administration improving oxygenation in the term baby even when treatment with nitric oxide (q.v.) had proved ineffective.

Pharmacology
Epoprostenol (PGI_2) is a prostaglandin-like substance first discovered in 1976. It is an extremely powerful inhibitor of platelet aggregation sometimes used during renal dialysis and in the management of haemorrhagic meningococcal purpura. Epoprostenol produces rapid, dose-related decreases in pulmonary arterial pressure and pulmonary vascular resistance and came to be used experimentally, therefore, in the management of babies with persistent pulmonary hypertension, or cyanosis due to a persisting transitional circulation. The drug is not metabolised during passage through the lung, but only has a 3-minute half life, making continuous infusion necessary. The drug's rapid action makes efficacy easy to judge but can also leave the baby very drug dependent. Tolazoline (q.v.) is much less expensive but has a much longer half life.

Early experience was encouraging, but a multicentre trial in the 1980s was discontinued because the results were so disappointing, and most experience since then has been equally discouraging. Systemic hypotension can also be a serious problem because of marked systemic vasodilatation. However, since it seems likely that persistent pulmonary hypertension can be caused in a number of different ways, and triggered by different factors, it remains possible that epoprostenol could help an occasional baby. More recently there have been three reports describing the management of seven babies where aerosolised epoprostenol improved oxygenation *without* affecting systemic blood pressure. A reduction in intrapulmonary shunting seemed to account for much of the improvement.

Treatment
Inhaled: Try giving 20 nanograms/kg per minute using a SPAG-2 aerosol generator. Double this dose has also been used with apparent safety. Tail off treatment gradually.
Intravenous: Try a continuous IV infusion of 8 nanograms/kg per minute of epoprostenol (0·2 ml/hour of a solution made up as specified below) to stimulate pulmonary artery vasodilatation, and watch carefully for systemic hypotension. If there is no response it is worth increasing the dose stepwise to no more than 20 nanograms/kg per minute, at least briefly. Even higher doses have been used anecdotally.

Supply and administration
Vials containing 500 micrograms of powder (costing £65), with 50 ml of glycine diluent buffer for reconstitution, are available from the pharmacy. Vials and diluent must be stored at 2–8°C, protected from light, and discarded promptly after use. To prepare epoprostenol for use draw 10 ml of sterile diluent (pH 10·5) into a syringe, inject into the epoprostenol vial, and dissolve the contents completely. Draw the epoprostenol back into the syringe and reunite the contents of the syringe with the residue of the original 50 ml of diluent. A filter is provided for use when drawing up the concentrate. Take 6 ml of the filtered concentrate for every kg the baby weighs, dilute to 25 ml with 0·9% sodium chloride, and infuse at 0·5 ml/hour to infuse 20 nanograms/kg per minute of epoprostenol. Do not employ a dilution of more than 1:6, or use any fluid other than 0·9% sodium chloride. Make up a fresh supply once every 24 hours (the manufacturer recommends once every 12 hours but potency only falls 5% in this time). Watch for tissue extravasation, and tail off any infusion over a number of hours.

References
Bindl I, Fahrenstick H, Peukert U. Aerosolised prostacyclin for pulmonary hypertension in neonates. *Arch Dis Child* 1994;**71**:F214–16.

Eronen M, Pohjavouri M, Andersson S, *et al*. Prostacyclin treatment for persistent pulmonary hypertension of the newborn. *Pediatr Cardiol* 1997;**18**:3–7.

Kaapa P, Koivisto M, Ylikorkala O, *et al*. Prostacyclin in the treatment of neonatal pulmonary hypertension. *J Pediatr* 1985;**107**:951–3.

Kelly LK, Porta NFM, Goodman DM, *et al*. Inhaled prostacyclin for term infants with persistent pulmonary hypertension refractory to inhaled nitric oxide. *J Pediatr* 2002;**141**:830–2.

Lock JE, Olley PM, Coceani F, *et al*. Use of prostacyclin in persistent fetal circulation. *Lancet* 1979;**1**:1343.

Pappert D, Busch T, Gerlach H, *et al*. Aerosolized prostacyclin *versus* inhaled nitric oxide in children with severe acute respiratory distress syndrome. *Anesthesiology* 1995;**82**:1507–11.

Soditt V, Aring C, Gronceck P. Improvement in oxygenation in a preterm infant with persistent pulmonary hypertension of the newborn. *Intensive Care Med* 1997;**23**:1275–8.

Use

Erythromycin, like azithromycin (q.v.), which only needs to be given once a day, is widely used to treat neonatal *Chlamydia*, *Mycoplasma* and *Ureaplasma* infections. Azithromycin is now more widely used to reduce whooping cough cross-infection. Erythromycin marginally, but usefully, delays delivery in a few women with preterm prelabour rupture of membranes (pPROM), and helps some babies with gut motility problems.

Pharmacology

This broad-spectrum macrolide antibiotic, first isolated in 1952, does not enter the CSF. A little crosses the placenta but the amount ingested in breast milk only exposes the baby (weight for weight) to 2% of the maternal dose. There is no evidence of teratogenicity. Erythromycin (1 gram IV every 8 hours) can be given in labour to mothers allergic to penicillin at risk of intrapartum group B streptococcal infection (see under penicillin). Giving mothers with pPROM 250 mg by mouth four times a day reduced delivery within 48 hours by 15% in the ORACLE trial, but delivered no long-term benefit and only delivered a significant reduction in neonatal problems in singleton pregnancy (which was not a prespecified trial outcome). More significantly predelivery use in preterm labour *not* associated with prelabour membrane rupture was associated with a greater risk of cerebral palsy.

Erythromycin is well absorbed by mouth and IV treatment is seldom necessary. The oral preparation (erythromycin ethylsuccinate) has to be hydrolysed to the active base after absorption, and the ester occasionally causes reversible liver toxicity. Sudden arrhythmia has occurred with rapid IV administration, and vomiting and diarrhoea (occasionally caused by pseudomembranous colitis) have been reported in older children, but the drug is, in most respects, one of the more innocuous antibiotics in current use. The serum half life is short (2–4 hours), is unaffected by renal function, and changes little during the neonatal period. Some of the drug appears in bile and urine but most is unaccounted for. Erythromycin is a motilin receptor agonist, but the value of use to speed full enteral feeding and reduce the incidence of TPN-associated cholestasis must be balanced against a knowledge that pyloric stenosis can occur after high-dose use.

Chlamydia infection

Chlamydiae are small intracellular bacteria that need living cells to multiply. Genitourinary infection is particularly common among young women who have had a new sexual partner in the last 12 months if they are not using barrier contraception. Some 5% of women of childbearing age are infected, but two-thirds have no symptoms and, since infection is responsible for two-thirds of all tubal infertility and nearly half of all tubal pregnancy, screening should be available to all high-risk groups. It should certainly be offered to all women requesting an abortion, and to all under 25 years booking for antenatal care. Babies often develop conjunctivitis at delivery, and a few develop an afebrile pneumonitis. Failure to recognise that this is due to *Chlamydia*, and to refer as appropriate, exposes the mother to all the risks associated with progressive unchecked pelvic inflammatory disease. Chronic eye infection (trachoma) causes progressive damage to the upper eyelid and the resultant corneal scaring is the commonest cause of preventable blindness in many countries.

Drug interactions

Erythromycin increases the half life of midazolam, theophylline and carbamazepine, producing potential toxicity. It also prolongs the QT interval and this effect can be dangerously potentiated by interaction with other drugs with a similar tendency such as cisapride. Its effect on the half life of caffeine has not yet been clarified. Increased oral bioavailability can also cause toxicity in a minority of patients on digoxin. Erythromycin also seems to potentiate the anticoagulant effect of warfarin. *Never* give erythromycin to a baby taking cisapride.

Treatment

Systemic infection: Give 12·5 mg/kg every 6 hours by mouth, or infuse IV over 1 hour (to avoid the risk of arrhythmia) as described below. There is no satisfactory IM preparation.
Conjunctivitis: A range of options are outlined in the monograph on eye drops but, where *Chlamydia* is suspected, the most effective treatment is almost certainly a single 20 mg/kg oral dose of azithromycin.
Gut dysmotility: Try 6 mg/kg by mouth once every 6 hours (12·5 mg/kg if TPN cholestasis is a concern).

Supply and administration

1 gram vials of the IV (lactobionate) salt cost £10. When made up with 20 ml of water for injection (not saline), the resultant stock solution contains 50 mg/ml. Individual doses containing 5 mg/ml can be prepared by drawing 5 ml of the stock solution into a syringe and diluting this to 50 ml with non-buffered 0·9% sodium chloride (or with buffered glucose previously prepared by adding 5 ml of 8·4% sodium bicarbonate to a 500 ml bag of 10% glucose or glucose saline). Give IV doses within 8 hours of preparation. The sugar-free oral suspension of erythromycin ethylsuccinate (25 mg/ml) costs 1p per ml and can be kept for up to 2 weeks after being reconstituted from the dry powder if stored at 4°C.

References

See also the relevant Cochrane reviews

Kenyon S, Pike K, Jones DR, *et al*. Childhood outcomes after prescription of antibiotics to pregnant women with spontaneous preterm labour: 7 year follow-up of the ORACLE II trial. *Lancet* 2008;**372**:1319–27. [RCT] (See also pp. 1310–18.)
Low N. Chlamydia (uncomplicated, genital). *BMJ Clinical evidence handbook*. London: BMJ Books, 2009: pp. 513–15 (and updates). [SR]
Ng PC. Use of oral erythromycin for the treatment of gastrointestinal dysmotility in preterm infants. *Neonatology* 2009;**95**:97–104. [SR]
Ng PC, Lee CH, Wong SPS, *et al*. High-dose oral erythromycin decreased the incidence of parenteral nutrition-associated cholestasis in preterm infants. *Gastroenterology* 2007;**132**:1726–39. [RCT]

Use
Erythropoietin stimulates red blood cell production, but has little impact on the need for blood transfusion if blood sampling is kept to a mimimum, and use within a week or so of birth seems to increase the risk of serious retinopathy of prematurity (ROP). High-dose use also increases mortality in adults in renal failure.

Pharmacology
Erythropoietin is a natural glycoprotein produced primarily in the kidneys, which stimulates red blood cell production, particularly when there is relative tissue anoxia. During fetal life it is mostly produced in the liver (which is presumably why babies with renal agenesis are not anaemic). Two commercial versions (epoetin alfa and epoetin beta), both synthesised using recombinant DNA technology, became available in 1986. They have identical amino acid sequences, but different glycosylation patterns. Epoetin alfa is the product most widely used in America, but epoetin beta is the product the manufacturer has been authorised to recommend for use in infancy in Europe. Progressive hypertension and severe red cell aplasia are the most serious adverse effects seen in adults, but they have not been reported in neonates to date. The platelet count may rise. Erythropoietin does not seem to cross the human placenta, and the amount absorbed from breast milk is not enough to affect haemopoiesis (although it could enhance gut maturity) so women should not be denied treatment just because they are pregnant or breastfeeding.

Numerous randomised and blinded, or placebo controlled, trials have now shown that early and sustained treatment with erythropoietin can stimulate red cell production in the very preterm baby, as long as supplemental iron is also given. However large doses have to be given because clearance, and the volume of distribution, are both 3–4 times as high as in adult life. Treatment certainly has a place in the early care of vulnerable babies born to families who are reluctant to sanction blood transfusion on religious grounds. Nevertheless, although early treatment reduces the need for replacement transfusion, especially in the smallest babies, it seldom eliminates it, and no response to treatment is generally seen for 1–2 weeks. In two controlled trials involving 391 babies weighing 1 kg or less at birth, high-dose treatment only marginally reduced the number of transfusions given (1·86 v. 2·66 in one study), and a recent meta-analysis suggests there may be one more case of grade 3 ROP for every 20 babies so treated. Attention to reducing loss into the placenta and loss from blood sampling, together with a more structured approach to transfusion policy, can be at least as effective as treatment with erythropoietin in reducing the need for blood transfusion. As long as the safety of donor blood can be assured, and care is taken to minimise the number of donors used using the strategies outlined in the monograph on blood, cost reduction is limited. Since treatment has to be started early to be effective, and because it is difficult to predict within a few days of birth *which* babies will later become anaemic, all those at high risk need treating, further limiting the drug's cost effectiveness.

Treatment
Give 250 units/kg by subcutaneous injection into the thigh three times a week for at least 3 weeks (treatment was continued for 6 weeks in many of the clinical trials). A higher weekly dose does not seem to be more effective.

Supplementary iron
Erythropoietin will fail to stimulate sustained red cell production if iron deficiency develops. A minimum of 3 mg/kg of elemental iron a day seems to be necessary in the neonatal period, which is more than in any UK formula milk (q.v.). Doubt has been cast over the common practice of giving twice as much as this. For very low birthweight babies supplementation can conveniently be achieved by giving 1 ml of oral sodium feredetate (5·5 mg of elemental iron) once a day, as outlined in the monograph on iron.

Compatibility
Erythropoietin seems equally effective given as a continuous (but not as a bolus) infusion in parenteral nutrition (q.v.), together with 1 mg/kg a day of parenteral iron if oral iron can not be given.

Supply
500 unit and 1000 unit prefilled syringes of recombinant human erythropoietin (epoetin beta) cost £3·90 and £7·80, respectively. The large multidose vials, which require water for reconstitution, should not be used when treating babies because they contain benzyl alcohol. Supplies should be stored at 4°C.

References
See also the relevant Cochrane reviews

Calhoun DA, Christensen RD. Hematopoietic growth factors in neonatal medicine: the use of enterally administered hematopoietic growth factors in the neonatal intensive care unit. *Clin Perinatol* 2004;**31**:169–82.

Franz AR, Pohlant F. Red cell transfusions in very and extremely low birthweight infants under restrictive transfusion guidelines: is exogenous erythropoietin necessary? *Arch Dis Child* 2001;**84**:F96–100.

Garcia MG, Hutson AD, Christensen RD. Effect of recombinant erythropoietin on "late" transfusions in the neonatal intensive care unit: a meta-analysis. *J Perinatol* 2002;**22**:108–11. [SR]

Kotto-Kome AC, Garcia MG, Calhoun DA, *et al*. Effect of beginning recombinant erythropoietin treatment within the first week of life, among very-low-birth-weight neonates, on "early" and "late" erythrocyte transfusions: a meta-analysis. *J Perinatol* 2004;**24**:24–9. [SR]

Ohls RK. Erythropoietin treatment in extremely low birth weight infants: blood in versus blood out. [Editorial] *J Pediatr* 2002;**141**:3–6.

Ohls RK. Human recombinant erythropoietin in the prevention and treatment of anemia of prematurity. *Pediatr Drugs* 2002;**4**:111–21.

Phrommintikul A, Haas SJ, Elsik M, *et al*. Mortality and target haemoglobin concentrations in anaemic patients with chronic kidney disease treated with erythropoietin: a meta-analysis. *Lancet* 2007;**369**:381–8. [SR] (See also pp. 346–50.)

Use

Antibiotic eye drops are used to treat acute bacterial conjunctivitis (ophthalmia neonatorum), and saline eye drops (or fresh tap water) are used to treat chemical conjunctivitis. Tropicamide and phenylephrine eye drops are used to dilate the pupil, proxymetacaine provides surface anaesthesia and hypromellose eye drops ('artificial tears') are used to moisten the cornea when tear production is inadequate, or the baby is paralysed or unconscious. Steroid drops are sometimes prescribed after surgery to the eye.

Pharmacology

Because penetration is limited and rather variable when antibiotics are prescribed topically as drops, a systemic antibiotic should always be given as well if there is serious deep-seated infection. Cyclopentolate is widely used to dilate the pupil but tropicamide may be a better choice because a less concentrated solution is available and the high-dose use of any mydriatic can cause adverse systemic side effects (including ileus). Atropine can be particularly troublesome in this regard. The routine, simultaneous use of phenylephrine, an α-adrenergic sympathomimetic, further improves pupilary dilatation. Proxymetacaine is a local anaesthetic of the ester type (like procaine) that acts by diminishing sensory nerve conduction. Hypromellose is a mixed ether of cellulose that forms a clear, viscous, slightly alkaline, colloidal solution in water. Steroid eye drops (such as betamethasone) with or without antibiotic (such as neomycin) are used to minimise inflammation and the risk of infection after ocular surgery.

Microbiology

Credé pioneered the prophylactic use of silver nitrate drops at birth to prevent blindness from gonococcal infection in 1881, and it had to be given by law for many years in some parts of America. Unfortunately it is not very effective against chlamydial infection, which is now commoner. In addition 1% drops cause a mildly irritating chemical conjunctivitis (a problem made worse if evaporation causes the baby to be exposed to a more concentrated solution). Tetracyline eye ointment is less irritant, but 2·5% povidone iodine drops (which briefly turn the cornea brown) may be a better option when routine prophylaxis is merited. Many of the 'sticky eyes' seen soon after birth are no more than a response to irritating vernix, and are best managed by bathing the eye regularly with fresh, clean tap water. The routine collection of swabs for bacteriology is expensive, and rarely influences management, but swabs *should* be collected to identify the causative agent when eye infection develops in a baby already on treatment. Swab collection when there is unusually severe or persistent inflammation also helps to identify gonococcal or chlamydial infection and the need for parental treatment. Mild conjunctivitis in young children usually clears within days without treatment.

Chloramphenicol eye drops are still widely used to deal with low-grade conjunctivitis (especially where this seems to be due to staphylococcal or coliform infection) except in America, where an unsubstantiated fear of aplastic anaemia, especially following prolonged use, has influenced prescribing. However, gonococcal infection is probably best treated with a single large IV or IM dose of ceftriaxone or ceftazidime (q.v.), while overt *Chlamydia* infection, which can cause inclusion conjunctivitis (or very rarely, if not treated, trachoma), is best managed with oral azithromycin (q.v.). Two weeks of either 1% chlortetracycline, or 0·5% erythromycin, eye ointment is also effective. *Pseudomonas* infection, which is potentially very dangerous but luckily very rare, except in the colonised preterm baby, should be treated with gentamicin eye drops and appropriate systemic antibiotics under the supervision of a consultant ophthalmologist. Look for keratitis or a corneal ulcer using fluorescein if in any doubt, after first anaesthetising the cornea. Herpes conjunctivitis as a first manifestation of generalised neonatal herpes infection requires equally expert management with topical and systemic aciclovir (q.v.). *Any* infection causing ophthalmia neonatorum in the UK is notifiable.

Swabs

Stop the use of antibiotic eye drops for a few hours before taking specimens for bacteriology and wash the eye with saline before swabbing the conjunctiva. Swabs of the purulent exudate may give negative results because the pus itself contains few viable organisms. Taking a second conjunctival swab and placing this in the transport medium provided by the Public Health Laboratory virology service will increase the chance of chlamydial infection being recognised. Smears can also be collected onto two plain glass slides for Gram stain testing to search for gonococci, and to look, by immunofluorescence, for *Chlamydia*, if the diagnosis proves elusive.

Differential diagnosis

It is important to differentiate conjunctivitis from orbital cellulitis associated with underlying ethmoiditis or maxillary osteomyelitis requiring urgent systemic treatment. A chronic watery discharge is usually due to congenital nasolacrimal duct obstruction (a very common condition that almost always cures itself and seldom needs treatment unless overt infection supervenes). The main need is to exclude congenital glaucoma, keratitis or uveitis. Pain, photophobia, corneal clouding and conjunctival injection are warning signs. Probing is only called for if problems persist for more than a year.

Contacts

The mother should always be seen and treated as well when venereally acquired neonatal gonococcal or chlamydial infection is encountered. It may also be important to trace the mother's contacts too.

Application

Antibiotic drops: Wait, if possible, until the baby is awake (e.g. immediately before a feed). Wash your hands before handling the baby and again after handling the baby if the eye is infected. Confine the baby's hands with a blanket or wrap

Continued on p. 106

the baby up. Start by using a fresh tissue moistened with clean tap water or normal saline to wipe away any accumulated discharge starting at the inner corner of the eye. Then place 1 drop of medication in the inner angle of the open eye. If the eyes do not open spontaneously it may be necessary to hold them open gently. Always treat **both** eyes unless expressly told not to. Finally wipe away any excess medication, if present, using a fresh swab or tissue for each eye. Make sure the drops do not themselves become infected by letting the pipette actually touch the eye when using a multidose container. Some authorities recommend the use of a separate bottle for each eye (but this is of more relevance following ophthalmic surgery than in the case of the otherwise healthy infant). Eye ointment should be squeezed as a thin ribbon into the gap between the lower lid and the white of the eye while the lower lid is held slightly everted. It is not enough to put ointment on the eyelid.

Screening for retinopathy: Dilate the pupils and anaesthetise the cornea (see web commentary). Gentle pressure on the duct in the inner corner of the eye may stop the drops draining into the nose and into the blood.

Routine prophylaxis at birth

A single drop of 2·5% povidone iodine is very effective. 1% chlortetracycline eye ointment is also an option when available (see the monograph on tetracycline). Squeeze a 1–2 cm ribbon of ophthalmic ointment onto the inside of the lower lid within an hour of birth, after allowing the baby a first breastfeed. Wipe any excess away with a clean swab.

Treatment

0·5% proxymetacaine hydrochloride: This provides corneal anaesthesia in half a minute. Just 1 or 2 drops will usually abolish all sensation for 15 minutes. The drug is called proparacaine hydrochloride in America. There is *no* evidence that use should be avoided in the preterm baby as some influential texts imply.

0·5% tropicamide and 2·5% phenylephrine: These eye drops are used to aid ophthalmic examination. Place 1 drop in each eye 30 minutes before examination is due. Do not be put off by the vasoconstrictive (blanching) seen in the skin round the eye.

0·5% atropine (q.v.): This is used as an eye drop twice a day to keep the pupil dilated after surgery to the eye.

0·3% hypromellose: These eye drops (1 drop in each eye every 6–8 hours) can help to prevent corneal damage in the unconscious or paralysed patient. They do not need a doctor's prescription.

Antibiotic eye drops: These should normally be instilled 6–8 times a day, although more frequent administration is sometimes indicated for the first 24 hours. It is often convenient to give the drops when the baby wakes for feeding and often appropriate to leave the medication for the mother to give (with a little supervision and help) if mother and child are both hospital inpatients. Eye ointments should be applied four times a day. Post-neonatal conjunctivitis is often viral rather than bacterial in origin, and even when it is bacterial there is little good evidence that it clears more rapidly as a result of treatment with antibiotic eye drops.

Steroid eye drops: Steroid eye drops with or without an antibiotic (such as Betnesol-N®) are given once every 6 hours for 5–7 days after ocular surgery to minimise inflammation and the risk of infection.

Saline: Saline (0·9% sodium chloride) eye drops (as minims) do not need a doctor's prescription. However they cost 25p each and their use is hard to justify in babies with a mild (probably chemical) conjunctivitis. Such eyes merely need to be bathed periodically with clean, fresh tap water.

Supply

0·5% tropicamide, 2·5% phenylephrine, 0·5% proxymetacaine, 0·5% chloramphenicol, and 0·9% sodium chloride, are all available as single-dose minims in the UK costing between 25p and 35p each. 0·3% hypromellose BPC eye drops should always be stocked in units undertaking intensive care (10 ml bottles cost 85p), while 0·5% atropine sulphate drops, 0·3% gentamicin drops, 1% fluorescein drops, Betnesol-N eye drops (a combination of 0·1% betamethasone sodium phosphate and 1·5% neomycin) and 3% aciclovir eye ointment are all immediately available on request. It is not normally necessary to use a different dropper bottle for each eye (except after surgery), but it is unnecessarily hazardous for two patients to share the same bottle. 0·5% erythromycin and 1% chlortetracycline eye ointment are no longer commercially available in the UK, but the former is available from Moorfields Eye Hospital, and the latter could be imported on request.

Chloramphenicol minims are now available 'off prescription' in the UK. They are best stored at 2–8°C, but are stable for a month at room temperature. Other minims do can be stored at room temperature.

References
See also the relevant Cochrane reviews ⏺

Epling J, Smucny J. Bacterial conjunctivitis. *Clin Evid* 2006;**15**:89–59 (and updates). [SR]

Isenberg SJ, Apt L, Del Signore M, *et al*. A double application approach to ophthalmia neonatorum prophylaxis. *Br J Ophthalmol* 2003;**87**:1449–52.

Isenberg SJ, Apt L, Wood M. A controlled trial of povidone-iodine as prophylaxis against ophthalmia neonatorum. *N Engl J Med* 1995;**332**:562–6. [RCT] (See also pp. 600–1.)

Rose PW, Harden A, Brueggemann AB, *et al*. Chloramphenicol treatment for acute infective conjunctivitis in children in primary care: a randomised double-blind placebo-controlled trial. *Lancet* 2005;**366**:37–43. (See also pp. 6–7 and 1431–2.) [RCT]

Wilholm B-E, Kelly JP, Kaufman D, *et al*. Relation of aplastic anemia to use of chloramphenicol eye drops in two international case–control studies. *BMJ* 1998;**316**:666. (See also p. 667.)

Use

Fentanyl is used to provide perioperative pain relief. Remifentanil (q.v.) is a very short-acting alternative. A continuous infusion will cause tolerance to develop, and exposes babies to symptoms of opiate withdrawal.

Pharmacology

Fentanyl citrate is a synthetic, fat-soluble opioid first developed as an analogue of pethidine and haloperidol in 1964 that is now widely used to provide rapid short-lived pain relief during surgery. It is also very widely used during epidural anaesthesia in childbirth. Neonatal administration can sometimes cause muscle rigidity and seizure-like activity, and rapid administration seems to make this more likely. Few haemodynamic effects are seen even with high-dose use, and the drug seems to be good at inhibiting the haemodynamic and metabolic effects of surgical stress. It is well absorbed from the gastrointestinal tract, but bioavailability is limited by rapid liver metabolism. Transdermal 'patch' administration can be a good way of managing chronic pain.

Fentanyl's reputation as a short-acting narcotic has tended to obscure the general recognition of its prolonged elimination half life. Significant doses rapidly cause respiratory depression. Its ability to limit pain peaks within 5 minutes (4–8 times sooner than morphine), but its ability to limit pain after a bolus dose may only last 30–60 minutes, because of rapid and cumulative redistribution into fat and muscle depots round the body (neonatal V_D 6–12 l/kg). Sustained use is, therefore, associated with all the problems seen in prolonged thiopental (q.v.) infusion. Elimination is controlled by N-dealkylation and hydroxylation in the liver, and is dose dependent. The half life, like the half life of morphine, is very variable in the neonate (6–30 hours) and only slightly influenced by gestation, but seems to approach that seen in adult life (2–7 hours) within 2–3 months of birth.

Tolerance starts to become progressively more likely in the neonate if fentanyl is used for more than 3 days – similar problems are only seen with morphine after a couple of weeks. A higher plasma level becomes necessary, and a higher dose has to be given. Unpleasant and potentially alarming withdrawal symptoms can then occur, with extreme irritability and hypertonia, unless use is stopped gradually. The drug also accumulates in body fat further delaying drug elimination. Alfentanil might, on theoretical grounds, be a useful alternative, because less tissue accumulation occurs, but muscle rigidity is even more common, and the shorter half life seen in adults is not replicated in infancy. Although fentanyl crosses the placenta moderately well, fetuses of more than 20 weeks' gestation should always be offered a direct 15 microgram/kg injection (based on the best estimate of fetal weight available) if subjected to any potentially painful procedure *in utero*. There is some evidence that epidural use (together with bupivacaine) during childbirth may make lactation rather harder to establish, but breastfed babies only ingest about 3% of the maternal dose on a weight-for-weight basis.

Pain relief

Short-term use: A 5 microgram/kg IV dose depresses respiration and provides good brief analgesia; twice this dose is effective for an hour. A smaller dose (2 micrograms/kg) is more often given, with a volatile agent such as isoflurane, as part of a 'balanced' general anaesthetic.

Sustained use: Give 10 micrograms/kg and then 1·5 micrograms/kg an hour. Tolerance (the need for a larger dose) and withdrawal symptoms become progressively more likely if treatment is continued for more than 3 days. Sustained use depresses gut motility and causes progressive drug accumulation in body fat.

Antidote

Bradycardia after excess fentanyl administration may respond to atropine. Muscle rigidity will respond to muscle relaxants. Naloxone (q.v.) is an effective fentanyl antidote.

Compatibility

Fentanyl can be added (terminally) to a line containing midazolam, milrinone or standard TPN (including lipid).

Supply and administration

2 and 10 ml ampoules containing 50 micrograms/ml cost 23p and £1·10, respectively. Take 0·2 ml (10 micrograms) and dilute to 1 ml with 5% glucose to obtain a solution containing 10 micrograms/ml for accurate low-dose administration. Storage and use are controlled under Schedule 2 of the UK Misuse of Drug Regulations (Misuse of Drugs Act 1971).

References

Arnold JH, Truog RD, Scavone JM, *et al*. Changes in the pharmacodynamic response to fentanyl in neonates during continuous infusion. *J Pediatr* 1991;**119**:639–43. (See also pp. 588–9.)

Fahnenstich H, Steffan J, Kau N, *et al*. Fentanyl-induced chest wall rigidity and laryngospasm in preterm and term infants. *Crit Care Med* 2000;**28**:836–9.

Fisk NM, Gitau R, Teixeira JM. Effect of direct fetal opioid analgesia on fetal hormonal and hemodynamic stress response to intrauterine needling. *Anesthesiology* 2001;**95**:828–35.

Frank LS, Naughton I, Winter I. Opioid and benzodiazepine withdrawal symptoms in pediatric intensive care patients. *Intensive Crit Care Nurs* 2004;**20**:344–51.

Frank LS, Vilardi J, Durand D, *et al*. Opioid withdrawal in neonates after continuous infusions or morphine or fentanyl during extracorporeal membrane oxygenation. *Am J Crit Care* 1998;**9**:364–9.

Jordan S, Emery S, Bradshaw C, *et al*. The impact of intrapartum analgesia on infant feeding. *Br J Obstet Gynaecol* 2005;**112**:927–34.

Saarenmaa E, Neuvonen PJ, Fellman V. Gestational age and birth weight effects on plasma clearance of fentanyl in newborn infants. *J Pediatr* 2000;**136**:767–70.

Taddio A. Opioid analgesia for infants in the neonatal period. [Review] *Clin Perinatol* 2002;**29**:493–509.

FIBRIN GLUE

Use
Fibrin glue, made by mixing bovine or human thrombin and fibrinogen (or cryoprecipitate), can secure haemostasis during surgery when blood oozes uncontrollably from multiple pinpoints on a large raw surface. The glue has also been used experimentally in a few patients with an intractable pneumothorax in order to achieve pleurodesis.

Product
Thrombin is currently available as a sterile freeze-dried powder prepared from bovine prothrombin by interaction with thromboplastin. Its main use is in the ***topical*** control of minor bleeding (as, for example, after dental treatment). It must not be injected or allowed to enter a large blood vessel because it could cause extensive, potentially lethal, intravascular clotting. An impregnated gelatin sponge was frequently used at one time to staunch extensive capillary bleeding, but the main commercial product once available (Sterispon®) has now been withdrawn. A commercial spray kit is also marketed.

Fibrin glue is made from fibrinogen and thrombin mixed in equal parts. The thrombin converts the fibrinogen to fibrin within 10–15 seconds depending on the concentration of thrombin employed. While the extrinsic and the intrinsic coagulation mechanisms are bypassed by this approach, the final common coagulation pathway is faithfully and physiologically replicated. A coagulopathy caused by antibody development has occurred on rare occasions when bovine thrombin is used. Anaphylaxis has also been reported. These hazards could be avoided by the use of human thrombin but no commercial preparation of human thrombin is currently available in the UK. The use of human fibrinogen also brings with it all the theoretical hazards associated with the use of a non-sterilised human product (as outlined in the monograph on fresh frozen plasma). The available products do not have a specific licence for use in children.

Treatment of pneumothorax
Pulmonary air leaks usually respond to drainage and expectant management within 2–3 days, but high-frequency ventilation, selective ventilation of a single lung and surgical exploration are occasionally called for. As a last resort, if all else fails, approximately 2 ml of reconstituted thrombin can be instilled into the pleural cavity followed, after 2 minutes, by 2 ml of fibrinogen or cryoprecipitate. The pleural drains need to be clamped for 3–5 minutes during this procedure. Such a strategy should not be adopted without first discussing the case with a paediatric or thoracic surgeon. Tetracycline and talc have been used successfully in much the same way to minimise the risk of a recurrence in adults. Some would have reservations over using either of these options in the neonate.

Treatment of chylothorax
Congenital chylothorax usually resolves over time with conservative management but carries a high mortality. Pleurodesis has seldom been attempted, but success has been claimed after the intrapleural instillation of 2 ml/kg of aqueous 4% povodine-iodine with opioid analgesia to control any resultant pain. Octreotide has also been used with apparent success when other measures fail. An IV infusion (1–3 micrograms/kg per hour) sustained for several days was used in the 12 reports published to date.

Supply and administration
Supplies of bovine thrombin could be made available by the pharmacy (as long as the request has first been authorised by a consultant), and commercial combination kits containing both bovine thrombin and fibrinogen in separate 2 ml vials (sold by Immuno for £1·40) for use on a 'named patient' basis could be obtained by the pharmacy on request. A second, rather similar product (Beriplast®) is available from Centeon Pharma GmbH, Marburg, Germany, and widely used in Europe. Neither of these products has been licensed for use in the UK or in America. Stocks must be stored at 4°C. The material should be reconstituted as described in the package insert and used within 4 hours. Reconstitution of the Immuno product requires access to a water bath maintained at 37°C.

References
Atrah HI. Fibrin glue. Topical use for areas of bleeding large and small. *BMJ* 1994;**308**:933–4.

Berger JT, Gilhooly J. Fibrin glue treatment of persistent pneumothorax in a premature infant. *J Pediatr* 1993;**122**:958–60.

Brissaud O, Desfrere L, Mohsen R, *et al*. Congenital idiopathic chylothorax in neonates: chemical pleurodesis with povodine-iodine (Betadine). *Arch Dis Child* 2003;**88**:F531–3.

Dunn CJ, Goa KL. Fibrin sealant. A review of its use in surgery and endoscopy. *Drugs* 1999;**58**:863–86. [SR]

Kuint J, Lubin D, Martinowitz U, *et al*. Fibrin glue treatment for recurrent pneumothorax in a premature infant. *Am J Perinatol* 1996;**13**:245–7.

Moront MG, Katz NM, O'Donnell J, *et al*. The use of topical fibrin glue at cannulation sites in neonates. *Surg Gynecol Obstet* 1988;**166**:358–9.

Pratap U, Sklavik Z, Ofoe VD, *et al*. Octreotide to treat postoperative chylothorax after cardiac operations in children. *Ann Thorac Surg* 2001;**72**:1740–2.

Wakai A. Spontaneous pneumothorax. *BMJ Clinical evidence handbook*. London: BMJ Books, 2009: pp. 500–1 (and updates). [SR]

Zeidan S, Delarue A, Rome A, *et al*. Fibrin glue application in the management of refractory chylous ascites in children. *J Pediatr Gastroenterol Nutr* 2008;**46**:478–81.

Use

Filgrastim (and lenograstim) enhance the production and release of white blood cells from bone marrow.

Physiology

Neutrophil white cells (so-called because they form a thin white line above the red cells when blood is spun, and turn neither red nor blue when stained) engulf and kill bacteria. They normally only remain in circulation for ~6 hours after leaving the bone marrow pool before entering other body tissues. Birth causes a transient increase in the number in circulation (Fig. 1), especially when this is stressful. Neonatal sepsis can rapidly *decrease* the number in circulation, because production is already close to its peak at birth. This, and functional immaturity, make babies more vulnerable to infection. Babies of <1·5 kg often have very low counts soon after birth (dotted line), and at 2–4 weeks of age when the marrow mounts its first response to the growing post-delivery anaemia.

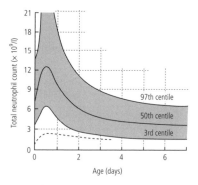

Fig. 1

Pharmacology

Marrow colony-stimulating factors are naturally occurring glycoprotein growth promoters (cytokines) that stimulate the proliferation and differentiation of red and white blood cell bone precursors in bone marrow. A number of these factors – including erythropoietin (q.v.) – have been produced by recombinant DNA technology in the last 15 years. Filgrastim (like lenograstim) is a recombinant version of the human granulocyte colony-stimulating factor (G-CSF), while sargramostim is a recombinant version of the granulocyte–macrophage colony-stimulating factor (GM-CSF). Both enhance the production and release of neutrophil white blood cells from bone marrow, and filgrastim is now being widely used to prevent chemotherapy-induced neutropenia and to speed neutrophil recovery after bone marrow transplantation.

Subcutaneous rather than IV use doubles the elimination half life to about 3 hours, and is believed to increase therapeutic efficacy while minimising the risk of toxicity associated with high peak blood levels. Adverse effects, including fever, dyspnoea, nausea and vomiting, have been very uncommon with neonatal use. Use during pregnancy is associated with increased fetal death in primates. Use during lactation has not been studied but seems unlikely, on theoretical grounds, to pose any serious risk.

The early postnatal and sepsis-induced neutropenia (<1500 neutrophils/mm³) often seen in the preterm baby can frequently be countered by giving G-CSF or GM-CSF, and these cytokines also augment neutrophil function. However, prophylactic use has not yet been shown to reduce the incidence of later infection in the neonatal trials completed to date, and the only trials of treatment have not yet been large enough to show whether treatment can convincingly improve outcome in babies with overt infection. More general use would, therefore, be premature. The one very small head-to-head neonatal trial undertaken to date suggests that treatment with G-CSF can sometimes generate a faster neutrophil response than treatment with GM-CSF. It was much too small to detect any difference in true therapeutic efficacy. The response to treatment is variable, and may turn out to be of least benefit where the need is greatest.

Treatment

Give 10 micrograms/kg of filgrastim (or lenograstim) subcutaneously into alternate thighs (or IV over 30 minutes) once a day for 3 days (0·1 ml/kg of either of the products made up as described below).

Supply and administration

Two very similar G-CSF products are available. Lenograstim is glycosylated, and filgrastim is not. Almost all the neonatal studies reported to date have used filgrastim, but the related product, lenograstim, comes in low-dose vials that can be more economical to use. The manufacturers have not yet endorsed the use of lenograstim in children less than 2 years old, or the use of filgrastim in neonates.

Filgrastim: Add 2 ml of 5% glucose to the 300 microgram (30 million-unit) 1 ml vials of filgrastim (costing £68), to obtain a preparation containing 100 micrograms/ml. Store all vials at 4°C, and do not keep material more than 24 hours once the vial has been opened, even if it is still stored at 4°C.

Lenograstim: 105 microgram (13·4 million-unit) 1 ml vials cost £42. Dissolve the lyophilisate with 1 ml of water for injection (as supplied). Agitate gently, but do not shake. Vials can be stored at room temperature. Reconstituted material should not be kept for more than 24 hours even if stored at 4°C.

References

See also the relevant Cochrane reviews

Ahmad A, Laborada G, Bussel J, *et al*. Comparison of recombinant granulocyte colony-stimulating factor, recombinant granulocyte-macrophage colony-stimulating factor and placebo for treatment of septic preterm infants. *Pediatr Infect Dis J* 2002;**21**:1061–5. [RCT]

Bernstein HM, Pollock BH, Calhoun DA, *et al*. Administration of recombinant granulocyte colony-stimulating factor to neonates with septicemia: a meta-analysis. *J Pediatr* 2001;**138**:917–20. [SR]

Carrison G, Ahlin A, Dahllöf G, *et al*. Efficacy and safety of two different rG-CSF preparations in the treatment of patients with severe congenital neutropenia. *Br J Haematol* 2004;**126**:1327–32.

Kuhn P, Paupe A, Espagne S, *et al*. A multicenter, randomized, placebo-controlled trial of prophylactic recombinant granulocycte-colony stimulating factor in preterm neonates with neutropenia. *J Pediatr* 2009;**155**:324–30. [RCT]

Use

Flecainide is increasingly replacing digoxin (q.v.) in the control of fetal and neonatal supraventricular arrhythmia. Amiodarone (q.v.) will usually work where flecainide does not. Because the manufacturer has not yet endorsed the use of either of these drugs in children, they should only be used under the direct supervision of a paediatric cardiologist.

Pharmacology

Flecainide is a class 1 antiarrhythmic agent that functions as a sodium channel blocker. It is a fluorinated derivative of procainamide, first synthesised in 1975. The drug is well absorbed by mouth, extensively metabolised to a range of non-active breakdown products in the liver, but also partly excreted by the kidney. There is one isolated report suggesting that diarrhoeal illness may actually cause blood levels to rise due to altered absorption. The half life in adults is about 14 hours, and such evidence as there is suggests that the half life is shorter than this in infancy. Tissue levels greatly exceed plasma levels (V_D ~10 l/kg).

The drug crosses the placenta and can be used to control any fetal supraventricular arrhythmia that does not respond to digitalisation. Indeed, it is increasingly being used from the outset where there is hydrops. It suppresses most re-entry tachycardias, and is also effective in atrial ectopic and His bundle tachycardia. Most children with tachycardia first manifesting itself in the perinatal period become symptom free within a year. Where problems persist or return 5–8 years later, radiofrequency catheter ablation of the offending pathways is becoming a progressively more effective long-term solution.

Teratogenic effects have been reported with high-dose treatment in laboratory animals: the relevance of this to the drug's use in early pregnancy remains to be established. The drug causes slowing of atrial, AV nodal and infranodal conduction, increasing the atrial and ventricular muscle's refractory period. The drug exerts little effect on sinus node function, but it increases the PR interval and the duration of the QRS complex. Few extracardiac adverse effects have been noted to date. Some caution should be exercised when the drug is used during lactation because the baby will receive 5–10% of the maternal dose when intake is calculated on a weight-for-weight basis.

The β blocker sotalol (q.v.) has sometimes been used as an alternative strategy for controlling supraventricular arrhythmia, but such comparative information as there is suggests that flecainide is probably the better drug to use both before and after birth. Sotalol may, however, be a better drug to use in the management of atrial flutter (a rare, and potentially lethal, fetal arrhythmia with an excellent long-term prognosis if identified in time).

Treatment

Oral treatment: Start by giving 2 mg/kg by mouth once every 8 hours, and monitor the ECG for at least the first 48 hours because, in one child in 20, this will trigger a slower but incessant form of supraventricular tachycardia. A broad P wave, widened QRS and prolonged PR interval provide early signs of toxicity.
IV treatment: Where other strategies fail a single 1–2 mg/kg dose given IV over about 10 minutes may successfully arrest a dangerous arrhythmia, but this should only be attempted by someone experienced enough to recognise and deal with any unexpected response. Oral treatment should then be started promptly.

Blood levels

The therapeutic plasma range in children is 0·25–0·75 mg/l (which is lower than the level sometimes needed in adults) (1 mg/l of flecainide acetate = 2·10 μmol/l). Trough drug levels can be measured in serum or plasma samples on request by the Analytical Unit, St Georges Hospital, Cranmer Terrace, London SW17 0RE (tel. 0208 672 1255, ext. 5345).

Supply

15 ml ampoules containing 10 mg/ml of flecainide acetate cost £4·40 each. An oral liquid containing 5 mg in 1 ml is available for 'named' patients from Penn Pharmaceuticals. It should *not* be refrigerated.

References

Fenrich AL, Perry JC, Freidman RA. Flecainide and amiodarone: combined therapy for refractory tachyarrhythmias in infancy. *J Am Coll Cardiol* 1995;**25**:1195–8.

O'Sullivan J, Gardiner H, Wren C. Digoxin or flecainide for prophylaxis of infant supraventricular tachycardia. *J Am Coll Cardiol* 1995;**26**:991–4.

Paul T, Bertram H, Bökenkamp R, *et al*. Supraventricular tachycardia in infants, children and adolescents. *Paediatr Drugs* 2000;**2**:171–81.

Perry JC, Garson A Jr. Flecainide acetate for treatment of tachyarrythmias in children: review of world literature of efficacy, safety and dosing. *Am Heart J* 1992;**124**:1614–21.

Use

Flucloxacillin is usually the drug of choice for penicillinase-resistant staphylococcal infection (unless the strain has also become meticillin resistant).

Pharmacology

Flucloxacillin is a non-toxic, semisynthetic, acid-resistant, isoxazolyl penicillin first developed in 1964. It has a side chain that protects the β-lactam ring from attack by staphylococcal (and some other) penicillinases, giving it properties similar to meticillin (known in the US as methicillin). Cloxacillin, nafcillin and oxacillin are closely related products, less well absorbed by mouth, but given in the same IV or IM dose as flucloxacillin. Cloxacillin is generally available in most parts of world, but flucloxacillin is the only product available in the UK. Dicloxacillin, which only differs from flucloxacillin in the substitution of a chlorine for a fluorine atom, is the product available in the US. Its properties very closely parallel those of flucloxacillin.

Flucloxacillin and dicloxacillin are both well absorbed by mouth and mostly inactivated within the body, although a third may appear in the urine. Because they are very non-toxic, the dose used only needs to be reduced when there is profound renal failure. Bioavailability approaches 50% when the drug is given by mouth both in babies and in adults, although the presence of food in the stomach delays absorption. The half life is only 1 hour in adults. It is five times longer than this at birth, but the half life falls rapidly during the first month of life. Drug penetration into the meninges and into bone is limited but, because of its lack of toxicity, high-dose treatment can be used safely in these situations. Anaphylaxis can occur (as with all penicillins) and patients who are hypersensitive to one product are often sensitive to others, but anaphylaxis is extremely uncommon in the neonatal period. Placental transfer is poor and little of the drug appears in breast milk (1 mg/l). Transient diarrhoea is quite common with oral flucloxacillin. While severe, delayed and occasionally lethal cholestatic jaundice has occasionally been seen in adults treated with flucloxacillin for more than 2 weeks, no such problem has yet been recognised with neonatal use.

Maternal mastitis

The main problem, especially in the early days, is usually local engorgement, and this can be overcome by relieving the obstruction and 'emptying' the breast. Recurrent trouble is almost always due to poor positioning, as is confirmed by the fact that the affected breast is nearly always on the side the mother less instinctively holds her baby. A red, swollen, tender area is *not* always a sign of bacterial infection, even if the temperature and pulse are up, or rigors appear, although this possibility always merits maternal treatment with oral flucloxacillin if symptoms persist, even if infection is only a secondary consequence of engorgement. Since infection is almost always staphylococcal in origin, the most appropriate treatment is oral flucloxacillin – 250 mg once every 6 hours by mouth. Cefalexin (q.v.) is a widely used alternative. Antibiotics are, however, no substitute for dealing with the engorgement and reviewing the mother's feeding technique. Never stop feeding just because antibiotics have been started – feed more often, offering the affected breast first. Ibuprofen (q.v.) may help both the pain and the inflammation. Localised *nipple* pain is usually traumatic, but can be due to *Candida* infection as discussed in the monographs on fluconazole and nystatin.

Treatment

Dose: A dose of 100 mg/kg IV or IM is the dose usually recommended locally when treating staphylococcal osteitis, meningitis or a cerebral abscess, but a dose of 50 mg/kg is adequate for most other purposes. These doses are higher than those usually recommended. A dose of 25 mg/kg by mouth is more than adequate when managing most minor infections.
Timing: Give one dose every 12 hours in the first week of life, one dose every 8 hours in babies 1–3 weeks old, and one dose every 6 hours in babies 4 or more weeks old. Treatment should be sustained for 2 weeks in proven septicaemia, for at least 3 weeks in babies with infections of the central nervous system, and for 4 weeks in babies with osteitis or proven staphylococcal pneumonia. Oral medication can often be used to complete a course of treatment, and the dosage recommended here allows for the fact that treatment may well need to be given to a baby who has recently been fed.

Supply and administration

Stock 250 mg flucloxacillin vials cost £1 each. Add 2·3 ml of sterile water for injection to get a solution containing 100 mg/ml. There is no published evidence to suggest that IV doses need to be injected slowly over more than 3–4 minutes. Vials should be discarded after use and never kept for more than 24 hours after reconstitution. A 100 mg/kg dose contains 0·23 mmol/kg of sodium. The stock oral suspension in syrup (25 mg/ml) costs £3·20 for 100 ml. Sustained IV treatment can cause a reactive phlebitis.

References

Adrianzen Vargas MR, Danton MH, Javaid SM, *et al*. Pharmacokinetics of intravenous flucloxacillin and amoxicillin in neonatal and infant cardiopulmonary bypass surgery. *Eur J Cardiothorac Surg* 2004;**25**:256–40.
Bergdahl S, Eriksson M, Finkel Y. Plasma concentration following oral administration of di- and flucloxacillin in infants and children. *Pharmacol Toxicol* 1987;**60**:233–4.
Inch S, Fisher C. Mastitis: infection or inflammation? *Practitioner* 1995;**239**:472–6.
Ladhani S, Garbash M. Staphylococcal skin infections in children: rational drug therapy recommendations. *Pediatr Drugs* 2005;**7**:77–102.
World Health Organisation. *Mastitis. Causes and management*. Geneva; World Health Organisation, 2000.

FLUCONAZOLE

Use
Fluconazole is the antifungal agent now very commonly used both to prevent and to treat invasive neonatal *Candida albicans* infection. Resistant strains respond to caspofungin (q.v.).

Pharmacology
Fluconazole is a potent, selective, triazole inhibitor of the fungal enzymes involved in ergosterol synthesis. The drug is reasonably effective against most *Candida* species, other than *C. krusei* and *C. glabrata*. It is also of value in the treatment of cryptococcal infection (although in this condition treatment needs to be sustained for several weeks). It was first synthesised and patented in 1982. It is water soluble, well absorbed by mouth even in infancy, and largely excreted unchanged in the urine. Penetration into the CSF is good. While high-dose systemic exposure (400 mg/day) in the first trimester of pregnancy can produce a constellation of serious fetal abnormalities, there are, as yet, no reports of teratogenicity with a single 150 mg dose in the first trimester, or with topical or oral use later in pregnancy. Fluconazole is probably the best antifungal to use when *Candida* infects the mother's milk ducts during lactation, even though the manufacturers have never endorsed such use, because the baby only gets ~10% of the weight-adjusted maternal dose.

Fluconazole is increasingly used, even in North America, in the treatment of babies with **invasive** (systemic) *Candida albicans* infection. Studies suggest that it is less toxic and at least as effective as amphotericin B. Liver function tests sometimes show a mild self-correcting disturbance, and rashes can occur, but serious drug eruptions have only been seen in immunodeficient patients. The half life is 40–60 hours at birth, but doubles within 2 weeks. It is 20 hours throughout infancy and childhood, but 30 hours in adults. There is no good reason to give amphotericin B as well as high-dose fluconazole, but there is evidence that effective treatment of all *Candida* species with a minimum inhibitory concentration of ≤8 μg/ml requires a higher dose than many reference texts currently quote (Wade *et al.* 2009). *In vitro* modelling also suggests that high-dose treatment makes the emergence of resistant strains less likely. Oral fluconazole is widely used to treat **superficial** (topical) infection in adults, and is now starting to be used for this purpose in babies. Prophylactic use has been widely studied in the last 10 years (as reviewed in the website commentary), but some prefer to use nystatin (q.v.), which is not systemically absorbed, to minimise the risk of fluconazole-resistant strains proliferating.

Diagnosing systemic candidiasis
Systemic candidiasis is difficult to diagnose, but not rare in colonised ill babies. The isolation of *Candida* from blood should never be ignored, especially if the patient has a long line in place, even if the child seems well. Unfortunately, blood cultures may take days to reveal evidence of infection and can be misleadingly negative, but *Candida* has a predilection for the urinary tract and the presence of budding yeasts or hyphae in freshly voided urine should lead to an immediate search for further evidence of infection. A suprapubic tap can be used to collect urine for microscopy and fungal culture to clinch any diagnosis and prove that treatment has been effective. Examination of the blood's buffy coat may show budding yeasts within phagocytic leucocytes. Check the CSF if *Candida* infection is suspected because blood cultures can be negative. Treatment should not necessarily await the outcome of laboratory studies. Congenital infection from ascending vaginal infection can occur. Tracheal colonisation frequently precedes systemic infection. Fungal and bacterial infection can coexist.

Candida infection of the breast
Give the mother a 150–300 mg loading dose by mouth, and then 100–200 mg once a day for at least 10 days. Treat the baby as well, and take steps to minimise the risk of reinfection as outlined in the web commentary.

Prophylactic use in the neonate
Giving 6 mg/kg of fluconazole twice a week is a strategy often used to prevent overt infection in very vulnerable babies (see web commentary). Give 6 mg/kg once every 2 days if prophylaxis is started in babies >6 weeks old.

Treatment in infancy
Systemic infection: Give a 12 mg/kg loading dose slowly IV followed by 6 mg/kg once a day by mouth or IV in babies less than 1–2 weeks old. Give 24 mg/kg and then 12 mg/kg once a day to babies older than this. Double the dosage interval after the first two doses if there is renal failure.
Thrush: Give a 6 mg/kg loading dose and then 3 mg/kg once a day by mouth. Many prefer to give nystatin.

Supply
25 ml bottles for IV use containing 2 mg/ml of fluconazole cost £7·30. A 12 mg/kg dose contains 0·92 mmol/kg of sodium. Packs for oral use costing £17 which, when reconstituted, contain 5·6 g/ml of sucrose, provide 35 ml of a solution containing 10 mg/ml. Do not dilute this further, or keep more than 2 weeks after reconstitution. 50, 150 and 200 mg capsules for adult use cost between 40p and 80p each.

References
See also the relevant Cochrane reviews

Driessen M, Ellis JB, Copper PA, *et al.* Fluconazole vs, amphotericin B for the treatment of neonatal fungal septicaemia: a prospective randomised trial. *Pediatr Infect Dis J.* 1996;**15**:1107–12. [RCT]
Long SS, Stevenson DK. Reducing *Candida* infections during neonatal intensive care: management choices, infection control, and fluconazole prophylaxis. [Editorial] *J Pediatr* 2005;**147**:135–41.
Manzoni P, Stolfi I, Pugni L, *et al.* A multi-center randomized trial of prophylactic fluconazole in preterm neonates. *N Engl J Med* 2007;**356**:2483–95. [RCT]
Schwarze R, Penk A, Pittrow L. Administration of fluconazole in children below 1 year. *Mycoses* 1998;**42**:3–16. [SR]
Wade KC, Benjamin CK, Kaufman DA, *et al.* Fluconazole dosing for the prevention or treatment of invasive candidiasis in young infants. *Pediatr Infect Dis J* 2009;**28**:717–23.

Use

Flucytosine is widely used, together with amphotericin B (q.v.), to treat respiratory and systemic fungal infection. This combination is used to treat aspergillosis, coccidioidomycosis and cryptococcosis, and is also often used to treat systemic *Candida* infection, although many now prefer to use fluconazole (q.v.) in this situation. Nystatin or miconazole (q.v.) are more appropriately used to treat superficial *Candida* infection.

Pharmacology

Flucytosine (previously called 5-fluorocytosine) is useful in the treatment of systemic infections due to *Candida* species and, because flucytosine penetrates the CSF and amphotericin and flucytosine are synergistic, combined treatment is increasingly advocated. Joint use may also make it possible to use a less toxic dose of amphotericin. While flucytosine has been used successfully on its own in the management of *Candida* renal tract infection, resistant strains have been reported with worrying frequency, and co-treatment with either amphotericin or fluconazole is now universally recommended to make the development of drug resistance less likely. *Candida* species are usually said to be resistant to flucytosine when the minimum inhibitory concentration (MIC) exceeds 60 μg/ml, and to *Cryptococcus* when the MIC exceeds 12·5 μg/ml.

Flucytosine is a fluorinated pyrimidine first developed in 1957 that acts as a competitive inhibitor of uracil metabolism. The drug is well absorbed by mouth and more than 90% is excreted unchanged in the urine. Renal clearance is about three-quarters that achieved for creatinine. The half life in the neonatal period is *very* variable, but usually about 8 hours. The drug is distributed widely through body tissues including the CSF. It is important to watch for leucopenia and thrombocytopenia with sustained use and, because co-treatment with amphotericin and the illness for which treatment is being given can both cause renal function to deteriorate, important to try and measure the trough blood level if the plasma creatinine level rises more than 40 μmol/l. Vomiting and diarrhoea can occur, and reversible liver function changes have been reported. Flucytosine has been given in pregnancy without seeming to cause any apparent harm to the baby, but the risk of teratogenicity cannot be discounted. It is not known whether the drug appears in breast milk.

Diagnosing fungal infection

Notes on the diagnosis of systemic candidiasis appear in the monograph on fluconazole.

Treatment

Neonatal use: Give 50 mg/kg by mouth or IV once every 12 hours for at least 10 days. Start with 50 mg/kg once every 24 hours if there is evidence of renal failure. Any IV infusion is probably best given using a 15 μm in-line filter to trap any possible drug crystals. The manufacturers also recommend slow infusion over at least 20 minutes, although they offer no reason for this recommendation.

Older children: A dose of 50 mg/kg every 6 or 8 hours is normally used in older children. Always check the blood level after 1–2 days if a dose as high as this is used in a young baby.

Blood levels

Marrow toxicity can occur when the blood level exceeds 100 mg/l for any length of time, so it is advisable to check the serum level when the fourth dose is due if renal function could be impaired. Most large hospitals now have access to a laboratory that can measure this, given at least 0·5 ml of whole blood. Peak levels occur a variable time after oral administration in young babies, so it is probably better to monitor the trough level, aiming for a level of 25–40 mg/l (1 mg/l = 7·75 μmol/l) because lower levels are sub-therapeutic.

Supply and administration

250 ml bottles of a 10 mg/ml IV formulation cost £30. This sugar-free IV product can be infused (terminally) into a line containing glucose or glucose saline. It can also be given by mouth. A 50 mg/kg dose contains 0·69 mmol/kg of sodium. Prefilled and sealed single-dose syringes can be dispensed on request in order to reduce costs, but this and the reserve stock *must* kept at room temperature and should be protected from light. Indeed crystals of flucytosine may precipitate out if the temperature falls below 18°C (which is why it is wise to use a 15 μm filter during IV administration). If precipitation is suspected, the bottle can be heated to 80°C for 30 minutes to redissolve the precipitate, but decomposition (and 5-fluorouracil formation) occurs with sustained storage at temperatures over 25°C. There is no IV product on the market in America, but an extemporaneous liquid that is stable for 2 weeks at room temperature can be prepared from the 250 or 500 mg oral capsules.

References

Baddley JW, Pappas PG. Antifungal combination therapy: clinical potential. *Drugs* 2005;**65**:1461–80.

Baley JE, Meyers C, Klegmann RM, *et al*. Pharmacokinetics, outcome of treatment, and toxic effects of amphotericin B and 5-fluorocytosine in neonates. *J Pediatr* 1990;**116**:791–7.

Butler KM, Baker CJ. Candida: an increasingly important pathogen in the nursery. *Pediatr Clin North Am* 1988;**35**:543–63.

Loke HL, Verber I, Szymonowicz W, *et al*. Systemic candidiasis and pneumonia in preterm infants. *Aust Paediatr J* 1988;**24**:138–42.

Pappas PG, Rex JH, Sobel JD, *et al*. Guidelines for treatment of candidiasis. *Clin Infect Dis* 2004;**38**:161–89.

Soltani M, Tobin CM, Bowker KE, *et al*. Evidence of excessive concentrations of 5-flucytosine in children below 12 years: a 12-year review of serum concentrations from a UK clinical assay reference laboratory. *Int J Antimicrob Agents* 2006;**28**:574–7.

Vermes A, Guchelaar H-J, Dankert J. Flucytosine: a review of its pharmacology, clinical indications, pharmacokinetics, toxicity and drug interactions. *J Antimicrob Chemother* 2000;**46**:171–9.

Use

Folic acid is necessary to prevent megaloblastic anaemia. Supplementation prior to conception can also reduce the risk of several fetal defects including anencephaly or spina bifida. Several uncommon conditions, including primary and secondary cerebral folate deficiency and folinic acid responsive seizures, result in progressive neurological deterioration after birth which, if unrecognised, can cause permanent brain damage.

Nutritional factors

Folic acid, first synthesised in 1945, is almost certainly the factor first identified in 1930 by the obstetrician Wills as the cause of prematurity and 'tropical macrocytic anaemia' among malnourished women in Bombay. Tetrahydrofolic acid, the metabolically active form of folic acid (one of the water-soluble B vitamins), participates in DNA synthesis and red cell maturation. Peas, beans, green vegetables, yeast extract, Bovril and fortified cereals are all good dietary sources. Excessive intake does not seem to be dangerous. Liver is a rich source of folate but this should be avoided in pregnancy because of its high vitamin A content.

Serum and red cell folate levels are higher in the infant than the mother at birth, and deficiency is only seen in the babies of grossly deficient mothers. Folate is actively excreted in breast milk and well absorbed in the duodenum and jejunum. Cow's milk contains as much as human milk ($3-6 \mu g/100$ ml) but folic acid is heat labile. All preterm formula milks in the UK contain $43-50 \mu g/100$ ml. It is often claimed that folate requirements in infancy are as high as $20-50 \mu g$ a day ($4-10$ times the adult requirement). This is more than most babies get by mouth for some months after birth. However, although serum and red cell folate levels fall after delivery, especially in babies of low birthweight, and urinary losses are high, symptomatic deficiency has not been observed in the absence of chronic infection, malabsorption (e.g. coeliac disease) or diarrhoea, and supplementary folic acid fails to produce any rise in haemoglobin in the absence of megaloblastic anaemia, even in babies with severe haemolytic disease. Many units still offer a routine supplement to every preterm baby, but there is no evidence that this is necessary.

Maternal prophylaxis

In countries that have not adopted a policy of food supplementation, as they have in North America, women should take 400 micrograms once a day *before* becoming pregnant and for the first 12 weeks of pregnancy to minimize the risk of fetal abnormality. Suitable tablets are available 'over the counter' in the UK without prescription. Three months of Preconceive® costs less £4, but the free 'Healthy Start' product (cf. vitamin D monograph) is only available to those already pregnant. Take 5 mg daily if there has been a previously affected pregnancy, if either parent has a neural tube defect, or if the woman is taking an anticonvulsant.

Treating folate deficiency diseases in infancy

Cerebral folate deficiency: Primary cerebral folate deficiency is a rare neurological disorder characterised by decreased CSF but normal serum 5-methyltetrahydrofolate levels that typically starts to affect a child's development after $4-6$ months. Further deterioration can be arrested by giving folinic acid. Start by giving 0·5 or 1 mg/kg a day and increase this slowly to no more than 2·5 mg/kg a day as advised by an experienced paediatric neurologist. A folate receptor-blocking antibody has sometimes been identified.

Folinic acid responsive seizures: This condition is due to mutations in the ALDH7A1 (antiquin) gene giving α-aminoadipic semialdehyde dehydrogenase (α-AASA) deficiency and is identical to the major form of pyridoxine-dependent epilepsy. Treatment with 2·5 mg/kg of folinic acid twice a day stops the seizures, but developmental delay persists. The optimum maintenance dose has not yet been established. The addition of pyridoxine has been suggested together with a lysine-restricted diet.

Megaloblastic anaemia: In the absence of vitamin B_{12} deficiency, infants are usually treated with 1 mg of folic acid daily by mouth, but they should respond rapidly to physiological doses of folic acid (50 micrograms a day) if a folate-deficient diet rather than malabsorption or a primary defect of uptake or cellular utilisation is causing the anaemia. Symptoms develop insidiously during the first months of life and deficiency can have permanent consequences unless the diagnosis is made before growth has already been affected.

Supply

Folic acid: 150 ml of an 80 microgram/ml sugar-free oral suspension costs £1·40. 1 ml (15 mg) ampoules cost £1·30. 400 microgram tablets (which need no prescription) and 5 mg tablets cost ~2p each.

Folinic acid: The product usually dispensed is calcium folinate (known as leucovorin in America). 30 mg (10 ml) vials suitable for IV, IM or oral administration cost £4·60, and 15 mg tablets cost £4.

References
See also the relevant Cochrane reviews

Cheriajn A, Seena S, Bullock RK, *et al*. Incidence of neural tube defects in the least-developed area of India: a population-based study. *Lancet* 2005;**366**:930−1. (See also pp. 871−2.)

De Wals P, Tairou F, Van Allen MI, *et al*. Reduction in neural-tube defects after folic acid fortification in Canada. *N Engl J Med* 2007;**357**:135−42.

Djukie A. Folate-responsive neurological diseases. [Review] *Pediatr Neurol* 2007;**37**:387−97.

Gallagher RC, Van Hove JL, *et al*. Folinic acid-responsive seizures are identical to pyridoxine-dependent epilepsy. *Ann Neurol*. 2009;**65**:550−6.

Gordon N. Cerebral folate deficiency. *Dev Med Child Neurol* 2009;**51**:180−2.

Ramaekers VT, Rothenberg SP, Sequeira JM, *et al*. Autoantibodies to folate receptors in the cerebral folate deficiency syndrome. *N Engl J Med*. 2005;**352**:1985−91.

Use

Fresh frozen plasma (FFP) and cryoprecipitate can be used to treat symptomatic coagulation factor deficiency. An exchange transfusion with freshly donated blood may sometimes be a better way of controlling early coagulation failure.

Product

Standard 200–250 ml packs of fresh plasma containing albumin, immunoglobulin and stable clotting factors are prepared and frozen at minus 30°C within 6 hours of collection from a single donation of whole blood. Cryoprecipitate, the precipitate formed during controlled thawing of fresh pooled frozen plasma, later resuspended in plasma, contains an eight-fold concentrate of fibrinogen together with a range of other coagulation factors (especially factor VIII) in 20 ml packs. Solvent/detergent treated (virally inactivated) packs of FFP are now becoming available that make HIV and hepatitis C transmission unlikely, but human parvovirus B19 and hepatitis A virus transmission could still occur – especially as most supplies come from pooled donors. Supplies of a methylene blue treated product (MB-FFP) from single donors who were never exposed to bovine spongiform encephalopathy (BSE) contaminated meat should also become available quite soon for children in the UK born after 1995.

Reports that the prophylactic use of FFP immediately after birth might reduce the risk of intraventricular haemorrhage in babies of less than 32 weeks' gestation were *not* confirmed by a multicentre trial involving more than 750 babies. Nor is it of value in managing sepsis or thrombocytopenia. A specific product of fraction III, plasminogen, was shown to reduce mortality from respiratory distress in a trial reported in 1977 (as briefly described in the monograph on urokinase), but no other studies of this strategy have appeared since then. Immunoglobulin (q.v.) concentrates may help where there is sepsis.

Assessment

Assessment of any bleeding tendency requires a knowledge of normal test ranges. Healthy babies have values in the range shown in Table 1 at birth. The normal prothrombin and activated partial thromboplastin times both decrease by about 10% in the first month of life. While D-dimer levels are usually below 250 µg/l, normal babies occasionally have values as high as 1000 µg/l.

Table 1 Coagulation screening tests (95% confidence intervals).

Test	Gestation (weeks)		
	24–29	30–36	37–41
Prothrombin time (seconds)	12·2–21·0	10·6–16·2	10·1–15·9
International normalised ratio (INR)	–	0·61–1·70	0·53–1·62
Activated partial thromboplastin time (seconds)	43·6–101+	27·5–79·4	31·3–54·5
Thrombin clotting time (seconds)	–	19·2–30·4	19·0–28·3
Fibrinogen (g/l)	0·69–4·12	1·50–3·73	1·67–3·99
Platelets (x 10^9/l)	150–350	150–350	150–350

Treatment

Infuse 20 ml/kg of blood group compatible FFP over 30–60 minutes. Use material from a group AB Rhesus negative donor or, failing this, blood of the same ABO group as the baby. Hypoglycaemia is possible if any existing glucose infusion is stopped during the administration of FFP.

Supply

Stocks of FFP and cryoprecipitate from the local blood bank cost £20 to prepare and dispense. 50 ml 'minipacks' are sometimes available. The packs should be thawed by the blood bank staff immediately prior to issue and used within 6 hours. Hold the material at 2–6°C if there is any unavoidable last minute delay in administration. A filter is not necessary. Commercial virus-inactivated products cost £45.

References See also the relevant Cochrane reviews and UK guideline

Buchanan GR. Coagulation disorders in the neonate. *Pediatr Clin North Am* 1986;**33**:203–20.
Cohen H. Avoiding the misuse of fresh frozen plasma. *BMJ* 1993;**307**:395–6.
Murray N, Roberts I. Neonatal transfusion of blood products. In: David TJ, ed. *Recent advances in paediatrics 23*. London: Royal Society of Medicine, 2006: pp. 139–53.
NNNI Trial Group. Randomised trial of prophylactic early fresh frozen plasma or gelatin or glucose in preterm babies: outcome at 2 years. *Lancet* 1996;**348**:229–32. [RCT]
Norfolk DR, Glaser A, Kinsey S. American fresh frozen plasma for neonates and children. *Arch Dis Child* 2005;**90**:89–91.
Seguin JH, Topper WH. Coagulation studies in very-lowbirthweight infants. *Am J Perinatol* 1994;**11**:17–19.

FUROSEMIDE = Frusemide (former BAN)

Use
Furosemide is a valuable, powerful and rapidly acting diuretic that can be particularly useful in the management of acute congestive cardiac failure. Alternatives (such as chlorothiazide with or without spironolactone) are cheaper and preferable for maintenance treatment.

Pharmacology
Furosemide was first marketed commercially in 1962. It crosses the placenta and increases fetal urine flow, but there is no good evidence that furosemide is teratogenic. It is also excreted into breast milk, but no adverse effects have ever been reported. Although it is protein bound in the plasma, normal doses do not significantly influence bilirubin-binding capacity. It is both filtered by the glomerulus and also actively excreted by the proximal renal tubule. The filtered drug then works from within the tubule inhibiting active chloride reabsorption and, as a result, passive sodium reabsorption from the thick ascending limb of the loop of Henlé and the distal tubule (hence the term 'loop' diuretic). While this can result in a six-fold increase in free water clearance in adults, its efficacy in the preterm baby remains less clearly quantified. Sustained use increases urinary sodium and potassium loss and can cause hypokalaemia. Urinary calcium excretion triples in the preterm baby, causing marked bone mineral loss, and renal and biliary calcium deposition.

Furosemide stimulates renal synthesis of prostaglandin E_2, thus enhancing, and modifying, renal blood flow. Early use is associated with some increase in the incidence of symptomatic patent ductus in babies requiring ventilation for respiratory distress, and this might be due to increased prostaglandin production. Furosemide also has a direct effect on lung fluid reabsorption, but there is no evidence that use speeds the resolution of transient tachypnoea of the newborn. Aerosol administration can transiently improve lung function, and sustained IV or oral use can improve oxygenation in babies over 3 weeks old with chronic lung disease, but there is no evidence, as yet, of sustained clinical benefit.

The half life is about 8 hours in the term baby at birth, but approaches adult values (2 hours) within a few months. It may be as long as 24 hours at first in the very preterm baby, making progressive drug accumulation possible with repeated use, and this may well be a factor in the increased risk of serious late-onset deafness seen in children exposed to sustained diuretic treatment in the neonatal period. The related diuretic bumetanide may be less ototoxic but neonatal use has not yet been fully evaluated; it might also be more effective in renal failure, because entry into the tubular lumen is less dependent on glomerular filtration and clearance less dependent on renal excretion. The usual dose of bumetanide in infancy is 20 micrograms/kg IV or IM once every 6 hours but, because of reduced clearance, drug accumulation must be a possibility if treatment is repeated more than once every 12 hours in the first month of life.

Drug interactions
Concurrent furosemide use significantly increases the risk of aminoglycoside ototoxicity.

Treatment
Use as a diuretic: Try 1 mg/kg of furosemide IV or IM, or 2 mg/kg by mouth, repeatable after 12–24 hours. The drug should not be given more than once every 24 hours to babies with a postconceptional age of less than 31 weeks. Patients on long-term treatment with furosemide may require 1 mmol/kg per day of oral potassium chloride (q.v.) to prevent hypokalaemia.

Renal failure: Give a single 5 mg/kg dose of furosemide IV as soon as renal failure is suspected to lower the metabolic activity of the chloride pump, minimise the risk of ischaemic tubular damage, and reduce the shut down in glomerular blood flow that follows from this. Consider giving 10 ml/kg of pentastarch (q.v.) or 5% albumin as well if hypovolaemia could be a contributory factor (as outlined in the monograph on water).

Chronic lung disease: 1 mg/kg of the IV preparation of furosemide added to 2 ml of 0·9% sodium chloride and given by nebuliser once every 6 hours may at least temporarily improve lung compliance (and therefore tidal volume) in some ventilator-dependent babies without affecting renal function.

Supply and administration
Furosemide: 2 ml (20 mg) ampoules cost 55p. Precipitation can occur when furosemide is mixed with any IV fluid (such as glucose and glucose saline) with a pH of <5·6, so it should *always* be separated by a 1 ml 'bolus' of 0·9% sodium chloride or water when given IV. The IV preparation can be given by mouth after dilution, but a cheaper, commercial, sugar-free, oral 4 mg/ml preparation in 10% alcohol is also available (100 ml costs £8).
Bumetanide: 4 ml (2 mg) ampoules of bumetanide cost £1·80.

References
See also the relevant Cochrane reviews

Borradori C, Fawer C-L, Buclin T, *et al*. Risk factors of sensorineural hearing loss in preterm infants. *Biol Neonat* 1997;**71**:1–10.
Karabayir N, Kavuncuoglu S. Intravenous frusemide for transient tachypnoea of the newborn. *J Paediatr Child Health* 2006;**42**:640–2. [RCT]
Moghal NE, Shenoy M. Furosemide and acute kidney injury in neonates. [Review] *Arch Dis Child* 2008;**93**:F313–16.
Pai VB, Nahata MC. Aerosolised furosemide in the treatment of acute respiratory distress and possible bronchopulmonary dysplasia in preterm neonates. *Ann Pharmacother* 2000;**34**:386–92. [SR]
Sullivan JE, Witte MK, Yamashita TS, *et al*. Dose-ranging evaluation of bumetanide pharmacodynamics in critically ill infants. *Clin Pharmacol Ther* 1996;**60**:424–34.

Use

Ganciclovir is a toxic antiviral agent used to treat of neonatal cytomegalovirus (CMV) infection, otherwise known as human herpes virus 5. It has to be given intravenously, but valganciclovir is a prodrug that can be given by mouth.

Pharmacology

Ganciclovir is a synthetic nucleoside with properties similar to aciclovir (q.v.) developed in 1980 that accumulates after phosphorylation in CMV-infected cells inhibiting virus replication. It is much more toxic than aciclovir, frequently causing neutropenia and thrombocytopenia, and treatment needs to be suspended (or the dose reduced) if the neutrophil counts falls below 750 cells/mm^3. Concurrent treatment with zidovudine (q.v.) increases the drug's toxicity. Both ganciclovir and valganciclovir are rapidly excreted by the kidney with an average half life of 3 hours. Animal studies suggest that both these drugs are not only fetal teratogens, but also potential mutagens and carcinogens. Fertility can be affected, and breastfeeding is inadvisable. Checking the amount of virus in the urine may help find a dose that minimises viral replication without causing toxicity.

Cytomegalovirus infection

Fifty per cent of all women of childbearing age in the UK have already had an asymptomatic infection before the start of pregnancy (often in early childhood), but primary or reactivated infection is thought to cause congenital or perinatal infection in about one in every 300 UK pregnancies. Most of these babies show few signs of overt infection, but about 5% develop disseminated cytomegalic inclusion disease with thrombocytopenic petechiae, hepatitis, chorioretinitis, intracranial calcification and/or microcephaly. Cerebral palsy can occur, and severe progressive deafness may develop even after an apparently asymptomatic infection especially when this occurred in the first trimester of pregnancy. Overt cytomegalic inclusion disease can also result from neonatal cross-infection, or exposure to CMV-infected blood or human milk; such babies often develop pneumonia as well as many of the symptoms listed above. Proof that infection was congenital requires the collection of a positive culture, or polymerase chain reaction (PCR) test, within 2 weeks of birth. Handwashing is important to prevent congenitally infected babies causing iatrogenic cross-infection. Staff are at little increased risk of personal infection as long as proper precautions against cross-infection are observed.

There is only limited evidence that any antiviral agent can alter the course of congenitally acquired infection, but ganciclovir can temporarily eradicate virus excretion, and sustained use after birth seems to reduce the risk of later progressive hearing loss. Giving the mother 8 grams of valaciclovir (a prodrug of aciclovir) daily may reduce fetal damage, but giving the mother 200 units/kg of hyperimmune globulin (with, on occasion, more of the same product into the fetal abdomen) is a strategy that has been better studied (Nigro *et al*. 2005).

Treatment

Seek expert advice. Explain that use seldom eliminates the virus, and that the manufacturer has not yet endorsed use in children. Watch for neutropenia, and increase the dosage interval if there is renal impairment.

IV treatment: Give symptomatic babies 6 mg/kg IV of ganciclovir (5 ml of the solution made up as described below) over 1 hour once every 12 hours until oral treatment is possible. Maintain hydration during IV use.

Oral treatment: Start by giving a 16 mg/kg dose of valganciclovir twice a day. Try to optimise dosing by monitoring urinary viral shedding if facilities exist. Some clinicians aim to sustain treatment for 2–4 months.

Supply and administration

Undiluted ganciclovir is very caustic (pH ~11). Both products are potential teratogens and carcinogens, so gloves and goggles should be used during reconstitution. Wash at once to limit accidental contact with skin.

Ganciclovir: 500 mg vials cost £32 each. The freeze-dried powder must be reconstituted with 9·7 ml of water for injection to give a solution containing 50 mg/ml (water containing a bacteriostatic such as *para*-hydroxybenzoate may cause precipitation). Shake to dissolve, and use promptly: do not use the vial if there is any particulate matter still present. To give 6 mg/kg of ganciclovir take 1·2 ml of this solution for each kg the baby weighs, dilute to 50 ml with 10% glucose or glucose saline, and infuse 5 ml over 1 hour.

Valganciclovir: 450 mg tablets of this prodrug (the L-valyl ester of ganciclovir) are available, cost £19 each, and Roche have developed an oral formulation with 50% bioavailablity (10 times more than for ganciclovir).

References

Capretti MG, Lanari M, Lazzarotto T, *et al*. Very low birth weight infants born to cytomegalovirus-seropositive mothers fed with their mother's milk: a prospective study. *J Pediatr* 2009;**154**:842–8.

Coll O, Benoist G, Ville Y, *et al*. for the WAPM Consensus Group. Guidelines on CMV congenital infection. *J Perinat Med* 2009;**37**:433–45.

Jacquemard F, Yamamoto N, Costa J-M, *et al*. Maternal administration of valaciclovir in symptomatic intrauterine cytomegalovirus infection. *Br J Obstet Gynaecol* 2007;**114**:1113–21.

Kimberlin DW, Acosta EP, Sánchez PJ, *et al*. Pharmacokinetic and pharmacodynamic assessment of oral valganciclovir in the treatment of symptomatic congenital cytomegalovirus disease. *J Infect Dis* 2008;**197**:836–45.

Kimberlin DW, Lin C-Y, Sanchez PJ, *et al*. Effect of ganciclovir therapy on hearing in symptomatic congenital cytomegalovirus disease involving the central nervous system: a randomized, controlled trial. *J Pediatr* 2003;**143**:16–25. [RCT] (See also pp. 4–6.)

Marshall BC, Koch WC. Antivirals for cytomegalovirus infection in neonates and infants: focus on pharmacokinetics, formulations, dosing and adverse events. [Review] *Pediatr Drugs* 2009;**11**:309–21.

Maruyama Y, Sameshima H, Kamitomo M, *et al*. Fetal manifestations and poor outcomes of congenital cytomegalovirus infection. *J Obstet Gynaecol Res* 2007;**33**:619–23.

Nigro G, Adler SP, La Torre R, *et al*. Passive immunisation during pregnancy for congenital cytomegalovirus infection. *N Engl J Med* 2005;**353**:1350–62.

GAVISCON®

Use

Infant Gaviscon may, by acting as an antacid, control some of the symptoms of gastro-oesophageal reflux.

Pharmacology

A range of antacid preparations containing magnesium salts (which have a mild laxative effect) and aluminium salts (which have the opposite tendency) are commercially available 'over the counter'. There is no contraindication to their use during pregnancy or lactation. Magnesium trisilicate and magnesium or aluminium hydroxide are commonly chosen, because they are retained rather longer in the stomach. Alginates are often added when reflux is a problem, because they react with gastric acid to form a viscous gel or 'raft' that then floats to the top of the stomach, acting as a mechanical barrier to oesophageal reflux. However, because Infant Gaviscon, the formulation most widely used in early infancy, lacks bicarbonate, this does not seem to be true of this product. Each single sachet of the latter contains 225 mg of sodium alginate and 87·5 mg of magnesium alginate, with colloidal silica and mannitol. Gaviscon is specifically contraindicated in the treatment of gastroenteritis and of suspected intestinal obstruction: even the infant formulation has a sodium content (21 mg or 0·9 mmol per dose) high enough to cause hypernatraemia if there is dehydration or poor renal function. Other formulations contain even more sodium. While Infant Gaviscon has, on occasion, been suspected of forming a solid intragastric mass or 'bezoar', it is now thought that this was probably caused by its (discontinued) aluminium content.

Gastro-oesophageal reflux

Art plays a larger role than science in the feeding of the small preterm baby, and experienced neonatal nurses are the acknowledged artists. Many babies 'posset' a few mouthfuls of milk quite regularly, and some swallow quite a lot of air while feeding and then bring back milk when winded. Many small babies regurgitate some milk back into the lower half of the oesophagus after feeding because of poor sphincter tone, but only a few aspirate, and very few develop a chemical oesophagitis because milk is an excellent antacid. Nevertheless, silent reflux can cause serious lung damage, and babies with a postconceptional age of less than 35 weeks have no effective cough reflex. Reflux must be distinguished from vomiting, which is characterised by reflex contraction of the stomach. Some preterm babies with reflux also have episodes of apnoea, but the few episodes of apnoea that are associated with reflux last no longer than those that are not. Placing the baby prone (face down), or on its left side, may help, but such a strategy should only be adopted with monitored babies in a hospital setting because of the increased risk of cot death. Tilting the head of the cot up 30° was once thought to help, but may increase abdominal pressure, and one trial suggests that a semi-upright posture can make matters worse. While severe symptoms may merit oesophageal pH monitoring, it is usually enough to test oropharyngeal secretions for acid with blue litmus paper once every 6–8 hours. Gaviscon only reduces reflux slightly but may be helpful where oesophagitis is suspected, or growth is affected, and probably works, in the main, like carob seed flour (q.v.), by thickening the feed. Oesophagitis, which is painful and can provoke apnoea, vomiting and/or food aversion, may require ranitidine or (rarely) omeprazole (q.v.). Cisapride was widely used for 10 years, although there was never any control trial evidence of efficacy. Many American clinicians currently use metoclopramide (q.v.) and Europeans use domperidone (q.v.), but there is no good evidence that either does any good. See the web commentary for a discussion of postural management.

Treatment

Term babies: Babies under 5 kg should be offered one dose of Infant Gaviscon with feeds. Babies over 5 kg may be offered a double dose (i.e. both sections of a paired sachet) with each feed.
Preterm babies: The manufacturer does not recommend the use of Infant Gaviscon, but it may, on occasion, be appropriate to give a proportionate dose (see below) regularly with each feed.

Supply and administration

Infant Gaviscon powder comes made up in paired sucrose- and lactose-free sachets, and each paired sachet contains enough powder for **two** standard doses of Gaviscon. Paired sachets cost 16p each. They can be purchased from community pharmacists without a doctor's prescription, but such use is not to be encouraged. Infant Gaviscon is one of the few commercial products, marketed specifically for use in the treatment of reflux vomiting in infancy, that can be prescribed on the NHS.

Take the powder from one section of a paired sachet of Infant Gaviscon, mix with 5 ml (1 teaspoon) of fresh tap water, and add 1 ml of this thin paste to each 25 ml of artificial milk. Breastfed babies can be offered a similar quantity after each feed on a spoon. Do not give the liquid formulation to babies.

References

See also the Cochrane review of reflux

Carroll AE, Garrison MM, Christakis DA. A systemic review of nonpharmacological and nonsurgical therapies for gastroesophageal reflux in infants. *Arch Pediatr Adolesc Med* 2002;**156**:109–13. [SR]

Del Buono R, Wenzl TG, Ball G, *et al*. Effect of Gaviscon Infant on gastro-oesophageal reflux in infants assessed by combined intraluminal impedance/pH. *Arch Dis Child* 2005;**90**:460–3. [RCT] (See also 2006;**91**:93.)

Hegar B, Dewanti NR, Kadim M, *et al*. Natural evolution of regurgitation in healthy infants. *Acta Paediatr* 2009;**98**:1189–93.

James ME, Ewer AK. Acid oro-pharyngeal secretions can predict gastro-oesophageal reflux in preterm infants. *Eur J Pediatr* 1999;**158**:371–4.

Kumar Y, Sarananthan R. Gastro-oesophageal reflux in children. *BMJ Clinical evidence handbook*. London: BMJ Books, 2009: pp. 88–9 (and updates). [SR]

Tighe MP, Afzal NA, Bevan A, *et al*. Current pharmacological management of gastro-esophageal reflux in children: an evidence-based systematic review. *Pediatr Drugs* 2009;**11**:185–202. [SR]

Use

Colloids can be used to expand intravascular volume in patients with shock or impending shock. Artificial products are generally as effective as 4·5% human albumin (see the monograph on plasma albumin) and significantly cheaper.

Pharmacology

Gelatin: Gelatin is a purified protein obtained by the partial hydrolysis of BSE-free bovine collagen. A sterile saline solution containing 40 g/l of modified gelatin has the same properties and uses as dextran 40 (a polymer of glucose) but gelatin, unlike dextran, does not interfere with subsequent blood grouping and compatibility testing procedures. A range of products, of which Gelofusine® is the best known, are available. Gelatin has also been used in some countries as a haemostatic film or sponge (Sterispon®) in surgical procedures. The gelatin in Gelofusine, with an average molecular weight (30,000) almost half that of human plasma albumin, only has a 4-hour half life and is rapidly excreted unchanged in the urine. Anaphylactic reactions have been described, but seem rare in young children. Immediate and delayed-type hypersensitivity reactions have sometimes occurred, however, after immunisation with vaccines containing gelatin in pre-sensitised children. The trivalent measles (MMR) vaccine is the only UK vaccine to contain gelatin. Prior exposure to gelofusine might nevertheless make a reaction to this vaccine marginally more likely.

Pentastarch: Penastarch and hexastarch are artificial colloids derived from etherified starch with a mean molecular weight (200,000) three times above that of plasma albumin. The glucagon-like polymerised glucose units are of variable size. While the smaller molecules are rapidly excreted in the urine, the larger molecules remain in the blood stream for some days undergoing slow enzymatic degradation. While use is thought to cause a sustained expansion of intravascular volume, even when endothelial damage causes increased capillary permeability allowing smaller molecules (such as plasma albumin) to leak rapidly out of the intravascular space, use of this product rather than gelatin was associated with an *increased* risk of transient renal failure in adults with septic shock in one recent trial. Large volumes reduce platelet aggregation, lower the factor VIII level and increase the bleeding time. The manufacturers stress that little in known about the use of any of these products during pregnancy or childhood.

Indications for use

A major systematic review in 1998 suggested that the indiscriminate use of *any* colloid in the management of hypo-volaemia actually does more harm than good. However, this may be because the product is being used inappropriately rather than because it is inherently dangerous. Gelatin can be used to reconstitute packed red cells. It may also be the best colloid to use during routine surgery because it has the least effect on *in vitro* tests of coagulation, but 20 ml/kg is the largest dose known to have been used in any 1 day in the neonatal period. Naturally, where blood has been lost, it will often be more appropriate to replace this as soon as practicable. Early neonatal hypotension without hypovolaemia is more appropriately treated with dobutamine and/or dopamine (q.v.), or hydrocortisone (q.v.), while fresh frozen plasma (q.v.) should be used where there is a significant clotting factor deficiency.

Treatment

20 ml/kg of gelatin infused over 5–15 minutes should correct all but the most severe hypovolaemia. The effect of giving more than a total of 30 ml/kg in the first week of life has not been studied.

Supply

500 ml bags of 4% gelatin (Gelofusine) in 0·9% sodium chloride cost £4·70. 500 ml bags of 6% pentastarch in 0·9% sodium chloride cost £16·50. Both products contain 154 mmol/l of sodium. They should not be kept once they have been opened because they contain no preservative. Do not use any material that looks cloudy or turbid.

References

See also the relevant Cochrane reviews

Boluyt N, Bollen W, Bos AO, *et al*. Fluid resuscitation in neonatal and pediatric hypovolaemic shock: a Dutch Pediatric Society evidence-based clinical practice guideline. *Intensive Care Med* 2006;**32**:995–1003.

Hope P. Pump up the volume? The routine early use of colloid in very preterm infants. [Commentary] *Arch Dis Child* 1998;**78**:F163–5.

NNNI Trial Group. A randomised trial comparing the effect of prophylactic early fresh frozen plasma, gelatin or glucose on early mortality and morbidity in preterm babies. *Eur J Pediatr* 1996;**155**:580–8. [RCT]

Roberts JS, Bratton SL. Colloid volume expanders. Problems, pitfalls and possibilities. *Drugs* 1998;**55**:621–30.

Schortgen F, Lacherade J-C, Bruneel F, *et al*. Effects of hydoxyethylstarch and gelatin on renal function in severe sepsis: a multicentre randomised study. *Lancet* 2001;**357**:911–16. [RCT] (See also **358**:581–3.)

Shierhout G, Roberts I. Fluid resuscitation with colloid or crystalloid solutions in critically ill patients: a systematic review of randomised trials. *BMJ* 1998;**316**:961–4. [SR]

Wilkes MM, Navickis RJ, Sibbald WJ. Albumin versus hydroxyethyl starch in cardiopulmonary surgery: a meta-analysis of postoperative bleeding. *Ann Thorac Surg* 2001;**72**:527–33. [SR]

Wills BA, Dung NM, Loan HT, *et al*. Comparison of three fluid solutions for resuscitation in dengue shock syndrome. *N Engl J Med* 2005;**353**:877–89. [RCT] (See also pp. 941–4.)

GENTAMICIN

Use

Gentamicin is very widely used to treat Gram-negative bacterial infection, but it is of variable efficacy (and not the treatment of choice) for known staphylococcal sepsis. It has to be given IV or IM.

Pharmacology

Gentamicin is a naturally occurring substance first isolated in 1963 and, like kanamycin and neomycin, it consists of a mixture of closely related compounds so it does not have a single quotable molecular weight. It crosses the placenta, producing fetal levels that are about half the maternal level, but it has never been known to have caused ototoxicity *in utero*. Absorption from the gut is too limited to make maternal use inappropriate during lactation (although the baby's gut flora could be altered). It undergoes no change in the body, but is passively filtered by the glomerulus and concentrated in the urine. As a result, the half life more than halves during the first 7–10 days after birth (unless function is compromised). Postconceptional age also affects the half life to a lesser extent. Damage to the renal tubules builds up with time, and can even produce a Bartter-like syndrome, and simultaneous treatment with vancomycin can increase these problems, but these changes are reversible when treatment is stopped and are seldom severe. Damage to the ear is uncommon in young children, but it can cause balance problems as well as high tone deafness, and these can become permanent if early symptoms go unrecognised (as they will in the neonatal period). While blood levels should always be measured therefore in order to minimise this risk where facilities exist, it is *at least* as important to avoid simultaneous treatment with furosemide, and to try to stop treatment after 7–10 days. There are theoretical reasons for not giving a β-lactam penicillin or cephalosporin at precisely the same time as an aminoglycoside (as outlined in the monograph on tobramycin), but the clinical relevance of this finding is not yet clear.

Therapeutic strategy

Aminoglycosides only become effective against many common bacteria when the serum level is high enough to be potentially toxic. A high peak level (at least eight times the minimum inhibitory dose) enhances the drug's bactericidal effect, but Gram-negative organisms stop taking up the drug after an hour, and only do so again 2–10 hours after exposure is over ('adaptive resistance'). Repeat treatment during this time is ineffective. However, serious toxicity is normally only seen with treatment lasting more than 7–10 days with sustained high trough serum levels and/or co-exposure to other ototoxic drugs (such as furosemide). These features suggest that treatment in patients with normal renal function will be optimised, and adverse effects minimised, by giving treatment once a day (a 'high peak, low trough' policy). Such controlled trial evidence as exists supports this conclusion in adults, and an increasing number of studies have now suggested that this is also the right strategy to adopt in children. When aminoglycosides *are* given more than once a day in children the serum level will remain sub-therapeutic for many hours if an initial loading dose is not given (because of the large V_D).

Preventing necrotising enterocolitis

Several small controlled trials have found that giving 2·5 mg/kg of gentamicin once every 6 hours **by mouth** for 7–10 days can reduce the risk of necrotising enterocolitis if prophylaxis is started before feeds are begun. A larger trial would be needed to show that this does not cause aminoglycoside-resistant organisms to proliferate.

Treating suspected sepsis

Dose: Give 5 mg/kg IV or IM to babies less than 4 weeks old, and 6 mg/kg to children older than this. A slow 30-minute infusion is *not* necessary when the drug is given IV.

Timing: Give a dose once every 36 hours in babies less than 32 weeks' gestation in the first week of life. Give all other babies a dose once every 24 hours unless renal function is poor.

Managing ventriculitis

CSF penetration is poor so it can *sometimes* be appropriate to give 1–2 mg of the ***intrathecal*** preparation once every 24–48 hours as a direct intraventricular injection, and to monitor the CSF drug level (aim for 5–10 mg/l) when treating chronic ventriculitis, especially when this complicates shunt surgery. Ceftazidime, cefotaxime, co-trimoxazole and chloramphenicol (q.v.) all achieve better CSF penetration when given IV.

Blood levels

Measure the trough level, if facilities exist, just before the fourth dose is given (or, preferably, before the third dose in babies less than a week old and in babies with poor renal function) aiming for a level of about 1 mg/l, and extend the dosage interval if this level exceeds 2 mg/l. Collect a minimum of 0·2 ml of serum and get the specimen spun and frozen if prompt analysis is not possible. The peak level only needs to be measured when using a non-standard treatment policy (as is discussed in the linked web commentary).

Supply

A 2 ml (20 mg) vial costs £1·40, and a 1 ml (5 mg) intrathecal ampoule costs 74p.

References

See also the relevant Cochrane reviews

English M, Mohammed S, Ross A, *et al*. A randomised, controlled trial of once daily and multi-dose daily gentamicin in young Kenyan infants. *Arch Dis Child* 2004;**89**:665–9. [RCT]

Nestaas E, Bangstad H-J, Sandvik L, *et al*. Aminoglycoside extended interval dosing in neonates is safe and effective: a meta-analysis. *Arch Dis Child* 2005;**90**:F294–300. [SR]

Thingvoll ES, Guillet R, Caserta M, *et al*. Observational trial of a 48-hour gentamicin dosing regimen derived from Monte Carlo simulations in infants born at less than 28 weeks' gestation. *J Pediatr* 2008;**153**:530–4.

Use

Glucagon can be useful in the management of neonatal hypoglycaemia.

Pharmacology

Glucagon is a polypeptide hormone produced by pancreatic α cells with a natural half life of 5–10 minutes. It used to be extracted from animal pancreatic islet cell tissue, but was synthesised in 1967, and a recombinant 29 amino acid product, identical to human glucagon, is now the main product available. Glucagon mobilises hepatic glycogen and increases hepatic glucose and ketone production, causing increased amino acid uptake and free fatty acid flux. It is also known to stimulate growth hormone release. Glucagon activates the adenyl cyclase system even when the β-adrenoreceptors are blocked, and a continuous infusion is of proven value in the management of unintentional overtreatment with β blockers such as atenolol, labetalol and propranolol (q.v.). Isoprenaline (q.v.) may be of value if glucagon is not effective. Glucagon does not cross the placenta, so there is no reason to suppose that its use would be hazardous during pregnancy. It is not known whether it appears in breast milk. However, it is difficult to see how maternal administration during lactation could have any effect on the baby because the drug has a very short half life and is inactivated when taken by mouth.

Glucagon is also useful in the management of hypoglycaemia. A single bolus injection can sometimes increase the blood glucose level enough to make further treatment unnecessary. It is not clear how this effect is achieved, but glucagon may act by inducing key gluconeogenic enzymes in the period immediately after birth. A subcutaneous or IM injection is sometimes used to counteract accidental hyperinsulinism in patients with diabetes. An IM injection can also be used as a temporary expedient to reduce the risk of reactive hypoglycaemia in an infusion-dependent baby when an IV drip suddenly 'tissues' and proves difficult to resite. Continuous infusions are not recommended by the manufacturer, but have sometimes been used in light-for-dates babies with persisting neonatal hypoglycaemia despite a substantial infusion of IV glucose (q.v.). They have also been used in the initial short-term management of babies with endogenous hyperinsulinism, sometimes in conjunction with octreotide (as outlined in the monograph on diazoxide), since glucagon can itself stimulate insulin production. High-dose infusion can cause nausea and vomiting.

Treatment

Single-dose treatment: Give 200 micrograms/kg of glucagon subcutaneously, IM or as a bolus IV. This can sometimes raise the blood glucose level permanently out of the hypoglycaemic range in the first few days of life (sometimes even making it unnecessary to erect an IV drip).
Continuous IV infusion: Start with 300 nanograms/kg per minute (0·3 ml/hour of a solution made up as described below) and increase this, if necessary, to a dose of not more than 900 nanograms/kg per minute. Prepare a fresh solution if treatment needs to be continued for more than 24 hours.

Supply and administration

Vials containing 1 mg of powder (1 mg = 1 unit), suitable for single-dose administration, are available costing £11·50 each. Reconstitute with the diluent provided to obtain a solution containing 1 mg/ml. To give an infusion of 100 nanograms/kg per minute, take 300 micrograms (0·3 ml) of this reconstituted material for each kg the baby weighs, dilute this to 5 ml with further 5% glucose to obtain a solution containing 60 micrograms/kg per ml, and infuse this at a rate of 0·1 ml/hour. Vials should be stored at 4°C and reconstituted immediately before use. The fluid has a pH of 2·5–3·0. Avoid co-infusion with any fluid containing calcium (to avoid immediate precipitation), and do not use the reconstituted solution if it is not clear.

References

Carter PE, Lloyd DJ, Duffty P. Glucagon for hypoglycaemia in infants small for gestational age. *Arch Dis Child* 1988;**63**:1264–5.

Charsha DS, McKinley PS, Whitfield JM. Glucagon infusion for treatment of hypoglycemia: efficacy and safety in sick preterm infants. *Pediatrics* 2003;**111**:220–1.

Hawdon JM, Aynsley-Green A, Ward Platt MP. Neonatal blood glucose concentrations: metabolic effects of intravenous glucagon and intragastric medium chain triglyceride. *Arch Dis Child* 1993;**68**:255–61.

Mehta A, Wootton R, Cheng KL, *et al*. Effect of diazoxide or glucagon on hepatic glucose production rate during extreme neonatal hypoglycaemia. *Arch Dis Child* 1987;**62**:924–30.

Miralles RE, Lodha A, Perlman M, *et al*. Experience with intravenous glucagon infusions as a treatment for resistant neonatal hypoglycemia. *Arch Pediatr Adolesc Med* 2002;**156**:999–1004.

Stevens TP, Guillet R. Use of glucagon to treat neonatal low-output congestive heart failure after maternal labetalol therapy. *J Pediatr* 1995;**127**:151–3.

GLUCOSE (Dextrose)

Use
Glucose given intravenously prevents and corrects hypoglycaemia, and provides calories for babies too ill to be fully fed by mouth. It is a key component of parenteral nutrition (q.v.).

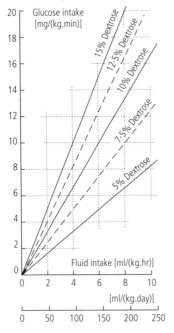

Fig. 1

Pharmacology
Dextrose is the naturally occurring D-isomer of glucose. A 5% solution is isotonic with blood; more concentrated solutions can cause thrombophlebitis due, in part, to the fact that autoclaved solutions have a relatively low pH – indeed, 50% dextrose has been used to sclerose varicose veins! A 'long line' with its tip in a large vessel is, therefore, the best way to deliver any solution containing more than 10% glucose (Fig. 1).

Hypoglycaemia: This is common shortly after birth, but monitoring is not necessary during the first postnatal hours because the brain is protected by a range of fuels. Subsequently a laboratory whole blood glucose of <2·5 mmol/l (45 mg/dl) is very unusual in any baby being maintained on a sustained infusion of 9 mg/kg per minute of 10% glucose within 48 hours of birth, and hyperinsulinism should be suspected if this level can only be sustained by giving more than 12 mg/kg per minute. Much asymptomatic hypoglycaemia is caused by delayed feeding, compounded by an inadequate (and frequently interrupted) glucose infusion rate. Never give oral glucose – milk is the best prophylaxis, and the best treatment, for any baby who is not too ill to absorb what is offered by mouth since milk has a calorie content 50% higher than that of 10% dextrose. Reagent-strip measurements should not be used. The HemoCue®, or Ames Glucometer®, can offer 'point-of-care' measurement with a precision comparable to any laboratory estimate, but even laboratory estimates are not very precise – results obtained by different, very well validated, techniques may vary by as much as ±30% (95% confidence interval). Sluggish homeostasis can cause a rebound that makes it difficult to interpret any measurement made soon after an infusion is stopped or reduced. Mild asymptomatic hypoglycaemia may respond to IM glucagon (q.v.), making IV glucose unnecessary. Sustained hypoglycaemia due to hyperinsulinism may respond to diazoxide or octreotide (q.v.). Hydrocortisone is of no proven value.

Hyperglycaemia: Although most healthy babies can metabolise at least 14 mg/kg of glucose per minute, small babies of under 1 kg are often relatively intolerant at first, and all babies spill small amounts of glucose in their urine for several days especially after any period of stress. Uptake saturation is best dealt with by reducing the rate of glucose infusion by 75% for 6–12 hours. Insulin (q.v.) is seldom needed. There is *no* good evidence that blood levels of up to 15 mmol/l (270 mg/dl) are dangerous, or that urinary loss can cause an osmotic diuresis (as is often feared) until the urine contains at least 1% glucose. Levels measured using any blood specimen taken from a line containing glucose will always be misleadingly high, even if a vigorous attempt was made to clear the 'dead space' first. Sudden hyperglycaemia in a previously stable baby may be caused by pain, infection, necrotising enterocolitis or an intracranial bleed. Very high plasma levels raise serum osmolality, but this does not cause the damaging transcellular shifts that are seen with high serum sodium levels because glucose can cross the cell membrane.

Treatment of hypoglycaemia
Starting a 5 ml/kg per hour infusion of 10% glucose will raise the blood sugar level out of the hypoglycaemic range within 10 minutes in 9 babies out of 10. A loading dose of 2·5 ml/kg over 5 minutes will speed the control of hypoglycaemic stupor or fits. The infusion must then be continued at a steady rate and only reduced slowly as the milk intake is increased. Avoid 'bolus' injections of any strength – they only destabilise the body's regulatory mechanisms. A maintenance infusion containing more than 10% glucose may be necessary where water intake has to be kept below 100 ml/kg per day.

Supply
500 ml bags containing 5%, 10% and 15% glucose, 4% glucose in 0·18% sodium chloride, and 10% glucose in 0·18% sodium chloride are available as stock, and cost 48p to 158p each. 25 ml ampoules of 25% glucose (costing £2·60 each) and 50 ml bags of 5% glucose are available on request.

References

Cornblath M, Hawdon JM, Williams AF, *et al*. Controversies regarding definition of neonatal hypoglycaemia. Suggested operational thresholds. *Pediatrics* 2000;**105**:1141–5.

Couthard MG, Hey EN. Renal processing of glucose in well and sick neonates. *Arch Dis Child* 1999;**81**:F92–8.

Hawdon JM, Modder J, eds. Glucose control in the perinatal period. *Semin Fetal Neonat Med* 2005;**10**:305–400. (Whole issue.)

Lilien LD, Grajwer LA, Pildes RS. Treatment of neonatal hypoglycaemia with continuous intravenous glucose infusions. *J Pediatr* 1977;**91**:779–82. (See also 1980;**97**:295–8.)

Rozance PJ, Hay WW. Hypoglycemia in newborn infants: features associated with adverse outcomes. [Review] *Biol Neonat* 2006;**90**:74–86. (See also pp. 87–8.)

Use
The main neonatal use of glyceryl trinitrate is in the management of low output cardiac failure. Topical use to counteract tissue ischaemia is discussed in the monograph on dopamine.

Pharmacology
The main use of glyceryl trinitrate (other than as an explosive!) is in the treatment of coronary heart disease. When it was first used for angina in 1879 it was presumed that it had a direct effect on the coronary arteries, but it is now recognised to have other systemic effects that help to reduce cardiac oxygen requirements. **Low** doses (between 500 nanograms and 3 micrograms/kg per minute) decrease ventricular filling pressure ('preload') by reducing venous tone. This decreases pulmonary artery pressure and increases cardiac output. It also improves coronary artery perfusion and decreases myocardial oxygen consumption, making secondary cardiac ischaemia less likely. **Moderate** doses (4–6 micrograms/kg per minute) cause pulmonary and systemic arteriolar dilatation, while **high** doses (7–10 micrograms/kg per minute) eventually cause hypotension and secondary tachycardia.

Glyceryl trinitrate is taken up avidly by vascular smooth muscle. Nitric oxide (q.v.) is then liberated causing a marked decrease in venous and arterial tone. It is also quickly metabolised (half life 1–4 minutes) by glutathione organic nitrate reductase in the liver and must, therefore, be given by continuous infusion. Therapy can be complicated by methaemoglobinaemia (an oxidation byproduct of the reaction between nitric oxide and haemoglobin) but this has not been described in neonates and children. It can also produce raised intracranial pressure although this has not been described in the newborn either. Nevertheless its use in children has not yet been endorsed by the manufacturers. There is no evidence of teratogenicity, and growing evidence that it can be used as a safe, rapid-onset, short-acting, tocolytic agent (one 100 microgram 'bolus' IV) to manage placental retention, or fetal entrapment during Caesarean section or vaginal twin delivery, or to control uterine tone during external cephalic version. While transdermal patch treatment has recently been used (as a nitric oxide 'donor') to control preterm labour, no trial has yet looked to see if this is as effective as atosiban or nifedipine (q.v.), and such treatment often causes headache. No information is available on use during lactation.

Treatment
Intravenous use: Continuous infusions have been used in the management of patients with systemic or pulmonary venous congestion due to poor ventricular function. Start with a low dose and increase as necessary. It is important to exclude hypovolaemia, and often appropriate to use an inotrope as well.

Topical use: Serious catheter-related vasospasm can sometimes be corrected by the application of 2% glyceryl trinitrate ointment. Papaverine (q.v.) may be an equally effective way of controlling vasospasm.

Compatibility
Glyceryl trinitrate can be added (terminally) to an IV line containing atracurium, dobutamine and/or dopamine, midazolam, milrinone or nitroprusside.

Supply and administration
10 ml ampoules containing 50 mg of glyceryl trinitrate are available costing £13. Most formulations contain some propylene glycol (a maximum of 30% v/v). To give an infusion of 1 microgram/kg per minute draw up 15 mg of glyceryl trinitrate for each kg the baby weighs, dilute to 25 ml with 10% glucose or glucose saline, and infuse at a rate of 0·1 ml/hour (a less concentrated solution of glucose or glucose saline can be used if necessary). Ampoules should be protected from strong light, discarded if the fluid is discoloured, and disposed of promptly after use. Check the strength of the ampoule carefully before use. Glyceryl trinitrate is absorbed by polyvinyl chloride and should only be given using syringes (Gillette Sabre®, BD Plastipack®, Monoject disposable®) and tubing (such as Vygon Lectrocath®) made of polyethylene. A fresh solution should be prepared every 24 hours.

An ointment containing 2% glyceryl trinitrate (60 grams costing £11) can be obtained on request. Transdermal patches are used in adults with coronary heart disease.

References
See also the relevant Cochrane reviews

Artman M, Graham TP. Guidelines for vasodilator therapy of congestive heart failure in infants and children. *Am Heart J* 1987;**113**:994–1004.

Baserga MC, Puri A, Sola A. The use of topical nitroglycerin ointment to treat peripheral tissue ischaemia secondary to arterial line complications in neonates. *J Perinatol* 2002;**22**:416–19.

Black RS, Lees C, Thompson S, *et al*. Maternal and fetal cardiovascular effects of transdermal glyceryl trinitrate and intravenous ritodrine. *Obstet Gynecol* 1999;**94**:572–6.

Keeley SR, Bohn DJ. The use of inotropic and afterload-reducing agents in neonates. *Clin Perinatol* 1988;**15**:467–89.

Smith GN, Walker MC, Ohlsson A, *et al*. Randomized double-blind placebo-controlled trial of transdermal nitroglycerin for preterm labour. *Am J Obstet Gynecol* 2007;**196**:37.e1–8 [RCT] (For full article see www.AJOG.org.)

Tamura M, Kawano T. Effects of intravenous nitroglycerin on hemodynamics in neonates with refractory congestive heart failure or PFC. *Acta Paediatr Jpn* 1990;**32**:291–8.

Wong AF, McCulloch LM, Sola A. Treatment of peripheral tissue ischaemia with topical nitroglycerin ointment in neonates. *J Pediatr* 1992;**121**:980–3.

Use

Glycine is used in the management of isovaleric acidaemia – a rare, autosomal recessive, inborn error of metabolism.

Biochemistry

Glycine is a naturally occurring amino acid. In isovaleric acidaemia, the administration of additional glycine greatly speeds the conversion of isovaleryl-CoA to isovalerylglycine, which is then excreted in the urine. Aspirin should be avoided as it is a competitive substrate for one of the essential metabolic steps involved.

Isovaleric acidaemia

Isovaleric acidaemia is a rare, inherited metabolic condition caused by a deficiency of the enzyme isovaleryl-CoA dehydrogenase, which controls an early step in the metabolism of the branch chain amino acid leucine. A range of metabolites, including isovaleric acid, then accumulate. Glycine and carnitine are conjugated to isovaleric acid and then excreted in the urine. Some patients present soon after birth (often within 3–6 days) with poor feeding, vomiting and drowsiness. Tremor, twitching and seizures may be seen before the child lapses into coma and death. Other patients present for the first time when rather older with similar symptoms precipitated by intercurrent illness. Symptoms are often accompanied by acidosis, ketosis and a high blood ammonia level (sometimes >500 µmol/l). There can often be neutropenia, thrombocytopenia and hypo- or hyperglycaemia when the condition first presents in the neonatal period. High isovaleric acid levels may give rise to a characteristic unpleasant odor, which has been likened to that of 'sweaty feet'. Patients present, very occasionally, with progressive generalised developmental delay. The condition is most easily diagnosed by detecting excess isovalerylglycine (and 3-hydroxyisovaleric acid) in the urine or abnormal acylcarnitines in the blood. Patients are generally treated with glycine and carnitine, a low protein diet, and measures to minimize catabolism during intercurrent illnesses. The prognosis can be good with early diagnosis but many patients suffer neurological damage prior to diagnosis. Symptomatic disturbance becomes less common in later childhood, and the condition is compatible with normal adult life (including a normal uneventful pregnancy). There is no reason to think that lactation would be unwise while the mother herself remains well.

Treatment

Acute illness: Withdraw all protein from the diet, and give IV glucose to minimise catabolism. Start treatment with oral glycine (see below). Urgent haemodialysis may be indicated if there is severe hyperammonaemia (>500 µmol/l) when the patient first presents.

Maintenance care: The usual maintenance dose is 50 mg/kg of glycine three times a day, although during acute illness the amount given can be increased to 100 mg/kg six times a day. The normal maintenance dose may need to be modified if there is liver or kidney impairment, and stopped if there is anuria. Long-term management involves dietary protein restriction supervised by someone experienced in the management of metabolic disease. L-carnitine is sometimes also given routinely by mouth (or IV if a metabolic crisis occurs).

Supply and administration

Glycine is available as a powder from SHS International, and a stable solution containing 50 or 100 mg/ml can be provided on request. 100 grams of power costs £5. No intravenous preparation is available, but glycine can be given by nasogastric tube, and the likelihood of vomiting can be reduced by giving small frequent doses.

References

Cohn RM, Yudkoff M, Rothman R, *et al*. Isovaleric acidemia: use of glycine therapy in neonates. *N Engl J Med* 1978;**299**:996–9.

Dixon MA, Leonard JV. Intercurrent illness in inborn errors of intermediary metabolism. *Arch Dis Child* 1992;**67**:1387–91.

Shih VE, Aubry RH, DeGrande G, *et al*. Maternal isovaleric acidemia. *J Pediatr* 1984;**105**:77–8.

Sweetman L, Williams JC. Branched chain organic acidurias. In: Scriver CR, Beaudet AL, Sly WS, *et al*., eds. *The metabolic and molecular bases of inherited disease*, 8th edn. New York: McGraw-Hill, 2001: pp. 2125–63.

Wendel U, de Baulny HO. Branched-chain organic acidurias/acidemias. In: Fernandes J, Saudubray J-M, van den Berghe G, *et al*., eds. *Inborn metabolic diseases. Diagnosis and treatment*, 4th edn. Berlin: Springer-Verlag, 2006: pp. 246–62.

Use

Glycopyrronium, like atropine (q.v.), can be used to combat vagal bradycardia and to control salivation and tracheal secretions during general anaesthesia. It is also given to control the muscarinic effect of neostigmine (q.v.) when this drug is used to reverse the effect of a non-depolarising muscle relaxant.

Pharmacology

Glycopyrronium bromide is a quarternary ammonium drug, with peripheral antimuscarinic effects similar to those of atropine, that is rapidly redistributed into the tissues after IV or IM injection. It was first introduced into clinical use in 1960. The full effect of IM administration is only seen after 15 minutes, and vagal blockade lasts about 3 hours. The plasma half life is only 5–10 minutes during childhood and adult life, with almost half the drug being excreted in the urine within 3 hours. The way that babies handle this drug when less than a month old has not yet been studied. Anaesthetists increasingly prefer glycopyrronium to atropine and the other belladona alkaloids, partly because very little glycopyrronium crosses the blood:brain barrier. Transplacental passage is also less than for atropine, and the amount detected in umbilical cord blood following use during Caesarean delivery is small. Rapid plasma clearance makes it extremely unlikely that use during lactation would pose any problem. Oral absorption is poor, but a 50 microgram/kg oral dose has been used with some success to control drooling in older children with severe cerebral palsy. A botulinum A toxin injection into the salivary gland may, however, be more effective.

Glycopyrronium, given with neostigmine, achieves an excellent controlled reversal of the neuromuscular blockade seen with the competitive muscle relaxant drugs such as pancuronium (q.v.), but it may take at least 30 minutes to effect the full reversal of deep blockade. A 1:5 drug ratio seems to minimise any variation in heart rate. The risk of dysrhythmia is lower with glycopyrronium, and the lack of any effect on the central nervous system speeds arousal after general anaesthesia.

Treatment

Premedication: The usual dose is 5 micrograms/kg IV shortly before the induction of anaesthesia. Oral premedication with 50 micrograms/kg 1 hour before surgery is not as effective as a 20 microgram/kg oral dose of atropine at controlling the bradycardia associated with anaesthetic induction.

Reversing neuromuscular block: 10 micrograms/kg of glycopyrronium and 50 micrograms/kg of neostigmine (0·2 ml/kg of a combined solution made up as described below), given IV, will reverse the muscle relaxing effect of pancuronium (and, where necessary, atracurium, rocuronium and vecuronium).

Drooling: 50 micrograms/kg by mouth 2–3 times a day may help control drooling in cerebral palsy.

Alternatives

Neuromuscular blockade can be reversed just as effectively with atropine and neostigmine if glycopyrronium is not available. Give 20 micrograms/kg of atropine IV followed by a 40 microgram/kg dose of IV neostigmine.

Toxicity

There are, as yet, few published reports of the effect of an excessive dose, but presentation and management would be the same as for atropine.

Supply and administration

Combined 1 ml ampoules containing 2·5 mg of neostigmine and 500 micrograms of glycopyrronium bromide are available costing £1. Take the content of the 1 ml ampoule, dilute to 10 ml with 0·9% sodium chloride, and give 0·2 ml/kg of this diluted solution to reverse the neuromuscular block caused by non-depolarising muscle relaxant drugs. Plain 1 ml ampoules simply containing 200 micrograms of glycopyrronium bromide are available for 60p. Dispersible 1 and 2 mg tablets for oral use could be imported into the UK on request.

References

Ali-Melkkilä T, Kaila T, Kanto J, *et al.* Pharmacokinetics of glycopyrronium in parturients. *Anesthesia* 1990;**45**:634–7.

Bachrach SJ, Walter RS, Trzeinski K. Use of glycopyrrolate and other anticholinergic medications for sialorrhea in children with cerebral palsy. *Clin Pediatr* 1998;**37**:485–90.

Cartabuke RS, Davidson PJ, Warner LO. Is premedication with oral glycopyrrolate as effective as oral atropine in attenuating cardiovascular depression in infants receiving halothane for induction of anaesthesia? *Anesth Analg* 1991;**73**:271–4. [RCT]

Goldhill DR, Embree PB, Ali HH, *et al.* Reversal of pancuronium. Neuromuscular and cardiovascular effects of a mixture of neostigmine and glycopyrronium. *Anaesthesia* 1988;**43**:443–6.

Jongerius PH, van den Hoogen FJA, van Limbeek J, *et al.* Effect of botulinum toxin in the treatment of drooling: a controlled clinical trial. *Pediatrics* 2004;**114**:620–7. [RCT]

Mirrkakhur RK, Shepherd WFI, Jones CJ. Ventilation and the oculocardiac reflex. Prevention of oculocardiac reflex during surgery for squints: role of controlled ventilation and anticholinergic drugs. *Anaesthesia* 1986;**41**:825–8. [RCT]

Rautakorpi P, Ali-Melkkila T, Kaila T, *et al.* Pharmacokinetics of glycopyrrolate in children. *J Clin Anesth* 1994;**6**:217–20.

van der Burg JJW, Jongerius PH, van Limbeek J, *et al.* Drooling in children with cerebral palsy: effect of salivary flow reduction on daily living and care. *Dev Med Child Neurol* 2006;**48**:103–7.

HAEMOPHILUS INFLUENZAE (Hib) VACCINE

Use

This vaccine, made from protein-conjugated polysaccharides, provides moderately well-sustained protection from type b *Haemophilus influenzae* (Hib) infection. Serious adverse reactions are rare.

Haemophilus infection

H. influenzae can be differentiated into six capsulated serotypes (Hia to Hif) and non-capsulated (ncHi) strains. Before immunisation, serotype b (Hib) accounted for >80% of invasive disease, mainly in children under 5, causing meningitis (60%), epiglottitis (15%), septicaemia (10%), septic arthritis, osteomyelitis, cellulitis and pneumonia. Hib vaccination, introduced in 1992, resulted in a rapid and sustained reduction in Hib disease. Hib cases increased between 1999 and 2003 but, since the introduction of a routine 12-month Hib booster in 2006, the incidence of Hib disease is very low. Other types of *H. influenzae* are now relatively more common. In 2008, only 20 cases of invasive Hib disease in children were reported, compared with 65 ncHi and 15 non-type b encapsulated *H. influenzae* cases. In the newborn, ncHi infections have a 10-fold higher incidence than Hib. They can be associated with septicaemia in the mother, increased complications during labour, and preterm delivery. Invasive ncHi infection usually develops within the first 48 hours of life, follows a fulminant clinical course and is associated with significantly higher case fatality than Hib infections. After the neonatal period, ncHi usually cause non-invasive respiratory tract infections, while invasive ncHi infection occurs mainly in children with significant co-morbidities. Invasive *H. influenzae* infections are notifiable – doctors in England and Wales can report cases via the HPA website (http://www.hpa.org.uk/; select H in topics A–Z: http://www.hpa.org.uk/Topics/InfectiousDiseases/InfectionsAZ/HaemophilusInfluenzae/).

Indications

All children should be offered immunisation against *Haemophilus* (Hib), preferably at the same time as they are immunised against *Meningococcus* (MenC) and against diphtheria, tetanus, pertussis and polio.

Contraindications

Immunisation should be delayed in any child who is acutely unwell, and not offered if a previous dose triggered an anaphylactic reaction. A minor non-febrile infection is no reason to delay immunisation, and the contraindications associated with the use of a live vaccine (cf. measles) do not apply.

Administration

Children under a year old: Give three 0·5 ml doses deep IM into the anterolateral aspect of the thigh at monthly intervals. The combined DTaP/IPV/Hib vaccine is used to offer simultaneous protection against diphtheria, tetanus, pertussis and polio in the UK. Use a different thigh when giving the pneumococcal or group C meningococcal vaccine simultaneously. Babies benefit from a further booster dose of the Hib vaccine at a year (especially if premature), and this became national policy in the UK in February 2006.

Older children: Give other previously unimmunised children under 10 a single 0·5 ml injection when opportunity arises. There is no contraindication to simultaneous immunisation with other routine vaccines, but use a different injection site. Older children only merit immunisation if they have sickle cell disease, asplenia or congenital or acquired immunodeficiency, because serious infection is uncommon.

Anaphylaxis

The management of anaphylaxis (which is very rare) is outlined in the monograph on immunisation.

Documentation

Tell the family doctor every time a child is immunised in hospital, and record what was done in the child's own personal health booklet. Community-based registers of vaccine uptake also need to be informed.

Supply

A product from Aventis Pasteur that combines the diphtheria, tetanus, acellular pertussis, inactivated polio and Hib (DTaP/IPV/Hib) vaccines in now used in the UK. Two companies also make 0·5 ml vials of the monovalent Hib vaccine; these products can be drawn up into the same syringe as the same company's DTP vaccine and given as a single 1 ml injection. Store vaccines at 2–8°C; do not freeze.

References

See also the relevant Cochrane reviews and UK guidelines

Adegbola RA, Secka O, Lahai G, *et al*. Elimination of *Haemophilus influenzae* type b (Hib) disease from The Gambia after the introduction of routine immunisation with a Hib conjugate vaccine: a prospective study. *Lancet* 2005;**366**:144–50. (See also pp. 101–2.)

Cowgill KD, Ndirity M, Nyiro J, *et al*. Effectiveness of *Haemophulus influenzae* Type b conjugate vaccine introduction into routine childhood immunization in Kenya. *JAMA* 2006;**296**:671–8.

Gessner BD, Sutanto A, Linchan M, *et al*. Incidences of vaccine-preventable *Haemophilus influenzae* type b pneumonia and meningitis in Indonesian children: hamlet-randomised vaccine-probe trial. *Lancet* 2005;**365**:43–52. [RCT] (See also pp. 5–7.)

Heath PT, Booy R, McVernon J, *et al*. Hib vaccination in infants born prematurely. *Arch Dis Child* 2003;**88**:206–10. (See also pp. 379–83.)

Ladhani S, Slack MP, Heys M, *et al*. Fall in *Haemophilus influenzae* serotype B disease following implementation of a booster campaign. *Arch Dis Child* 2008;**93**:665–9.

McVernon J, Trotter CL, Slack MPE, *et al*. Trends in *Haemophilus influenzae* group b infections in adults in England and Wales: surveillance study. *BMJ* 2004;**329**:655–8.

Peltola H, Salo E, Saxén H. Incidence of *Haemophilus influenzae* type b meningitis during 18 years of vaccine use: observational study using routine hospital data. *BMJ* 2005;**330**:18–19.

Watt JP, Wolfson LJ, O'Brien KL, *et al*. Burden of disease caused by *Haemophilus influenzae* type b in children younger than 5: global estimates. *Lancet* 2009;**374**:903–11. (See also pp. 854–6.)

Use

Heparin can help maintain catheter patency, and is used during and after cardiovascular surgery. Low molecular weight heparins, such as enoxaparin (q.v.), are now generally used to prevent and manage venous thromboembolism but there is, as yet, little experience of their use in the neonate.

Pharmacology

Heparin is an acid mucopolysaccharide of variable molecular weight (4000–40,000 Daltons) that was first obtained from the liver (hence its name) in a form pure enough to make clinical trials possible in 1935. While it has some thrombolytic action it is mostly used to prevent further blood clot formation rather than to lyse clots that have already formed. The higher molecular weight heparins also inhibit platelet activity. Heparin works *in vitro* by activating plasma antithrombin inhibitor, which then deactivates thrombin and factor Xa. It is metabolised by *N*-desulfation after IV administration and then rapidly cleared from the body. The half life of conventional unfractionated heparin is dose dependent, increasing as the plasma level rises. It averages 90 minutes in adults, but may be less at birth. Fractionated low molecular weight (4000–6000 Dalton) heparins, such as enoxaparin, have a much longer half life. They do not cause osteopenia during long-term use, show much greater bioavailability when given subcutaneously, and are mostly excreted by the kidneys. All products occasionally cause an immune-mediated thrombocytopenia, most commonly 5–10 days after the start of treatment. Because this can, paradoxically, cause a major thromboembolic event, the platelet count *must* be monitored. Stop treatment at once if thrombocytopenia develops, and do not give platelets. Heparin does not cross the placenta, is not teratogenic, and can be given with complete safety during lactation.

Women at high risk of thromboembolism because of immobility, obesity, high parity, previous deep vein thrombosis or an inherited thrombophilia are now increasingly given enoxaparin during pregnancy and, more particularly, operative delivery and the early pueperium. Warfarin (q.v.) continues to be used to anticoagulate women with pulmonary vascular disease, and patients with an artificial heart valve or atrial fibrillation, but time may show that they, too, can be protected with low molecular weight heparin.

Indications for neonatal use

Although one small study has suggested that full *heparinisation* may reduce the formation of arterial thrombi, the effect of any such approach on the risk of intraventricular haemorrhage remains uncertain. Three observational studies (one only reported in abstract) even suggest a correlation between total heparin exposure and the risk of intraventricular haemorrhage in babies of under 1·5 kg in the first week of life. However, this may merely mean that some babies got more heparin because they were already less well. No adequate sized trials have ever been done, and neonatal use has never been subjected to serious study (Newall *et al.* 2009). However, while adverse effects of heparin are rare, heparinised babies can bleed unpredictably, so it is probably unwise to use in heparin in babies with intracranial or gastrointestinal haemorrhage. Uncorrected thrombocytopenia ($<50 \times 10^9/l$) is also a contraindication, and IM injections should not be given to any heparinised patient. Lumbar puncture can also be hazardous. Alteplase and streptokinase (q.v.) are almost certainly better at removing clots that have already formed. Prophylactic *low-dose* use to maintain catheter patency is much better established (see below).

Prophylactic strategies

Monitoring lines: Intravascular catheters are often used to monitor blood pressure and to make blood sampling possible without disturbing the patient. A steady 0·5 or 1·0 ml/hour infusion containing 1–2 units of heparin for each ml of fluid prolongs catheter patency. Glucose shortens the line's life and makes it impossible to monitor blood glucose levels. The use of 0·45% rather than 0·9% sodium chloride reduces the risk of sodium overload. Clear the 1 ml catheter 'dead space' carefully after sampling and consider using water rather than dextrose or saline for this in order to avoid sudden swings in blood glucose and the infusion of further unmeasured quantities of sodium chloride. Any water or saline used to 'flush' the dead space does not need to contain further heparin and should not, when treating a small baby, come from an ampoule containing a bacteriostatic for the reasons outlined in the archived monograph on benzyl alcohol.

'Stopped off' lines and cannulas: 'Normal' saline containing 10 units/ml of heparin is commonly flushed through and left in 'stopped off' cannulas after use, but the addition of heparin does little to prolong patency. Central venous long lines are often left primed with a fluid containing 5000 units/ml of heparin, but a solution containing 1 mg/ml of alteplase (q.v.) seems to be a better way of keeping the catheter patent.

Cardiac catheterisation: A 100 unit/kg IV bolus at the start of the procedure greatly reduces the risk of symptomatic thromboembolism.

Intravascular infusions: Neonatal trials have shown that adding heparin to the infusate prolongs the patency, not only of arterial catheters, but also of peripherally inserted central venous lines. The most recent trial in babies with a central venous line in place used a dose of 0·5 units/kg per hour. Such use caused a five-fold reduction in the number of catheters needing replacement because of blockage, but it did not reduce the number needing replacement because of extravasation or suspected sepsis (an equally common reason for replacement), or the risk of a clot forming close to where the tip of the catheter was (or had been). Only two small trials have yet been done (involving just 200 children) to see whether the use of a heparin-bonded catheter helps to sustain catheter patency.

Full anticoagulation

The indications for this in the neonate remain unclear. There is no good evidence that anticoagulation reduces the risk of an existing clot enlarging, fragmenting and shedding emboli, or reforming after lysis. Neither is heparinisation called for in

Continued on p. 128

most cases of disseminated intravascular coagulation (DIC). If treatment *is* indicated start by giving a loading dose of 75 units/kg IV over 10 minutes (a loading dose of 50 units/kg may be safer in babies with a postconceptional age of less than 35 weeks). Maintenance requirements vary – start with a continuous IV infusion of 25 units/kg per hour (1 ml/hour of a solution made up as described below) and assess the requirement by measuring the activated partial thromboplastin time (APTT) after 4 hours. Monitor the platelet level weekly.

Dose monitoring

The anticoagulant dose used during extracorporeal membrane oxygenation (ECMO) and to lyse thrombi is one that raises the APTT to 1·8–2·0 times the normal level. Never take blood for this test from an intravascular line that has *ever* contained heparin: sufficient heparin will remain to invalidate the laboratory result even if the line is flushed through first. Normal neonatal APTT times are given in the monograph on fresh frozen plasma.

Antidote

Protamine sulphate is a basic protein that combines with heparin to produce a stable complex devoid of anticoagulant activity. The effect of heparin can, therefore, be neutralised by giving 1 mg of protamine sulphate IV over about 5 minutes for every 100 units of heparin given in the previous 2 hours. Excess protamine is dangerous because it binds platelets and proteins such as fibrinogen producing, in itself, a bleeding tendency.

Compatibility

It is known that adrenaline, atracurium, fentanyl, glyceryl trinitrate, insulin, isoprenaline, lidocaine, midazolam, milrinone, morphine, nitroprusside, noradrenaline, propofol, prostaglandin E_1, ranitidine, streptokinase, TPN (the standard formulation with or without lipid) and urokinase can be added (terminally) to a line containing heparin. So can plain amphotericin (but not the liposomal formulation because of concern that this may destabilise the colloid). So, too, can dopamine, but there are reports suggesting that although heparin is compatible with dobutamine when suspended in 0·9% sodium chloride, precipitation may occur (somewhat unpredictably) when the two drugs are mixed, even briefly, in a glucose solution.

Supply and administration

Heparin is stable in solution so IV lines do not need to be replaced after some set time on these grounds.

Multidose vials: 5 ml multi-use vials containing 1000 units/ml of standard, unfractionated heparin sodium cost 92p, and 5 ml 5000 unit/ml vials cost £2·10. Vials can be stored at room temperature (5–25°C) for 18 months, but are best not kept more than 28 days once open. These vials contain 50 mg of benzyl alcohol.

Single-dose ampoules: 5 ml vials containing 1000 and 5000 units/ml of single-use, preservative-free, unfractionated heparin calcium cost 93p and £1·90 respectively.

Full anticoagulation: To give 25 units/kg of heparin per hour, take 1·25 ml (1250 units) from the multidose vial for each kg the baby weighs into a syringe, dilute this to 50 ml with 0·9% sodium chloride, and infuse at a rate of 1 ml/hour.

Flush solution: Accurate dilution is best achieved by making any syringe containing 1 unit/ml of heparin 'flush' solution up from a 500 ml bag of 0·9% (or 0·45%) IV sodium chloride freshly prepared by the prior addition of 0·5 ml (500 units) of heparin. Small 5 ml preservative-free ampoules of Hep-Lock® and Hepsal® flush solution (costing 25p) contain 0·75 mmol of sodium and 50 units of unfractionated heparin.

Protamine sulphate: 5 ml ampoules containing 10 mg/ml cost 96p each.

References   See also the relevant Cochrane reviews and UK guideline on thromboembolic disease in pregnancy

Hecker JF. Potential for extending survival of peripheral intravenous infusions. *BMJ* 1992;**304**:619–24. [SR]

Horgan MJ, Bartoletti A, Polansky S. Effect of heparin infusates on umbilical arterial catheters on frequency of thrombolic complications. *J Pediatr* 1987;**111**:774–8.

Monagle P, Chalmers E, Chan A, *et al*. Antithrombotic therapy in neonates and children: American College of Chest Physicians evidenced-based clinical practice guidelines (8th edition). *Chest* 2008;**133**(suppl 6):887S–968S.

Newall F, Barnes C, Igjatovic V, *et al*. Heparin-induced thrombocytopenia in children. *J Paediatr Child Health* 2003;**39**:289–92. [SR]

Newall F, Johnston L, Ignjatovic V, *et al*. Unfractionated heparin therapy in infants and children. [Review] *Pediatrics* 2009;**123**:e510–18.

Pierce CM, Wade Amok Q. Heparin-bonded central venous lines reduce thrombotic and infective complications in critically ill children. *Intensive Care Med* 2000;**26**:967–72. [RCT]

Pryce R. Cannula patency: should we use flushes or continuous fluids, or heparin? *Arch Dis Child* 2009;**94**:992–4. [SR]

Randolph AG, Cook DJ, Gonzales CA, *et al*. Benefit of heparin in peripheral venous and arterial catheters: systematic review and meta-analysis of randomised controlled trials. *BMJ* 1998;**316**:969–75. [SR]

Shah PS, Kalyn A, Satodia P, *et al*. A randomized, controlled trial of heparin versus placebo infusion to prolong the usability of peripherally placed percutaneous central venous catheters (PCVCs) in neonates: the HIP (Heparin Infusion for PCVC) study. *Pediatrics* 2007;**119**:e284–91. [RCT].

Silvers KM, Darlow BA, Winterbourn CC. Pharmacological levels of heparin do not destabilise neonatal parenteral nutrition. *J Parent Ent Nutr* 1998;**22**:311–14.

Use
Hepatitis B vaccine provides active lasting immunity to the hepatitis B virus (HBV); a specific immunoglobulin (HBIg) can be used to provide immediate short-lasting passive immunity.

Hepatitis B
Hepatitis B is a major worldwide problem. Illness starts insidiously and is of variable severity. Infection can result from sexual contact, from contaminated blood or a blood-contaminated needle. Some 2–10% of the adults so infected become chronic carriers, and nearly a quarter of these eventually develop chronic disease (with possible cirrhosis or hepatocellular carcinoma). Infection can also pass from mother to child. Transplacental passage is rare, but 80% of babies become infected during delivery, and 90% of those so infected become chronic carriers. Universal early immunisation is the policy recommended by WHO, and the approach now being adopted in most parts of the world. Maternal screening and selective neonatal immunisation remains the approach still being adopted in Scandinavia and the UK, but this is only going to be effective if robust steps are taken to make sure that the babies so identified get the treatment they need. The present vaccines contain 10 or 20 micrograms/ml of hepatitis B surface (Australian) antigen (HBsAg) adsorbed on an aluminium hydroxide adjuvant. Hepatitis B, like any form of hepatitis, is a notifiable infection.

Indications
Babies born to mothers with the hepatitis B surface (s) antigen (HBsAg) need prompt active immunisation. Babies born to mothers developing hepatitis B during pregnancy, or born to mothers who are both surface and core (e) antigen (HBeAg) positive are at particularly **high risk** and need immediate bridging protection with specific hepatitis B immunoglobulin as well. Where the mother's 'e' marker status is unknown, or the baby weighs <1·5 kg at birth, the baby should be treated as if it were at high risk. The UK's current policy of selective immunisation can only be made to work if the policy of universal antenatal screening is fully implemented, and there is a fail-safe call back system so that those identified get all the treatment recommended. Active immunisation is also offered to all health care staff, and to all children on haemodialysis, requiring frequent or large blood transfusions or repeated factor concentrates.

Contraindications
Side effects of immunisation (other than local soreness) are rare, and contraindications to immunisation are almost non-existent (although vaccination should be delayed in the face of intercurrent illness). Vaccination should not be withheld from a high-risk woman because she is pregnant since infection in pregnancy can result in severe illness and chronic infection in the baby.

Administration
Universal vaccination: Doses are usually given at 0–2, 1–4 and 6–18 months. Premature babies given their first dose within a month of birth benefit from a fourth dose. Protection wanes over time.

Selective vaccination: At-risk babies need a first 0·5 ml IM injection of hepatitis B vaccine within 24 hours of birth, and booster injections 1, 2 and 12 months later. High-risk babies (as defined above) also need 200 units of hepatitis B specific immunoglobulin (HBIg) IM into the other thigh within 24 hours of birth (irrespective of birthweight). Breastfeeding can safely continue. This policy provides 95% protection, but it is wise to check that the baby is not surface antigen (HBsAg) positive at 12 months.

Anaphylaxis
The management of anaphylaxis (which is very rare) is outlined in the monograph on immunisation.

Supply
Vaccine: Give a 0·5 ml injection irrespective of which product is used. The SmithKline Beecham (Engerix B®) vaccine comes in 0·5 ml (10 microgram) vials; Aventis-Pasteur produce an interchangeable product (HBvaxPRO®) in 0·5 ml (5 microgram) vials. Both cost £9·10 each. Store at 2–8°C but do not freeze. Shake before use. *Always* record administration in the child's personal health record.

Immunoglobulin: Ampoules containing 200 or 500 units of HBIg prepared by the Blood Products Laboratory are available in the UK from most Health Protection Agency laboratories. HBIg is expensive and only limited supplies are available. Store all ampoules at 4°C.

References
See also the full UK website guidelines

Aggarwal R, Ranjan P. Preventing and treating hepatitis B infection. *BMJ* 2004;**329**:1080–6. (See also pp. 1059–60.)

Lee C, Gong Y, Brok J, *et al*. Effect of hepatitis B immunisation in newborn infants of mothers positive for hepatitis B surface antigen: systematic review and meta-analysis. *BMJ* 2006;**332**:328–31. [SR]

Lin Y-C, Chang M-H, Ni Y-H, *et al*. Long-term immunogenicity and efficacy of universal hepatitis B virus vaccine vaccination in Taiwan. *J Infect Dis* 2003;**187**:134–8.

Norris S, Siddiqi K, Mohsen A. Hepatitis B (prevention). *Clin Evid* 2006;**15**:1049–60 (and updates). [SR]

Petersen KM, Bulkow LR, McMahon BJ, *et al*. Duration of hepatitis B immunity in low risk children receiving hepatitis B vaccinations from birth. *Pediatr Infect Dis J*.2004;**23**:650–5.

Zanetti AR, Mariano A, Romanò L, *et al*. Long-term immunogenicity of hepatitis B vaccination and policy for booster: an Italian multicentre study. *Lancet* 2005;**366**:1379–84. (See also pp. 1337–8.)

Use

Extravasation can cause severe tissue injury when irritant fluid leaks from a vein during infusion, and hyaluronidase can, if started promptly, be used to limit such damage. It can also be used to aid subcutaneous rehydration ('hypodermoclysis') when venous access proves difficult.

Pharmacology

Hyaluronidase is a naturally occurring enzyme that has a temporary and reversible depolymerising action on the polysaccharide hyaluronic acid present in the intercellular matrix of connective tissue. It can be used to enhance the permeation of local anaesthetics, subcutaneous infusions and intramuscular injections into the body tissues. It can also aid the resorption of excess tissue fluid. The product mostly used since 1980 is a purified extract of sheep semen. The dose recommended here (the dose usually employed in the UK) is five times the dose generally used in the United States. Hyaluronidase was initially used on its own in an attempt to disperse damaging extravasated fluid, but immediate irrigation (with or without prior infiltration with hyaluronidase) with a view to washing away any irritant fluid is probably a much more effective strategy. There is still, regrettably, almost no good controlled trial evidence on which to base the management of extravasation injury.

Treating IV extravasation tissue damage

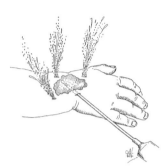

Clean the damaged area of skin and then infiltrate it immediately with a 0·3 ml/kg of 1% lidocaine (q.v.). (Bupivacaine (q.v.) could, alternatively, be used to provide a more sustained pain relief although it takes longer to become effective.) Then inject 500–1000 units of hyaluronidase into the subcutaneous tissues under the area of damaged skin. The simplest approach is merely to inject some hyaluronidase into the cannula through which extravasation occurred (if this is still in place), but it is said to be better, especially with large lesions, to make three or four small 'incisions' into the skin with a sharp scalpel round the edges of the area to be treated (Fig. 1), insert a blunt Verres needle into each incision in turn, inject the hyaluronidase and then irrigate the damaged tissue with 25–100 ml of 0·9% saline using the needle and three-way tap (i.e. a total of 100–400 ml of irrigating fluid in all, depending on the size of the lesion). Saline should flow freely out of the other incisions. Excess fluid can be massaged out of the incisions by gentle manipulation. The damaged area is probably then best kept reasonably moist. A paraffin gauze (tulle gras) dressing is commonly employed, but a hydrocolloid dressing may be better at facilitating auto-debridement (a very poorly researched topic).

Fig. 1 Reproduced with permission from Davies *et al.* (1994).

Extravasation of vasoconstrictive drugs

It has been traditional to manage the dangerous ischaemia and the dermal necrosis that can result from the extravasation of fluid containing vasoconstrictive drugs such as adrenaline, dopamine and noradrenaline (q.v.) by prompt infiltration with not more than 5 mg of phentolamine mesilate in 5 ml 0·9% sodium chloride using a fine needle. There is, however, some evidence that the application of 25 mm (16 mg) of topical 2% glyceryl trinitrate ointment (q.v.) may prove a simpler and equally effective strategy. Infusions of dopamine in particular seem capable of causing ischaemic tissue damage even when there has been no visible extravasation, and staff may sometimes need to stop the infusion if there is significant blanching along the side of the vein.

Emergency rehydration when venous access is difficult

A similar initial dose of hyaluronidase can be used to speed the subcutaneous delivery of any isotonic fluid.

Supply

Hyaluronidase: Ampoules containing 1500 units of hyaluronidase injection BP cost £7·60 each. Dissolve the contents in 3 ml of water for injection to give a solution containing 500 units per ml just before use.
Phentolamine mesilate: 1 ml ampoules containing 10 mg of phentolamine mesilate (Rogitine® or Regitine®) cost £1·70 each.
Needles: Verres needles are obtainable in the UK from Downes Surgical Ltd, Sheffield. They are widely used to insufflate air during laparoscopy.

References

Allen CH, Etzwiler LS, Miller MK, *et al.* Recombinant human hyaluronidase-enabled subcutaneous pediatric rehydration. *Pedatrics* 2009;**124**:e858–67.
Camp-Sorrell D. Developing extravasation protocols and monitoring outcomes. *J Intraven Nurs* 1998;**21**:232–9.
Casanova D, Bardot J, Magalon G. Emergency treatment of accidental infusion leakage in the newborn: report of 14 cases. *Br J Plast Surg* 2001;**54**:396–9.
Davies J, Gault D, Buchdahl R. Preventing the scars of neonatal intensive care. *Arch Dis Child* 1994;**70**:F50–1.
Lehr VT, Lulic-Botica M, Lindblad WJ, *et al.* Management of infiltration injury in neonates using DuoDerm Hydroactive gel. *Am J Perinatol* 2004;**21**:409–14.
Ramasethu J. Pharmacology review: prevention and management of extravasation injuries in neonates. *Neoreviews* 2004;**5**:e491–7.
Raszka WV, Kueser TK, Smith FR, *et al.* The use of hyaluronidase in the treatment of intravenous extravasation injuries. *J Perinatol* 1990;**10**:146–9.
Subhani M, Sridhar S, DeCristofaro JD. Phentolamine use in a neonate for the prevention of dermal necrosis caused by dopamine: a case report. *J Perinatol* 2001;**21**:324–6.
Wilkins CE, Emmerson AJB. Extravasation injuries on regional neonatal units. *Arch Dis Child* 2004;**89**:F274–5.

Use

Hydralazine has long been used to control severe hypertension in pregnancy. It is also still sometimes used in the long-term management of neonatal hypertension together, if necessary, with propranolol (q.v.).

Hypertension in the first year of life

Systolic blood pressure at rest varies with postmenstrual (that is gestational plus postnatal) age during the first year of life (Fig. 1). Dark lines show the level usually seen in the term baby and dashed lines the normal range for a baby of 24–26 weeks' gestation at birth. Systolic pressure in those less immature than this seldom exceeds that shown for a 24–26-week gestation baby. See the monograph on labetalol for general guidance on the measurement of blood pressure.

Serious hypertension is rare in the neonatal period, but can present with signs of congestive cardiac failure. The cause is most often renal in origin, and can follow silent embolic arterial damage (hypertension due to renal vein thrombosis usually only occurs after a longer latent phase). Hydralazine, with or without propranolol, was often used for maintenance in the past, once any acute crisis was under control, but nifedipine (q.v.) is now increasingly the

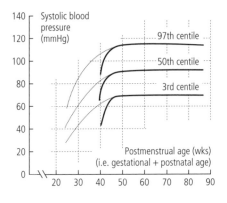

preferred option. The response to captopril (q.v.) and enalapril is too unpredictable to make either of these drugs easy to use. Unilateral nephrectomy occasionally merits consideration.

Pharmacology

Hydralazine became the first effective oral antihypertensive when it was patented in 1949. It is well absorbed by mouth but rapid metabolism within the liver as the drug passes up the portal vein halves bioavailability when the drug is given by mouth. Hydralazine is eliminated by acetylation at a very variable rate ('fast acetylation' being an inherited characteristic). The drug causes vasodilatation, drug retention in the vascular wall making it unnecessary to prescribe the drug more than once every 8–12 hours despite a variable plasma half life. The side effects of acute use can mimic those seen in deteriorating pre-eclampsia. Vomiting, diarrhoea and postural hypotension are relatively common adverse effects in older subjects, but little is known about the side effects associated with treatment in the first year of life. Reflex tachycardia is sometimes a problem but this can be controlled with a β-blocker drug such as propranolol. Salt and water retention, as a result of increased renal medullary blood flow, can be counteracted by prescribing a diuretic. Hepatitis, oedema and paralytic ileus have occasionally been reported following long-term administration. There is no evidence of teratogenicity, but trials suggest that labetalol or nifedipine may be better drugs to use in pregnancy. Hydralazine appears in human milk but, weight for weight, a breastfed baby only ingests about 1% of the maternal dose. The manufacturer has not endorsed the use of hydralazine in children.

Drug interactions

Severe hypotension has been described when a patient on hydralazine is given diazoxide.

Treatment

Use in pregnancy: 5–10 mg given slowly IV will usually bring serious hypertension under control, while for maintenance an IV dose of 50–150 micrograms/min is usually effective. For oral maintenance a 25 mg (or occasionally 50 mg) dose twice a day is commonly used.

Use in the first year of life: Try 500 micrograms/kg once every 8 hours by mouth and increase, as necessary, to a maximum of 2–3 mg/kg every 8 hours. Intravenous labetalol hydrochloride (q.v.) is more effective in the initial urgent control of any acute hypertensive crisis, and nifedipine may provide better long-term control.

Supply and administration

Ampoules containing 20 mg of hydralazine, costing £1·60, are available for IV use. Reconstitute the powder with 1 ml of water and then dilute the required amount in 10 ml of 0·9% sodium chloride. Hydralazine is rapidly inactivated by contact with solutions contained glucose. 25 and 50 mg tablets are available for 5p. An oral suspension can also be prepared from a dispersible 12·5 mg tablet.

References

See also the relevant Cochrane reviews

Fried R, Syeinherz LJ, Levin AR, et al. Use of hydralazine for intractable cardiac failure in childhood. J Pediatr 1980;**97**:1009–11.

Magee LA, Cham C, Waterman EJ, et al. Hydralazine for treatment of severe hypertension in pregnancy: meta-analysis. BMJ 2003;**327**:955–60. [SR]

Northern Neonatal Nursing Initiative. Systolic blood pressure in babies of less than 32 weeks gestation in the first year of life. Arch Dis Child 1999;**80**:F38–42.

Rasoulpour M, Marinelli KA. Systemic hypertension. Clin Perinatol 1992;**19**:121–37.

Watkinson M. Hypertension in the newborn baby. [Review] Arch Dis Child 2002;**86**:F78–81.

HYDROCORTISONE

Use
Hydrocortisone has been in use to manage congenital adrenal abnormality and adrenal insufficiency due to hypopituitarism since 1949. Hypotension in the preterm baby often responds to low-dose IV hydrocortisone. Trials of use to prevent bronchopulmonary dysplasia (BPD) have not delivered much consistent benefit.

Pathophysiology
The adrenal cortex normally secretes hydrocortisone (cortisol), which has glucocorticoid activity and weak mineralocorticoid activity. It also secretes the mineralocorticoid aldosterone. Physiological replacement in adrenal insufficiency is best achieved by a combination of hydrocortisone and the artificial mineralocorticoid fludrocortisone (Table 1) but, where the problem is secondary to pituitary failure, mineralocorticoid replacement is not required because aldosterone production is primarily controlled by the rennin–angiotensin system.

Various recessively inherited enzyme deficiencies can cause congenital adrenal hyperplasia, but nearly 95% are due to 21-hydroxylase deficiency, and most of the others to 11-hydroxylase deficiency. Diagnosis is relatively easy in girls because of virilisation and sexual ambiguity, but less easy in boys until the child presents with vomiting, failure to thrive and (ultimately) circulatory collapse; some boys are initially misdiagnosed as having pyloric stenosis. Pelvic imaging, an urgent karyotype, 17-hydroxyprogesterone (17-OHP) measurement and a urinary steroid profile confirm the diagnosis. Congenital adrenal *hypo*plasia can also present in a similar manner, or with hypoglycaemia. It is diagnosed by the presence of salt wasting in the presence of a normal urinary tract, the lack of a significant cortisol response to tetracosactide (q.v.) and a normal 17-OHP level.

Table 1

Drug	Equivalent activity (mg)		Biological half life (hours)
	Glucocorticoid	Mineralocorticoid	
Fludrocortisone	0	20	–
Cortisone acetate	25	0·8	8–12
Hydrocortisone	20	1	8–12
Prednisolone	5	<1	12–36
Betamethasone	0·75	0	36–54
Dexamethasone	0·75	0	36–54

Treatment
Early neonatal hypotension: Hydrocortisone (like dexamethasone (q.v.)) often increases blood pressure as effectively as dopamine (q.v.), and may work when a catecholamine does not. A 1 mg/kg dose IV once every 8 hours is usually enough to reduce the need to use other vasopressor drugs. Try and withdraw treatment within 2–4 days because steroid use increases the risk of fungal infection and also seems to increase the risk of focal gut perforation, especially if the baby is also given ibuprofen or indometacin.

Preventing BPD: Low-dose trials (0·5 mg/kg IV twice a day for 12 days, and half this for 3 days) delivered no benefit except to a subgroup with chorioamnionitis. Later development was not affected by such treatment.

Treating BPD: 2·5 mg/kg twice a day for 7 days, and a reducing dose for a further 2 weeks, was as effective as dexamethasone in one study, and did not have the latter's detrimental effect on later development.

Congenital adrenal hyperplasia: 5–7 mg/m^2 of hydrocortisone once every 8 hours, plus at least 200 micrograms of fludrocortisone once a day, provides a good starting point for neonatal care. Babies with 21-hydroxylase deficiency usually need an additional 2–4 mmol/kg of sodium a day.

Adrenal hypoplasia: Production of cortisol normally averages 6–9 mg/m^2 per day and, making allowance for absorption, 8–10 mg/m^2 of hydrocortisone by mouth will meet normal replacement needs (although need may rise several fold during any acute illness).

Addisonian crisis: This requires IV glucose and a 10 mg bolus followed by a continuing 100 mg/m^2 a day infusion of hydrocortisone. Rapid fluid replacement may be necessary with 0·9% sodium chloride. The high serum potassium almost always corrects itself, but 2 ml/kg of 10% calcium gluconate and/or an infusion of glucose and insulin (q.v.) may be needed if a cardiac arrhythmia develops.

Steroid induced adrenal suppression: See the monograph on dexamethasone.

Supply
100 mg vials of hydrocortisone (as the sodium succinate powder) cost 93p each. Reconstitute with 2 ml of water. An oral suspension can also be provided. Scored 100 microgram fludrocortisone tablets cost 5p each, and small doses can be given with relative ease because the tablets disperse readily in water.

References
See also the relevant Cochrane reviews

Ng PC, Lee CH, Bnur FL, *et al*. A double-blind, randomized, controlled study of a "stress dose" of hydrocortisone for rescue treatment of refractory hypotension in preterm infants. *Pediatrics* 2006;**117**:367–75. [RCT] (See also pp. 516–18.)

Noori S, Friedlich P, Wong P, *et al*. Hemodynamic changes after low-dosage hydrocortisone administration in vasopressor-treated preterm and term neonates. *Pediatrics* 2006;**118**:1456–66.

Rademaker KJ, de Vries LS, Uiterwaal CSPM, *et al*. Postnatal hydrocortisone treatment for chronic lung disease in the preterm newborn and long-term neurodevelopmental follow-up. *Arch Dis Child* 2008;**93**:F58–63. [SR]

Use

Early controlled hypothermia can reduce the long-term disability caused by serious intrapartum asphyxia in the term and near term baby, but it does not reduce the number who are so seriously affected that they die.

Pathophysiology

One of the first major advances in neonatal care came with the recognition that allowing a small baby to become cold greatly decreases the chance of survival – a lesson driven home by the late Bill Silverman's early ground-breaking randomised controlled trials. Now, after another 50 years, we finally have equally good evidence that deliberate cooling can *improve* the chance of disability-free survival in the term baby who has suffered serious intrapartum asphyxia. Hypothermia was long used, before the development of heart–lung bypass technology, to double the time the heart could be stopped to make complex surgery possible without damaging the brain. However, the recognition that much of the damage caused by asphyxia only occurs during the recovery phase eventually sparked a search for ways to mitigate this *secondary* damage.

No drug has yet been shown to be of benefit, but we do now know that some combination of respiratory support with sedation or paralysis, anticonvulsant treatment and a controlled lowering of body temperature to 33–34°C for 3 days can reduce the secondary damage done by acute neonatal anoxic or asphyxial cerebral injury, and that an attempt should be made to stop deep body temperature from rising above 37·5°C even if active cooling is not attempted. Animal evidence suggests that cooling should be started within 3 hours if possible, but clinical trials have shown clear benefit as long as cooling is started within 6 hours of birth. However, cooling does little to help neonates with really severe injury, and does *not* improve outcome in older children suffering brain trauma or a stroke. The first trial tried to selectively cool the head, but whole body cooling is now known to be safe and more effective. Continuous aEEG (amplitude integrated EEG) analysis using a cerebral function monitor is one established way to identify babies justifying such intervention. A two-channel bedside monitor may offer improved discrimination, but monitoring does not pick up all seizure activity. Term babies with a flat trace, a continuous low voltage or a burst suppression pattern that persists for more than 24–36 hours who survive are nearly always left with severe spastic quadriplegia.

One early 8 mg/kg IV dose of theophylline (q.v.) seems to reduce some of the adverse renal consequences of perinatal asphyxia. The use of magnesium sulphate (q.v.) has shown promise, and a range of antioxidant drugs are currently being studied in animal models. Babies who display clinically obvious seizure activity have a much worse long-term outcome than those who do not seem to fit, over and above what can be predicted from damage visible on an MRI scan at 4–6 days. There may not be a causal link here but, because there is good animal evidence that seizure activity can itself be damaging, the search is now on for better ways to prevent or control seizure activity. Giving phenobarbital (q.v.) before seizures occurred seemed to show benefit in one small trial but not another, while a study using thiopental (q.v.) also delivered little benefit. Hypocapnia and hyperoxia seem to be harmful, and respiratory support needs to be managed with this in mind.

Indications

Cooling is indicated in babies of ≥36 weeks' gestation who remain hypotonic or stuporose or who fit after a delivery where sustained resuscitation was needed *or* who have a pH of <7·0 or a base deficit of ≥16 mmol/l within an hour of birth.

Management

Cooling is best achieved using a servo-controlled body wrap, but can be managed with covered ice packs or a fan. Aim to lower body temperature to 33·5°C within 2 hours and hold it there to within ±0·5°C for 72 hours, and then let temperature rise gently over 12 hours. Such moderate cooling does not cause a fall in cardiac output. The later phases of care are best managed in a unit with ready access to neuroimaging and EEG facilities.

Case notification

More will be learnt if all UK use is reported to the TOBY register (www.npeu.ox.ac.uk/tobyregister/contact).

Hypothermia can affect drug clearance

Many drugs mainly metabolised in the liver, such as the barbiturates and opiates, are cleared more slowly during hypothermia. This is also likely to be true of carbamazepine, phenytoin and the benzodiazepines, but we know much less about whether cooling also alters the effectiveness of many of these drugs. The clearance of renally excreted antibiotics will only be affected if hypothermia is severe enough to reduce cardiac output.

References

See also the Cochrane review

Azzopardi DV, Strohm B, Edwards AD, et al. Moderate hypothermia to treat perinatal asphyxial encephalopathy. *N Engl J Med* 2009;**361**:1349–58. [RCT]

Glass HC, Glidden D, Jeremy RJ, et al. Clinical neonatal seizures are independently associated with outcome in infants at risk of hypoxic-ischaemic brain injury. *J Pediatr* 2009;**155**:318–23. (See also pp. 305–6.)

Klinger G, Beyene J, Shah P, et al. Do hyperoxaemia and hypocapnia add to the risk of brain injury after intrapartum asphyxia? *Arch Dis Child* 2005;**90**:F49–52.

Liu Z, Xiong T, Meads C. Clinical effectiveness of treatment with hyperbaric oxygen for neonatal hypoxic-ischaemic encephalopathy: systematic review of Chinese literature. *BMJ* 2006;**333**:374–6. [SR]

Polderman KH. Induced hypothermia and fever control for prevention and treatment of neurological injuries. *Lancet* 2008;**371**:1955–69. [SR]

Shellhaas RA, Soaita AI, Clancy RR. Sensitivity of amplitude-integrated electroencephalography for neonatal seizure detection. *Pediatrics* 2007;**120**:770–7.

Thoresen M. Supportive care during neuroprotective hypothermia in the term newborn: adverse effects and their prevention. *Clin Perinatol* 2008;**35**:74963. (See also the article by Barks on pp. 765–75.)

Tortorici MA, Kochanek PM, Poloyac SM. Effects of hypothermia on drug disposition, metabolism and response: a focus on hypothermia-mediated alterations of the cytochrome P450 enzyme system. *Crit Care Med* 2007;**35**:2196–204.

IBUPROFEN

Use
Ibuprofen is an effective alternative to indometacin (q.v.) in the management of patent ductus arteriosus, and is now widely used instead of paracetamol (q.v.) to control fever in babies over 3 months old.

Pharmacology
Aspirin (q.v.) is the most widely used non-steroidal anti-inflammatory drug (NSAID), but many other drugs with similar properties are now marketed. Different drugs seem to suit different patients best, but ibuprofen (another commonly used NSAID first patented in 1964) seems, in general, to have been associated with the fewest reported adverse effects when used in adults with rheumatoid arthritis. Using ibuprofen in a child who is dehydrated can cause acute severe renal failure. Gastrointestinal complications are, however, the most common problem, making NSAID treatment inappropriate in any patient with a history of peptic ulceration.

Ibuprofen is generally well absorbed when taken by mouth and is excreted in the urine part metabolised. The half life is extremely variable at birth (10–80 hours) but is similar to that seen in adults (~90 minutes) within 3 months of birth. Oral ibuprofen has a useful role in the management of postoperative pain in childhood, but it interferes with bilirubin binding to albumin, and its variable half life precludes its use as a neonatal analgesic. Ibuprofen is the most widely used NSAID in children with rheumatoid arthritis, but the manufacturers do not recommend use for *any* reason in children weighing less than 5 kg.

All NSAIDs inhibit prostaglandin synthesis to some degree. There is, therefore, at least a theoretical risk that high-dose use in the third trimester of pregnancy could cause premature closure of the ductus arteriosus before birth, could prolong or delay labour, or affect post-delivery pulmonary vascular tone (see website commentary). Use around the time of conception doubles the risk of miscarriage, and there may be a marginal increase in the risk of malformation. Manufacturers remain reluctant to recommend the use of any NSAID in pregnancy, and information on recently introduced products is limited. The amount present in breast milk is undetectably small, and there is no contraindication to maternal use during lactation.

The NSAID indometacin has been used for nearly 30 years to induce ductal closure in preterm babies because of its ability to inhibit prostaglandin synthesis. However, indometacin also causes a more marked fall in cerebral, renal and gut blood flow than other NSAID. While there is no evidence that these changes are of any clinical significance, ibuprofen rather than indometacin is now widely used to effect duct closure in Europe. Like indometacin, early prophylactic ibuprofen reduces the number of very preterm babies eventually undergoing duct ligation. However, there is no evidence that early prophylactic use of either drug improves the long-term prognosis for survivors.

Drug interactions
Babies given steroids while on ibuprofen are at increased risk of focal ischemic gut perforation.

Treatment
Patent ductus: 10 mg/kg IV, traditionally infused over 15 minutes, should be followed by 5 mg/kg 24 and 48 hours later. Some studies suggest that oral treatment is just as effective. A second course of treatment may be effective when the first course is not.

Fever: An oral dose of 5–8 mg/kg, repeatable after 6 hours, is widely used to control fever in children over 3 months old (and is slightly more effective than paracetamol). Avoid use in any child who is dehydrated.

Supply
IV preparations vary greatly in price. The 10 mg/ml preparation used in all the trials published to date was obtained by asking a local pharmacy to reconstitute one of the 300 mg vials of the lysine salt marketed by Merckle in Germany for IM use with 23·4 ml of water for injection. Such vials cost £1·75 each. Formulations containing lidocaine cannot be substituted for this product. Ovation Pharmaceuticals market an IV product in America. The 20 mg vials cost $60 each. Orphan Europe have marketed an IV product dissolved in trometamol, although a trial of prophylactic use raised safety issues. The 10 mg (2 ml) ampoules cost £62. A sugar-free 20 mg/ml oral suspension is available from community pharmacists without prescription (100 ml costs £1·60).

References
See also the relevant Cochrane reviews and UK guideline

Cherif A, Khrouf N, Jabnoun S, *et al*. Randomized pilot study comparing oral ibuprofen with intravenous ibuprofen in very low birth weight infants with patent ductus arteriosus. *Pediatrics* 2008;**122**:e1256–61. [RCT]

Dani C, Bertini G, Pezzati M, *et al*. Prophylactic ibuprofen for the prevention of intraventricular hemorrhage among preterm infants: a multicenter, randomised study. *Pediatrics* 2005;**115**:1529–35. [RCT]

Li D-K, Liu L, Odouli R. Exposure to non-steroidal anti-inflammatory drugs during pregnancy and risks of miscarriage: population based cohort study. *BMJ* 2003;**327**:367–71.

Richards J, Johnson A, Fox G, *et al*. A second course of ibuprofen is effective in the closure of a clinically significant PDA in ELBW infants. *Pediatrics* 2009;**124**:e287–93.

Su B-H, Chiu H-Y, Hsieh H-Y, *et al*. Comparison of ibuprofen and indometacin for early targeted treatment of patent ductus arteriosus in extremely premature infants: a randomised trial. *Arch Dis Child* 2008;**93**:F94–9. [RCT]

Thomas RL, Parker GC, Van Overmeire B, *et al*. A meta-analysis of ibuprofen versus indomethacin for closure of patent ductus. *Eur J Pediatr* 2005;**164**:135–40. [SR]

Van Overmeire B, Touw D, Schepens PJC, *et al*. Ibuprofen pharmacokinetics in preterm infants with patent ductus arteriosus. *Clin Pharmacol Ther* 2001;**70**:336–43.

Use

Imipenem is a useful reserve antibiotic that is active against a very wide range of bacteria. Cilastatin is always administered as well. Meropenem (q.v.) is more appropriate where meningitis is suspected, has fewer adverse effects and is easier to give, but little information on neonatal use is yet available.

Pharmacology

This β-lactam antibiotic, developed in 1983, is active against a very wide range of Gram-positive and Gram-negative aerobic and anaerobic bacteria. Some meticillin-resistant staphylococci, group D streptococci and *Pseudomonas* species are resistant to imipenem. The drug acts synergistically with the aminoglycosides *in vitro*, and is sometimes prescribed with an aminoglycoside in the treatment of *Pseudomonas* infection in order to prevent emergence of drug resistance. Imipenem is a valuable reserve antibiotic that should only be used on the advice of a consultant microbiologist.

Because imipenem can cause renal toxicity, and because it is partially inactivated within the kidney, it is always given in combination with cilastatin, a specific dehydropeptidase enzyme inhibitor that blocks imipenem's renal breakdown. Imipenem is widely distributed in many body tissues and crosses the placenta, but CSF levels are low, and the drug is not recommended for CNS infection. Both imipenem and cilastatin are rapidly eliminated by a combination of glomerular filtration and tubular secretion into the urine in adults, the plasma half life being under 1 hour. Less is known about drug handling in the neonatal period; the half life of imipenem is increased three-fold, but that of cilastatin increases 11-fold in the first week of life. As a result any dose regimen that is appropriate for the bactericidal ingredient imipenem will result in the progressive accumulation of cilastatin when the standard product containing equal amounts of both products is used. Whether this matters is not known. A 4:1 imipenem:cilastatin formulation might be better. In its absence prolonged, or high-dose, treatment should be employed with caution. Both drugs are rapidly cleared from the body during haemodialysis.

Adverse effects include localised erythema and thrombophlebitis. Neurotoxic reactions including a progressive encephalopathy with seizures have been seen, sometimes preceded by myoclonic twitching, especially in patients with an existing CNS abnormality. Rapid infusion may cause nausea and vomiting. Diarrhoea can occur and this may, on occasion, be the first sign of pseudomembranous colitis. Superinfection with a non-susceptible organism is an ever present possibility. The manufacturers have advised against the use of imipenem with cilastatin in pregnancy because of increased embryonic loss in animal studies, and have not, as yet, been ready to recommend their use in children less than 3 months old. Substantial placental transfer occurs, but there is no evidence of teratogenicity. Treatment during lactation also seems safe since the baby receives less than 1% of the weight-related maternal dose and the drug is largely inactivated in the gut.

Drug prescribing

The drug should technically be referred to as 'imipenem with cilastatin', but omitting the words 'with cilastatin' is unlikely to cause misunderstanding since all commercial preparations contain both drugs. Record merely the dose of imipenem required.

Treatment

Give 20 mg/kg of imipenem IV over 30 minutes once every 12 hours in the first week of life, every 8 hours in babies 1–3 weeks old, and every 6 hours in babies 4 or more weeks old. Use with caution in patients with any suspected CNS abnormality. Dosage frequency should be reduced if there is any evidence of renal failure, and treatment stopped altogether if there is anuria, unless dialysis is instituted.

Supply and administration

Vials suitable for IV use contain 500 mg of imipenem monohydrate, with an equal quantity of the sodium salt of cilastatin, as a powder ready for reconstitution. Vials cost £12 each. Dilute the content of the 500 mg vial with 100 ml of 10% glucose or glucose saline immediately before use to obtain a solution containing 5 mg/ml. (The drug can be prepared using a less concentrated solution of glucose or glucose saline where necessary.) Shake the vial well until the powder is all dissolved and then infuse the prescribed dose slowly over 30 minutes. Discard the remaining unused solution promptly. Avoid IM use in young children. A 20 mg/kg dose contains 0·07 mmol/kg of sodium.

References

Lau KK, Kink RJ, Jones DP. Myoclonus associated with intraperitoneal imipenem. *Pediatr Nephrol* 2004;**19**:700–1.
Matsuda S, Suzuki M, Oh K, *et al*. Pharmacokinetic and clinical studies on imipenem/cilastatin sodium in the perinatal period. *Jpn J Antibiot* 1988;**41**:1731–41.
Mouton JW, Touzw DJ, Horrevorts AM, *et al*. Comparative pharmacokinetics of the carbapenems: clinical implications. *Clin Pharmacokinet* 2000;**39**:185–201.
Reed MD, Kleigman RM, Yamashita TS, *et al*. Clinical pharmacology of imipenem and cilastatin in premature infants during the first week of life. *Antimicrob Agents Chemother* 1990;**34**:1172–7.
Stuart RL, Turnidge J, Grayson ML. Safety of imipenem in neonates. *Pediatr Infect Dis J* 1995;**14**:804–5.

IMMUNISATION

Aim

National policies now exist in most countries to provide protection against a range of potentially serious infectious illnesses. Separate monographs are available in this manual for BCG vaccination (against TB) and for immunisation against: *Haemophilus influenzae*; hepatitis B; measles, mumps and rubella (MMR: see the rubella vaccine monograph); meningococcal infection; pneumococcal infection; polio; and diphtheria, tetanus and pertussis (DTP: see the whooping cough vaccine monograph). All the above products (other than the hepatitis B vaccine) are available free of charge in the UK and in many other countries.

Basic schedule

UK schedules were simplified in 2004 with the introduction of a new five-in-one vaccine, and augmented in 2006 with the addition of the pneumococcal vaccine (a vaccine first introduced into America 6 years earlier). Immunisation should never be delayed because of prematurity or low body weight. Indeed, it should always be started before discharge in babies spending more than 7 weeks in hospital after birth.

Birth	Give selected babies BCG, and start 'at-risk' babies on a course of hepatitis B vaccination (q.v.)
8 weeks	Combined diphtheria, tetanus, pertussis, polio and *Haemophilus* (DTaP/IPV/Hib) vaccine *and* pneumococcal vaccine
12 weeks	Combined DTaP/IPV/Hib vaccine *and* meningococcal (MenC) vaccine
16 weeks	Combined DTaP/IPV/Hib, MenC *and* pneumococcal vaccines (three injections)
12 months	Combined Hib and MenC vaccine
13 months	Combined measles, mumps and rubella (MMR) *and* pneumococcal vaccine
3·5–5 years	Preschool booster vaccination with the combined DTaP/IPV (or dTaP/IPV) *and* MMR vaccine
12–13 years (girls)	Human papilloma virus vaccination (HPV 16,18) or (HPV 6,11,16,18)
13–18 years	Booster vaccination with a combined tetanus, low-dose diphtheria and polio (Td/IPV) vaccine

Foreign travel

Advice for families on immunisation prior to foreign travel is given in a UK Department of Health leaflet obtainable from the web (www.dh.gov.uk), pharmacies, GP surgeries, post offices and travel agents, or by telephoning 0800 555 777. See also the Department's website: www.travax.nhs.uk/ and www.fitfortravel.scot.nhs.uk. More detailed advice on this, and on malaria prophylaxis, is also given in the *British National Formulary for Children*. Professionals can also get advice from the National Travel Health Network and Centre in the UK by ringing 0845 602 44006712 during normal office hours.

Reactions to immunisation

Most reactions to immunisation are not serious. Older children sometimes faint, and a few hyperventilate. Even quite young infants sometimes respond to pain or sudden surprise with a syncopal attack. Blue breath-holding attacks, in which a child cries and then stops breathing, turning limp and unconscious can occur, and can end with a seizure. Attacks of stiffness and pallor, with self-limiting bradycardia or asystole (reflex anoxic seizures), are less common but well documented. Infants prone to these may also have a seizure if they become feverish after immunisation. Sudden brief loss of consciousness and body tone a few hours after vaccination for pertussis is another well described, but poorly understood, clinical entity (the hypotonic–hyporeflexic episode (HHE) syndrome). Such events should *not* be interpreted as anaphylactic or encephalopathic. Loss of consciousness should only last 5–10 minutes, and recovery is complete without treatment. Such episodes should be managed as though they were a fainting attack.

Anaphylaxis in children under 1 year: True anaphylactic reactions after immunisation are *very* rare and seldom severe. A single 10 microgram/kg dose of adrenaline (q.v.) given deep IM (not subcutaneously) serves to contain most reactions, and is all that can realistically be made available in most community settings. Only a rough estimate of weight is ever needed when giving adrenaline – a standard 150 microgram dose, repeatable once after 5 minutes, is widely recommended. A 1 microgram/kg dose can be given as an IV bolus.

Where urticaria or slowly progressive peripheral oedema is all that develops, it can help to give 250 micrograms/kg of the H_1 histamine antagonist chlorphenamine maleate (chlorpheniramine maleate (former BAN)) promptly IM (even though the manufacturers have not yet endorsed its use in children). If there is *serious* stridor, breathing difficulty or progressive angio-oedema, some advocate giving 0·4 ml/kg of a 1 mg/ml (1:1000) solution of L-adrenaline by nebuliser after administering a first IM dose. Then give 250 micrograms/kg of chlorphenamine IM or, preferably, IV diluted in 5 ml of 0·9% sodium chloride. Give oxygen and take whatever steps are necessary to ensure that the airway can be secured should this become necessary. The dose of nebulised adrenaline can be repeated after 30 minutes.

Wheeze and bronchospasm (seen particularly in patients with a past history of asthma) respond best to nebulised salbutamol (q.v.); 4 mg/kg of IV hydrocortisone (q.v.) may also be of benefit. Use 0·9% sodium chloride rather than colloid if circulatory collapse makes volume expansion appropriate. Lay the child flat, raise the legs and send for help, but never leave the patient unattended. While severe anaphylactic shock, with hypotension, tachycardia and rapid cardiovascular collapse, can cause death, there has not been a single death using any of these products in the UK since formal monitoring began 25 years ago. Notify all untoward events in the UK to the Medicines and Health Products Regulatory Agency.

Problems in the preterm baby

Irrespective of weight or gestation at birth, a course of primary immunisation should be started in *every* baby after 8 weeks.

Continued

While this seems to trigger a marginal increase in self-limiting apnoea for the next 2–3 days, no such increase could be detected in a recent controlled trial involving 190 babies. Although very preterm babies mount a less vigorous antibody response, and those on dexamethasone for chronic lung disease mount a particularly limited response to the several vaccines, immunisation should not be delayed because such children are likely to become seriously ill if they encounter whooping cough infection in the first year life. The suggestion that the most vulnerable children should be given a fourth dose of the DTP vaccine at a year has now been discounted, except in countries where diphtheria still occurs with any frequency.

Managing fever
Although giving prophylactic paracetamol (three 15 mg/kg doses over 24 hours) reduces the risk of fever after immunisation, high fever (<39°C) is very uncommon, and such treatment often reduces the antibody response.

Measles
In communities where measles is still prevalent, a case can be made for offering two doses of the combined measles (MMR) vaccine 4 months apart to all at serious risk once they are 4–5 months old. If an *unimmunised* child ≥6 months old *does* come into contact with a case of measles (and infectivity lasts from 4 days before to 4 days after the rash appears), a single dose of MMR or measles vaccine will usually prevent overt illness if given within 3 days of exposure. These babies should still be given two further doses of the MMR vaccine at the normal time. Babies <6 months old are probably best offered 250 mg of normal human immunoglobulin (q.v.).

HIV infection
Babies with suspected or proven human immunodeficiency virus (HIV) infection need protection from diphtheria, tetanus and whooping cough, and from *Haemophilus*, pneumococcal and meningococcal infection like any other child. Consider annual vaccination again the influenza virus. These children should be given the inactivated, rather than the live (oral), polio vaccine, and only given the MMR vaccine if the CD4 count is above 500 cells/μl. They also merit co-trimoxazole prophylaxis (q.v.). Babies in the UK are not given BCG.

Patients with sickle cell disease or no spleen
Babies with situs ambiguus and certain cardiac syndromes are often born without a spleen, making them dangerously prone to infection. While haematological features (Howell–Jolly bodies, etc.) are suggestive, imaging is essential for diagnosis. Give amoxicillin (125 mg twice a day) (q.v.) until the baby is immunised against *Haemophilus influenzae*, and a similar dose of phenoxymethylpenicillin (penicillin V) once immunised. Such babies benefit from being offered the flu vaccine, and should eventually receive both the available pneumococcal vaccines (q.v.), as well as all the other usual vaccines. Do the same for children with homozygous (SS or Sb0Thal) sickle cell disease.

Babies with a serious lung or heart problem
Consider winter prophylaxis against respiratory syncytial virus (RSV) infection with palivizumab (q.v.), and take steps to minimize the risk of influenza, as outlined in the monograph on the influenza vaccine.

Consent
Time must be taken to ensure that parents have had all their questions answered. A record of any issues raised, and of any verbal consent given, should then be placed in the case notes. Prior written consent implies general agreement to the child's inclusion in an immunisation programme, but does not address the issue of current fitness and is no substitute for the presence and involvement of a parent when any vaccine is actually given.

Documentation
Record the batch number and the site of vaccination in the case notes, and also record what has been done in the family copy of the child's personal health folder. Always tell the family doctor of every vaccination undertaken in a hospital setting as well, in the UK, as those who maintain the community child health register.

References See also the UK 2002 guideline on immunising immunocompromised children **DHUK**

American Academy of Pediatrics. *Red book. 2009 report of the Committee on Infectious diseases*, 28th edn. Elk Grove Village, IL: American Academy of Pediatrics, 2009.

Carbone T, McEntire B, Kissin D, *et al*. Absence of an increase in cardiorespiratory events after diphtheria-tetanus-acellular pertussis immunisation in preterm infants: a randomised, multicenter study. *Pediatrics* 2008;**121**:e1085–90. [RCT]

Department of Health. Joint Committee on Vaccination and Immunisation. *Immunisation against infectious disease*, 3rd revised edn. London: The Stationary Office, 2006 (and subsequent web updates).

Klein NP, Massolo ML, Greene J, *et al*. Risk factors for developing apnea after immunisation in the neonatal intensive care unit. *Pediatrics* 2008;**121**:463–9.

Manillavasagan G, Ramsay M. Protecting infants against measles in England and Wales: a review. *Arch Dis Child* 2009;**94**:681–5.

Martins CL, Garly M-L, Balé C, *et al*. Protective efficacy of standard Edmonston-Zagreb measles vaccination in infants aged 4·5 months: interim analysis of a randomised controlled trial. *BMJ* 2008;**337**:a661. [RCT]

Pourcyrous M, Korones SB, Arheart KL, *et al*. Primary immunisation of premature infants with gestational age <35 weeks: cardiorespiratory complications and C-reactive protein responses associated with administration of single and multiple separate vaccines simultaneously. *J Pediatr* 2007;**151**:167–72.

Prymula R, Siegrist C-A, Chlibek R, *et al*. Effect of prophylactic paracetamol administration at time of vaccination on febrile reactions and antibody responses in children: two open-label, randomised controlled trials. *Lancet* 2009;**374**:1339–50. [RCT] (See also pp. 1305–6)

Tse Y, Rylance G. Emergency management of anaphylaxis in children and young people: new guidance from the Resuscitation Council (UK). *Arch Dis Child Educ Pract Ed* 2009;**94**:97–101.

IMMUNOGLOBULIN (Gamma globulin)

Use

An immediate IV dose of immunoglobulin (Ig) may reduce mortality in patients with a severe infection. It can also modify the effects of several severe alloimmune illnesses.

Physiology

Immunoglobulin antibodies help ward off infection. Babies produce few antibodies until they are 3–4 months old, although they acquire maternal gamma globulin transplacentally in the last 3 months of pregnancy. Preterm babies have low levels at birth which can decline further, and this seems to be one reason why they are at particular risk of nosocomial (hospital-acquired) infection in the first few weeks of life. Large trials have shown that the benefit of *prophylaxis* (often 700 mg/kg IV every 2 weeks), though significant, only reduces the risk of infection by 3–4%. However, a meta-analysis of a number of small trials suggests that the same dose used *therapeutically* may reduce mortality in babies with clinical evidence of severe early sepsis. The neutrophil white cells are of equal importance in defending the body against infection, but whether the prophylactic or therapeutic use of the marrow-stimulating factors filgrastim (q.v.) or molgramostim is of any value in the neutropenic preterm baby is not yet clear.

Pharmacology

Human normal immunoglobulin (HNIG) contains IgG prepared from pooled human plasma collected during blood donation. It contains antibodies against a range of common infectious diseases including measles, mumps, varicella, hepatitis A and other common viruses, and can be used to provide immediate but short-lasting passive immunity to a range of viral and bacterial illnesses. Products vary in potency. Special products such as Rhesus and varicella-zoster immunoglobulin (q.v.) also exist. Donor and PCR screening, heat treatment and alcohol fractionation combine to make HNIG safer than fresh frozen plasma (q.v.) or cryoprecipitate. The process also removes IgM, the main source of anti-T antibody that some have claimed could be a cause of haemolysis in patients with necrotising enterocolitis and *Clostridium difficile* infection. Infusion not infrequently causes a headache and generalised discomfort.

A large MRC funded trial (the International Neonatal Immunotherapy Study – INIS) is currently testing whether normal polyclonal immunoglobulin can reduce mortality and improve the long-term outcome in proven (or suspected) neonatal sepsis (as a recent meta-analysis suggests it does in adults). It closed to recruitment in June 2007 after recruiting almost 3500 babies, and the outcome will be known in 2 years.

Treatment

Fetal thrombocytopenia: Some treat severe alloimmune disease by giving the mother 1 gram/kg of IV human immunoglobulin weekly. Very severe disease may make fetal platelet transfusions necessary.

Neonatal thrombocytopenia: Babies with immune thrombocytopenia who fulfil the criteria given in the monograph on platelets should be given 400 mg/kg (or even 1 gram/kg) of human immunoglobulin IV once a day for 1–3 days. Some give oral prednisolone (2 mg/kg every 12 hours for 4–6 days) instead.

Neonatal haemochromatosis: Give women who have had a previously affected child 1 gram/kg IV once a week from 18 weeks to prevent the liver damage caused by a materno-fetal alloimmune reaction. Exchange transfusion and then 1 gram/kg of immunoglobulin IV may improve the prognosis for babies diagnosed at birth.

Rhesus haemolytic disease: 500 mg/kg IV given over 2 hours reduces the need for phototherapy and exchange transfusion, but increases the likelihood that the baby will need a 'top up' transfusion.

Neonatal sepsis: Give an immediate 500 mg/kg dose of human immunoglobulin IV to babies with signs of severe sepsis, and another dose after 1–2 days if the serum IgG level is still less than 5 grams/l.

Supply and administration

A range of IV preparations are available, but all UK use has to be registered (see website commentary) because preparations of reliable quality are currently in short supply. A 2·5 or 3 gram pack typically costs about £35; other pack sizes are also produced. Storage at 4°C is recommended for some products. Preparations designed for IM use, though cheaper, must *not* be given IV. Reconstitute where necessary by adding 20 ml of 0·9% sodium chloride or diluent (as provided) to each gram of lyophilisate immediately before use to obtain a preparation containing 50 mg/ml. Do not shake; wait until the solution is clear. Start to infuse at a rate of 30 mg/kg per hour (that is at 0·6 ml/kg per hour when using the 50 mg/ml solution), and double the rate twice at half-hourly intervals to a maximum rate of 120 mg/kg per hour, unless there is a systemic reaction (usually vomiting or hypotension). Discard all unused material.

References

See also the relevant Cochrane reviews

Gill KK, Kelton JG. Management of ideopathic thrombocytopenic purpura in pregnancy. *Semin Hematol* 2002;**37**:275–89.

Jolly MC, Letsky EA, Fisk NM. The management of fetal thrombocytopenia. *Prenat Diag* 2002;**22**:96–8.

Nasseri R, Mamouri GA, Babaei H. Intravenous immunoglobulin in ABO and Rh haemolytic disease of the newborn. *Saudi Med J* 2006;**27**:1827–30. [RCT]

Rand ER, Karpen SJ, Kelly S, *et al*. Treatment of neonatal haemochromatosis with exchange transfusion and intravenous immunoglobulin. *J Pediatr* 2009;**155**:566–71.

Roifman CM, ed. Intravenous immunoglobulin treatment of immunodeficiency. *Immunol Allergy Clin North Am* 2009;**28**(issue 4).

Turgeon AF, Hutton B, Fergusson DA, *et al*. Meta-analysis: intravenous immunoglobulin in critically ill adult patients with sepsis. *Ann Intern Med* 2007;**146**:193–203. [SR]

Whitington PF, Kelly S. Outcome of pregnancies at risk for neonatal hemochromatosis is improved by treatment with high-dose intravenous immunoglobulin. *Pediatrics* 2008;**121**:e1615–21.

Use
Indometacin causes effective patent ductus arteriosus (PDA) closure, as does ibuprofen (q.v.).

Pharmacology in pregnancy
Indometacin is an inhibitor of prostaglandin synthesis, widely used as an analgesic anti-inflammatory drug in rheumatoid arthritis and gout. It is normally well absorbed by mouth, but neonatal oral absorption is sometimes unpredictable. The neonatal half life averages 16 hours (nearly seven times the half life in adults). Indometacin crosses the placenta and is excreted in the urine. There is no evidence of teratogenicity. Maternal treatment (25 mg by mouth every 6 hours after a loading dose of 50 mg) can be used to treat polyhydramnios, but the use of double this dose to control premature labour has now declined because there are better alternatives. Some recent studies have suggested such use may also increase the risk of the baby developing necrotising enterocolitis and focal gut perforation. A recent meta-analysis did not find any increase in the risk of treatment-resistant PDA, but it did find that periventricular leukomalacia was more common. Breastfeeding is quite safe because the baby gets less than 1% of the weight-adjusted maternal dose.

Pharmacology in the neonate
Indometacin was first used experimentally to effect ductal closure in 1976, and some centres still use the dose used in the early studies (three 200 microgram/kg doses 12 hours apart). This dose is of proven value in the *treatment* of symptomatic patent ductus, especially when used within 2 weeks of birth, but more sustained treatment is measurably more effective in the very preterm baby (where the risk of treatment failure is highest), as is the use of a higher dose. A left atrium to aortic root (LA:Ao) ratio of 1·5 or more, a ductal diameter on colour Doppler of over 1·3 mm/kg, and descending aortic flow reversal in diastole on ultrasound after the first 2 days of life, all suggest the presence of a haemodynamically significant duct. Babies offered early *prophylaxis* (as in the TIPP trial) had less ultrasound evidence of serious intraventricular haemorrhage, but cerebral palsy and other disability was *no* less common; nor was bronchopulmonary dysplasia (BPD) less common. However, for every 20 babies of under 1 kg so treated, five avoided prolonged duct patency and one avoided duct ligation. Evaluation at school entry has failed to confirm an earlier report that early prophylaxis reduces the number of survivors with speech and language problems. Nor, however, is there any evidence that early low-dose use increases the risk of necrotising enterocolitis or ischaemic brain damage — an issue of real concern since even slow infusion causes a brief drop in cerebral, renal and gut blood flow.

Serious coagulation problems are traditionally considered a contraindication to neonatal treatment, because of the effect of indometacin on platelet function, as is necrotising enterocolitis. Jaundice is not a contraindication. The decrease in urine flow is transient even with sustained treatment, so indometacin can still be given even when there are early signs of renal failure, and *no* adjustment needs to be made in the dosage of other renally excreted drugs. Focal ischaemic gut perforation is the most dangerous, and gastrointestinal haemorrhage the commonest, complication (even with IV administration). Whether sustained, or high-dose, treatment increases the risk of these complications is not yet clear. Ligation is only justified if the duct remains symptomatic as well as patent, since there are suggestions that ligation may occasionally make any existing BPD worse.

Drug interactions
Babies given steroids while on indometacin are at increased risk of focal ischemic gut perforation.

Treatment
Early pre-emptive treatment: Give babies under 28 weeks' gestation three 100 microgram/kg doses IV (traditionally over 20 minutes) at daily intervals starting 12 hours after birth (as in the TIPP trial).

Haemodynamically significant ducts: Give 200 micrograms/kg IV, and then a 100 microgram/kg dose 24 and 48 hours later. In very preterm babies with residual patency after this, a further 3 days' treatment can halve the number eventually judged to need surgical ligation. A higher dose is no more effective, and seems to exacerbate any coexistent retinopathy of prematurity.

Supply
1 mg vials of the IV preparation cost £7·50. They should be reconstituted just before use with 2 ml of sterile water for injection to give a solution containing 500 micrograms/ml. The IV formulation can also be given by mouth. A 5 mg/ml oral suspension (containing 1% alcohol) is available in North America.

References
See also the relevant Cochrane reviews

Ami SB, Sinkin RA, Glantz JC. Metaanalysis of the effect of antenatal indomethacin on neonatal outcomes. *Am J Obstet Gynecol* 2007;**197**:486.e1–496.e10. [SR]

Bose CL, Loughon MM. Patent ductus arteriosus: lack of evidence for common treatments. [Review] *Arch Dis Child* 2007;**92**:F498–502. (See also pp. F424–7.)

Clyman R, Cassady G, Kirklin JK, *et al.* The role of patent ductus arteriosus ligation in bronchopulmonary dysplasia: reexamining a randomized controlled trial. *J Pediatr* 2009;**154**:873–6. [RCT]

Jegatheesan P, Ianus V, Buchh B, *et al.* Increased indomethacin dosing for persistent patent ductus arteriosus in preterm infants: a multi-center, randomized, controlled trial. *J Pediatr* 2008;**153**:1839. [RCT]

Kabra NS, Schmidt B, Roberts RS, *et al.* Neurosensory impairment after surgical closure of patent ductus arteriosus in extremely low birth weight infants: results from the trial of indomethacin prophylaxis in preterms. *J Pediatr* 2007;**150**:229–34. (See also pp. 216–19.)

Sperandio M, Beedgen B, Feneberg R, *et al.* Effectiveness and side effects of an escalating, stepwise approach to indomethacin treatment of symptomatic patent ductus arteriosus in premature infants below 33 weeks gestation. *Pediatrics* 2005;**116**:1361–6. (See also **117**:1863–4.)

Use

The influenza virus is an important worldwide cause of serious upper and lower respiratory tract infection which can occur at any time of year, but peaks in the winter months. It is a rare cause of CNS infection.

Influenza

Epidemics of influenza, or flu, occur every winter, and the most prevalent subtype varies from year to year making annual immunisation the only way to provide near-certain protection. Currently available vaccines are trivalent, containing two subtypes of influenza A plus one type B virus. These have provided 70–80% protection, after 10–14 days, from strains that are well matched for those in the vaccine in recent years, and have provided protection that lasts about a year. Should a new A subtype emerge with epidemic potential, a monovalent vaccine against that strain might be thought necessary. Children under 5 (and especially under 2) years old are the most likely to become infected, but it is adults over 65 who are more likely to become seriously ill if they do become infected – the risk being 18-fold higher for those over 85. Women are at slightly more risk during pregnancy, and can occasionally become rapidly unwell. A live attenuated vaccine and an intranasal product are available in some countries but not, as yet, in the UK. Vaccination is not contraindicated during lactation.

Indications for giving the inactivated vaccine

Pregnant women: There is good evidence that vaccination is safe during pregnancy and can also provide the baby with significant short-term protection from infection by viral strains against which the vaccine is active.
Children at least 6 months old: These children can be offered the current trivalent inactivated vaccine just before each annual epidemic begins. Ideally two 0·25 ml doses should be given at least 4 weeks apart the first year that vaccination is offered. A single dose is adequate in subsequent years. All such children are considered eligible for annual vaccination in America, but in the UK annual vaccination is usually only offered to children if they have asthma or some other major long-term medical problem, or are the sibling of such a child.

Contraindications

Flu vaccine can be given at the same time as other live or inactivated vaccines, but preferably into a different limb, and certainly at least 2·5 cm away from any other injection site. Minor illness, with or without fever, does not make vaccination unwise. Anaphylactic reactions are rare, but a mammalian cell-based, and *not* a hen's egg-based, product *must* be used if there is a history of egg allergy or of an adverse reaction to any earlier vaccine product.

Documentation

Record the batch number and the site of vaccination in the case notes, and tell the family doctor as well if vaccination is undertaken in a hospital setting.

Protecting children under 6 months old

The manufacturer has not yet sought permission to advocate use in children less than a year old, but there is growing experience of its use in the most vulnerable 6–12-month-old babies. Efficacy is likely to be progressively more limited in babies younger than this. Maternal vaccination during pregnancy provides some short-term protection. The most effective oral antiviral drug currently available is oseltamivir, the usual adult dose being one 75 mg capsule twice a day for 5 days, to be started just as soon as there are clear symptoms. Pregnancy is *not* a contraindication. If the aim is to offer **treatment** start this within 48 hours of the onset of symptoms regardless of vaccination status, and give a dose twice a day for 5 days, the generally recommended dose being 2 mg/kg (often simplified to 12 mg in children less than 3 months old, 18 mg in babies 3–5 months old, and 24 mg at 6–12 months). Reduce the dose in renal failure. There is also some limited support for **prophylactic** use in particularly vulnerable unvaccinated babies who are known to have been exposed to the virus. Give these babies the same dose of oseltamivir once a day for 10 days.

Supply and administration

A range of vaccines become available annually for about £5 in 0·5 ml prefilled syringes (and 0·25 ml syringes in America). Shake well before use, and give deep IM into the anterolateral aspect of the thigh (or deltoid in adults). The recommended dose for children less than 3 years old is 0·25 ml. Store all products in the dark at 2–8°C.
　　Oseltamivir (Tamiflu®) comes in 75 mg capsules (costing £1·60) and 75 ml bottles suitable for reconstitution with water to give a 12 mg/ml sugar-free suspension (costing £16). Use is considered safe during pregnancy.

References

See also the relevant Cochrane reviews and UK guidelines

American Academy of Pediatrics. Committee on Infectious Diseases. Policy statement – recommendations for the prevention and treatment of influenza in children 2009–10. *Pediatrics* 2009;**124**:1216–26.

Centers for Disease Control and Prevention. Prevention and control of seasonal influenza with vaccines. *MMWR* 2009;**58**:RR-8. (See www.cdc.gov/mmwr.)

Eisenberg KW, Szilagyi PG, Fairbrother N, *et al.* Vaccine effectiveness against laboratory-confirmed influenza in children 6 to 59 months of age during the 2003–2004 influenza seasons. *Pediatrics* 2008;**122**:911–19.

Erlewyn-Lajeunesse M, Braithwaite N, Lucas JSA, *et al.* Recommendations for the administration of influenza vaccine in children allergic to egg. *BMJ* 2009;**339**:912–15. (*BMJ* 2009;**339**:b3680.) (See also correspondence on p. 1100.)

Szilagi PG, Fairbrother G, Griffin MR, *et al.* Influenza vaccine effectiveness among children 6 to 59 months of age during 2 influenza seasons. *Arch Pediatr Adolesc Med* 2008;**162**:943–51.

Zaman K, Roy E, Arifeen SE, *et al.* Effectiveness of maternal influenza immunisation in mothers and infants. *N Engl J Med* 2008;**358**:1555–64. [RCT]

Use

Insulin, the hormone first isolated from β cells in the islets of the pancreas in 1922, is used to treat diabetes mellitus. It can also be used to correct unusually high blood glucose levels (hyperglycaemia) in the neonate and to counteract any dangerous rise in the blood potassium level (hyperkalaemia).

Pathophysiology

Inadequate insulin production and abnormal resistance to its secretion cause type 1 and type 2 diabetes, respectively (a condition in which glucose draws a dangerous excess of fluid into the urine). All women with diabetes need to optimise glucose homeostasis during conception and pregnancy, aiming for a glycated haemoglobin (HbA_{1c}) level below 7·5% to minimise the risk of congenital malformation and miscarriage, and, since it does not cross the placenta or appear in human milk, insulin is the drug of choice. Some women also become less able to stabilise their blood glucose levels during pregnancy ('gestational' diabetes), and insulin, or a sulfonylurea drug such as glibenclamide, will reduce the risk of fetal macrosomia (usually defined as a >4 kg baby) if dietary advice alone does not suffice.

Newborn babies are relatively intolerant of glucose and the pancreatic response to an IV load is relatively sluggish. Giving 10% glucose at a rate appropriate to normal fluid and calorie needs may sometimes exceed the very preterm child's ability to metabolise glucose, or turn glucose into glycogen, and a glucose uptake of more than 14 mg/kg per minute is not called for in the first week of life. Similarly, while the use of a continuous IV infusion of insulin to increase total calorie intake in babies on parenteral nutrition yet also *prevent* high glucose levels developing did result in babies getting 20% more glucose in one recent trial, more babies had occasional low levels and there were more deaths in the first 28 days of life, so this strategy cannot be endorsed. Nevertheless, although high levels usually fall quickly if less glucose is given for 6–12 hours, it can be appropriate to give insulin for a time to *correct* high blood levels (>12 mmol/l) if they persist once sepsis or some other intercurrent illness has been ruled out. Note that glucose in the *urine* (glycosuria) will not cause excess water loss until the *blood* glucose level exceeds 15 mmol/l.

Arrhythmia due to sudden unexplained neonatal hyperkalaemia (K^+ >7·5 mmol/l) is occasionally seen in very preterm babies especially in the first 3 days of life. A continuous infusion of glucose and insulin can be used to control this, and will usually work quicker than a polystyrene sulphonate resin enema (q.v.). Salbutamol (q.v.) and correction of acidosis with sodium bicarbonate (q.v.) may also help.

Treatment

Hyperglycaemia: Giving 0·05 units/kg of insulin per hour for a few hours IV can be used to bring down the worryingly high blood glucose levels (>12 mmol/l) sometimes caused by giving IV glucose.

Hyperkalaemia: Infuse 0·5 units/kg of insulin per hour IV in 10% glucose – and watch glucose levels closely.

Neonatal diabetes: This rare condition, which presents with acidosis, dehydration and hyperglycaemia (usually >20 mmol/l), but little ketosis, responds to a very low dose of insulin. Giving 0·5–3·0 units/kg per *day* is usually adequate. Try giving this subcutaneously instead of IV if problems persist for more than 2 weeks. Treatment can usually be tailed off within 4–6 weeks and, if evidence of type 1 diabetes does re-emerge, this can usually be controlled by giving 0·1–0·4 mg/kg of glibenclamide by mouth twice a day.

Compatibility

Insulin can be added (terminally) to a line containing TPN (with or without lipid), or containing dobutamine (but not dopamine), glyceryl trinitrate, heparin, midazolam, milrinone, morphine, nitroprusside or propofol.

Supply and administration

10 ml multidose vials of human soluble insulin containing 100 units/ml cost approximately £15 each. They are best stored at 4°C, but contain m-cresol as a preservative and can be kept for a month at room temperature. Do not freeze. Any short-acting soluble product (such as Humulin S®) can be used for IV or subcutaneous administration. These products should not be used if they appear hazy or coloured. Long-acting slow-release products, containing a cloudy zinc suspension are only suitable for subcutaneous use.

Take 0·25 ml (25 units) from the vial and dilute to 50 ml with 0·9% sodium chloride to obtain a preparation containing 0·5 units/ml. The IV solution is stable and does not need to be changed daily, but insulin adheres to plastic and consistent IV delivery will not be achieved for several hours unless the delivery tubing is first flushed with at least 20 ml of fluid. It is also more consistent if the set is left standing with fluid in it for an hour before it is flushed through. While this is less essential when treatment is first started because the response will determine the initial infusion rate, failure to prime any *replacement* set could well destabilise glucose control. Pharmacies can provide an oral suspension of glibenclamide on request.

References

See also the relevant Cochrane reviews ◗

Beardsall K, Vanhaesebrouck S, Ogilvy-Stuart AL, *et al*. Early insulin therapy in very-low-birth-weight infants. *N Engl J Med* 2008;**359**:1873–84. [RCT] (See also pp. 1951–3.)

Cody D. Infant and toddler diabetes. *Arch Dis Child* 2007;**92**:716–19.

Crowther CA, Hiller JE, Moss JR. Effect of treatment of gestational diabetes mellitus on pregnancy outcomes. *N Engl J Med* 2005;**352**:2477–86. [RCT] (See also pp. 2544–6.)

Hey E. Hyperglycaemia and the very preterm baby. [Review] *Semin Neonatol* 2005;**10**:377–87.

Pearson ER, Flechter I, Njølstrad PR, *et al*. Switching from insulin to oral sulphoneas in patients with diabetes due to Kir6·2 mutations. *N Engl J Med* 2006;**355**:467–77. (See also pp. 507–10.)

Use

Interferon alfa-2 has been used to induce the early regression of life-threatening corticosteroid-resistant haemangiomas of infancy. Combined treatment with ribavirin (q.v.) can control hepatitis C infection.

Vascular birth marks

Haemangiomas are common in infancy. Seldom noticed at birth, they grow rapidly for 6–9 months and then gradually involute during early childhood. Bleeding is uncommon. Usually solitary and superficial, they are most often found on the head and neck. They are particularly common in preterm babies, and occur in almost a quarter of babies of less than 28 weeks' gestation. Superficial dermal haemangiomas are fleshy and bright red ('strawberry naevi'), but deeper ones only show surface telangiectasia or a bluish hue. Lesions around the eye can cause amblyopia (a 'lazy eye'), while sublaryngeal lesions can cause serious bidirectional stridor as they grow. Children with multiple lesions sometimes have visceral haemangiomas. Large lesions can cause thrombocytopenia from platelet trapping (Kasabach–Merritt syndrome) and high output heart failure. Treatment is mainly used for lesions causing airway or visual obstruction, facial distortion or thrombocytopenia: 1 mg/kg of prednisolone twice a day for 3 months is usually very effective if started promptly in the early proliferative phase. Most dermatologists recommend slow weaning after that to minimise 'rebound'. Some start with a higher dose than this for 4–8 weeks, although this causes greater adrenal suppression. There is one report of treatment with propranolol (1 mg/kg three times a day for up to 6 months). While pulsed dye laser treatment can render port wine stains less noticeable, it is little used in the treatment of haemangiomas.

Other vascular malformations, in contrast, do not generally increase in size disproportionately after birth. Although by definition congenital, they may not be noticed for some months. Capillary and venous malformations lose their colour on compression (unlike strawberry naevi). Most capillary malformations ('port wine stains') are flat and sharply demarcated. The paler salmon-coloured patches, often seen on the forehead, nose and eyelids always fade with time, although patches on the nape of the neck ('stork bites') sometimes persist. Lymphatic and mixed malformations are usually noticed within a few months of birth. Venous and arteriovenous lesions are seldom suspected at birth.

Pharmacology

Interferons are proteins or glycoproteins produced by the body in response to viral and other stimuli. Interferon alfa is derived from leukocytes, interferon beta from fibroblasts and interferon gamma from stimulated T-lymphocytes. Human alfa interferon was first manufactured artificially from bacteria in 1980 using recombinant DNA technology (as indicated by the use of the suffix 'rbe'). It has since been used to treat chronic hepatitis B and C, and certain types of leukaemia, myeloma and lymphoma. Flu-like symptoms and fever are the only common problems, but nausea, lethargy and depression can occur with high-dose treatment. Motor problems have been seen with use in young children, but these usually seem to resolve when treatment is stopped. Little is known about use during pregnancy, but it does not seem to pose a toxic or teratogenic threat. Only small amounts appear in breast milk. The fact that interferon alfa is of benefit in the management of Kaposi sarcoma, an endothelial cell tumour associated with HIV infection, has led to its use to suppress the endothelial proliferation that forms the cellular basis of other haemangiomatous lesions.

Treatment

Serious haemangiomatous lesions that fail to respond to prednisolone (see above) are sometimes treated with interferon alfa-2a. The usual dose is 3 million units/m^2 subcutaneously once a day (i.e. 600,000 units for an average baby of 3 kg). Serious side effects of such treatment seem to be rare, even though treatment may need to be continued for several months.

Supply

A range of products are available, but there is no convenient low-dose preparation suitable for neonatal use. One preparation suitable for use in older infants is Intron-A® (interferon alfa-2b (rbe)) which is available as an injection pen with a multidose cartridge that can deliver six 0·2 million unit doses (at a cost of £16 per dose). A 10 million unit vial containing powder requiring reconstitution with water (as supplied) costs £54. The alternative product, Roferon-A® (interferon alfa-2a (rbe)), is best avoided when treating babies because it contains benzyl alcohol as an excipient. The products should be stored at 4°C, but *not* frozen.

References

Atherton D, Infantile haemangiomas. *Early Hum Dev* 2006;**82**:789–95.

Batta K, Goodyear HM, Moss C, *et al*. Randomised controlled trial of early pulsed dye laser treatment of uncomplicated childhood haemangiomas: results of a 1-year analysis. *Lancet* 2002;**360**:521–7. [RCT] (See also **361**:348–9.)

Chang LC, Haggstrom AN, Drolet BA, *et al*. Growth characteristics of infantile hemangiomas: implications for management. *Pediatrics* 2008;**122**:360–7.

Dubois J, Hershon L, Carmant L, *et al*. Toxicity profile of interferon alfa-2b in children: a prospective evaluation. *J Pediatr* 1999;**135**:782–5.

Gruinwald JH, Burke DK, Bonthius DJ, *et al*. An update on the treatment of haemangiomas in children with interferon alfa-2. *Arch Otolaryngol Head Neck Surg* 1999;**125**:21–7.

Lopriore E, Markhorst DG. Diffuse neonatal haemangiomatosis: new views on diagnostic criteria and prognosis. *Acta Paediatr* 1999;**88**:93–9.

Pope E, Krafchik BR, Macarthur C, *et al*. Oral versus high-dose corticosteroids for problematic hemangiomas: a randomized, controlled trial. *Pediatrics* 2007;**119**:e1239–47. [RCT]

Sans V, de la Roque ED, Berge J, *et al*. Propranolol for severe infantile hemangiomas: follow-up report. *Pediatrics* 2009;**124**:e423–31.

Use

Intralipid is the most widely studied of the lipid products used to give fat (and the associated essential fatty acids) to children requiring parenteral nutrition (q.v.). No other IV fluid is as calorie rich.

Pharmacology

Intralipid is an emulsion of soy bean oil stabilised with egg phospholipid. It is approximately isotonic, and is available as a 10% solution providing 1·1 kcal/ml and as a 20% solution providing 2 kcal/ml (1 kcal = 4·18 kJ). It contains 52% linoleic acid, 22% oleic acid, 13% palmitic acid and 8% linolenic acid (and so lacks the best linoleic:linolenic ratio for brain growth). Metabolism is the same as for chylomicrons. When first introduced it was often only infused for 4–20 hours a day, so that lipaemia could 'clear', but continuous infusion has been shown to improve tolerance and seems more 'physiological'. The 20% product is tolerated better than 10% Intralipid, possibly because the phospholipid content is lower. Infection with *Malassezia* can occur, and this lipid-dependent fungus may escape detection if specific culture techniques are not used, but the fungaemia usually clears if administration is stopped. Intralipid can cause the blood glucose level to rise. It can also cause a ten-fold increase in the risk of coagulase-negative staphylococcal bacteraemia. The amount given is often limited in babies with serious unconjugated jaundice, but there is no evidence that use interferes with the protein binding of bilirubin. Early use does not increase the risk of chronic lung disease developing.

Nutritional factors

The use of Intralipid enhances protein utilisation, and considerably increases calorie provision in babies receiving total parenteral nutrition (TPN). The co-infusion of 0·8 ml/kg of 20% Intralipid per hour with an infusion of 6 ml/kg per hour (i.e. 144 ml/kg per day) of an amino acid solution containing 10% glucose increases total calorie intake from 60 to 100 kcal/kg per day. By way of comparison, 160 ml/kg per day of one of the high-calorie preterm milk formulas provides an intake of 130 kcal/kg per day (if no allowance is made for incomplete intestinal absorption). An infusion of 0·1 ml/kg per hour (0·5 grams/kg per day) is the minimum needed to meet essential fatty acid needs. Gluconeogenic metabolic pathways also seem to utilise the glycerol generated to make glucose and improve glucose homeostasis.

Intake

Policies still vary widely (a sure sign of continued uncertainty), but it seems quite safe to start infusing at least 0·4 ml/kg of 20% Intralipid (0·08 g of fat) per hour through a peripheral, central or umbilical line within a day or two of birth once it is clear that the baby is stable (as this *Formulary* has recommended for more than 14 years). There is no evidence that stepped introduction improves tolerance, but good evidence that many babies will develop hyperlipidaemia when intake exceeds 0·8 ml/kg per hour (3·8 g/kg of fat a day). Babies less than a week old, or less than 28 weeks' gestation at birth, may be marginally less tolerant. Septic, acidotic and postoperative babies should probably not be offered more than 2 g/kg a day.

Administration

1·2 μm lipid filters exist, but Intralipid cannot be infused through the 0·2 μm filter normally used for TPN, so lipid is best only allowed to mix with TPN just before it enters the baby. Protection from light may limit hydroperoxide production, but this has not yet been shown to deliver clinical benefit. Some units change the syringe and giving set daily because of concern that Intralipid can leach the chemical plasticiser out of syringes.

Blood levels

Serum triglycerides can be measured in 50 μl plasma (~150 μl of heparinised whole blood). A level much above 2 mmol/l (the highest level seen in the breastfed baby) suggests early lipid overload. Plasma turbidity is a much less satisfactory test. Re-emergent lipaemia may suggest early sepsis.

Supply

Stock 100 ml bags of 20% Intralipid (0·2 grams of fat per ml) cost £5·80, and 10 ml ampoules of Vitlipid N® infant cost £2·20. Store below 25°C, but do not freeze. Children requiring sustained parenteral nutrition should have Vitlipid N infant (containing vitamins A, D_2, E and K_1) added to their Intralipid by the pharmacy prior to issue (as outlined in the monograph on multiple vitamins), and material so primed should then be used within 24 hours. Never add anything else to Intralipid or co-infuse it with a fluid containing any drug other than heparin, insulin or isoprenaline. Discard all open bags.

References

See also the relevant Cochrane reviews

Avila-Figueroa C, Goldmann DA, Richardson DK, *et al*. Intravenous lipid emulsions are the major determinant of coagulase-negative staphylococcal bacteremia in very low birth weight newborns. *Pediatr Infect Dis J* 1998;**17**:10–17.

Cairns PA, Wilson DC, Jenkins J, *et al*. Tolerance of mixed lipid emulsion in neonates: effect of concentration. *Arch Dis Child* 1996;**75**:F113–16. [RCT]

Drenckpohl D, McConnell C, Gaffney S, *et al*. Randomized trial of very low birth weight infants receiving higher rates of infusion of intravenous fat emulsions during the first week of life. *Pediatrics* 2008;**122**:743–51. [RCT]

Driscoll DF, Bistrian BR, Demmelmair H, *et al*. Pharmaceutical and clinical aspects of parenteral lipid emulsions in neonatology. *Clin Nutr* 2008;**27**:497–503.

Matlow AG, Kitai I, Kirpalani H, *et al*. A randomised trial of 72- versus 24-hour intravenous tubing changes in newborns receiving lipid therapy. *Infect Control Hosp Epidemiol* 1999;**20**:487–93. [RCT]

Sherlock R, Chessex P. Shielding parenteral nutrition from light: does the available evidence support a randomized, controlled trial? *Pediatrics* 2009;**123**:1529–33.

Use

The main use of oral iron in the first year of life is to prevent iron deficiency anaemia during growth in babies fed breast milk who weighed less than 2·3 kg at birth. It is also used after birth to correct the iron loss that a few babies suffer as a result of chronic fetal blood loss before birth. Routine supplementation during pregnancy serves no useful purpose for most women, but is of real value in countries where their nutritional status is poor.

Nutritional factors

Iron is a major constituent of the haemoglobin molecule and routine supplementation is traditional in pregnancy, although the scientific basis for this is far from convincing and the practice is now actively discouraged except in developing countries where the nutritional status of many women is poor. Here the baby clearly benefits if the mother takes a regular daily supplement (60 mg of iron and 400 micrograms of folic acid) during pregnancy. The value of adding other micronutrients is, at the moment, much less clear. Iron tablets can, however, pose a very real hazard to young children because they are often mistaken for sweets, and the ingestion of as little as 3 grams of ferrous sulphate can kill a small child. We also know that maternal iron deficiency has to be very severe before it causes neonatal anaemia or iron deficiency during infancy. However, all babies need to acquire a further 0·4−0·7 micrograms of iron a day to maintain their body stores because the circulating blood volume triples during the first year of life, and this requires a diet containing 1−2 mg/kg of iron a day.

While babies normally have substantial iron stores at birth even when born many weeks before term (and even in the face of severe maternal iron deficiency), these stores start to become depleted unless dietary intake is adequate by the time the child's blood volume has doubled. Microcytosis (MCV <96 μm^3) at birth is **never** a sign of iron deficiency, but can be due to a haemoglobinopathy (usually some form of thalassaemia). The iron in breast milk is extremely well absorbed (as long as the baby is not also being offered solid food), but absorption from artificial feeds is only a fifth as good, and the use of unmodified cow's milk in the first 12 months of life is particularly likely to cause iron deficiency anaemia. It used to be thought that this might be due to iron loss as a result of occult gastrointestinal bleeding, but recent studies have failed to confirm this. It is possible that the high phosphate content of whole cows' milk may interfere with iron absorption.

Haemoglobin and haematocrit levels change rapidly during the first 2−4 weeks of life, as outlined in the monograph on blood, but these changes are *not* due to iron deficiency and cannot be influenced by iron supplementation. While 'anaemia of prematurity' can be modified using recombinant human erythropoietin (q.v.) as long as the baby is also given at least 3 mg/kg of supplemental iron, it is doubtful whether such treatment is justified given the cost and the evidence that it may increase the risk of retinopathy of prematurity. The commonest cause of iron deficiency in the first year of life is iatrogenic because, if the cord is clamped early before the uterus contracts again after birth, this can deprive the baby of 20% of the elemental iron normally present in the body after an intervention-free delivery. Similarly, the commonest cause of neonatal anaemia is also iatrogenic − from doctors taking blood for laboratory analysis! Such babies should be offered a replacement transfusion: they do not respond to supplemental iron.

The fortification of artificial feeds with 0·6 mg iron/100 ml is enough to prevent iron deficiency in babies of normal birthweight and it is now reasonably clear, despite official advice to the contrary, that this is also enough for the preterm baby. Almost all the commonly used formula milks in current use contain at least as much iron as this (as outlined in the monograph on milk formulas) making the widespread practise of further supplementation quite unnecessary. There is rather more uncertainty as to how well the iron in most fortified infant cereal foods is absorbed. Wholegrain cereals and some tannins (as found in tea) bind iron and prevent absorption. The most easily assimilated form of iron is haem iron. Some vegetarian diets, therefore, may increase the risk of iron deficiency. Children on a poor diet often become anaemic during the second year of life, especially if they are given cows' milk rather than a fortified formula, but randomised trials have yet to confirm observational studies (and animal studies) suggesting that iron deficiency at a critical time during the brain's growth can cause sustained psychomotor delay. Of equal concern is the finding that routine supplements during the first 3 years of life can actually *increase* mortality in an area where malaria is rife, and that it may be the babies who are not iron deficient who are placed most at risk by routine prophylaxis.

Breastfed babies weighing less than about 2·3 kg at birth are, however, at some risk of developing iron deficiency anaemia 2−3 months after birth, as a result of the rapid expansion of their circulating blood volume with growth, and these babies benefit from supplemental iron started within 4−6 weeks of birth. There is no good reason for starting supplemental iron before this because there is some doubt whether the gut absorbs iron in excess of immediate requirement, and some reason for believing that the iron-binding protein, lactoferrin, present in milk (and particularly in breast milk), only inhibits bacterial growth when not saturated with iron. Some think that early supplementation of breast milk with iron might also unmask latent vitamin E deficiency.

Assessment

A serum ferritin of less than 20 µg/l is considered diagnostic of iron deficiency in a 4-month-old child, especially if the transferrin saturation is below 10%. A 10 µg/l 'cut off' can be used after 6 months. Anaemia in young children is very seldom due to iron deficiency, and most babies who are iron deficient are not anaemic. Send 1 ml of blood in a plain tube or EDTA tube to the Department of Haematology. An attempt was made to keep the serum ferritin level above 100 µg/l in some neonatal trials of erythropoietin use.

Prophylaxis and treatment

Normal babies: Breastfed babies benefit from supplementation if no other source of iron is introduced into the diet by about 6 months. Term babies fed one of the standard, artificially fortified, neonatal milk formulas (q.v.) never require further supplementation.

Continued

Preterm babies: Iron deficiency anaemia can be avoided in babies fed ***breast*** milk who weigh less than 2·3 kg at birth by giving them a single daily dose of sodium feredetate (Sytron®). Prophylaxis is most logically started 6–8 weeks after birth (or, more simply, at discharge) and sustained until mixed feeding is established. The precise dose of Sytron necessary to meet the nutritional guideline is 0·4 ml/kg (2·2 mg/kg of elemental iron) once a day, but for most babies over 3 kg it is probably enough to tell the parents to give half a teaspoon (2·5 ml) once a day. Although it is traditional to offer all preterm babies further supplemental iron after discharge, this advice is a 'hang over' from the days when the powdered artificial milks used for infant feeding were not specially fortified. There is no good evidence that ***formula***-fed babies benefit from further supplementation after discharge (unless they are still on Osterprem®), and excess intake can have disadvantages.

Babies with anaemia at birth (Hb <120 g/l): Babies who have suffered *chronic* blood loss from feto-maternal bleeding or twin-to-twin transfusion benefit from supplemental iron once their initial deficit has been corrected by transfusion. Babies with anaemia due to *acute* blood loss at birth do not usually become iron deficient. Neither do babies with haemolytic anaemia.

Babies on parenteral nutrition: Babies unable to tolerate even partial enteral feeding by 3 months benefit from 100 micrograms/kg of iron a day IV (most conveniently given as iron chloride). Babies on erythropoietin (q.v.) also need IV supplementation if they can not be given oral iron.

Toxicity

Get the stomach emptied and organise prompt lavage if oral ingestion is suspected. Activated charcoal is of no value, but an attempt should be made to identify the amount ingested, and treatment started by giving 15 mg/kg of desferrioxamine mesilate (deferoxamine mesilate (pINNM)) per hour IV for 5 hours if the ingested dose is thought to exceed 30 mg/kg. No universally agreed treatment protocol exists and advice should be sought from the local Poisons Centre. Acute toxicity is likely if the serum iron level exceeds 90 μmol/l 4 hours after ingestion. A leukocytosis of over 15×10^9/l, or a blood glucose of over 8·3 mmol/l, also suggests serious toxicity. Early symptoms include diarrhoea and vomiting followed, after 12–48 hours, by lethargy, coma, convulsions, intestinal bleeding and multiorgan failure. Intestinal strictures may develop 2–5 weeks later.

Supply

It is best to choose a sugar-free preparation requiring no further dilution. Sodium feredetate (previously known as sodium ironedetate) is widely used in the UK. Each ml of the commercial elixir (Sytron) contains 5·5 mg of elemental iron (38 mg of sodium feredetate). 500 ml bottles cost £5, but smaller volumes can be dispensed on request. Ferrous fumarate is one alternative for those concerned that Sytron contains 96% ethanol. Each ml of the commercial syrup (Galfer®) contains 9 mg of elemental iron (28 mg of ferrous fumarate). Ferrous sulphate (still widely used in North America) is a second alternative – two widely used commercial formulations (Ironorm® and Fer-Gen-Sol®) come in dropper bottles containing 25 mg/ml of iron (~1 mg per drop). Parents can obtain all these similarly priced products from any community pharmacist without a doctor's prescription.

10 ml ampoules of iron chloride for IV use containing 1 mg (17·9 micromol) of iron are obtainable through the pharmacy from the Queens Medical Centre, Nottingham.

Vials containing 500 mg of desferrioxamine mesilate powder (costing £4·30) suitable for reconstitution with 5 ml of water for injection could be provided by the pharmacy on request.

References

See also the relevant Cochrane reviews

Domellöf M, Dewey KG, Lönnerdal B, *et al*. The diagnostic criteria for iron deficiency in infants should be reevaluated. *J Nutr* 2002;**132**:3680–6.
Domellöf M. Iron requirements, absorption and metabolism in infancy and childhood. *Cur Opin Clin Nutr Metab Care* 2007;**10**:329–35.
Friel JK, Andrews WL, Aziz K, *et al*. A randomized trial of two levels of iron supplementation and developmental outcome in low birth weight infants. *J Pediatr* 2001;**139**:254–60. [RCT]
Griffin IJ, Cooke RJ, Reid MM, *et al*. Iron nutritional status in preterm infants fed formulas fortified with iron. *Arch Dis Child* 1999;**81**:F45–9. [RCT]
Hutto EK, Hassan ES. Late vs early clamping of the umbilical cord in full-term neonates: systematic review and meta-analysis of controlled trials. *JAMA* 2007;**297**:1241–52. [SR]
Iannotti LL, Tielsch JM, Black MM, *et al*. Iron supplementation in early childhood: health benefits and risks. *Am J Clin Nutr* 2006;**84**:1261–76. [SR]
Rao R, Georgieff MK. Iron therapy for preterm infants. *Clin Perinatol* 2009;**36**:27–42.
Sankar MJ, Renu S, Kalaivani K, *et al*. Early iron supplementation in very low birth weight infants – a randomized controlled trial. *Acta Paediatr* 2009.**98**:953–8. [RCT]
Sazawal S, Lack RE, Ramsan M, *et al*. Effects of routine prophylactic supplemental with iron and folic acid on admission to hospital and mortality in preschool children in a high malaria transmission setting: community-based, randomised, placebo-controlled trial. *Lancet* 2006;**367**:133–43. [RCT]
White KC. Anemia is a poor predictor of iron deficiency among toddlers in the United States: for heme the bell tolls. *Pediatrics* 2005;**115**:315–20.
Zeng L, Dibley MJ, Cheng Y, *et al*. Impact of micronutrient supplementation during pregnancy on the birth weight, duration of gestation, and perinatal mortality in rural west China double blind cluster randomised controlled trial. *BMJ* 2008;**337**:1211–15. [RCT] (See also pp. 1180–1.)
Ziaei S, Norrosi M, Faghigzadeh S, *et al*. A randomised placebo-controlled trial to determine the effect of iron supplementation on pregnancy outcome in pregnant women with haemoglobin ≥13·2 g/dl. *Br J Obstet Gynaecol* 2007;**114**:684–8. [RCT] (See also p. 1308.)

ISONIAZID

Use
Isoniazid is used, with pyrazinamide (q.v.), in the primary treatment and retreatment of tuberculosis (TB), which remains a serious notifiable disease. Guidance on dosing in children varies widely (see website commentary). Babies who come into contact with a case of active TB also merit prophylaxis.

Pharmacology
Isoniazid (INH) was first isolated in 1912 and found to be bacteriostatic and, in high concentrations, bactericidal against *Mycobacterium tuberculosis* in 1952. It is active against both intracellular and extracellular bacilli, but because resistance develops when given on its own, when *active* infection is suspected, at least one other drug is always given as well. A 9-month course of isoniazid on its own has long been the standard approach for *latent* infection, but studies in adults and children now suggest that a 3- or 4-month course of isoniazid and rifampicin (q.v.) may be better tolerated and better adhered to. There is no evidence that isoniazid is teratogenic, but treatment does increase the excretion of pyridoxine (vitamin B_6) and, to counter the risk of peripheral neuropathy, women should take 10 mg of pyridoxine (q.v.) once a day if pregnant or breastfeeding. Malnourished children also benefit from prophylactic pyridoxine, especially in the first year of life. Treatment during lactation will result in the baby receiving up to a fifth of the maternal dose of the drug, and of the drug's main metabolite, on a weight-for-weight basis. However, toxicity has not been seen, and breastfeeding should only be discouraged if the mother is still infectious (i.e. sputum positive).

Isoniazid is well absorbed by mouth and excreted in the urine after inactivation in the liver. The half life is long at birth, but is substantially shorter in early childhood than it is in adult life (2–5 hours). However, inactivation is by acetylation, the speed of which is genetically determined (fast acetylators eliminating the drug twice as fast as slow acetylators). Liver toxicity is not common in children but appears related to high-dose treatment, and to combined treatment with rifampicin (q.v.). It is probably commoner in slow acetylators, but this has yet to be established. Haemolytic anaemia and agranulocytosis are rare complications, while a lupus-like syndrome, liver damage and gynaecomastia have been reported in adults. Treatment should be stopped and reviewed if toxicity is suspected. Use is usually contraindicated in patients with drug-induced liver disease and porphyria.

Maternal tuberculosis
Mothers found to have TB during pregnancy need expert management: they usually get a 10-month course of isoniazid and rifampicin, along with 6 months of pyrazinamide. Some may need 2 months of ethambutol. Fetal infection is only likely if the mother has an extrapulmonary infection, but the baby is vulnerable to infection after birth from any care giver with open untreated pulmonary disease, and remains at risk of serious generalised ('miliary') infection. Patients are not likely to pass infection to others after they have been on effective treatment for at least 2 weeks, so babies born into such a household only need prophylactic isoniazid as indicated below. Where there is a real possibility that the baby has become infected give both isoniazid and 10 mg/kg of rifampicin (q.v.) once a day for at least 6 months. Pyrazinamide (q.v.) should also be given for the first 2 months under expert supervision (30 mg/kg once a day), especially if there is a possible non-pulmonary focus of infection. Possible meningeal involvement calls for at least a year's expert treatment using four drugs.

Drug interactions
Isoniazid can potentiate the effect of carbamazepine and phenytoin to the point where toxicity develops.

Prophylaxis and treatment
Neonatal prophylaxis: Give babies exposed to infection 5 mg/kg once a day by mouth. Dose adjustment is not necessary for poor renal function. If the baby is tuberculin negative at 3 months, treatment can be stopped and BCG (q.v.) given. Treat for 6 months (as outlined above) if the tuberculin test is positive.
Treating latent infection: Give 10 mg/kg of isoniazid *and* 10 mg/kg of rifampicin once a day for 3 months.
Treating overt infection: Give babies over a month old 10 mg/kg once a day by mouth.

Toxicity
Treat any encephalopathy due to an overdose by giving 1 mg of pyridoxine IV (or by mouth) for every mg of excess isoniazid ingested. Control seizures, acidosis and respiration as necessary.

Supply
An inexpensive sugar-free oral elixir of isoniazid containing 10 mg/ml is available, as are 2 ml ampoules containing 50 mg (costing £7·40 each) suitable for IM or IV injection.

References

Adhikari M. Tuberculosis and tuberculosis/HIV co-infection in pregnancy. [Review] *Semin Fetal Neonat Med* 2009;**14**:234–40.

Page KR, Sifakis F, de Oca, *et al*. Improved adherence and less toxicity with rifampin vs isoniazid for treatment of latent tuberculosis. *Arch Int Med* 2006;**166**:1863–70.

Roy V, Tekur U, Chopra K. Pharmacokinetics of isoniazid in pulmonary tuberculosis – a comparative study at two dose levels. *Indian Pediatr* 1996;**33**:287–91.

Schaaf HS, Parkin DP, Seifart HI, *et al*. Isoniazid pharmacokinetics in children treated for respiratory tuberculosis. *Arch Dis Child* 2005;**90**:614–18. (See also pp. 551–2.)

Spyridis NP, Spyridis PG, Gelseme A, *et al*. The effectiveness of a 9-month regimen of isoniazid alone versus 3- and 4-month regimens of isoniazid plus rifampin for treatment of latent tuberculosis infection in children: results of an 11-year randomized study. *Clin Infect Dis* 2007;**45**:715–22. [RCT]

Use
Isoprenaline is a sympathomimetic drug sometimes used in the management of haemodynamically significant bradycardia or heart block.

Pharmacology
Isoprenaline is a synthetic sympathomimetic related to noradrenaline (q.v.) with potent β-adrenergic receptor activity that was first brought into clinical use in 1951. This adrenergic agonist has virtually no effect on α receptors. Gastrointestinal absorption is unpredictable but sublingual administration is effective and the drug was widely given by aerosol as a bronchodilator for asthma in the 1960s. Continuous IV infusion can cause marked vasodilatation and a significant increase in cardiac output, an effect further potentiated by the drug's inotropic and chronotropic action, and by an increase in cardiac venous return. It has more effect on heart rate than on stroke volume, and has relatively little effect on renal blood flow. Isoprenaline is known to be of value in the management of low cardiac output with or without pulmonary hypertension in older children and adults; it is probably under-utilised in the neonatal period. While a high dose can cause hypotension, this is usually transient. There is also some risk of tachycardia and cardiac arrhythmia, but these toxic effects usually subside very rapidly as soon as treatment is stopped.

Treatment with isoprenaline is still sometimes appropriate in the initial management of complete AV heart block until such time as a permanent pacemaker can be implanted.

Treatment
Start with a continuous IV infusion of 20 nanograms/kg per minute (0·2 ml/hour of a solution made up as described below), and increase as necessary. Use the lowest possible effective dose and never use a dose of more than 200 nanograms/kg per minute (2 ml/hour of the standard dilution recommended below).

Compatibility
Isoprenaline can be added (terminally) into a line containing standard TPN (with or without lipid) when absolutely necessary, and into a line containing dobutamine, heparin or milrinone. Isoprenaline is only stable in acid solutions, and should never, therefore, be infused into the same line as sodium bicarbonate.

Supply and administration
2 ml ampoules containing 2 mg of isoprenaline (costing ~£2) are now only available in the UK on special order. Protect the ampoules from light prior to use. To give an infusion of 10 nanograms/kg per minute place 300 micrograms (0·3 ml) of isoprenaline for each kg the baby weighs in a syringe, dilute to 50 ml with 10% glucose or glucose saline and infuse at a rate of 0·1 ml/hour. (A less concentrated solution of glucose or glucose saline can be used where necessary.) The drug is relatively stable in solutions with a low pH such as glucose and does not need to be prepared afresh every 24 hours.

References
Driscoll DJ. Use of inotropic and chronotropic agents in neonates. *Clin Perinatol* 1987;**14**:931–49.
Drummond WH. Use of cardiotonic therapy in the management of infants with PPHN. *Clin Perinatol* 1984;**11**:715–28.
Fukushige J, Takahashi N, Ingasashi H, *et al*. Perinatal management of congenital complete atrioventricular block: report of nine cases. *Acta Paediatr Jpn* 1998;**40**:337–40.

IVERMECTIN

Use

Ivermectin has revolutionised the treatment of several chronic, and potentially debilitating, parasitic infections in the last 25 years. Little is known about use in babies weighing less than 15 kg because the manufacturer has never supported such use, but there is no good reason to suppose use would be hazardous if called for.

Pharmacology

Ivermectin was isolated from a mixture of macrolide antibiotics found in *Streptomyces avermitilis* in 1980. It is well absorbed when taken by mouth and was found to prevent the reproduction of the nematode worm that causes 'river blindness' (see below). A closely related antibiotic abamectin is used in animals. The plasma half life is ~12 hours, and the metabolites are eventually excreted is the stool over the next 2 weeks. It is only teratogenic in animals in near toxic doses and, even though whole communities have been treated with the drug once every 6–12 months for nearly 20 years now, no adverse effect has yet been detected after unintended exposure during pregnancy. The drug appears in breast milk but, despite a milk:plasma ratio of 0·5, the baby is unlikely to ingest more than 2% of the weight-adjusted maternal dose.

Parasitic infections

The filariform larvae of three relatively common tropical nematode roundworms can cause human infection.

Onchocerciasis: Infection caused by the larvae of *Onchocerca volvulus* transmitted between individuals by the black flies that are common round many fast flowing rivers in Africa and in Central and South America can, if untreated for long enough, eventually cause blindness ('river blindness'). Some 15 million are currently affected and several hundred thousand have been rendered blind. Ivermectin kills the larvae but cannot kill adult worms (which can live for a decade) so repeat dosing is often needed every 6 months.

Filariasis: The larvae of the nematodes *Wuchereria bancrofti*, *Brugia malayi* and *B. timori* are transmitted between individuals by mosquito bites. Chronic infection is often unnoticed until it causes lymphadenopathy. Ivermectin only kills the larvae, so a cure requires treatment with diethylcarbamazine citrate (1 mg/kg three times a day for 1–2 weeks, but less at first because larval death can trigger a hypersensitivity reaction).

Strongyloidiasis: Infection by larvae of the nematode *Strongyloides stercoralis* is usually asymptomatic. Larvae in infected soil can enter the skin before migrating elsewhere, even eventually turning into adult worms (sometimes called threadworms in America) in the small intestine – so maintaining the life cycle by auto-reinfection. Treatment with ivermectin may need to be repeated more than once.

Treatment

The generally recommended treatment for all the above conditions is a single 150–200 microgram/kg dose of ivermectin, but in babies weighing 15–25 kg it seems to be acceptable, in practice, to give a single 3 mg dose. The WHO campaign funded by Merck since 1987 has done much to eliminate 'river blindness', but the parasite's extermination still seems a long way off even though man seems to be the parasite's only host.

Management of scabies

The mite *Sarcoptes scabiei* is another parasite that can only survive in contact with man. Covering the whole body overnight with 5% permethrin cream (a potent but poorly absorbed insecticide) will nearly always eradicate infection and seems safe even in the neonate (even though the manufacturer does not recommend use in children less than 2 months old). It can also be used to kill head lice, although wet combing should suffice in a small child. Ivermectin should be used, along with topical treatment, to treat hyperkeratotic 'crusted' scabies – severe infection may need several doses at weekly intervals as the drug is not ovicidal.

Supply and administration

Ivermectin is available in America as a 3 mg tablet. Supplies can be imported into the UK on request, although the manufacturers have not sought permission to market the product in the UK. A 30 gram tube of 5% permethrin cream is available without prescription for £5·60.

References

See also the relevant Cochrane reviews

Gann PH, Nreva FA, Gam AA. A randomized trial of single- and two-dose ivermectin versus thiobendazole for treatment of strongyloidiasis. *J Infect Dis* 1994;**169**:1076–9. [RCT]

Gyopong JO, Chinbuah MA, Gyapong M. Inadvertent exposure of pregnant women to invermectin and albendazole during mass drug administration for lymphatic filariasis. *Trop Med Int Health* 2003;**8**:1093–101.

Karthikeyan K. Scabies in children. *Arch Dis Child* 2007;**92**:ep65–9.

Katabarwa M, Eyamb A, Hsabomugisha P, *et al*. After a decade of annual dose mass ivermectin treatment in Cameroon and Uganda, onchocerciasis transmission continues. *Trop Med Int Health* 2008;**13**:1196–203.

Ndyomugyenyi R, Kabatereine N, Olsen A, *et al*. Efficacy of ivermectin and albendazole alone and in combination for treatment of soil-transmitted helminths in pregnancy and adverse events: a randomized open label controlled intervention in Masindi district, western Uganda. *Am J Trop Med Hyg* 2008;**79**:856–63. [RCT]

Nwaorgu OC, Okeibunor JC. Onchocerciasis in the pre-primary school children in Nigeria: lessons for onchocerciasis county control programme. *Acta Trop* 1999;**73**:211–15.

Ogbuokiri JE, Ozumba BC, Okonkwo PO. Ivermectin levels in human breast milk. *Eur J Clin Pharmacol* 1994;**46**:89–90.

Quarteman MJ, Lesher JL. Neonatal scabies treated with 5% permethrin cream. *Pediatr Dermatol* 1994;**11**:264–6.

Ramaiah KD, Das PK, Vanamail P, *et al*. Impact of 10 years of diethylcarbamazine and ivermectin mass administration on infection and transmission of lymphatic filariasis. *Trans R Soc Trop Med Hyg* 2007;**101**:555–63.

Roberts LJ, Huffam SE, Walton SF, *et al*. Crusted scabies: clinical and immunological findings in seventy-eight patients and a review of the literature. *J Infect* 2005;**50**:375–81.

Use

Ketamine given IV or IM produces a short-lasting, trance-like state with profound analgesia and amnesia.

Pharmacology

Ketamine was first developed in 1970, but its mode of action is complex and still unclear. IV administration produces an immediate feeling of dissociation followed, after 30 seconds, by a trance-like state that lasts 8–10 minutes. It produces marked amnesia but is devoid of hypnotic properties. The eyes often remain open, and nystagmus may develop. Functional and electrophysiological dissociation seem to occur between the brain's cortical and limbic systems. Respiration is not depressed, but salivation may increase and laryngeal stridor is occasionally encountered. Muscle tone increases slightly, and random limb movements occasionally require restraint. Serious rigidity is sometimes seen in adults. Tachycardia, systemic hypertension and increases in pulmonary vascular resistance have been reported in adults, but such problems have not been encountered in children. Analgesia persists for a sustained period after the anaesthetic effect has worn off. These characteristics make ketamine a particularly useful drug to give during painful but short-lasting procedures that do not require muscle relaxation. Full recovery can take 2–3 hours, and signs of distress and confusion are sometimes seen in adults during this time. Nightmares and hallucinations have been reported. Midazolam (q.v.) may help if this happens, but these problems are uncommon in children, and there is no evidence that they are common enough to make routine combined use appropriate. Nausea and vomiting are the commonest problems. Excessive salivation is only common in children more than a year old. The IV anaesthetic propofol (q.v.) provides an alternative strategy, and is also associated with quicker recovery.

Oral administration has been used in older children needing many invasive procedures, but plasma levels only peak after 30 minutes and a 10 mg/kg dose is necessary because bioavailability is low (~16%) because of first pass liver metabolism. Ketamine is rapidly redistributed round the body (V_D ~2·5 l/kg) after an IV dose and then cleared from the plasma with a terminal half life of 3 hours. Clearance is slightly faster in children than in adults. Neonatal clearance has not been studied. Ketamine undergoes extensive metabolism in the liver before excretion in the urine, and the metabolic product norketamine has analgesic properties. An overdose may make respiratory support necessary, but has no adverse long-term consequences. Doses lower than those quoted here are adequate when a volatile anaesthetic is also administered. While ketamine crosses the placenta when given in induction doses, its use during Caesarean delivery does not sedate the baby. There are no clear reports of teratogenicity or suggestions that ketamine is incompatible with lactation.

Anaesthesia

'Bolus' IV administration: A 2 mg/kg IV dose administered over at least 1 minute will provide about 10 minutes of surgical anaesthesia after about 30 seconds. Have either atropine or glycopyrronium (q.v.) available for prompt IV use because excessive secretions can, just occasionally, become troublesome.

Sustained IV administration: Give a loading dose of 1 mg/kg IV followed by an infusion of 500 micrograms/kg per hour (2 ml of the dilute preparation described below, followed by 1 ml/hour). Four times this dose can be used to produce *deep* anaesthesia when few other options exist.

IM administration: 4 mg/kg given IM will provide dissociative anaesthesia for about 15 minutes after a latent 5–10-minute period. Recovery will usually be complete after 2–3 hours.

Precautions

There are very few reports of neonatal use (see website commentary). Complications are uncommon in older children, but stridor and laryngospasm can be encountered, especially in response to pharyngeal or laryngeal stimulation. Prolonged apnoea has also been encountered. Because of this, ketamine should ***only*** be given by an experienced intensivist who is ready and equipped to take immediate control of the airway should this prove necessary (and any such clinician might prefer some other anaesthetic option). Monitoring is essential until recovery is complete. Use is not unwise in patients with head injury as was once thought.

Supply and administration

Ketamine is available in 20 ml vials containing 10 mg/ml costing £4·20 each. To give a continuous infusion of 500 micrograms/kg of ketamine per hour take 0·5 ml of the 10 mg/ml preparation for each kg the baby weighs, dilute to 10 ml with 5% glucose or glucose saline, and infuse at a rate of 1 ml/hour. Multidose vials containing 50 or 100 mg/ml are also manufactured.

References

See SIGN guideline on sedation of children for procedures

Green SM, Roback MG, Krauss B, *et al*. Predictors of airway and respiratory adverse events with ketamine sedation in the emergency department: an individual-patient meta-analysis of 8282 children. *Ann Emerg Med* 2009;**54**:158–68. [SR] (See also pp. 169–70 and 171–80.)

Howes MC. Ketamine for paediatric sedation/analgesia in the emergency department. *Emerg Med J* 2004;**21**:275–80. [SR]

Lin C, Durieux ME. Ketamine and kids: an update. *Pediatr Anaesth* 2005;**15**:91–7.

Mistry RB, Nahata MC. Ketamine for conscious sedation in pediatric emergency care. *Pharmacotherapy* 2005;**25**:1104–11. [SR]

Morton NS. Ketamin for procedural sedation and analgesia in pediatric emergency medicine: a UK perspective. *Pediatr Anesth* 2008;**18**:25–9.

Pun MS, Thakur J, Poudyal G, *et al*. Ketamine anaesthesia for paediatric ophthalmology surgery. *Br J Ophthalmol* 2003;**87**:535–7.

Wathen JE, Roback MG, Mackenzie T, *et al*. Does midazolam alter the clinical effects of intravenous ketamine sedation in children? A double-blind, randomised, controlled emergency department trial. *An Emerg Med* 2000;**36**:579–88. [RCT]

LABETALOL HYDROCHLORIDE

Use
Labetalol is the best drug for achieving quick but safe control over high blood pressure in infancy.

Pathophysiology
Judge the need for treatment by measuring the systolic blood pressure in a quiet baby, using a Doppler flow probe or stethoscope, a close fitting cuff that is as wide as possible, and an inflatable section that more than surrounds the arm. Resting systolic pressure at 2 weeks varies with gestation at birth as shown in Fig. 1. Ninety five per cent of babies have a systolic pressure of between 72 and 112 mmHg throughout the first year of life (as summarised in the monograph on hydralazine) once they reach a postmenstrual age of 46 weeks.

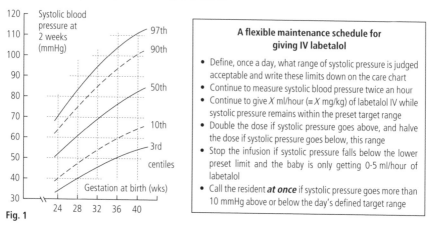

Fig. 1

A flexible maintenance schedule for giving IV labetalol

- Define, once a day, what range of systolic pressure is judged acceptable and write these limits down on the care chart
- Continue to measure systolic blood pressure twice an hour
- Continue to give X ml/hour ($\equiv X$ mg/kg) of labetalol IV while systolic pressure remains within the preset target range
- Double the dose if systolic pressure goes above, and halve the dose if systolic pressure goes below, this range
- Stop the infusion if systolic pressure falls below the lower preset limit and the baby is only getting 0·5 ml/hour of labetalol
- Call the resident **at once** if systolic pressure goes more than 10 mmHg above or below the day's defined target range

Serious hypertension in any young child is an emergency. It can be difficult to treat, and overtreatment can cause dangerous hypotension and potentially lethal β blockade. Treatment should always be discussed with a consultant therefore, and with a paediatric nephrologist where possible, because the cause is often renal.

Pharmacology
Labetalol is a non-selective α blocker (causing some decrease in peripheral vascular tone) with additional β-blocking properties like propranolol (q.v.). It was patented in 1971. It is rapidly effective, but rapidly metabolised by the liver (adult half life 4–8 hours), so any reactive hypotension quickly corrects itself once the infusion is stopped even though tissue levels exceed plasma levels (V_D ~9 l/kg). The neonatal half life may be rather longer, making reactive hypotension more hazardous. The benefit achieved by controlling hypertension usually outweighs the risk of use in cardiac failure. Glucagon (q.v.) may be of help following an overdose. Hydralazine (q.v.), with or without propranolol, used to be given once the acute situation was under control, but oral nifedipine (q.v.) is now more commonly given. Oral labetalol is sometimes used to control severe maternal hypertension although it can sometimes make the baby mildly hypotensive, hypoglycaemic and even bradycardic if used shortly before delivery. Use during lactation only exposes the baby to ~1% of the maternal dose on a weight-for-weight basis, although there is one isolated report of this appearing to cause sinus bradycardia. The manufacturers have not yet endorsed the drug's use in children.

Treatment
Initiating treatment: Start by giving 0·5 mg/kg of labetalol per hour (0·5 ml/hour of the dilute solution described below). Measure systolic pressure at least once every 15 minutes, and double the dose given once every 3 hours until an acceptable reduction in pressure has been achieved. The maximum safe dose is 4 mg/kg per hour (4 ml/hour). Once pressure has been reduced as much as seems immediately safe, write down the dose currently being given (X ml/kg) and the pressure limits currently considered acceptable, and initiate a flexible graded maintenance schedule for the next 24 hours using the strategy summarised in the box above.
Lowering blood pressure gradually: Modify the defined target range daily, aiming to take 3 days to bring the pressure down to normal, as discussed in the website commentary, unless hypertension is known to be of very recent onset. Start an oral drug and wean from labetalol as soon as practicable.

Supply and administration
20 ml ampoules containing 5 mg/ml of labetalol cost £2·10. Take 10 ml of labetalol for each kg the baby weighs from several such ampoules and dilute to 50 ml with 10% glucose or glucose saline to give a solution containing 1 mg/kg per ml of labetalol. Then pick-aback this infusion into an IV glucose line. The drug is stable in solution and does not need to be prepared afresh every 24 hours. Neat labetalol is irritant to veins.

References
See also the relevant Cochrane reviews

Bunchman TE, Lynch RE, Wood EG. Intravenously administered labetalol for treatment of hypertension in children. *J Pediatr* 1992;**120**:140–4.
Crooks BNA, Deshpande SA, Hall C, *et al.* Adverse neonatal effects of maternal labetalol treatment. *Arch Dis Child* 1998;**79**:F150–1.
Deal JE, Barratt TM, Dillon MJ. Management of hypertensive emergencies. *Arch Dis Child* 1992;**67**:1089–92.
Mirpuri J, Patel H, Rhee H, *et al.* A case of bradycardia in a premature infant on breast milk. *J Invest Med* 2008;**56**:409. (Abstract 203.)

Use

Lamivudine is used, in combination with other antiviral drugs, in the control of human immunodeficiency virus (HIV) infection. Short-term use, together with zidovudine and nevirapine (q.v.), in women who are infected but not on any long-term treatment, will minimise viral transmission from mother to child.

Pharmacology

Lamivudine (or 3TC) is an antiviral drug first introduced in 1992 that works, like zidovudine, after intracellular conversion to the triphosphate form, as a nucleoside reverse transcriptase inhibitor (NRTI) to halt retroviral DNA synthesis. Resistance quickly develops if it is used on its own to treat HIV infection, and it is unclear whether sustained low-dose treatment is any better than interferon alfa (q.v.) in the management of chronic hepatitis B infection. Indeed there is no good information on the use of this drug in young children with hepatitis B infection. Oral uptake is good and is not reduced (although it is delayed) by ingestion with food. Bioavailability seems, nevertheless, to be rather lower in children than in adults. Most of the drug is rapidly excreted, unchanged, in the urine, ($t_{1/2}$ ~2 hours in children) making dosage reduction necessary when there is serious renal failure. It is usually well tolerated, though adverse effects include nausea, vomiting and diarrhoea, malaise, muscle pain and a non-specific rash. All the NRTI drugs occasionally cause liver damage with hepatomegaly, hepatic steatosis and potentially life-threatening lactic acidosis. Neuropathy and pancreatitis are only common in children with advanced disease on many other drugs. Lamivudine crosses the placenta. It does not seem to be teratogenic but there is not enough information to exclude the possibility that it could be embryotoxic if taken at the time of conception. The baby of a mother on treatment with lamivudine would only get about 4% of the weight-related dose in breast milk.

Managing overt HIV infection

New information on optimum management becomes available so frequently that anyone treating this condition *must* first familiarise themselves with the latest available posted website information (as outlined in the monographs on zidovudine and didanosine). Diagnosis and management must also be discussed with, and supervised by, someone with extensive experience of this condition. Treatment will be influenced by any prior treatment that the mother has received, but will normally include zidovudine and lamivudine together with *either* a protease inhibitor (such as lopinavir or nelfinavir) *or* nevirapine. Other drug strategies can be difficult to use in young babies because no suitable liquid formulation exists.

Emergency intrapartum prophylaxis

Give any previously untreated mother 150 mg of lamivudine by mouth at the onset of labour, and repeat this once every 12 hours until delivery; also give zidovudine, either IV as outlined in the zidovudine monograph, or as a 600 mg oral loading dose at the start of labour and then 300 mg every 3 hours until delivery. (In the main trial of this strategy low-dose maternal treatment was continued for a week after delivery.) Give the baby 4 mg/kg of zidovudine and 2 mg/kg of lamivudine by mouth once every 12 hours for at least 1, and preferably 4, weeks. Give the baby 2 mg/kg of nevirapine once a day for 1 week and then 4 mg/kg once a week for 1 week as well.

Treating known HIV infection in infancy

The standard dose is 4 mg/kg by mouth twice a day alone if appropriate, or with two or more other antiviral drugs. In the rare situation where treatment is called for in the first month of life give 2 mg/kg twice a day.

Supply

150 mg lamivudine tablets cost £2·50 each. Stable oral solutions (banana and strawberry flavoured) containing 5 and 10 mg/ml are available costing £9 and £17 per 100 ml, respectively. The oral syrups contain 0·2 g/ml of sucrose, and also contain propylene glycol. Lamivudine can not be given IV or IM.

References

American Academy of Pediatrics. Human immunodeficiency virus infection. In: Pickering LK, ed. *Red book*. *2003 report of the Committee on Infectious Diseases*, 26th edn. Elk Grove Village, IL: American Academy of Pediatrics, 2003: pp. 360–82.

Capparelli E, Rakhamanina N, Mirochnick M. Pharmacotherapy of perinatal HIV. *Semin Fetal Neonat Med* 2005;**10**:161–75.

Johnson MA, Moore KHP, Yuen GJ, *et al*. Clinical pharmacokinetics of lamivudine. *Clin Pharmacokinet* 1999;**36**:41–66.

Moodley D, Moodley J, Coovadia H, *et al*. A multicenter randomised controlled trial of nevirapine versus a combination of zidovudine and lamivudine to reduce intrapartum and early postpartum mother-to-child transmission of human immunodeficiency virus type 1. *J Infect Dis* 2003;**187**:725–35. [RCT]

Moodley JO, Moodley D, Pillay K, *et al*. Pharmacokinetics and antiretroviral activity of lamivudine alone or when coadministered with zidovudine in human immunodeficiency virus type 1-infected pregnant women and their offspring. *J Infect Dis* 1998;**178**:1327–33.

Panburana P, Sirinavin S, Phuapradit W, *et al*. Elective cesarean section plus short-course lamivudine and zidovudine for the prevention of mother-to-child transmission of human immunodeficiency virus type 1. *Am J Obstet Gynecol* 2004;**190**:803–8.

Shetty AK, Coovadia HM, Mirochnick M, *et al*. Safety and trough concentrations of nevirapine prophylaxis given daily, twice weekly, or weekly in breast-feeding infants from birth to 6 months. *J Acquir Immune Defic Syndr* 2004;**34**:482–90.

UK Group on Transmitted HIV Drug Resistance. Time trends in primary resistance to HIV drugs in the United Kingdom: multicentre observational study. *BMJ* 2005;**331**:1368–71.

Use

Lamotrigine is increasingly used to improve seizure control in children already taking one anticonvulsant drug, but experience with use in young children is still very limited. The fact that treatment has to be introduced gradually is often seen as something of a disadvantage.

Pharmacology

Lamotrigine is a phenyltriazine, and structurally unrelated to any other established antiepileptic drug. It first came into clinical use in 1987, and may work as a sodium channel blocker, or by inhibiting excitatory (glutamate) neurotransmitter release. It is well absorbed when taken by mouth and mostly metabolised by the liver. The half life in adults taking no other drug is 24−36 hours, but it is shorter than this in pregnancy, and in children. Tissue levels are high (V_D >1·2 l/kg). A measles-like skin rash is the commonest adverse effect. It is usually seen if the dose is too high or is increased too quickly, and usually occurs within a few weeks of starting treatment. Combined use with valproate also makes it more likely. More serious toxic skin changes may make it necessary to stop treatment quickly. Fulminant hepatic failure is a further rare hazard.

Lamotrigine has only been formally approved for 'adjunctive' use in young children with refractory partial and general tonic-clonic seizures who are also taking some other anticonvulsant, but it may occasionally be effective in controlling infantile spasms and absence seizures. It is also effective in Lennox−Gastaut syndrome (a severe form of epilepsy in early childhood associated with multiple seizure types in which the waking EEG shows interictal slow, spike-wave activity). Lamotrigine is now increasingly thought to be the first anticonvulsant to try when managing partial (focal) epilepsy, not only in adults but also in children 5 or more years old. It may reduce seizure activity in juvenile myoclonic epilepsy, but is of no help in severe myoclonic epilepsy of infancy (Dravet syndrome). The risk of malformation with maternal use seems to be dose related, but is generally quite low. Such use does not render the baby vitamin K deficient, and adverse effects have not been seen in breastfed babies even though the blood level is about a tenth of that present in the mother.

Drug interactions

All the drugs that increase liver enzyme activity (such as carbamazepine, phenobarbital and phenytoin) greatly speed the elimination of lamotrigine. The dose given often needs to be *increased* as a result. Combined treatment with carbamazepine may increase the risk of toxicity. Combined treatment with valproate, in contrast (which may confer synergistic benefit), doubles the half life, probably because both drugs compete for glucuronidation in the liver. A *lower* dose needs to be used in consequence, especially when treatment is first started. The valproate dose will also need to be lowered by 25−35%.

Treatment

Monotherapy: Start by giving 300 micrograms/kg once a day by mouth for 2 weeks, and then twice a day for a further 2 weeks. Treatment can then be further 'titrated' upwards as necessary to maximise seizure control, to a dose that should not, initially, exceed 2 mg/kg twice a day.

Adjunctive (combined) therapy: Children taking other enzyme-inducing drugs (see above) often require double the usual dose, while those on valproate usually only need a third to a half the usual dose.

Blood levels

A knowledge of the blood level does not help to optimise management, but may reveal failure to take medicine as prescribed. Effective levels are usually 1−4 mg/l (1 mg/l = 3·9 μmol/l) but can be higher.

Case notification

A voluntary, confidential, UK-based register continues to collect *prospective* information on anticonvulsant use during pregnancy. For further information ring 0800 389 1248.

Supply

Scored dispersible 5 mg tablets of lamotrigine cost 30p each. Although they are only semisoluble, small doses can be given with reasonable accuracy by adding a tablet to 10 ml of tap water − 1 ml of liquid will then contain approximately 500 micrograms of lamotrigine as long as the particulate matter is kept in suspension. The same dose can also be given into the rectum if oral treatment is not possible. A stable suspension with a 4-week shelf life can be prepared, but it has a very unpleasant taste.

References

See also the relevant Cochrane reviews

Frank LM, Enlow T, Holmes GL, *et al*. Lamictal (lamotrigine) monotherapy for typical absence seizures in children. *Epilepsia* 1999;**40**:973−9. [RCT]

Marson AG, Al-Kharusi A, Alwaidh M, *et al*. The SANAD study of the effectiveness of carbamazepine, gabapentic, lamotrigine, oxarbazepine, or topiramate for treatment of partial epilepsy: an unblended randomised trial. *Lancet* 2007;**369**:1000−15. [RCT]

Meador KJ, Baker GA, Finnell RH, *et al*. In utero antiepileptic drug exposure. Fetal death and malformations. *Neurology* 2006;**67**:407−12.

Morrow J, Russell A, Guthrie E, *et al*. Malformation risks of antiepileptic drugs in pregnancy: a prospective study from the UK epilepsy and pregnancy register. *J Neurol Neurosurg Psychiatry*. 2006;**77**:193−8. (See also the editorial on p. 145.)

Newport DJ, Pennell PB, Calamaras MR, *et al*. Lamotrigine in breast milk and nursing infants: determination of exposure. *Pediatrics* 2008;**122**:e223−31.

Pennell PB, Peng L, Newport DL, *et al*. Lamotrigine in pregnancy: clearance, therapeutic drug monitoring and seizure frequency. *Neurology* 2008;**70**:2130−6.

Piña-Garza JE, Levisohn P, Gucuyener K, *et al*. Adjunctive lamotrigine for partial seizures in patients aged 1 to 24 months. *Neurology* 2008;**70**:2099−108.

Use

Thyroid extracts have been used to treat hormone deficiency since 1890.

Pathophysiology

Thyroid-stimulating hormone (TSH) produced by the pituitary regulates the release of levothyroxine (T_4) and (to a lesser extent) liothyronine (T_3) from the thyroid gland. T_4 is then converted to T_3 in the tissues. Significant amounts of maternal T_4 (but not TSH and T_3) cross the placenta – explaining the relatively normal appearance of the baby at birth. Subclinical maternal hypothyroidism in early pregnancy may increase the risk of spontaneous abortion and has a deleterious effect on the child's neurodevelopment; the aim of treatment should therefore be to keep maternal TSH ≤2·5 mU/l. Antithyroid drugs and maternal thyroid receptor antibodies can cross the placenta, causing fetal hypo- and hyperthyroidism. Fetal goitre can now be detected by antenatal ultrasound. The mother can be offered an antithyroid drug if the fetus is thyrotoxic, while hypothyroidism has, occasionally, been managed by inserting 250–500 micrograms of thyroxine into the amniotic cavity once every 10–14 days (so it can be swallowed by the fetus). Mothers taking thyroxine may breastfeed. The management of neonatal thyrotoxicosis is discussed in the monograph on propranolol.

Hypothyroidism at birth

Congenital hypothyroidism occurs in about 1 in 3500 babies, and is due to thyroid dysgenesis (~85%) and dyshormono-genesis (~15%). There is considerable clinical and biochemical heterogeneity but treatment should be started within 2 weeks of birth if outcome is to be optimised. Babies in the UK are screened for hypothyroidism using the Guthrie card at a week of age. Confirmation requires the demonstration of a high TSH and, usually, also a low T_4 in a serum sample. This programme has been very successful, but thyroid function should still be measured if hypothyroidism is suspected because false negatives can occur and because hypothyroidism can evolve.

The normal TSH surge and the rise in T_3 and T_4 after birth are less marked in the preterm infant. These babies often have low thyroid hormone levels, a trend that may be exacerbated by exposure to the iodine in antiseptics and X-ray contrast media. The risk of developmental delay and cerebral palsy also seems to be increased in preterm babies who had transient low thyroxine levels after birth, but trials have not shown that correction improves long-term outcome.

Guthrie screening

TSH screening for hypothyroidism is generally performed on dried (Guthrie) blood samples. Quantitative TSH assays are undertaken by the UK Supra-Regional Assay Service on 200 µl of serum (~600 µl of whole blood). T_4 assays can be undertaken on 50 µl of serum (~150 µl of whole blood).

Treatment

Neonatal treatment: The usual starting dose is 10–12 micrograms/kg of levothyroxine by mouth once a day. Smaller doses may be needed in babies with significant endogenous thyroid hormone production. Monitor the thyroid hormone and TSH levels after 2 and 4 weeks and then every 1–2 months during the first year of life, aiming for a TSH in the normal range and a free T_4 level in the upper part of the normal range. Because hypothyroidism is occasionally transient it is usual to reassess the requirement for continued treatment when the child is 2 or 3 years old.

Older children: In older children a starting dose of 50–100 micrograms/m² per day has been suggested.

Blood levels

Early levels vary, but serum TSH levels above 10 mU/l are rare after the first week of life. Free T_4 levels are typically higher in neonates than in adults but this is not always reflected in local reference ranges.

Supply

25, 50 and 100 microgram tablets of levothyroxine cost between 2p and 3p each. A sugar-free suspension, which is stable for 3 months, can be provided on request. If treatment has to be given IV or IM, and no suitable T_4 product is available (as in the UK), treatment with a 2 microgram/kg dose of liothyronine (T_3) twice a day should be considered (although experience with such an approach is very limited).

References

See also the relevant Cochrane reviews

American Academy of Pediatrics. Update on newborn screening and therapy for congenital hypothyroidism. *Pediatrics* 2006;**117**:2290–303.

Biswas S, Buffery J, Enoch H, *et al*. A longitudinal assessment of thyroid hormone concentrations in preterm infants younger then 30 weeks' gestation during the first 2 weeks of life and their relationship to outcome. *Pediatrics* 2002;**109**:222–7.

Glinoer D, Abalovich M. Unresolved questions in managing hypothyroidism during pregnancy. *BMJ* 2007;**335**:300–2.

Hrytsiuk I, Gilbert R, Logan S, *et al*. Starting dose of levothyroxine for the treatment of congenital hypothyroidism. *Arch Pediatr Adolesc Med* 2002;**156**:485–91. [SR]

Kloostra L, Crawford S, van Baar AL, *et al*. Neonatal effects of maternal hypothyroxinemia during early pregnancy. *Pediatrics* 2006;**117**:161–7.

Korada M, Pearce MS, Ward Platt MP, *et al*. Difficulties in selecting an appropriate neonatal TSH screening threshold. *Arch Dis Child* 2009; published online as 10.1136/adc.2008.147884. Aug 12 2009.

Neale DM, Cootauco AC, Burrow G. Thyroid disease in pregnancy. *Clin Perinatol* 2007;**34**:54–357.

Valerio PG, van Wassenaer AG, Vijlder JJM, *et al*. A randomized masked study of triiodothyronine plus thyroxine administration in preterm infants less than 28 weeks of gestational age: hormonal and clinical effects. *Pediatr Res* 2004;**55**:248–53. [RCT]

Williams FL, Simpson J, Delahunty C, *et al*. Collaboration from the Scottish Preterm Thyroid Group. Developmental trends in cord and postpartum serum thyroid hormones in preterm infants. *J Clin Endocrinol Metab* 2004;**89**:5314–20.

LIDOCAINE = Lignocaine (former BAN)

Use
Lidocaine is a widely used local anaesthetic. A short infusion can sometimes stop neonatal fits resistant to phenobarbital and the benzodiazepines, and is occasionally used to control arrhythmia.

Pharmacology
Systemic and subcutaneous use: Lidocaine hydrochloride is a local anaesthetic of the amide group with effects on the central nervous system (where it acts as a sedative in low doses and a stimulant in high doses), on peripheral nerves (where it decreases conduction) and on the heart (where it shortens the duration of the action potential). It was first marketed in Sweden in 1948. Lidocaine is metabolised by the liver, but some of the intermediary breakdown products are metabolically active as well as potentially toxic; up to a third is excreted unchanged by the neonatal kidney. Oral administration fails to produce adequate blood levels because of rapid first pass liver metabolism. The terminal half life is about 100 minutes in adults, and at least twice this in the newborn. Intravenous infusion produces high drug concentrations in those organs with a high blood flow, with later redistribution throughout the body. This volume of distribution is particularly high in the neonatal period (V_D >1 l/kg). Drowsiness is a common side effect, while overtreatment can cause irritability and fits, but the amount required to cause neonatal depression is above the level required to treat arrhythmia. Use in pregnancy seems safe, and use during lactation only exposes the baby to 2% of the weight-related maternal dose.

Analgesic cream: Plain (30%) lidocaine ointment is ineffective when applied to the skin, but a eutectic mixture of local anaesthetics (EMLA) as a cream (Emla® cream), containing 2·5% lidocaine and 2·5% prilocaine, provides good surface anaesthesia for 1–2 hours in children if applied under an occlusive dressing at least 1 hour in advance of venepuncture, but seems less effective in babies (possibly because of rapid skin clearance). Tetracaine gel (q.v.) may provide quicker and marginally better pain relief for venepuncture in infancy. The manufacturers have been reluctant to endorse the use of Emla cream in children less than a year old, but the prilocaine it contains does not seem to cause significant methaemoglobinaemia (at least in babies of 30 or more weeks' gestation with a reasonably mature epidermis) as had once been feared.

Treatment
Surface anaesthesia: Apply 1 gram of Emla cream to a 2 × 2 cm area of undamaged skin, and cover with an occlusive dressing for 1 hour. Keep away from the eyes. Tetracaine gel may be a better alternative.

Mucosal anaesthesia: Use no more than 0·1 ml/kg of a 4% lidocaine spray or 0·3 ml/kg of a 2% lidocaine gel on mucosal surfaces. Experience with the spray in small children is limited and a randomised study showed that use did not reduce the distress displayed by 1–5-year-old children during nasogastric tube insertion.

Infiltrative local anaesthesia: 0·3 ml/kg of 1% plain lidocaine provides excellent anaesthesia for 1–2 hours after 1–2 minutes. Take care not to inject anything into a blood vessel and give no further lidocaine for 4 hours. A 0·6 ml/kg dose of 1% lidocaine in adrenaline will offer pain relief for 3 hours. Bupivacaine (q.v.) can provide pain relief for at least 6 hours, but only after a half hour latent period.

Fits and arrhythmia: Give a 2 mg/kg dose (0·2 ml/kg of a 1% solution of adrenaline-free lidocaine IV over 10 minutes) followed by a maintenance infusion of 6 mg/kg per hour for 6 hours. Then tail treatment off over the next 24 hours (4 mg/kg for 12 hours followed by 2 mg/kg for 12 hours). A marginally lower dose may be better in the very preterm baby.

Toxicity
Accidental infiltration of the fetal scalp during the injection of lidocaine into the maternal perineum can cause toxic apnoea, bradycardia, hypotension and fits – a cluster of features that can be mistaken for intrapartum asphyxia. Some babies have required ventilatory support, but most have made a complete recovery. Management is as discussed in the monograph on bupivacaine.

Compatibility
Compatibility with other continuously infused drugs is noted, where known, in the monograph for the second product. It can also be added (terminally) to TPN and lipid. It is not compatible with phenytoin.

Supply
Ampoules of adrenaline-free 1% (10 mg/ml) lidocaine cost between 21p and 35p each. 20 ml ampoules of 1% lidocaine with adrenaline (10 mg of lidocaine and 5 micrograms of adrenaline per ml) cost 76p. 5 gram tubes of Emla cream cost £1·70. Anhydrous lidocaine as a 2% gel is available in 20 gram tubes costing £1 each. A 4% lidocaine jet-spray (Celltech) delivery system for use during laryngoscopy costs £5.

References
See also the relevant Cochrane reviews

Babl FE, Goldfinch CM, Mandrawa C, *et al*. Does nebulized lidocaine reduce the pain and distress of nasogastric tube insertion in young children? A randomized, double-blind, placebo-controlled trial. *Pediatrics* 2009;**123**:1548–55. [RCT]

Boylan GB, Rennie JM, Chorley G, *et al*. Second-line anticonvulsant treatment of neonatal seizures: a video-EEG monitoring study. *Neurology* 2004;**62**:486–8. [RCT]

Malingré MM, van Rooij LGM, Rademaker CMA, *et al*. Development of an optimal lidocaine infusion strategy for neonatal seizures. *Eur J Pediatr* 2006;**165**:598–604.

Shany E, Banzagen O, Watemberg N. Comparison of continuous drip of midazolam or lidocaine in the treatment of intractable neonatal seizures. *J Child Neurol* 2007;**22**:255–9.

Van Rooij LGM, Toet MC, Rademaker KMA, *et al*. Cardiac arrhythmias in neonates receiving lidocaine as anticonvulsive treatment. *Eur J Pediatr* 2004;**163**:637–41.

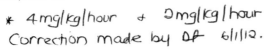
* 4 mg/kg/hour & 2 mg/kg/hour
Correction made by OF 6/1/12.

Use

This expensive new antibiotic should be kept in reserve and only used, on microbiological advice, to treat meticillin-resistant *Staphylococcus aureus* (MRSA) and vancomycin-resistant enterococcal infection. There is, as yet, little published information on neonatal use and almost none on use in the preterm baby.

Pharmacology

Linezolid is an oxazolidinone antibiotic, first marketed in 2000, that inhibits bacterial protein synthesis in a new and unique way. The drug is active against a range of Gram-positive bacteria, including both MRSA and glycopeptide intermediate-resistant *Staph. aureus*. MRSA is becoming increasingly common in young children. It is also active against vancomycin-resistant enterococci, and strains of *Streptococcus pneumoniae* resistant to a range of other antibiotics, and against some anaerobes including *Clostridium perfringens, C. difficile* and *Bacteroides fragilis*. Enterobacteriaceae and *Pseudomonas aeruginosa* are not susceptible to linezolid, but it has occasionally been used to treat multidrug-resistant TB. Linezolid is rapidly and completely absorbed when given by mouth, and it penetrates the meninges well when these are inflamed. Thirty per cent is excreted, unchanged, in the urine; the remainder is excreted as inactive metabolites (which could accumulate in severe renal failure). The half life in children 1 week to 10 years old (2–3 hours) is half what it is at birth and in adults.

Generally, reversible thrombocytopenia can occur when treatment is given for more than 10–14 days. More serious temporary marrow depression, similar to that seen with chloramphenicol, has also (rarely) been reported, and a full blood count should probably be performed once a week if treatment becomes necessary for longer than this. Severe optic neuropathy has also, very rarely, been encountered, especially with sustained use. There is also concern that prolonged low-dose use could lead to the development of bacterial resistance (especially with *Enterococcus faecium*). Linezolid is a weak, reversible, non-selective, monoamine oxidase (MAO) inhibitor, and it has been suggested that this makes its use at the same time as – or within 2 weeks of treatment with – a MAO antidepressant unwise. Similarly, combined use with a range of other antidepressants could cause a 'serotonin syndrome' with hyperpyrexia and cognitive dysfunction.

No information is available as yet on use during pregnancy, but placental transfer is to be expected, because the drug has a low molecular weight. Indeed, the drug should only be used during pregnancy for the moment when no other good option exists because, although there is no evidence of teratogenicity, increased embryo death, decreased litter size, decreased fetal weight and costal cartilage abnormalities were reported during drug testing in mice. Nothing is known about use during lactation either but, based on extrapolated animal data, a baby might be expected to ingest a little under 10% of the weight-related maternal dose. Manufacturers have not yet recommended use in children under 18 years.

Drug interactions

Use with care and monitor blood pressure during co-administration with any sympathomimetic drug (such as dopamine or dobutamine).

Treatment

Dose: Give 10 mg/kg IV. Oral absorption is good in adults, but has not yet been studied in children. Treatment is usually continued for 2 weeks.
Timing: Give once every 12 hours in children less than a week old, and once every 8 hours after that.

Supply and administration

300 ml bags containing 2 mg/ml of linezolid suitable for IV administration cost £44 each. Do not mix linezolid with, or infuse it into the same line as, any other drug. Do not dilute further before administration. The manufacturers say that adults should receive any IV infusion over at least 30 minutes, but that is because the volume of fluid involved is considerable. Bags should be stored at room temperature, protected from light during storage in the foil overwrap provided, and inverted gently 2–3 times before use. The fluid slowly turns yellow with time, but this does not affect potency. No IM preparation exists, but an oral suspension containing 20 mg/ml is now available (100 ml costs £150).

References

Jungbluth GL, Welshman IR, Hopkins NK. Linezolid pharmacokinetics in pediatric patients: an overview. *Pediatr Infect Dis J* 2003;**22**:S153–7.
Kaplan SL, Deville JG, Yogev R, *et al*. Linezolid *versus* vancomycin for treatment of resistant Gram-positive infections in children. *Pediatr Infect Dis J* 2003;**22**:677–85.
Kearns GL, Andersson T, James LP, *et al*. Impact of ontogeny on linezolid disposition in neonates and infants. *J Clin Pharmacol* 2003;**43**:840–8.
Khairulddin N, Bishop L, Lamagni TL, *et al*. Emergence of methicillin resistant *Staphylococcus aureus* (MRSA) bacteraemia among children in England and Wales, 1990–2001. *Arch Dis Child* 2004;**89**:378–9.
Langgartner M, Mutenthaler A, Haiden N, *et al*. Linezolid for treatment of catheter-related cerebrospinal fluid infections in preterm infants. [Letter]. *Arch Dis Child* 2008;**93**:F397.
Schaaf HS, Willemse M, Donald PR. Long-term linezolid treatment in a young child with extensively drug-resistant tuberculosis. *J Pediatr Infect Dis* 2009;**28**:748–50.
Stalker DJ, Jungbluth GL. Clinical pharmacokinetics of linezolid, a novel oxazolidinone antibacterial. *Clin Pharmacokinet* 2003;**42**:1129–40.
Tan TQ. Update on the use of linezolid: a pediatric perspective. *Pediatr Infect Dis J* 2004;**23**:955–6.

LOPINAVIR with RITONAVIR (LPV/r)

Use

Protease inhibitors are used with other drugs, to control human immunodeficiency virus (HIV) infection.

Pharmacology

Lopinavir (LPV) and ritonavir (RTV) are protease inhibitors that bind to HIV-protease, causing the formation of immature viral particles that are incapable of infecting other cells. Both first came into general clinical use in the late 1990s. Giving a low, and in itself subtherapeutic, 1:4 dose of ritonavir with lopinavir boosts the effectiveness of lopinavir. Both are well absorbed by mouth, especially when given with food, metabolised by the liver and excreted in the faeces, the half life in adults being about 4 hours. Diabetes can develop or be exacerbated in patients taking a protease inhibitor. Placental transfer is very limited but, because there is some animal evidence of teratogenicity, all use in pregnancy should be reported (anonymously) to the Antiretroviral Pregnancy Register as outlined in the monograph on zidovudine. It is not yet known how much is excreted into breast milk. Because trials are still underway the manufacturers have not yet recommended the use of any protease inhibitor in children less than 2 years old (<6 months in the US).

Nelfinavir (NFV) is a related protease inhibitor with many of the same properties. Early studies used too low a dose – infants probably need at least 75 mg/kg twice by mouth, but the optimum dose is not yet clear.

Principles of overt HIV management

Combined treatment with several drugs, or **h**ighly **a**ctive **a**nti-**r**etroviral **t**herapy (HAART), is now widely used to control overt HIV infection. Such a strategy optimises the suppression of viral replication and reduces the risk of drug resistance developing. The commonest strategy (where it can be afforded) is a combination of two nucleoside reverse transcriptase inhibitor (NRTI) drugs (the best known of which is zidovudine) with either a *non*-NRTI drug such as nevirapine (q.v.) or a protease inhibitor such as lopinavir or nelfinavir. Such treatment should not be modified during pregnancy – to do so risks jeopardising the mother's health. Opinion is more divided as to the best management of infection in early infancy. Vigorous treatment is clearly indicated where there is a high HIV RNA viral load, because there is a high risk of rapid disease progression. The best strategy where there is only a low viral load is less clear. Since no strategy seems capable of eliminating all virus from the body, some clinicians would prefer to use as little potentially toxic drug treatment as is compatible with inhibiting all detectable virus replication. Major collaborative trials comparing various drug combinations have been under way since 2001. For further information contact the MRC Clinical Trials Unit in the UK (tel: +44 207 670 4700; email: PENTA@ctu.mrc.ac.uk). PENTA members can access a wealth of authoritative, up to date, information on *all* aspects of HIV care in children on the Paediatric European Network for Treatment of Aids website www.pentatrials.org.

Drug interactions

The protease inhibitors are best given with food, but didanosine is best given on an empty stomach, so simultaneous administration should be avoided. Since lopinavir, ritonavir and nelfinavir are all part metabolised by the liver's P450 cytochrome enzyme system, their clearance is increased by co-treatment with a wide range of other drugs including cabamazepine, dexamethasone, phenobarbital, phenytoin, rifampicin and theophylline. Protease inhibitors also inhibit the clearance of other drugs. Co-treatment with a narrow therapeutic range such as antihistamines, benzodiazepines, cisapride, rifampicin and a range of cardiac drugs (including amiodarone and flecainide) is discouraged because clearance is unpredictably decreased. Digoxin levels are variably affected. See www.hiv-druginteractions.org.

Treatment

Little information is available on the best dose of lopinavir (with ritonavir) to use in the first month of life. A starting dose of 300 mg/m^2 twice a day is currently under investigation. Older children are usually given 230 mg/m^2 of lopinavir by mouth twice a day (or 300 mg/m^2 if taking nevirapine).

Supply

These drugs can not be given IV or IM, and are best taken with a little food to minimise gastric irritation.

Lopinavir with ritonavir: A solution is available containing 80 mg/ml of lopinavir and 20 mg/ml of ritonavir (100 ml costs £45). It contains 43% alcohol, propylene glycol and fructose corn syrup. The bitter taste can be disguised by giving it with chocolate-flavoured milk. It must *not* be mixed with water, and is best kept at 4°C, but is stable at room temperature for a month.

Nelfinavir: This available as 50 mg/g powder that can be mixed, just before use with water, milk, ice cream or puddings, but crushed 250 mg tablets (costing £1 each) are more palatable.

References

Chadwick EG, Rodman JH, Britto P, *et al*. Ritonavir-based highly active antiretroviral therapy in human immunodeficiency virus type 1-infected infants younger than 24 months. *Pediatr Infect Dis J* 2005;**24**:793–800.

Microchnick M, Capparelli E. Pharmacokinetics of antiretrovirals in pregnant women. *Clin Pharmacokinet* 2004;**43**:1071–87.

Oldfield V, Plosker GL. Lopinacir/ritonavir: a review of its use in the management of HIV infection. *Drugs* 2006;**66**:1275–99. [SR]

Resino S, Bellón JM, Ramos JT, *et al*. Salvage lopinavir-ritonavir therapy in human immunodeficiency virus-infected children. *Pediatr Infect Dis J* 2004;**23**:923–30.

Sáez-Llorens X, Violair A, Deetz CO, *et al*. Forty-eight-week evaluation of lopinavir/ritonavir, a new protease inhibitor, in human immuno-deficiency virus-infected children. *Pediatr Infect Dis J* 2003;**22**:216–23.

Use
Several benzodiazepine drugs have been used to arrest seizure activity. Of these lorazepam would seem at the moment to be the product of choice. When sustained seizure activity ('status epilepticus') in older children does not respond to this drug, an infusion of thiopental sodium (q.v.) is probably the most effective option.

Pharmacology
Sales of chlordiazepoxide (or Librium®) rose so fast when Hoffman-La Roche put the first benzodiazepine on the market in 1960 that many other products soon followed. Diazepam, a structurally simpler analogue, was licensed in 1963, and lorazepam was synthesised 1 year later. These, and a range of other products, were widely used to treat anxiety, but it is now generally accepted that such use should always be limited to the lowest possible dose for the shortest possible time. Dependence can become a serious problem, even with careful prescribing, particularly in patients with a history of alcohol or drug abuse, or a personality disorder.

Lorazepam readily crosses the placenta, but there is no clear evidence of teratogenicity. Respiratory depression, hypothermia, lethargy and poor feeding have all been observed, however, when a mother is given high-dose medication shortly before delivery. Breastfeeding may further sedate the baby in the period immediately after birth, even though the baby only receives 5–10% of the maternal dose on a weight-for-weight basis, but sustained use during lactation does not seem to cause noticeable drowsiness. The drug is well absorbed when taken by mouth, is conjugated to an inactive glucuronide in the liver and then excreted in the urine by glomerular filtration. The half life in the neonatal period is 30–50 hours (2–3 times as long as in adult life). Tissue drug levels slightly exceed plasma levels ($V_D \sim 1\cdot3$ l/kg).

Most benzodiazepines are of limited value in the long-term treatment of epilepsy, but they have an important role in acute seizure management. Diazepam was the first to be widely used. Clonazepam, lorazepam and midazolam (q.v.) have all been used more recently to control serious persisting seizures that fail to respond to phenobarbital. There is, however, continuing concern that, while sedation with a benzodiazepine may well abolish the abnormal movements that are the outward sign of cerebral seizure activity, electrical seizure activity may still sometimes persist. For a review of the various treatment options see the web commentary linked to the monograph on phenobarbital. Rapid IV administration in the neonate can sometimes precipitate hypotension, respiratory depression and abnormal seizure-like movements, especially in response to the first dose given. Withdrawal symptoms are also very common after sustained use (as they are with midazolam) even if the dose given is lowered slowly ('tapered' dosing).

Treatment
Dose: A single 100 microgram/kg dose will usually stop all visible seizure activity within 10 minutes. The drug's long half life in early infancy makes repeat dosing unwise for 24 hours.
Route of administration: Lorazepam is normally given IV, but mucosal absorption is rapid enough to make delivery into the nose, or under the tongue, almost equally effective (at least in babies more than a few weeks old). Lorazepam can also be given by mouth, but IM administration is painful and best avoided. Sustained infusion can cause a progressive accumulation of the potentially toxic excipient propylene glycol.

Antidote
Flumazenil is a specific antidote (as described in the monograph on midazolam).

Supply and administration
1 ml ampoules containing 4 mg of lorazepam cost 37p each. These contain 1 ml of propylene glycol and 0·02 ml of benzyl alcohol, should be protected from light, and are best stored at 4°C. For accurate neonatal administration it is best to draw the content of the ampoule into a large syringe immediately before use, and then dilute this to 40 ml with 0·9 sodium chloride (producing a solution that contains 100 micrograms/ml). For intranasal use, dilution to 8 ml is more appropriate (producing a 500 microgram/ml solution). Absorption after IM administration is not only slow but also rather unpredictable. A sugar-free oral suspension can be provided.

References
See also the relevant Cochrane reviews

Ahmad S, Ellis JC, Kamwendo H, *et al*. Efficacy and safety of intranasal lorazepam versus intramuscular paraldehyde for protracted convulsions in children: an open randomised trial. *Lancet* 2006;**367**:1591–7. [RCT]

Appleton R, Sweeney A, Choonara I, *et al*. Lorazepam *versus* diazepam in the acute treatment of epileptic seizures and status epilepticus. *Dev Med Child Neurol* 1995;**37**:682–8.

Chess PR, D'Angio CT. Clonic movements following lorazepam administration in full-term infants. *Arch Pediatr Adolesc Med* 1998;**152**:98–9.

Chicella M, Jansen P, Parthiban A, *et al*. Propylene glycol accumulation associated with continuous infusion of lorazepam in pediatric intensive care patients. *Crit Care Med* 2002;**30**:2752–6.

Dominquez KD, Crowley MR, Colemen DM, *et al*. Withdrawal from lorazepam in critically ill children. *Ann Pharmacother* 2006;**40**:1035–9.

Maytal J, Novak GP, King KC. Lorazepam in the treatment of refractory neonatal seizures. *J Child Neurol* 1991;**6**:319–23.

McDermott CA, Kowalczyk AL, Schritzler ET, *et al*. Pharmacokinetics of lorazepam in critically ill neonates with seizures. *J Pediatr* 1992;**120**:479–83.

Muchohi SN, Obiero K, Newton CRJC, *et al*. Pharmacokinetics and clinical safety of lorazepam in children with severe malaria and convulsions. *Br J Clin Pharmacol* 2008;**65**:12–21.

Sexson WR, Thigpen J, Stajich GV. Stereotypic movements after lorazepam administration in premature neonates: a series and review of the literature. *J Perinatol* 1995;**15**:146–9.

MAGNESIUM SULPHATE

Use
Magnesium sulphate is used to prevent or control eclampsia, and to treat neonatal hypomagnesaemia and late neonatal hypocalcaemia. Use does *not* prevent preterm labour, but it can, when given to the mother before delivery, reduce the risk of cerebral palsy in babies of less than 30 weeks' gestation.

Pharmacology
Magnesium sulphate is the treatment of choice for the mother if she has eclampsia, and for *pre*-eclampsia that is severe enough for urgent delivery to be contemplated; follow-up studies show that there are no long-term disadvantages associated with the obvious short-term benefit. Use reduces the risk of maternal seizures and probably lowers maternal mortality, but it does nothing to lower blood pressure or reduce perinatal mortality. Treatment with magnesium sulphate is still widely used to inhibit preterm labour in North America, although there is no controlled trial evidence of benefit, and increasing evidence that high-dose treatment may have adverse consequences for the baby. Even short-term use increases the fetal as well as the maternal plasma magnesium level, causing hypotonia, reduced gastrointestinal motility and mild respiratory depression, and treatment with gentamicin after birth could exacerbate this hypotonia. Five trials have, however, now found that brief use reduces the risk of severe cerebral palsy when given for just 12–24 hours to mothers in strong, well-established preterm labour (see web commentary). Two small trials also suggest that use may lessen the early symptoms of perinatal asphyxia in the term baby. Breastfeeding does not need to be discouraged because of maternal treatment.

Magnesium is a smooth muscle relaxant, causing significant pulmonary and systemic vasodilatation and, following a number of encouraging observational studies, continuous infusions are now sometimes used in ventilated babies with persistent pulmonary hypertension unresponsive to tolazoline (q.v.). No controlled trial of this strategy has yet been mounted, and babies showing no sustained response should be transferred to a unit able to offer treatment with nitric oxide (q.v.). A similar strategy seems to reduce the need for other medication in adults with severe tetanus. High serum levels (>4 mmol/l) cause generalised hypotonia.

Symptomatic neonatal hypocalcaemia (a serum calcium less than 1·7 mmol/l) is now rare, and usually associated with hypomagnesaemia. Empirical data suggest that children treated with IM magnesium sulphate improve more quickly than children given calcium gluconate (q.v.).

Maternal use
Preventing or treating eclampsia: Give 4 grams IV over 15 minutes followed by 1 gram/hour IV for up to 24 hours. In countries where sustained IV treatment could be problematic give 5 grams IM once every 4 hours.
Reducing the risk of cerebral palsy: Giving mothers facing imminent delivery before 30 weeks' gestation a 4 gram IV loading dose and then a 1 gram/hour infusion until delivery (but for no more than to 24 hours) has no impact on perinatal mortality, but does significantly reduce the risk of the baby developing serious cerebral palsy.

Neonatal use
Hypocalcaemia: Giving 100 mg/kg of magnesium sulphate (0·2 ml/kg of a 50% solution) deep IM on two occasions 12 hours apart will control most cases of symptomatic late neonatal hypocalcaemia.
Hypomagnesaemia: The same dose every 6–12 hours can also be used to treat primary neonatal hypomagnesaemia irrespective of the cause (normal plasma level: 0·75–1·0 mmol/l). This is usually given IV or IM because it is a purgative (like Epsom salts) when given by mouth.
Persistent pulmonary hypertension: Give a loading dose of 250 mg/kg of magnesium sulphate IV over 10–15 minutes. If a clinical response is obtained once the serum magnesium level exceeds 3·5 mmol/l, give between 20 and 75 mg/kg an hour for 2–5 days, while maintaining a blood level of between 3·5 and 5·5 mmol/l. This strategy has not yet been subjected to controlled trial evaluation.
Intrapartum asphyxia: Try a 250 mg/kg dose IV once a day for 3 days. Watch for respiratory depression.

Supply and administration
Magnesium sulphate is conventionally prescribed as the heptahydrate; 2 ml ampoules of 50% magnesium sulphate contain 1 gram (4·1 mmol) of magnesium, and cost £2·90. To give a baby a 250 mg/kg IV 'stat' dose, draw 1 gram of magnesium sulphate (2 ml of the 50% solution) for each kg the baby weighs into a syringe, dilute to 20 ml with 10% glucose saline to obtain a solution containing 50 mg/kg per ml, and give 5 ml of this solution slowly over 10–15 minutes. To then continue delivering 20 mg/kg per hour, give 0·4 ml/hour of the same solution. 20 ml (4 gram) ampoules of a 20% solution costing £2·80 are available for use in adults.

References
See also relevant Cochrane reviews and UK guideline on pre-eclampsia

Bhat MA, Charoo BA, Bhat JI, *et al*. Magnesium sulfate in severe perinatal asphyxia: a randomized, placebo-controlled trial. *Pediatrics* 2009;**123**:e764–9. [RCT]

Duley L. Pre-eclampsia and hypertension. *BMJ Clinical evidence handbook*. London: BMJ Books, 2009: pp. 481–3 (and updates). [SR]

Grimes DA, Nanda KK. Magnesium sulfate tocolysis. Time to quit. *Obstet Gynecol* 2006;**108**:986–9.

Gurner TL, Cockburn F, Forfar JO. Magnesium therapy in neonatal tetany. *Lancet* 1977;**i**:283–4. [RCT]

Magpie Trial Follow-up Study Collaborative Group. The Magpie trial: a randomised trial comparing magnesium sulphate with placebo for pre-eclampsia. Outcome for children at 18 months. *Br J Obstet Gynaecol* 2007;**114**:300–9. [RCT] (See also pp. 289–9.)

Rouse DJ, Hirtz DG, Thom E, *et al*. A randomized controlled trial of magnesium sulfate for the prevention of cerebral palsy. *N Engl J Med* 2008;**359**:895–905. [RCT] (See also pp. 962–4.)

Tolsa J-F, Cotting J, Sekarski N, *et al*. Magnesium sulphate as an alternative and safe treatment for severe persistent pulmonary hypertension of the newborn. *Arch Dis Child* 1995;**72**:F184–7.

Use

Spaced doses of sulfadoxine and pyrimethamine (q.v.) have been shown to reduce the risk of an overt attack of malaria in countries where young children are at high risk, but mefloquine, given the same way, is probably more effective in areas where resistance to this drug combination is now high. Visitors to areas of high resistance to chloroquine (q.v.) are also now, similarly, advised to take a weekly dose of mefloquine.

Pharmacology

Mefloquine hydrochloride is an amino alcohol with a half life of 2–3 weeks that is concentrated in the red cells. It was developed by the US military as an antimalarial in the 1960s, and became generally available in 1986. High-dose treatment can provoke nausea, vomiting, loose stools, headache, abdominal pain and somnolence – symptoms that can be hard to distinguish from malaria itself. It is also teratogenic in animals and high-dose use should probably be avoided during pregnancy. There have been few published studies of the regular use of mefloquine in pregnancy, but a review of the available unpublished evidence in 1993 found nothing to suggest that prophylactic use was hazardous and all visitors to an area where malaria is prevalent should certainly adopt one of the available prophylactic strategies. Little of the drug seems to appear in breast milk, and the baby is not likely to be exposed to more than 10% of the weight-adjusted maternal dose during lactation, even after allowance is made for the drug's long half life. However, the amount ingested from breast milk is certainly not enough to reduce the risk of the child becoming infected and does not make it necessary to modify any dose given to the child by way of prophylaxis. It should be noted, however, that the manufacturer has not yet recommended use during pregnancy, or in children less than 3 months old.

Drug resistance

WHO advice on how drug resistance to malaria varies in different parts of the world can be found on http://www.who.int/ith/ITH2009Chapter7.pdf, and very similar advice from the CDC in America is available on http://www.cdc.gov/malaria/. Similar advice can also be found in the *British National Formulary* and the related children's formulary *BNF-C*. Multiple drug resistance is sufficiently common in Southeast Asia to require specialist advice.

Prophylactic strategies

See the monograph on proguanil with atovaquone.

Treatment options in infancy

Intermittent prevention: A single dose every 2–4 months in the first year of life (as for example when seen for vaccination) can substantially reduce the risk of overt infection. A 125 mg dose at 2 months, or 250 mg at 9 months, seems safe.

Sustained prevention: Visitors to any area where malaria is endemic should take 5 mg/kg of mefloquine by mouth once a week. Start treatment ideally 3 weeks before entering any endemic area (since most adverse effects will manifest themselves within 3 weeks of starting treatment), and continue treatment for 4 weeks after leaving. There is little experience with sustained use for more than a year, and use is not advised in children with a history of seizures.

Cure: Give 15 mg/kg of mefloquine by mouth followed, after 12 hours, by one further 10 mg/kg dose.

Supply

Scored 250 mg tablets of mefloquine cost £1·80 each. They have a bitter taste, making administration difficult in small children (although the crushed tablet can be mixed with honey, jam or other food). In addition, no low-dose tablet or liquid formulation exists, making accurate administration to a small baby extremely problematic. Protect from sunlight and humidity once removed from the foil wrapping.

References

Croft AM. Malaria: prevention in travellers. *BMJ Clinical evidence handbook*. London: BMJ Books, 2009: pp. 269–73 (and updates). [SR] (See also pp. 276–7.)

Edstein MD, Veenendaal JR, Hyslop R. Excretion of mefloquine in human breast milk. *Chemotherapy* 1988;**34**:165–9.

Gosling PD, Gesase S, Mosha JF, *et al*. Protective efficacy and safety of three antimalarial regimens for intermittent preventive treatment for malaria in infants: a randomised, double blind, placebo controlled trial. *Lancet* 2009;**374**:1521–32. [RCT] (See also pp. 1480–2.)

Nosten F, ter Kuile F, Maelankiri L, *et al*. Mefloquine prophylaxis prevents malaria during pregnancy: a double-blind placebo-controlled study. *J Infect Dis* 1994;**169**:595–603. [RCT]

Palmer KJ, Holliday SM, Brogden RN. Mefloquine. A review of its antimalarial activity, pharmacokinetic properties and therapeutic efficacy. *Drugs* 1993;**45**:430–75.

Radloff PD, Phillips J, Nkeyi M, *et al*. Atovaquone and proguanil for Plasmodium falciparum malaria. *Lancet* 1996;**347**:1511–14. [RCT]

Smoak BL, Writer JV, Keep LW, *et al*. The effects of inadvertent exposure of mefloquine chemoprophylaxis on pregnancy outcomes and infants of US army servicewomen. *J Infect Dis* 1997;**176**:831–3.

Vamhauwere B, Maradit H, Kerr L. Post-marketing surveillance of prophylactic mefloquine (Lariam®) use in pregnancy. *Am J Trop Med Hyg* 1999;**58**:17–21.

Use
Vaccines offer protection from some, but not all, forms of meningococcal meningitis and septicaemia.

Meningococcal disease
Meningococcal infection is a notifiable illness caused by the Gram-negative diplococcus *Neisseria meningitides*. Group A strains are common in sub-Saharan Africa and the Indian subcontinent. Group B strains have a low case fatality rate. Before the introduction of the conjugate vaccine, the group C strain accounted for 40% of all meningococcal infection in the UK, but a much higher proportion of all meningococcal deaths. Travel to the Hajj is causing the group W_{135} strain to be seen more widely. Half the population carry meningococci in the nose. Infection is spread by droplet and direct contact, the incubation period being 2–7 days. Babies usually present with pyrexia, irritability, vomiting, limpness, palor and cold extremities; older children with headache, drowsiness and limb pain. The petechial or purpuric rash, which fails to blanch on pressure (best tested using a glass slide or tumbler), is seldom an early feature. Infection is commonest in children less than 4 years old, with a second small peak at 15–20 years. Preventive measures are important, since one in ten will die despite prompt treatment with benzylpenicillin. Contacts are normally given rifampicin (q.v.), but ciprofloxacin (q.v.) is equally effective, and less likely to cause a resistant strain to emerge. Vaccines can, as yet, only provide protection from serogroup A, C, W_{135} and Y infection.

Indications
Group C conjugate vaccine (MenC): This vaccine, first introduced in 1999, using the same technology as was used to produce the very safe and effective *Haemophilus* (Hib) vaccine (q.v.), should be used to offer babies early and lasting protection from group C disease.
Group ACWY polysaccharide vaccine: This plain vaccine generates little response to the group C, W_{135} and Y polysaccharides in infants less than 18 months old, or to the group A polysaccharide in babies less than 3 months old. It provides 3–5 years of immunity in older children, but should only be offered to those planning to travel abroad or in contact with a case of W_{135}.

Contraindications
Immunisation should not be offered to any child who is acutely unwell, or has had a severe, proven, reaction to a previous injection. Minor infections unassociated with fever are not a reason to delay immunisation, however, and the contraindications associated with the use of a live vaccine (cf. polio vaccine) do not apply.

Administration
MenC for children under 1 year old: Three 0·5 ml doses are currently given in the UK at monthly intervals starting at 2 months. Give the IM injection deep into the anterolateral aspect of the thigh using a 25 mm, 23 gauge needle, using a different limb from that used for any simultaneous DTP, Hib and inactivated polio vaccines. This policy provides good short-term and herd immunity, but lasting immunity may turn out to require that at least one more dose is given when the child is rather older.
MenC for older children: Offer previously unimmunised children just one 0·5 ml intramuscular, or deep subcutaneous, injection when opportunity arises. There is no contraindication to simultaneous immunisation with other routine vaccines, but it is best to use a different injection site.
ACWY vaccine: Give a single 0·5 ml deep subcutaneous injection.

Anaphylaxis
The management of anaphylaxis (which is very rare) is outlined in the monograph on immunisation.

Documentation
Tell the family doctor every time a child is immunised in hospital, and record what was done in the child's own personal health booklet. Community-based registers of vaccine uptake also need to be informed.

Supply
Free supplies of the conjugate group C (MenC) vaccine in 0·5 ml vials are available in the UK from three firms through Farrillon. The products are interchangeable. They must be stored at 2–8°C, but stability is probably unaffected if they are allowed to reach a temperature not exceeding 25°C on the day of use. Do not freeze. Vaccine remaining unused should only be re-refrigerated once. Single-dose 0·5 ml vials of the lyophilised ACWY vaccine, with diluent for reconstitution, cost approximately £7 each. Do not let the diluent become frozen. Use within an hour of reconstitution.

References
See also the relevant Cochrane reviews and UK guidelines

American Academy of Pediatrics. Committee on Infectious Diseases. Prevention and control of meningococcal disease: recommendations for use of meningococcal vaccines in pediatric patients. *Pediatrics* 2005;**116**:496–50.
Hart CA, Thomson APJ. Meningococcal disease and its management in children. *BMJ* 2006;**333**:685–90. [SR]
Purcell B, Samuelsson, Hahné SJM, *et al*. Effectiveness of antibiotics in preventing meningococcal disease after a case: systematic review. *BMJ* 2004;**328**:1339–42. [SR]
Stephens DS, Greenwood B, Brandtzaeg P. Epidemic meningitis, meningococcaemia, and *Neissria meningitidis*. *Lancet* 2007;**369**:2196–210. [SR]
Thompson MJ, Ninis N, Perera R, *et al*. Clinical recognition of meningococcal disease in children and adolescents. *Lancet* 2006;**367**:397–403. (See also pp. 371–2.)

Use

Meropenem is a very valuable, recently introduced, broad-spectrum antibiotic. There remains an agreement in many units that it should be held in reserve at present, and only used in consultation with a microbiologist or in a research context, when no other satisfactory alternative exists.

Pharmacology

Meropenem is a carbapenem β-lactam antibiotic active against a very wide range of Gram-positive and Gram-negative aerobic and anaerobic bacteria that first came into general clinical use in 1985. Meticillin-resistant staphylococci and *Enterococcus faecium* are resistant to meropenem, as are some strains of *Pseudomonas aeruginosa*. Meropenem is excreted in the urine, mostly unchanged, but partly as an inert metabolite. The elimination half life in adults is only 1 hour, but a little longer in children 2–6 months old. The initial half life in the term baby is 2 hours, and in the preterm baby 3 hours, but the half life falls significantly, irrespective of gestation, within 10–14 days of birth.

Meropenem has many of the same properties, and most of the same adverse effects, as imipenem (q.v.), but it seems to cause less nausea. It is also stable to the renal enzyme that inactivates imipenem and does not need, therefore, to be given with cilastatin. It has not been in use as long as imipenem, and has not been as extensively studied, but the evidence to date suggests that meropenem is less likely to induce seizures than imipenem/cilastatin (which is not licensed for the treatment of CNS infection). Meropenem can also, unlike imipenem/cilastatin, be given as a standard slow IV bolus injection. It penetrates the CSF of patients with bacterial meningitis, and most other body fluids, well. It crosses the placenta, but there is (as yet) no evidence of teratogenicity. Only a small amount of meropenem appears in animal milk, and its use during lactation is unlikely to be hazardous. There is too little published experience for the manufacturers to have yet recommended the use of meropenem in children less than 3 months old.

Treatment   12 hrs in the 1st week

Give 20 mg/kg slowly IV once every ~~8 hours in the first 10 days~~ of life, and once every 8 hours for babies older than that. Give double this dose where meningitis or *Pseudomonas aeruginosa* infection is suspected. Intramuscular use is not recommended. Dosage frequency should be halved if there is evidence of renal failure, and treatment stopped altogether if there is anuria unless dialysis is instituted.

Supply

Vials suitable for IV use containing 500 mg of meropenem as a powder cost £14·30 each. Vials should be reconstituted with 9·6 ml of water for injection to give a solution containing 50 mg/ml. The manufacturers recommend prompt use after reconstitution, and say that vials are for 'single use only', but they also say that the preparation can be kept for up to 24 hours after reconstitution if kept at 4°C. A 20 mg/kg dose contains 0·08 mmol/kg of sodium.

References

Baldwin CM, Lyseng-Williamson KA, Keam SJ. Meropenem. A review of its use in the treatment of serious bacterial infections. *Drugs* 2008;**68**:803–38. [SR]
Blumer JL. Pharmacokinetic determinants of carbapenem therapy in neonates and children. *Pediatr Infect Dis J* 1996;**15**:733–7.
Bradley JS. Meropenem: a new, extremely broad spectrum beta-lactam antibiotic for serious infections in pediatrics. *Pediatr Infect Dis J* 1997;**16**:263–8.
Bradley JS, Sauberan JB, Ambrose PG, *et al*. Meropenem pharmacokinetics, pharmacodynamics, and Monte Carlo simulation in the neonate. *Pediatr Infect Dis J* 2008;**27**:784–9.
Klugman KP, Dagan R and the Meropenem Meningitis Study Group. Randomised comparison of meropenem with cefotaxime for treatment of bacterial meningitis. *Antimicrob Agents Chemother* 1995;**39**:1140–6. [RCT]
Mouton JW, Touzw DJ, Horrevorts AM, *et al*. Comparative pharmacokinetics of the carbopenems: clinical implications. *Clin Pharmacokinet* 2000;**39**:185–201.
Odio CM, Puig JR, Ferris JM, *et al*. Prospective randomised investigator-blinded study of the efficacy and safety of meropenem vs. cefotaxime in bacterial meningitis in children. *Pediat Infect Dis J*. 1999;**18**:581–90. [RCT]
Schuler D and the Meropenem Paediatric Study Group. Safety and efficacy of meropenem in hospitalised children: randomised comparison with cefotaxime, alone and combined with metronidazole or amikacin. *J Antimicrob Chemother* 1995;**36**(suppl A):99–108. [RCT]
van Enk JG, Touw DJ, Lafeber HN. Pharmacokinetics of meropenem in preterm neonates. *Ther Drug Monit* 2001;**23**:198–201.

Use

Methadone is used in the management of opioid addiction, and to control the more severe withdrawal ('abstinence') symptoms seen in some babies born to mothers with such an addiction.

Pharmacology

Methadone hydrochloride is a useful synthetic opioid analgesic, developed in Germany during the 1939–45 war, that is capable of providing sustained pain relief. It is usually taken by mouth, and is less sedating than morphine. Opiate addiction may be associated with reduced fetal growth (as outlined in the monograph on diamorphine (heroin)), but there is no evidence of teratogenicity. Methadone is well absorbed when taken by mouth (90% bioavailability) and largely metabolised by the liver, the neonatal half life being about 20 hours. Tissue levels exceed plasma levels (V_D ~6 l/kg). Arrhythmia due to the long QT syndrome is a rare complication, and has been seen at birth in the baby of a mother stabilised on methadone. Excessive doses can cause ileus and respiratory depression. Use during lactation only results in the baby receiving about 3% of the weight-adjusted maternal dose, so breastfeeding does not need to be discouraged once HIV infection has been excluded. Indeed there is evidence that breastfed babies show fewer symptoms of withdrawal, and seem less likely to require medication irrespective of the nature of the mother's addiction.

Opiate addiction

Mothers with an opiate addiction are often placed on methadone before delivery in an attempt to reduce illicit opioid usage. Methadone is useful because it can be taken orally, only needs to be taken once or twice a day and has a long-lasting effect. Maternal blood levels are therefore more stable, reducing some of the intoxicating (and potentially damaging) 'swings' to which the fetus of an addicted mother is otherwise exposed. Weaning should not be attempted during pregnancy and, because of increased clearance, the dose may need to be increased in the last 3 months of pregnancy. Because of this, babies often start to show some signs of an abstinence syndrome 1–3 days after birth, with restlessness, irritability, rapid breathing, vomiting and intestinal hurry, especially where the mother was on a dose of more than 20 mg per day. Feeding problems may exacerbate weight loss. Swaddling and the use of a dummy or pacifier should be enough to control the symptoms in up to half the babies of drug-dependent mothers, but a rapidly reducing dose of methadone can be given to babies with severe symptoms. Fits are uncommon, seldom seen in the first few days, and more suggestive of a non-opiate drug dependency. Symptoms coming on after 2·5 days are usually mild and more typically seen where the mother is dependent on a hypnotic or sedative (barbiturates, diazepam, etc.). A mixed picture due to the abuse of several drugs is not uncommon, and may justify giving phenobarbital (q.v.) as well as methadone (or morphine). Chlorpromazine (q.v.) is an understudied alternative. The web commentary reviews the care of the drug-dependent mother and her baby.

Managing neonatal opiate withdrawal

Achieving control: Give one dose every 6 hours by mouth. Start with 100 micrograms/kg, and increase this by 50 micrograms/kg each time a further dose is due until symptoms are controlled.
Maintaining control: Calculate the total dose given in the 24 hours before control was achieved, and give half this amount by mouth once every 12 hours.
Weaning: Once control has been sustained for 48 hours, try and reduce the dose given by 10–20% once each day. Treatment can usually be stopped after 7–10 days although mild symptoms may persist for several weeks. Scoring systems are interpreted too inconsistently by different members of staff to be of much use.
Seizures: Give 250 micrograms/kg IM, and monitor for possible apnoea.

Antidote

Naloxone (q.v.) is effective, but may unmask withdrawal symptoms in an opiate-dependent patient.

Supply and administration

A clear yellow-green non-proprietary oral mixture of this controlled drug, containing 1 mg/ml of methadone hydrochloride, can be provided on request (100 ml costs £1·50). A more dilute solution (100 micrograms/ml) with a month shelf life could be provided by the pharmacy for neonatal use on request. An IM preparation containing 10 mg/ml is also available; to obtain a 1 mg/ml solution for accurate neonatal administration, take 1 ml of this and dilute to 10 ml with sterile water for injection. Storage and administration of methadone is controlled under Schedule 2 of the UK Misuse of Drugs Regulations 1985 (Misuse of Drugs Act 1971).

References

See also the Cochrane reviews of opiate withdrawal

Abdel-Latif ME, Pinner J, Clews S, *et al*. Effects of breast milk on the severity and outcome of neonatal abstinence syndrome among infants of drug-dependent mothers. *Pediatrics* 2006;**117**:e1163–9.
Bell J, Harvey-Dodds L. Pregnancy and injecting drug use. [Review] *BMJ* 2008;**336**:1303–5.
Dryden C, Young D, Hepburn M, *et al*. Maternal methadone use in pregnancy: factors associated with the development of neonatal abstinence syndrome and implications for healthcare resources. *Br J Obstet Gynaecol* 2009;**116**:665–71.
Hussain T, Ewer AK. Maternal methadone may cause arrhythmias in neonates. *Acta Paediatr* 2007;**96**:768–9.
Jansson LM, Choo R, Valez ML, *et al*. Methadone maintenance and breastfeeding in the neonatal period. *Pediatrics* 2008;**121**:106–14.
Jarvis M, Schnoll S. Methadone treatment in pregnancy. *J Psychoactive Drugs* 1994;**26**:155–61.
Johnson K, Gerada C, Greenough A. Treatment of neonatal abstinence syndrome. *Arch Dis Child* 2003;**88**:F2–5. [SR]
Kandall SR, Doberczak TM, Jantunen M, *et al*. The methadone-maintained pregnancy. *Clin Perinatol* 1999;**26**:173–83.

Use

Methyldopa is the best studied of all the antihypertensive drugs used in pregnancy. It was also used for some years, often with hydralazine (q.v.), in cases of resistant neonatal hypertension. It is now only rarely used to treat hypertension children.

Pharmacology

Methyldopa interferes with the normal production of the neurotransmitter noradrenaline (norepinephrine), but also seems to have direct effects on arterioles and on the central vasomotor centre. Methyldopa was first shown to be of use in the management of hypertension in 1960. It causes a fall in blood pressure and a reduction in total peripheral vascular resistance without any change in cardiac output or renal blood flow. It has been widely used in the management of maternal hypertension and in patients with pre-eclamptic toxaemia. It readily crosses the placenta, but fetal side effects have not been identified, and the only neonatal effects ever noted have been occasional transient tremor and an equally transient lowering of blood pressure. Neither is there any known contraindication to use during lactation because the baby receives less than 5% of the maternal dose when this comparison is made on a weight-for-weight basis.

Oral absorption is variable and incomplete, much of the drug is eliminated by the kidney, and there is some evidence that treatment should be modified in the presence of serious renal failure. The way drug elimination varies with age has not been well studied, but is known to have a biphasic profile: the initial half life is only about 2 hours, but there is a second much more prolonged second phase. The drug's therapeutic action is not, however, related to this half life: even with IV use the full effect only becomes apparent after 4 hours and some effect can still be detected for 10–15 hours, while with oral administration twice a day the drug's ability to lower blood pressure may not become fully apparent for 2–3 days. Long-term medication induces salt and water retention unless a diuretic is prescribed. Side effects include haemolytic anaemia, thrombocytopenia and gastrointestinal disturbances. Large doses have a sedative effect. If treatment is stopped suddenly there may be a hypertensive rebound crisis.

Hypertension in pregnancy

The management of a woman already on treatment for hypertension prior to conception does not usually need to be changed because none of the commonly used drugs are teratogenic. Diuretic treatment can also be continued if considered appropriate, although continued use does carry disadvantages should pre-eclampsia supervene. If serious hypertension (a blood pressure of 170/110 mmHg or more) is found at booking it merits immediate treatment, but there is no evidence that early pre-emptive intervention in women with hypertension less serious than this does anything to reduce the eventual incidence of superimposed pre-eclampsia. Hydralazine and, more recently, nifedipine (q.v.) have been the drugs most often used when other symptoms of proteinuric pre-eclampsia become apparent. Short-term atenolol (see Part 3) use does not inhibit fetal growth. Labetalol (q.v.), given IV, is probably the drug of choice when it becomes necessary to lower blood pressure in a rapid but controlled way, while magnesium sulphate (q.v.) can be given to minimise the risk of an eclamptic seizure. The only *definitive* treatment for severe pre-eclampsia is delivery, and even after delivery blood pressure often continues to rise for another 3–5 days before finally returning to normal 2–3 weeks later.

Treatment

Use in pregnancy: Start by giving 250 mg two or three times a day and increase the dose incrementally as necessary not more frequently than once every 3 days. A first 1 gram oral loading dose can be given when hypertension needs to be controlled quickly. Doses as high as 1 gram four times a day have been used on occasion. Nifedipine is sometimes used as well in patients with pre-eclamptic hypertension.

Use in infancy: Start with 2·5 mg/kg of methyldopa by mouth once every 8 hours, together with a diuretic, and increase the dose as required once every 3–5 days to a maximum of no more than 15 mg/kg once every 8 hours. The same dose of methyldopate can be given as a slow infusion over 30–60 minutes where oral treatment is not possible.

Supply and administration

5 ml (250 mg) ampoules of methyldopate for IV use are still available in North America and in some other countries but are no longer immediately available from any UK pharmaceutical company (although the product could be imported on request). When last available in the UK they cost £2·30 each. In order to ensure accuracy, dilute 1 ml (50 mg) from the ampoule with 9 ml of 5% glucose to provide a solution containing 5 mg/ml prior to oral or IV administration. 125 and 250 mg tablets (costing 2–3p each) remain widely available, and a low-dose oral suspension could be prepared, on request, with a 7-day shelf life.

References

See also the relevant Cochrane reviews

Anon. Managing high blood pressure in pregnancy. *Drug Ther Bull* 1993;**31**:53–6.
Cockburn J, Moar VA, Ounsted M, *et al.* Final report of study of hypertension during pregnancy: the effects of specific treatment on the growth and development of the children. *Lancet* 1982;**i**:647–9. (See also p. 1237.)
Jones HMR, Cummings AJ, Setchell KDR. Pharmacokinetics of methyldopa in neonates. *Br J Clin Pharmacol* 1979;**8**:433–40.
White WB, Andreoli JW, Cohn RD. Alpha-methyldopa disposition in mothers with hypertension and their breast-fed infants. *Br J Pharmacol* 1985;**37**:387–90.

METHYLENE BLUE = Methylthioninium chloride (rINN)

Use

Methylene blue is used to treat methaemoglobinaemia. It has also been used experimentally to treat the refractory hypotension sometimes associated with septic shock.

Methaemoglobinaemia

Methaemoglobin is the oxidised (ferric) form of the haemoglobin molecule, lacking the normal molecule's ability to carry oxygen to the tissues. The condition can be inherited (as a recessive reductase enzyme deficiency, or as a dominantly inherited haemoglobinopathy) or occur briefly as a result of drug exposure. Babies are at particular risk because reductase enzyme levels are initially low. Nitric oxide is rapidly inactivated by the haemoglobin molecule forming nitrosyl-haemoglobin, which is then converted to methaemoglobin. It is for this reason that excess inhaled nitric oxide (q.v.) can cause methaemoglobinaemia. Aniline dyes (even when absorbed through the skin) can have the same effect, as can the local anaesthetic prilocaine (see the monograph on lidocaine). Excess nitrates in drinking water were once a common cause. If a drop of suspect blood turns chocolate brown rather than red over 30 seconds, when compared to a control sample, as it dries on a filter paper, the suspect specimen almost certainly contains more than 10% of methaemoglobin.

Pharmacology

Methylene blue is a basic dye first synthesised in 1876. Histologists have used it for more than a century to dye living nerve tissue. It is reduced in the red cell to leucomethylene blue where it then acts to convert methaemoglobin back to haemoglobin. It is therefore used in the treatment of both congenital and acquired methaemoglobinaemia. It has also been used as a dye to monitor reflux, trace fistulas, position tubes, identify premature rupture of membranes, and to 'mark' the different amniotic sacs in multiple pregnancy, although this last use can cause serious haemolytic anaemia and neonatal jaundice and is claimed to be associated with a high risk of jejunal atresia. Recently there has been experimental interest in the use of the same drug to control the severe hypotension seen in septic shock when this fails to respond to inotropes and hydrocortisone (q.v.), because this condition seems to be mediated, at least in part, by excess tissue nitric oxide synthesis. Nitric oxide causes vasodilatation by activating soluble guanylate cyclase in smooth muscle cells to produce cyclic guanosine monophosphate, and methylene blue inhibits this activation.

Methylene blue is moderately well absorbed when given by mouth and slowly excreted in the urine, after partial conversion to leucomethylene blue. Repeated use may be hazardous if renal function is poor. Intravenous administration can cause a number of adverse reactions including pain, nausea, vomiting, confusion, dizziness, sweating and hypotension. Repeated treatment, or an overdose, can actually *cause* methaemoglobinaemia, haemolysis and hyperbilirubinaemia, and there is no effective treatment for this other than exchange transfusion. Infants with G6PD deficiency are at particular risk in this regard. Long-term treatment has been known to cause haemolytic anaemia. Heinz body formation has also been reported. Methylene blue turns the urine, stools and body secretions blue. The skin also becomes discoloured. Nothing is known about the safety of giving IV treatment to a mother during pregnancy or lactation.

Treatment

Give 1 mg/kg IV (1 ml of a solution made up as described below) over 1 hour. A repeat dose can be given if necessary after a few hours. Oral treatment has occasionally been used to manage serious congenital methaemoglobinaemia, even though this tends to make the cyanosed patient blue for a different reason! Doses of up to 2 mg/kg once a day by mouth have been used. Oral ascorbic acid (500 mg once a day) may also be effective.

Supply and administration

Methylene blue trihydrate USP is available as a 1% solution in 5 ml ampoules costing £5·60 each; to give 1 mg/kg IV take 1 ml from the 1% ampoule for each kg the baby weighs, dilute to 10 ml with 5% glucose immediately before use and infuse 1 ml of the resultant solution over 1 hour. More rapid infusions have been given with apparent safety on occasion. Take care to avoid tissue extravasation as this can cause necrotic ulceration.

References

Allergaert K, Miserez M, Naulaers G, *et al*. Enteral administration of methylene blue in a preterm infant. [Abstract] *Pediatr Perinat Drug Ther* 2004;**6**:70.
Driscoll W, Thurin S, Carrion V, *et al*. Effect of methylene blue on refractory neonatal hypotension. *J Pediatr* 1996;**129**:904–8. (See also pp. 790–3.)
Ofoegbu BN, Agrawal RP, Lewis MA. Methylene blue irrigation-treatment of renal fungal balls causing acute renal failure in a preterm infant. *Acta Paediatr* 2005;**96**:939–40.

Use

Metoclopramide is a safe and effective drug to use to when gastro-oesophageal reflux (GOR) complicates nausea and vomiting in pregnancy. Meclozine (see Part 3) is a better studied alternative where there is no reflux. There are conflicting reports as to its ability to enhance breast milk production. There is some evidence that use reduces symptomatic reflux in children a few months old, but no neonatal studies have been published.

Pharmacology

Metoclopramide hydrochloride is a substituted benzamide related to procainamide which stimulates motility in the upper gastrointestinal tract without affecting gastric, biliary or pancreatic secretion. It was being evaluated as a possible antiarrhythmic agent when its antiemetic properties came to light in 1964. It is rapidly absorbed from the intestinal tract, but plasma levels are rendered unpredictable by variable first pass hepatic metabolism. Metoclopramide possesses parasympathomimetic activity. It has been used to control some forms of nausea and vomiting (particularly in cancer patients undergoing cytotoxic treatment or radiotherapy), and in the management of gastric stasis and GOR, but there is good evidence that ondansetron (q.v.) is a better drug to use to control nausea and vomiting in young children. Metoclopramide is a dopamine-receptor antagonist, and idiosyncratic dystonic and dyskinetic extrapyramidal signs are not infrequently seen in children, even at the normally recommended dose. For these reasons the manufacturers only recommend use in patients under 20 years old to prevent postoperative vomiting, to control the nausea caused by chemotherapy and as an aid to gastrointestinal intubation. Domperidone (q.v.) is a related drug that causes fewer dystonic problems. Erythromycin (q.v.) is sometimes used in the neonatal period to stimulate gastrointestinal motility. In America, however, metoclopramide is now being used to manage minor reflux in preterm babies even more frequently than cisapride was before it was abruptly removed from the market on safety grounds in 1999.

Metoclopramide has also been used to treat the severe nausea and vomiting that occasionally occurs during pregnancy (hyperemesis gravidarum) and a study of the outcomes of these pregnancies found no evidence of teratogenicity. It has also been given to speed gastric emptying during labour, or as a pre-anaesthetic medication to reduce the risk of vomiting. Metoclopramide, like domperidone, stimulates prolactin secretion from the anterior pituitary but there are conflicting reports as to its ability to enhance lactation (see website commentary). It does not work in all women (possibly because they already have raised prolactin levels) and side effects, such as cramp and diarrhoea, sometimes limit compliance. The drug accumulates in breast milk, but ingestion by the baby would be unlikely to exceed 50 micrograms/kg per day – one-tenth the maximum dose used for medicinal purposes.

Treatment

Mother: Giving 10 mg (or even 15 mg) to the mother by mouth three times a day stimulated milk production in some studies. Taper treatment off over 5–10 days to limit the risk of milk production declining again later.
Baby: 100 micrograms/kg every 8 hours by mouth (or IV) speeds gastric emptying, and has some effect on reflux, but higher doses can cause increased general irritability and may even make reflux worse. Thickening the milk with carob seed flour (q.v.) is probably a better first strategy in the term baby.

Toxicity

The therapeutic dose is only slightly less than the toxic dose in children. Tachycardia, agitation, hypertonia, feeding problems and diarrhoea have all been reported following a neonatal overdose, together with methaemoglobinaemia that responded to treatment with methylene blue (q.v.).

Supply and administration

2 ml ampoules containing 10 mg of metoclopramide (costing 26p) are also available for IV or IM use. For IV use take 1 ml of the liquid formulation in the ampoule, dilute to 50 ml with 0·9% sodium chloride to provide a solution containing 100 micrograms/ml, and give as a slow bolus infusion. Discard discoloured ampoules.

10 mg tablets cost 3p. Metoclopramide is also available as a liquid containing 1 mg/ml (100 ml costs £2·50) which *must* be protected from light. This can be further diluted with an equal quantity of pure water, but should be used within 2 weeks of being dispensed. A sugar-free formulation can be provided on request.

References

See also the Cochrane review of GOR in infancy

Bellisant E, Duhamel JF, Guilot M, *et al*. The triangular test to assess the efficacy of metoclopramide in gastroesophageal reflux. *Clin Pharmacol Ther*, 1997;**61**:377–84. [RCT]

Berkovitch M, Elbirt D, Addis A, *et al*. Fetal effects of metoclopramide therapy for nausea and vomiting in pregnancy. *N Engl J Med* 2000;**343**:445–6.

Hibbs M, Lorch SA. Metoclopramide for the treatment of gastroesophageal reflux disease in infants: systematic review. *Pediatrics* 2006;**118**:746–52. [SR] (See also pp. 793–4.)

Machida HM, Forbes DA, Gall DG, *et al*. Metoclopramide in gastroesophageal reflux in infancy. *J Pediatr* 1988;**112**:483–7.

Sørensen HT, Nielsen GL, Christensen K, *et al*. Birth outcome following maternal use of metoclopramide. *Br J Clin Pharmacol* 2000;**49**:264–8.

Tolia V, Calhoun J, Kuhns L, *et al*. Randomised, prospective double blind trial of metoclopramide and placebo for gastroesophageal reflux in infants. *J Pediatr* 1989;**115**:141–5. [RCT]

Toppare MF, Laleli Y, Senses DA, *et al*. Metoclopramide for breast milk production. *Nutr Res* 1994;**14**:1019–23.

Use

Metronidazole is used in the management of anaerobic bacterial infection (including meningitis), and in the treatment of a range of protozoal infections such as amoebiasis, giardiasis and trichomoniasis. It is also widely used in the UK after intestinal surgery and in the management of necrotising enterocolitis.

Pharmacology

Metronidazole is a unique bactericidal antibiotic that first came into clinical use in 1960 and is a 5-nitroimidazole derivative. It is particularly useful in the treatment of dental, surgical and gynaecological sepsis because of its activity against obligate anaerobes such as *Bacteroides* and *Clostridium* species, and facultative anaerobes such as *Gardnerella* and *Helicobacter*. It seems rare for bacterial resistance to develop. Both partners should be treated when trichomonal infection is suspected. Short prophylactic courses, with or without ampicillin, are frequently given during abdominal and pelvic surgery in Europe, but cefoxitin (q.v.) is more often used for this purpose in North America (where metronidazole is still seldom used in children). A reversible sensory neuropathy has been seen in adults after prolonged treatment. Mild gastrointestinal symptoms can occur.

Metronidazole can be given IV, but is very well absorbed by mouth. Rectal bioavailability is about 60%. The drug has a large volume of distribution (V_D ~0·8 l/kg), penetrates most body fluids (including CSF and ascitic fluid) well, and is excreted in the urine after partial breakdown to a product that also has some antimicrobial activity. The plasma half life is long, and inversely related to gestational age at birth, but soon approaches that seen in adults (7–10 hours). The dosage interval may need to be increased where there is hepatic failure, but does not usually require modification in renal failure although some metabolites may accumulate.

Use in pregnancy was long considered controversial because the drug crosses the placenta with ease, is mutagenic to bacteria and seems to produce tumours in rodents. However, there is no evidence that the drug is a carcinogen in man. Nor is there any evidence to suggest it is a teratogen, although it can increase the fetotoxic and teratogenic effect of alcohol in mice. More recently it has been widely used with apparent safety to treat trichomonal and bacterial vaginitis both during pregnancy and during lactation. However, while the increased vaginal discharge and the characteristic odour (vaginosis) caused when anaerobic bacteria replace lactobacilli can certainly merit treatment, the PREMET trial recently suggested that treatment with metronidazole might actually *increase* the risk of preterm birth. Oral or vaginal clindamycin (q.v.) seems to be a better alternative. Some other strategies are reviewed in the monograph on erythromycin.

The breastfed baby of any mother on the dose usually used to treat urogenital trichomoniasis (400 mg twice a day for 7 days) will end with a blood level about a quarter of that seen during treatment. While this is said to affect the milk's taste, it seems otherwise harmless. Women can, however, suspend lactation for 24 hours and request the well-recognised alternative treatment – a single high (2 gram) oral dose of metronidazole.

Amoebiasis

Asymptomatic infection is common, and it is difficult to distinguish *Entamoeba histolytica*, which is a worldwide tissue-invasive pathogen, from *E. dispar* – a mere commensal. Intestinal amoebiasis can cause abdominal pain and bloody diarrhoea, while invasive infection can invade the liver, chest or brain. Metronidazole for 5–10 days will deal with invasive infection, but diloxanide will be necessary to clear the bowel (6·6 mg/kg by mouth three times a day for 10 days) even though the manufacturer has not yet endorsed use in young children.

Drug interactions

Concurrent barbiturate use can decrease the half life in children, making a higher daily dose necessary. Steroids and rifampicin may have a similar but less marked effect.

Treatment

Give a 15 mg/kg IV loading dose. Then give 7·5 mg/kg, orally or IV, once every 12 hours in babies less than 4 weeks old, and every 8 hours in older babies. Higher doses have been used in meningitis. Slow IV administration is only necessary in older children and adults because of the volume of fluid involved.

Supply

A 20 ml (5 mg/ml) IV ampoule of metronidazole costs £1·50. A 7·5 mg/kg dose contains 0·2 mmol/kg of sodium. Limited solubility precludes IM use – the volume involved would be too large. A 40 mg/ml oral suspension in sucrose is available (100 ml costs £8·50) and a more dilute suspension can be prepared with a 2-week shelf life. 500 mg tablets of diloxanide cost £1·40, and an oral suspension can be prepared from these.

References

See also the relevant Cochrane reviews

Burtin P, Taddio A, Ariburna O, *et al*. Safety of metronidazole in pregnancy: a meta-analysis. *Am J Obstet Gynecol* 1995;**172**:525–9. [SR]
Escobedo AA, Almirall P, Alfonso M, *et al*. Treatment of intestinal protozoan infections in children. *Arch Dis Child* 2009;**94**:478–82.
Joesoef MR, Schmid G. Bacterial vaginosis. *BMJ Clinical evidence handbook*. London: BMJ Books, 2008: pp. 527–8 (and updates). [SR]
Morency A-M, Bujold E. The effect of second trimester antibiotic therapy on the rate of preterm birth. *J Obstet Gynaecol Can* 2007;**29**:35–44. [SR]
Shennan A, Crawshaw S, Briley A, *et al*. A randomised controlled trial of metronidazole for the prevention of preterm birth in women positive for cervicovaginal fibronectin: the PREMET study. *Br J Obstet Gynaecol* 2006;**113**:65–74. [RCT] (See also pp. 976–7.)
Simcox R, Sin WA, Seed PT, *et al*. Prophylactic antibiotics for the prevention of preterm birth in women at risk: a meta-analysis. *Aust NZ J Obstet Gynaecol* 2007;**47**:368–77. [SR]

Use

Miconazole and nystatin (q.v.) are both widely used in the treatment of topical *Candida* infection. There is good controlled trial evidence that miconazole is better than nystatin at eliminating oral thrush.

Pharmacology

Miconazole is an artificial imidazole agent first developed in 1969 that is active against a wide range of pathogenic yeasts and dermatophytes, as well as a range of Gram-positive bacteria (staphylococci and streptococci). These properties make it particularly useful in the treatment of oral and vaginal thrush, *Candida* nappy rash, intertrigo, paronychia, ringworm and athlete's foot. It seems to work by interfering with ergosterol synthesis, damaging fungal cell wall permeability. It is moderately well absorbed when given by mouth (unlike nystatin) and then inactivated by the liver before excretion in the urine, but much of any oral dose is excreted unchanged in the stool. It was, for some years, given IV or by mouth in the treatment of a range of systemic fungal infections, but is now only used topically to treat infection of the skin, gut or mucous membranes. Miconazole seems to eliminate vaginal candidiasis in pregnancy better then nystatin, and there is no evidence that topical use by the mother during pregnancy or lactation poses any hazard to the baby.

Candida dermatitis

Candida can be found in the vagina of 1 in 4 pregnant women – a fifth of these babies become colonised at birth, and more over the next month. *Candida* proliferates in moist skin, but overt infection is seldom seen except in babies with excessive intestinal colonisation. It is not surprising therefore, that overt skin damage (dermatitis) usually starts in the perianal region, especially if the skin is already damaged. Prior prolonged and broad-spectrum antibiotic use makes overt infection more likely.

Use of gentian violet

Gentian violet (otherwise known as crystal violet), a triphenylmethane antiseptic dye, is an old-fashioned treatment for *Candida* infection of the skin that is also active against a range of Gram-positive organisms including staphylococci. Although it is at least as effective as its colour is alarming, it is no longer used in the UK (especially on broken skin or mucous membranes) because of theoretical concern about carcinogenicity in mice. However a 0·5% aqueous solution is still sometimes used to treat *Candida* infection of the skin elsewhere in the world (including North America), and it is often thought to be the most effective topical product currently available because of its deep penetration. It is probably not wise to apply the solution to mucosal surfaces more than twice a day for 3–4 days. It stains everything it touches – including clothing and skin. It is worth treating the gut with miconazole or nystatin at the same time. Little is known about use during pregnancy or lactation.

Drug interactions

Never give *oral* miconazole to a patient taking cisapride (see archived monograph) because of the risk of arrhythmia.

Treatment

Oral thrush: Smear 1 ml of miconazole oral gel round the mouth and gums with a finger after feeds four times a day, and take steps to prevent reinfection as outlined in the monograph on nystatin. Continue treatment for at least 2 days after all the signs of infection have gone (usually 7–10 days in all).
Candida (Monilia) dermatitis: Use miconazole nitrate as a cream twice a day for at least 10 days, even if the rash improves quickly. There is a real risk of the problem recurring if treatment is stopped too soon. It may be advisable to treat the gastrointestinal tract as well as the skin if there is evidence of stubborn infection (and nystatin may be better at eradicating *Candida* from the lower bowel).

Supply

One 30 g tube of miconazole skin cream (2% w/w) costs £2. One 80 g tube of the sugar-free oral gel (24 mg/ml) costs £4·80. The gel has not been licensed for use in the USA, but small (15 g) quantities are available in the UK without prescription (although the manufacturer does not recommend use in babies less than 4 months old because excessive administration could cause the baby to choke). The cream, and a dusting powder, are also available 'over the counter' without prescription.

Inexpensive crystal violet paint (as a 0·5% aqueous preparation) is dispensable on request. Avoid the use of alcoholic solutions, and solutions that are more concentrated than this, especially when treating the mouth and tongue.

References

See also the relevant Cochrane reviews

Ainsworth SB, Jones W. It sticks in our throats too. *BMJ* 2009;**338**:a3178.
Drinkwater P. Gentian violet: is it safe? *Aust NZ J Obstet Gynaecol* 1990;**30**:65–6.
Hoppe JE. Treatment of oropharyngeal candidiasis and candidal diaper dermatitis in neonates and infants: review and reappraisal. *Pediatr Infect Dis J* 1997;**16**:885–94. [SR]
Piatt JP, Bergeson PS. Gentian violet toxicity. *Clin Pediatr* 1992;**31**:756–7.
Rosa FW, Baum C, Shaw M. Pregnancy outcomes after first-trimester vaginitis drug therapy. *Obstet Gynecol* 1987;**69**:751–5.

MIDAZOLAM

Use

Midazolam is an effective sedative, and a useful first line anticonvulsant, but it does not relieve pain. 'One off' use does not cause any of the unpleasant withdrawal symptoms commonly seen after use for several days.

Pharmacology

Midazolam hydrochloride is a short-acting benzodiazepine with hypnotic, anxiolytic, muscle relaxant and anticonvulsant activity, now most widely used to generate antegrade amnesia, and was first patented in 1976. Bioavailability is about 35% when given as an oral syrup, and 50% when absorbed through the mucosa of the mouth or nose. It is cleared from the body 20 times more quickly than diazepam, the half life being 2 hours in adults (but 12 hours in the neonate). Although use during pregnancy should be approached with the same caution as the use of diazepam (q.v.), rapid clearance means that very little appears in breast milk. Midazolam is now increasingly used to stop prolonged seizures in children – the rapidity of mucosal absorption from the nose or mouth ('buccal' administration) making IV administration less necessary.

Unfortunately any first IV 'loading' dose in a preterm baby not infrequently causes respiratory depression, with hypotension and a fall in cerebral blood flow. Myoclonus unassociated with any EEG abnormality is sometimes seen, and paradoxical agitation has been reported. Sustained use causes drug accumulation, with tissue levels that variably exceed plasma levels (V_D 1–3 l/kg), and withdrawal symptoms have been reported in up to a quarter of all children. Severe encephalopathic features have sometimes been reported 1–2 days after treatment was stopped, with drowsiness and dystonic posturing, and choreoathetosis. The manufacturer does not recommend use as a sedative or anticonvulsant in any child less than 6 months old and the Cochrane overview found inadequate evidence to support neonatal use (see website commentary).

Treatment

Short-term sedation: A 500 microgram/kg dose by mouth is often used to premedicate children prior to anaesthesia. A 300 microgram/kg dose into the nose can provide sedation during investigational procedures, and 500–700 micrograms/kg into the nose (monitored, ideally, with an oximeter) relieves stress during suturing.

Continuous sedation: Some units give 60 micrograms/kg per hour to sedate the ventilated newborn baby for 2–4 days after birth, but this strategy is now increasingly questioned. The rate of infusion **must** be halved after 24 hours in babies of less than 33 weeks' postconceptional age to prevent drug accumulation.

Controlling seizures: A 200 microgram/kg dose given IV over 2 minutes stops most fits in infancy, but giving 500 micrograms/kg of the IV preparation into the nose or under the tongue will usually achieve this just as quickly (and this can be done outside hospital). How often midazolam really stops neonatal seizures not controlled by _henobarbital (q.v.) is not entirely clear. Lorazepam (q.v.) is a slightly better studied alternative.

Antidote

All benzodiazepines cause hypotonia, hypotension and coma in excess, but these effects can be reversed by flumazenil, a competitive antagonist with a relatively short (50 minute) half life first synthesised in 1979. High-dose use also causes respiratory depression. While the manufacturers are not yet ready to recommend such use, there are several reports of flumazenil being used in children. Give one (or even two) 10 microgram/kg IV doses and assess the effect. If there is a definite but unsustained response start a continuous IV infusion with 10 micrograms/kg per hour for 6–12 hours. Use may unmask fits suppressed by benzodiazepines.

Compatibility

Compatibility with other continuously infused drugs is noted, where known, in the monograph for the second product. Midazolam can also be added (terminally) to an IV line containing standard TPN (but not lipid).

Supply and administration

Midazolam: 5 ml ampoules containing either 5 or 10 mg of midazolam cost about 60p. To give 60 micrograms/kg of midazolam per hour as a continuous IV infusion, place 3 mg of midazolam for each kg the infant weighs in a syringe, dilute to 50 ml with 10% glucose or glucose saline, and infuse at a rate of 1 ml/hour. (A less concentrated solution of dextrose or dextrose saline can be used where necessary.) The drug is stable in solution so it is not necessary to change the infusate daily. It is a schedule 4 controlled drug in the UK. Most North American products contain 1% benzyl alcohol.

Flumazenil: 5 ml, 500 microgram, ampoules of flumazenil cost £14·50. Dilute with 5% glucose.

References

See also the relevant Cochrane reviews

Anand KJS, McIntosh N, Lagercranz H, *et al*. Analgesia and sedation in neonates who require ventilatory support – results from the NOPAIN trial. *Arch Pediatr Adolesc Med* 1999;**153**:331–8. [RCT]

Aviram EE, Ben-Abraham R, Weinbrioum AA. Flumazenil use in children. *Paed Perinatal Drug Ther* 2004;**5**:202–9.

de Wildt SN, Kearns GL, Hop WCJ, *et al*. Pharmacokinetics and metabolism of intravenous midazolam in preterm infants. *Clin Pharmacol* 2001;**70**:525–31.

Hellström-Westas L. Midazolam and amplitude-integrated EEG. [Commentary] *Acta Paediatr* 2004;**93**:1153–5.

Ista E, van Diik M, Gamei C, *et al*. Withdrawal symptoms in critically ill children after long term administration of sedatives and or analgesics: a first evaluation. *Crit Care Med* 2008;**36**:2427–32.

McIntyre J, Robertson S, Norris E, *et al*. Safety and efficacy of buccal midazolam versus rectal diazepam for emergency treatment of seizures in children: a randomised controlled trial. *Lancet* 2005;**366**:205–10. [RCT] (See also pp. 182–3.)

Shany E, Benzaqen O, Watemberg N. Comparison of continuous drip of midazolam or lidocaine in the treatment of intractable neonatal seizures. *J Child Neurol* 2007;**22**:255–9.

Use

Artificial milks designed to approximate human breast milk have been commercially available for 30 years. Modified formulas designed for use in preterm babies have been developed more recently, while formulas have now been designed for children over 6 months old with a higher casein:whey ratio. Fortifying powders are also available for use when breast milk (q.v.) is used to feed the very preterm baby.

Nutritional factors

Most milk formulas are made from demineralised protein-enriched whey, skimmed milk, vegetable oils and milk fat, glucose, lactose and/or maltodextrin, with mineral and vitamin supplements (Table 1).

Table 1 Composition per 100 ml of various neonatal milks available in the UK.

	Protein (g)	Fat (g)	Carbohydrate (g)	Energy (kcal)	Na (mmol)	Ca (mmol)	P (mmol)	Fe (mg)	Vit D (µg)
Neonatal milks									
Farleys First milk®	1·5	3·6	7·0	68	0·8	0·9	0·9	0·6	1·0
Cow & Gate Premium®	1·4	3·5	7·5	67	0·8	1·4	0·9	0·5	1·4
SMA Gold®	1·5	3·6	7·2	67	0·7	1·2	1·1	0·8	1·1
Milupa Aptamil First®	1·5	3·6	7·2	67	0·8	1·5	1·1	0·7	1·0
Preterm milks									
Farleys Osterprem®	2·0	4·6	7·6	80	1·8	2·8	2·0	<0·1	2·4
Cow & Gate Nutriprem®	2·4	4·4	7·9	80	1·8	2·5	1·6	0·9	5·0
SMA LBW Formula®	2·0	4·4	8·6	82	1·5	2·0	1·4	0·8	1·5
Milupa Pre-Apamil®	2·4	3·5	7·8	80	1·2	1·2	1·3	0·9	2·4
Hydrolysed protein milks with MCT									
Mead Johnson Pregestimil®	1·9	3·8	6·9	68	1·4	1·6	1·4	1·2	1·1
Cow & Gate Peptijunior®	1·8	3·6	6·6	66	0·9	1·4	0·9	0·5	1·3
Mature human breast milk									
Widdowson (1977)	1·3	4·2	7·4	70	0·7	0·9	0·5	0·1	<0·1

A low lactose product will minimise intolerance in the very preterm baby. Specialised formulas where the protein is provided as 'pre-digested' hydrolysed peptides and amino acids derived from casein (Pregestimil) or whey (Peptijunior) are also available. In these two products half the fat is provided as medium chain triglyceride (MCT). Advice on special products is available from hospital dietitians.

While breast milk is the food of choice for almost every baby, most grow very well on 130–150 kcal/kg a day of any one of these formulas in the neonatal period, and can accept an oral intake of 200 ml/kg a day once feeding is fully established. In some babies of less than 2 kg, growth can be enhanced by using a nutrient-enriched preterm formula. Details of four different low birth weight (LBW) formulas widely used in the UK are shown in Table 1. All have a potassium content of between 1·4 and 2·0 mmol/100 ml. With the exceptions noted below, artificial milk formulas contain adequate quantities of all the nutrients, trace elements and vitamins known to be necessary for growth in the neonatal period. In particular there is no evidence that babies ever need further supplemental vitamin K (q.v.) once established on an artificial milk formula. Nor do babies need more folic acid (q.v.) than is provided by every one of the artificial infant milk products currently on sale in the UK, even when born preterm.

Further supplements

Sodium: Most babies of less than 30 weeks' gestation require further routine sodium with their milk to bring their total intake up to between 4·5 and 6·0 mmol/kg a day (the equivalent to the intake provided by 150–200 ml/kg of 10% glucose in 0·18% sodium chloride). This high need is caused by the immature kidney's limited ability to conserve sodium. The necessary extra sodium is best provided by adding a further 2 mmol of sodium chloride to every 100 ml of preterm milk formula or breast milk fed to all babies of less than 30 weeks' gestation (for details see the monograph on sodium chloride). Loss should also be monitored intermittently because some very preterm babies require more supplemental sodium than most, especially in the first 2 weeks of life. If the sodium content of a 'spot' urine sample is high, something is limiting renal tubular reabsorption, unless intake has been abnormally high.

Vitamin D: Babies are known to require 10 micrograms of vitamin D a day irrespective of their weight. The content of most artificial milk only averages 1 microgram/100 ml (with an agreed maximum of 5 micrograms/100 ml because of the risk associated with excessive intake). All preterm babies should therefore have supplemental vitamin D drops once a day until they weigh at least 3 kg. For further details see the monograph on vitamin D.

Iron: All babies have reasonable iron stores at birth even if born prematurely, but dietary iron becomes necessary within 2–3 months of birth to provide the additional iron needed by the child's growing red cell mass. Repeated blood sampling may further reduce available body iron if the blood taken is not replaced by transfusion. All standard artificial UK milk

Continued on p. 170

formulas contain enough iron to provide for the needs of babies born at term, being formulated to contain much more iron than breast milk in order to compensate for poor iron absorption. The same is not true in all countries.

Most of the preterm formulas available in the UK (other than Osterprem) contain similar supplements of iron, but there is no evidence that babies absorb this iron in the first month of life, even when they are offered it, and there are theoretical reasons for limiting early supplementation because this interferes with the antimicrobial activity of lactoferrin in the gut. However, all babies who are not breastfed should certainly be on a milk containing at least 500 micrograms/100 ml of iron by the time they are 2 months old. While it has long been traditional to provide preterm babies with further supplementation, it is now clear that this routine is quite unnecessary. For further details see the monograph on iron.

Phosphate: Human milk is capable of sustaining excellent bone growth in the full term baby, but bone growth and increased bone mineralisation is so rapid in the preterm baby that babies weighing <1·3 kg at birth are at serious risk of osteopenia and of spontaneous pathological fractures in the second and third month of life if not offered further supplementation. Both calcium and phosphorus are usually provided, and all artificial preterm milk formulas provide some supplementation. Calcium and phosphorus absorption are linked and a calcium:phosphorus ratio of between 1·4:1 and 2:1 seems to optimise absorption and minimise the risk of late neonatal hypocalcaemia. Phosphorus is well absorbed and its availability seems to limit calcium absorption. It is now thought that optimum phosphorus intake in the growing preterm baby is probably provided by a milk containing between 1·3 and 2·3 mmol of phosphorus per 100 ml. Human milk only contains a third of this and requires regular supplementation (see the monograph on phosphate). Additional calcium is probably not necessary if adequate phosphorus is provided. Most commercial preterm milks contain at least the minimum amount of phosphorus now recommended (Table 1).

Bicarbonate: Some preterm babies develop a late metabolic acidosis on formula feeds due to the neonatal kidney's limited ability to excrete acid. Oral bicarbonate will relieve this, improving weight gain and nitrogen retention, as described in the monograph on sodium bicarbonate.

Supply

Hospital catering departments are responsible for the supply and distribution of artificial milks. Manufacturers are now banned from subsidising the cost of pre-packed milk supplied to hospitals or from providing free samples in an attempt to increase their share of the market with newly delivered mothers (the practice has been shown in nine controlled trials to reduce the number of mothers achieving a sustained lactation). Most pre-packed neonatal milks cost about 25p per bottle. Equivalent volumes of Pregestimil and Peptijunior can be made up for 30p per feed. Individually packed sterile disposable teats cost about 14p each.

References   See also the relevant Cochrane reviews

American Academy of Pediarics. Committee on Nutrition. Iron fortification of infant formulas. *Pediatrics* 1999;**104**:119–23.
American Academy of Pediatrics. Committee on Nutrition. Use of soy protein-based formulas in infant feeding. *Pediatrics* 2008;**121**:1062–8.
Edmond K, Bahl R. Optimal feeding of low-birth-weight infants. [WHO technical review] Geneva: World Health Organisation, 2006.
European Society of Paediatric Gastroenterology and Nutrition (ESPGAN) Committee on Nutrition of the Preterm Baby. Nutrition and feeding of preterm infants. *Acta Paediatr Scand* 1987;suppl 336.
Hays T, Wood RA. A systematic review of the role of hydrolyzed infant formulas in allergy prevention. *Arch Pediatr Adolesc Med* 2005;**159**:810–16. [SR]
Klein CJ. Nutrient requirements for preterm infant formulas. *J Nutr* 2002;**132**:1395S–1577S.
McGuire W, Anthony MY. Donor human milk versus formula for preventing necrotising enterocolitis in preterm infants: systematic review. *Arch Dis Child* 2003;**88**:F11–14. [SR]
Radde IC, Chance GW, Bailey K, *et al*. Growth and mineral metabolism 1. Comparison of the effects of two modes of NaHCO$_3$ treatment of late metabolic acidoses. *Pediatr Res* 1975;**9**:564–8. [RCT]
Steer PA, Lucas A, Sinclair JC. Feeding the low birthweight infant. In: Sinclair JC, Bracken MB, eds. *Effective care of the newborn infant*. Oxford: Oxford University Press, 1992: pp. 94–140. [SR] (See also pp. 161–77.)
Tsang RC, Uauy R, Koletzko B, *et al*., eds. *Nutrition of the preterm baby: scientific basis and practical guidelines*, 2nd edn. Cincinnati, OH: Digital Educational Publishing, 2005.

Use

Milrinone lactate is mainly used in the management of septic shock and in the short-term support of patients after cardiac surgery. There is some evidence that it can further reduce pulmonary vascular tone in babies with persistent pulmonary hypertension severe enough to merit treatment with nitric oxide (q.v.).

Pharmacology

Milrinone is a selective phosphodiesterase inhibitor first developed in 1981 with the same properties as enoximone. There is good evidence that combined short-term use with adrenaline or dobutamine (q.v.) can reduce systemic vascular resistance and increase cardiac output in babies suffering septic shock. The mode of action has not been fully determined, but seems to involve an increase in cyclic adenosine monophosphate concentration secondary to inhibition of phosphodiesterase leading to an increase in the contractile force of cardiac muscle. A trial of long-term oral use in patients with heart failure in 1991 found an unexpected, and unexplained, increased mortality in those taking milrinone. Sustained use has been avoided ever since, although recent studies have reported safe IV use for up to 8 weeks in both in children and in adults with end-stage heart failure awaiting a heart transplant.

Milrinone is actively excreted (largely unmetabolised) by the kidney, the half life being rather variable (usually 1–2 hours), but five times as long as this immediately after birth. The volume of distribution in young children ($V_D > 1$ l/kg) is substantially more than in adult life, making it important to administer an initial loading dose if an early response to treatment is required. An optimal response seems to be achieved when the blood level is approximately 200 ng/ml. Mild thrombocytopenia is common when milrinone is infused for more than 24 hours. Other complications, such as arrhythmia, are rare in children. Those ill enough to require treatment with milrinone after surgery almost certainly merit central venous pressure monitoring. Milrinone crosses the placenta. There is no evidence of teratogenicity in animals, but no published reports relating to use during human pregnancy or lactation. The manufacturers have not yet endorsed the use of milrinone in children.

Treatment

Neonatal treatment: A recent study used 0·75 micrograms/kg per minute IV for 3 hours and then 0·2 micrograms/kg per minute for 18 hours to sustain stable blood levels. (This is 1·5 ml/hour of a solution prepared as described below for 3 hours followed by 0·4 ml/hour for 18 hours.) However, early *preventive* use did not improve systemic (superior vena caval) blood flow or outcome in a trial in very preterm babies.

Older children: Give 60 micrograms/kg IV over 15 minutes, and then 0·5 micrograms/kg per minute (2·0 ml of a solution made up as described below over 15 minutes, and then 1 ml/hour) for up to 2 days. Babies with septic shock sometimes need rather more than this. Reduce the maintenance dose if there is renal failure.

Watch for hypotension: Mild hypotension may occur while the loading dose is being given because the drug causes some vasodilatation. Volume expansion and/or low-dose dopamine will usually counteract this.

Compatibility

Milrinone can be added (terminally) to a line containing adrenaline, atracurium, dobutamine, dopamine, fentanyl, glyceryl trinitrate, heparin, insulin, isoprenaline, midazolam, morphine, nitroprusside, noradrenaline, propofol, ranitidine or standard TPN (but not furosemide). Compatibility with IV lipid has not been assessed.

Supply and administration

10 ml ampoules containing 10 mg of milrinone (as lactate) cost £16·60. Take 0·6 ml (0·6 mg) of milrinone for each kg the baby weighs, and dilute this to 20 ml with 10% glucose, or glucose saline. To give 0·5 micrograms/kg per minute infuse this dilute solution at a rate of 1 ml/hour. Less concentrated solutions of dextrose or dextrose saline can be used. The drug is stable in solution, so a fresh infusion does not need to be prepared every 24 hours. Injecting furosemide into a line containing milrinone will cause precipitation.

References

Bailey JM, Hoffman TM, Wessel DL, *et al*. A population pharmacodynamic analysis of milrinone in pediatric patients after cardiac surgery. *J Pharmacokinet Pharmacodyn* 2004;**31**:43–59.

Barton P, Garcia J, Kouatli A, *et al*. Hemodynamic effects of IV milrinone lactate in pediatric patients with septic shock. A prospective, double-blinded, randomized, placebo-controlled, interventional study. *Chest* 1996;**109**:1302–12. [RCT]

Bassler D, Choong K, McNamara P, *et al*. Neonatal persistent pulmonary hypertension treated with milrinone: four case reports. *Biol Neonat* 2006;**89**:1–5.

Cai J, Su Z, Shi Z, *et al*. Nitric oxide and milrinone: combined effect on pulmonary circulation after Fontan-type procedure: a prospective randomized study. *Ann Thorac Surg* 2008;**86**:882–8. [RCT]

Hoffman TM, Wernovsky G, Atz AM, *et al*. Efficacy and safety of milrinone in preventing low cardiac output syndrome in infantts and children after corrective surgery for congentialheart disease. *Circulation* 2003;**107**:995–1002. [RCT]

McNamara PJ, Laique F, Muang-In S, *et al*. Milrinone improves oxygenation in neonates with severe persistent pulmonary hypertension of the newborn. *J Crit Care* 2006;**21**:217–22.

Paradisis M, Evans NJ, Kluckow MR, *et al*. Randomised trial of milrinone versus placebo for prevention of low systemic blood flow in very preterm infants. *J Pediatr* 2009;**154**:189–95. [RCT]

Paradisis M, Jiang X, McLachlan AJ, *et al*. Population pharmacokinetics and dosing regimen design of milrinone in preterm infants. *Arch Dis Child* 2007;**92**:F204–9.

Ramamoorthy C, Andersib GD, Williams GD, *et al*. Pharmacokinetics and side effects of milrinone in infants and children after open heart surgery. *Anesthg Analg* 1998;**86**:283–9.

Zuppa AF, Nicolson SC, Adamson PC, *et al*. Population pharmacokinetics of milrinone in neonates with hypoplastic left heart syndrome undergoing stage I reconstruction. *Anesth Analg* 2006;**102**:1062–9. (A report of management during and after cardiopulmonary bypass.)

MISOPROSTOL

Use

Although gastric ulcer prevention is currently the only marketed indication for misprostol in most countries, it is now widely used to terminate pregnancy, and is a valuable alternative to oxytocin (q.v.) in the control of serious postpartum bleeding (a problem that currently kills one woman every 4 minutes in resource-poor countries) and does not need refrigeration. It also has a role (if the dose is kept low) in the induction of labour.

Pharmacology

The only officially recognised use of misoprostol, an orally active prostaglandin E_1 analogue first synthesised in 1973, is to prevent and treat the gastric ulcers that are sometimes caused by non-steroidal anti-inflammatory drug (NSAID) use. The drug's original manufacturer (Searle Pharmaceuticals) has never recommended use for any other purpose, or supported the studies needed to evaluate any other use, and only makes the drug available in 100 and 200 microgram tablets (a higher dose than is usually appropriate when attempting to induce labour in late pregnancy). It is, however, widely accepted that a 400 microgram vaginally administered dose of misoprostol is an effective way of preparing the first trimester cervix for suction termination, while an 800 microgram dose given 48 hours after a 200 mg dose of oral mifepristone will effect non-surgical termination of pregnancy in any woman less than 8 weeks' pregnant. Nausea, abdominal pain, diarrhoea, shivering and fever are the commonest transient, dose-dependent side effects.

Much lower doses usually suffice to induce labour at term, and dangerous uterine hyperstimulation was a common problem before this was recognised. Indeed uterine rupture has been reported so often in women with a uterine scar that any such use is now considered very unwise. In fact there is probably nothing specifically dangerous about the use of misoprostol in this situation – it is probably the dose used that has been the problem, because other strategies for induction can also cause uterine rupture. The active metabolite, misoprostol acid, is rapidly cleared by the liver, and the half life with oral administration is less than an hour. Placing a tablet in the posterior fornix of the vagina increases the drug's bioavailability, and its half life, but most women prefer oral treatment and, while the optimum oral dose still requires further study, a recent systematic review found the two approaches to be of comparable efficacy. Misoprostol should never be used for other reasons during pregnancy, not just because it stimulates uterine activity, but because high-dose first trimester use can cause fetal deformity. There are no reports of complications with use during lactation.

Treatment

Inducing labour: One approach is to give up to three 25 microgram oral (or sublingual) doses once every 2 hours, doubling the dose to 50 micrograms every 2 hours if necessary after 6 hours. Treatment is stopped once the uterus is contracting regularly (three 30-second contractions every 10 minutes). An alternative strategy has been to give up to five 100 microgram doses at 4-hourly intervals. The existence of a uterine scar is a contraindication to *either* of these strategies, as is the simultaneous use of IV oxytocin.

Postpartum haemorrhage: While IV oxytocin is the drug of choice to control early postpartum bleeding, 600 micrograms of oral (or sublingual) misoprostol is (once absorbed) extremely effective at controlling serious, sustained and life-threatening postpartum bleeding because of its longer half life.

Supply and administration

The only product currently available in the UK is a 200 microgram tablet that costs 17p. Smaller doses can, however, be given by crushing the tablet and dissolving it in tap water. Any such solution must then be used within 12 hours. Misoprostol has not yet been licensed for obstetric use but, unlike oxytocin, it does not have to be stored in the dark, or kept at 4°C, to maintain its potency. It is also much cheaper than dinoprostone vaginal gel. The pharmaceutical industry needs to shoulder much of the blame for the fact that legal supplies are still hard to obtain in most resource-poor countries, even though the drug's patent has now expired.

References

See also the relevant Cochrane reviews and UK guideline on induction of labour

Bregstrom S, Aronsson A. Misoprostol in resource poor countries. [Editorial] *BMJ* 2008;**336**:1032.

Crane JMG, Butler B, Young DC, *et al*. Misoprostol compared with prostaglandin E_2 for labour induction in women at term with intact membranes and unfavourable cervix: a systematic review. *Br J Obstet Gynaecol* 2006;**113**:1366–76. [SR] (See also pp. 1431–7.)

Derman RJ, Kodkany BS, Goudar SS, *et al*. Oral misoprostol in preventing postpartum haemorrhage in resource-poor communities: a randomised controlled trial. *Lancet* 2006;**368**:1248–53. [RCT] (See also pp. 1216–8.)

El-Refaey H, Rodeck C. Post-partum haemorrhage: definitions, medical and surgical management. Time for change. [Review] *Br Med Bull* 2005;**67**:205–17.

Hofmeyr GJ, Walraven G, Gülmezoglu AM, *et al*. Misoprostol to treat postpartum haemorrhage: a systematic review. *Br J Obstet Gynaecol* 2005;**112**:547–53. [SR]

Høj L, Cardoso P, Nielsen BB, *et al*. Effect of sublingual misoprostol on severe postpartum haemorrhage in a primary health centre in Guinea-Bissau: randomised double blind clinical trial. *BMJ* 2005;**116**:753–7. [RCT]

Langenbach C. Misoprostol in preventing postpartum hemorrhage: a meta-analysis. *Int J Gynaecol Obstet* 2006;**92**:10–18. [SR]

Pagel C, Lewycka S, Colbourn T, *et al*. Estimation of potential effects of improved community-based drug provision, to augment health-facility strengthening, on maternal mortality due to post-partum haemorrhage and sepsis in sub-Saharan Africa: an equity effectiveness model. *Lancet* 2009;**374**:1441–8. (See also pp. 1400–2.)

Prager M, Eneroth-Grimfors E, Edlund M, *et al*. A randomised controlled trial of intravaginal dinoprostone, intravaginal misoprostol and transcervical balloon catheter for labour induction. *Br J Obstet Gynaecol* 2008;**115**:1443–50. [RCT]

Souza ASR, Amorim MMR, Feitosa FEL. Comparison of sublingual versus vaginal misoprostol for the induction of labour: a systematic review. *Br J Obstet Gynaecol* 2008;**115**:13409. [SR]

Vargas FR, Schuler-Faccini L, Brunoni D, *et al*. Prenatal exposure to misoprostol and vascular disruption defects: a case–control study. *Am J Med Genet* 2000;**95**:302–6. (See also pp. 297–301.)

Use
Mivacurium is a useful, quick-acting, alternative to atracurium (q.v.) when short-term muscular paralysis is required. It does not blunt the perception of pain.

Pharmacology
Mivacurium, like atracurium and pancuronium, is a non-depolarising muscle relaxant that works by competing with acetylcholine at the neuromuscular junction's receptor site – an effect that can be reversed with anticholinesterases such as neostigmine (q.v.). It was developed as an analogue of atracurium, and first brought into clinical use in 1988. The drug, as prescribed, is actually a mixture of three stereoisomers; only two seem to cause much neuromuscular blockade, but all three are inactivated by plasma cholinesterase. Paralysis is dose related but, after a single bolus dose, seldom lasts more than 20 minutes (30 minutes in older children). Activity is, however, prolonged by volatile anaesthetics such as isoflurane, and recovery can take 2–4 hours in some patients who have inherited one of the genes associated with deficient cholinesterase production (about 0·04% of the population) – a problem not encountered with atracurium. The manufacturers have not yet endorsed the use of mivacurium in children less than 2 months old, partly because of concern about possible increased sensitivity, but extensive clinical experience suggests that such caution may be unnecessary. There is no contraindication to use during pregnancy or labour, and use during lactation is also almost certainly safe given the drug's short half life and probable poor oral absorption.

Atracurium and mivacurium are benzylisoquinolinium non-depolarising muscle relaxants. All drugs in this class (other than cisatracurium) can cause histamine release with flushing, tachycardia, hypotension and (very rarely) an anaphylactoid reaction. Such problems seem less common in children. The risk can also be _inimized by avoiding unnecessarily rapid administration.

Treatment
Single-dose administration: A 200 microgram/kg IV injection provides almost complete muscle relaxation after 1–2 minutes, that lasts for about 10–15 minutes. Only flush this bolus dose through into the vein slowly over a period of 10–20 seconds to minimise the risk of histamine release. A smaller dose is often enough to achieve relaxation prior to tracheal intubation. Paralysis can be sustained longer if necessary by giving further IV doses once every 5–10 minutes.

Continuous infusion: Sustained paralysis generally requires a continuing infusion of about 10 micrograms/kg per minute in early infancy (only slightly more than the amount generally needed in adult life), but some older children require almost twice as much as this. The amount needed is not always predictable and may require individual titration. Recovery is usually rapid once the infusion is stopped.

Antidote
Most of the effects of mivacurium could be reversed by giving a combination of 10 micrograms/kg of glycopyrronium (or 20 micrograms/kg of atropine), and 50 micrograms/kg of neostigmine as outlined in the glycopyrronium monograph, but reversal should seldom be called for given atracurium's short half life.

Supply and administration
5 ml ampoules are available containing 10 mg of mivacurium chloride (costing £2·80). Multidose vials are available in North America, but these should be avoided when treating young children because they contain benzyl alcohol. Store all products below 25°C, but do not freeze. Protect from light.

Bolus administration: Take 1 ml of mivacurium from a 2 mg/ml ampoule and dilute to 10 ml with 5% glucose or glucose saline to obtain a preparation containing 200 micrograms/ml.

Continuous infusion: To give 10 micrograms/kg per minute, draw 6 mg (3 ml) of mivacurium for each kg the baby weighs from the ampoule into a syringe, dilute to 10 ml with 5% dextrose in 0·18% sodium chloride, and infuse at 1 ml/hour. A less concentrated solution of dextrose or dextrose saline can be used if appropriate.

References

Atherton DPL, Hunter JM. Clinical pharmacokinetics of the newer neuromuscular blocking drugs. *Clin Pharmacokinet* 1999;**36**:169–89.

Cerf C, Mesuish M, Gabriel I, *et al*. Screening patients for prolonged neuromuscular blockade after succinylcholine and mivacurium. *Anesth Analg* 2002;**94**:461–6.

Dempsey EM, Al Hazzani F, Faucher D, *et al*. Facilitation of neonatal endotracheal intubation with mivacurium and fentanyl in the neonatal intensive care unit. *Arch Dis Child* 2006;**91**:F279–82.

Guay J, Grenier Y, Varin F. Clinical pharmacokinetics of neuromuscular relaxants in pregnancy. *Clin Pharmacokinet* 1998;**34**:483–96.

Meakin GH. Recent advances in myorelaxant therapy. *Paediatr Anaesth* 2001;**11**:5623–31.

Nauheimer D, Fink H, Fuchs-Buder Th, *et al*. Muscle relaxant use for tracheal intubation in pediatric anaesthesia: a survey of clinical practice in Germany. *Pediatr Anesth* 2009;**19**:225–31.

Plaud B, Goujard E, Orliaguet G, *et al*. Pharmacodynamie et tolérance du mivacurium chez le nourrisson et l'enfant sous anesthésie par halothane-protoxyde d'azote. *Ann Fr Anesth Reanim* 1999;**18**:1047–53.

Rashid A, Watkinson M. Suxamethonium is safe in safe hands: mivacurium should also be considered. *Arch Dis Child* 2000;**83**:F160–1.

Roberts KD, Leone TA, Edwards WH, *et al*. Premedication for nonemergent neonatal intubations: a randomized, controlled trial comparing atropine and fentanyl to atropine, fentanyl, and mivacurium. *Pediatrics* 2006;**118**:1583–91. [RCT]

Use

Morphine is the best studied neonatal analgesic. Use a loading dose and continuous infusion.

Pharmacology

Morphine, the principle alkaloid of opium, has been used for over 2000 years and a pure extract was obtained from poppy heads in 1805. It is well absorbed when taken by mouth but undergoes rapid first pass metabolism in the liver (bioavailability about 30%). The half life in the preterm baby is 6–12 hours and **very** variable, but inversely related to gestational age, at birth. Some tissue accumulation occurs with sustained use (V_D ~2 l/kg). Elimination is delayed during therapeutic hypothermia, but is much more rapid in babies more than 2 months old, the half life in 1–6-year-old children (about 1 hour) being less than in adults. Ordinary doses cause constipation, urinary retention and respiratory depression, and an overdose can cause hypotension, bradycardia and even (rarely) fits. One study suggests that neonatal pain relief may require a blood level of ~120 ng/ml, while adverse effects start to appear at levels exceeding 300 ng/ml. Lower levels (20–40 ng/ml) seem adequate in older children. The high levels required in the newborn may reflect drug-receptor differences, and low glucuronide (M6G) metabolite levels. It has been hard to show that ventilated babies benefit from routine treatment with morphine. Tolerance may develop with prolonged treatment, and withdrawal symptoms can also occur. Addiction has not been seen with neonatal use for pain relief. Morphine crosses the placenta, causing some neonatal depression (as discussed in the monograph on pethidine), but use during lactation probably only exposes the baby to a tenth of the maternal dose on a weight-for-weight basis. Maternal addiction is discussed in the monograph on diamorphine.

Treatment

Opioid withdrawal: Give 40 micrograms/kg by mouth once every 4 hours. Double the dose interval as soon as symptoms are controlled, and then reduce the dose. Aim to stop treatment after 6–10 days.

Severe or sustained pain: Provide ventilatory support, give a loading dose of 240 micrograms/kg and then a maintenance infusion of 20 micrograms/kg per hour (12 ml/hour of a solution prepared as described below **for 1 hour**, followed by a maintenance infusion of 1 ml/hour). While this will usually control even severe pain in the first 2 months of life, providing a plasma morphine level of 120–160 ng/ml, treatment *has* to be individualised (as discussed in the web commentary). Staff need discretion to give a further 20 microgram/kg bolus up to once every 4 hours to control any 'break through' pain.

Sedation while ventilated: Babies given both a loading dose and a maintenance dose that are **half** as large as those used for managing severe pain seldom breathe out of phase with the ventilator.

Short-term pain relief: Give 100 micrograms/kg IM or IV (or twice this by mouth). Rapid IV administration does *not* cause hypotension but may cause respiratory depression. A further 50 microgram/kg dose can usually be given after 6 hours without making ventilator support necessary.

Older children: Drug clearance is more rapid in babies more than 2 months old, but the plasma morphine level needed to provide pain relief seems to fall. The interplay between these factors has not yet been studied. Use the above guidance as a starting point and then individualise treatment.

Compatibility

Compatibility with other continuously infused drugs is noted, where known, in the monograph for the second product. Morphine can also be added (terminally) to an IV line containing standard TPN and lipid.

Antidote

Naloxone (q.v.) is a specific opioid antagonist.

Supply and administration

Ampoules of morphine sulphate containing 10 mg in 1 ml are available at a cost of 72p each. The use of a preservative-free ampoule will reduce the risk of phlebitis. **Always** start by diluting the contents ten-fold for accurate neonatal administration. For single bolus doses 0·1 ml of morphine can be made up to 1 ml with 0·9% sodium chloride, giving a solution of 1 mg/ml. To set up a continuous infusion, dilute the 1 ml of fluid from the ampoule to 10 ml with 0·9% sodium chloride (as above), place 1 ml of this diluted preparation for each kg the baby weighs in a syringe, dilute to 50 ml with 10% glucose or glucose saline, and infuse at 1 ml/hour to provide an infusion of 20 micrograms/kg per hour. The drug is chemically stable in solution so the infusate does not need to be changed daily.

The storage and administration of morphine (other than as an oral solution containing <2·6 mg/ml) is controlled under Schedule 2 of the UK Misuse of Drugs Regulations 1985 (Misuse of Drugs Act, 1971).

Reference

See also the relevant Cochrane reviews

Anand KJS. Pharmacological approaches to the management of pain in the neonatal intensive care unit. *J Perinatol* 2007;**27**:S4–11.

Anand KJS, Whit Hall R, Desai N, *et al*. Efects of morphine analgesia in ventilated preterm neonates: primary outcomes from the NEOPAIN randomised trial. *Lancet* 2004;**363**:2673–82. [RCT] (See also **364**:498.)

Carbajal R, Lenclen R, Jugie M, *et al*. Morphine does not provide adequate analgesia for acute procedural pain among preterm neonates. *Pediatrics* 2005;**115**:1494–500.

Menon G, McIntosh N. How should we manage pain in ventilates neonates? [Review] *Neonatology* 2008;**93**:316–23.

Olkkola KT, Hamunen K, Maunuksela E-L. Clinical pharmacokinetics and pharmacodynamics of opioid analgesics in infants and children. *Clin Pharmacokinet* 1995;**28**:385–403.

Use

This antibiotic ointment is sometimes used to treat staphylococcal skin infection and, more importantly, to control surface colonisation by meticillin-resistant staphylococci.

Pharmacology

This unusual antibiotic, a fermentation product of the bacterium *Pseudomonas fluorescens*, was formerly called pseudomonic acid. It is structurally unlike any other antibiotic, containing a unique hydroxynonanoic acid linked to monic acid. It is bacteriostatic in low concentrations and slowly bactericidal at high concentrations against *Mycoplasma* and most Gram-positive aerobes in an acid environment such as that provided by the skin (pH 5·5). It is non-toxic but rapidly de-esterified and rendered inert by the tissues after parenteral injection, making the drug only suitable for topical use. The drug first came into clinical use in 1988. Microbiological advice should be taken before using mupirocin, and the product should only be used for a limited period to minimise the risk of drug resistance developing. There has been one report suggesting that mupirocin may be more effective in treating candidal skin infection than *in vitro* assessments of its sensitivity would suggest, and further controlled studies seem called for. The drug has sometimes, but not always, proved of value in eliminating the chronic nasal carriage of pathogenic staphylococci by staff. Transient stinging and localised skin reaction can occur. There is no evidence of teratogenicity, and nothing to suggest that mupirocin needs to be avoided during pregnancy in situations where its use seems otherwise justified on clinical grounds. Breastfeeding is not contraindicated, because absorption is minimal after topical administration, and any of the drug that is ingested is very rapidly metabolised to monic acid.

Hospital-acquired staphylococcal infection

The general public has long thought that babies were only taken to 'intensive care' if they were ill – it is not surprising that they become angry if admission causes a previously healthy child to pick up a potentially life-threatening infection. Although staphylococcal infection can occur soon after birth (since the organism is a common vaginal commensal), 95% of invasive staphylococcal infection in the newborn occurs in babies more than 48 hours old, making it the commonest infection acquired *after* admission to intensive care (a nosocomial infection), and the frequency with which such infection occurs is a good measure of the attention a unit pays to skin care (q.v.), and to the proper management of intravascular long lines (as outlined in the monograph on skin sterility). The problem is made much worse if infection is caused by a strain resistant to most commonly used antibiotics. Such resistance is increasingly common; and a quarter of those acquiring a meticillin-resistant *Staphylococcus aureus* (MRSA) infection currently die. Vancomycin-resistant enterococci can be equally lethal. Without routine screening, contact tracing and cohorting (see website commentary), and the selective use of mupirocin to control carriage by clinical staff, such organisms can soon become endemic in a unit.

Treatment

Use mupirocin on the skin (avoiding the eyes) three times a day for not more than 10 days.

Supply

Mupirocin ointment (2% w/w) is available in 15 g tubes costing £4·40 each. This formulation uses a macrogol (polyethylene glycol) base, and it is possible that renal toxicity could result from macrogol absorption through mucous membranes, or through extensive application to thin or damaged neonatal skin. In that situation the equivalent paraffin-based formulation of calcium mupirocin might be preferable; this is currently marketed as an ointment officially designed for nasal use in 3 g tubes costing £5·80. A cream is also available, but this is probably best avoided in the preterm baby because it contains benzyl alcohol.

References

See also the relevant Cochrane reviews

Davies EA, Emmerson AM, Hogg GM, *et al*. An outbreak of infection with a methicillin resistant staphylococcus aureus in a special care baby unit: value of topical mupirocin and traditional methods of infection control. *J Hosp Infect* 1978;**10**:120–8.

Fortunov RM, Hulten KG, Hammerman WA, *et al*. Community-acquired *Staphylococcal aureus* infections in term and near-term previously healthy neonates. *Pediatrics* 2006;**118**:874–81.

Gemmell CG, Edwards DI, Fraise AP, *et al*. Guidelines for the prophylaxis and treatment of methicillin-resistant *Staphylococcus aureus* (MRSA) infections in the UK. *J Antimicrob Chemother* 2006;**57**:589–608. [SR]

Graham PL, Morel A-S, Zhou J, *et al*. Epidemiology of methicillin-susceptible *Staphylococcus aureus* in the neonatal intensive care unit. *Infect Control Hosp Epidemiol* 2002;**23**:677–82.

Grundmann H, Aires-de-Sousa M, Tiemersma E. Emergence and resurgence of meticillin-resistant *Staphylococcus aureus* as a public health threat. *Lancet* 2006;**368**:874–85. [SR]

Helai N, Carbonne A, Naas T, *et al*. Nosocomial outbreak of staphylococcal scalded skin syndrome in neonates: epidemiological investigation and control. *J Hosp Infect* 2005;**61**:130–8.

Isaacs D, Fraser S, Hogg G, *et al*. *Staphylococcus aureus* infections in Australian neonatal nurseries. *Arch Dis Child* 2004;**89**:F331–5.

Lally RT, Lanz E, Schrock CG. Rapid control of an outbreak of *Staphylococcus aureus* on a neonatal intensive care department using standard infection control practices and nasal mupirocin. *Am J Infect Control* 2004;**32**:44–7.

Muto CA, Jernigan JA, Ostrowsky BE, *et al*. Guideline for preventing nosocomial transmission of multidrug-resistant strains of *Staphylococcus aureus* and *Enterococcus*. *Infect Control Hosp Epidemiol* 2003;**24**:362–86. [SR]

Rode H, de Wet PM, Millar AJW, *et al*. Efficacy of mupirocin in cutaneous candidiasis. *Lancet* 1991;**338**:578.

Saiman L, Cronquist A, Wu F, *et al*. An outbreak of methicillin-resistant *Staphylococcus aureus* in a neonatal intensive care unit. *Infect Control Hosp Epidemiol* 2003;**24**:317–21. (See also pp. 314–16.)

Tan KW, Tay L, Lim SH. An outbreak of methicillin-resistant staphylococcus aureus in a neonatal intensive care unit in Singapore: a 20 month study of clinical characteristics and control. *Singapore Med J* 1994;**35**:277–82.

Zakrzewska-Bode A, Mujtjens HL, Liem KD, *et al*. Mupirocin resistance in coagulase-negative staphylococci, after topical prophylaxis for the reduction of colonisation of central venous lines. *J Hosp Infect* 1995;**31**:189–93.

NALOXONE

Use

Naloxone reverses the respiratory depression that can be caused by the use of opioids such as codeine, dextro-propoxyphene, diamorphine (heroin), fentanyl, meptazinol, methadone, morphine, nalbuphine and pethidine. Use, however, inevitably interferes with their ability to reduce pain. Naloxone can only partly reverse the effects of buprenorphine and pentazocine (which have both agonist and antagonist properties).

Pharmacology

Naloxone is a potent pure opioid antagonist first discovered in 1961. It crosses the placenta rapidly but is not known to be teratogenic. Large doses can be given without apparent toxicity (except in patients dependent on opioids) and repeated use does not cause dependence or tolerance. The drug is largely metabolised by glucuronide conjugation. The plasma half life is 1–3 hours immediately after birth but approaches that seen in adults (65 minutes) within a few days of birth (V_D ~2·5 l/kg). The drug is widely used, but even more widely abused, in the 'resuscitation' of babies at birth. Since it is a specific opioid antagonist it can have no place whatsoever in the resuscitation of a baby who has not been rendered drowsy by maternal analgesia. Even in these babies the only role of this drug is to check that opioid depression is not causing continued respiratory depression *after* breathing has been established (artificially if necessary) and *after* a reliable sustained cardiac output has been established. However, if the potential for opiate use (including epidural use) during labour to depress respiration has been exaggerated in the past, there is also evidence that its sedative effect may have more of an effect on the ability of the baby to play its part in the successful establishment of lactation than has been generally appreciated to date. This certainly remains an under-researched issue. A 3 microgram/kg oral dose of naloxone four times a day may help to reduce some of the constipation caused by morphine analgesia.

Neonatal opioid depression can certainly last quite a long time. A large maternal dose of pethidine (q.v.) during labour can sometimes make a baby drowsy and reluctant to feed for 2 days. While a single IV dose of naloxone will immediately reverse this depression, the benefit will only be transient because pethidine has such a long half life and naloxone such a short half life. Luckily a single 100 microgram/kg IM dose of naloxone seems to produce a drug 'depot' at the site of the injection that generates an effective plasma level of naloxone for at least 24 hours. Only occasionally is a second IM dose necessary.

A continuous infusion of naloxone is the best way to counteract accidental opiate poisoning in infancy. Such babies present with drowsiness, respiratory depression and pinpoint pupils. Hypotension is not uncommon and fits may occur. Similar infusions have also been used, anecdotally, to counteract the effect of the body's own endogenous opioids (β-endorphins) when their excessive release in severe septic shock lowers blood pressure and reduces cardiac output. Try the effect of a 50 microgram/kg IV bolus dose first. Methylene blue (q.v.) has also been used experimentally for the same purpose.

Treatment

Opioid sedation at birth: 100 micrograms/kg (0·25 ml/kg of 'adult' naloxone) IM has a gradual effect as an opioid antagonist, but an effect that is sustained for 24 hours. Treatment may be repeated if necessary. It is not necessary to calculate a precise weight-related dose – an initial 200 microgram dose, irrespective of weight, provides a pragmatic delivery room approach suitable for most babies.

Intravenous use: A 100 microgram/kg dose is of diagnostic help in opioid poisoning, and a continuous infusion of 50–100 micrograms/kg per hour in glucose or glucose saline will control stupor if it re-emerges.

Contraindications

Administration to the baby of an opiate-dependent mother could precipitate withdrawal symptoms. Nevertheless there is, at the moment, still only one published report of this precipitating seizures during resuscitation (see web commentary). The mother had taken a very high dose of methadone (60 mg) 8 hours earlier and documented fetal distress complicates the interpretation of this isolated case report.

Supply

1 ml (400 microgram) ampoules of naloxone marketed for 'adult' use are available costing £6·90 each. 40 microgram 'neonatal' ampoules are also available but not as useful. Midwives can give 100 micrograms/kg IM on their own authority to counteract the depressive effect of maternal opioid medication if the baby remains sleepy after neonatal resuscitation is complete.

References

See also the relevant Cochrane reviews

Akkawi R, Eksborg S, Andersson Å, *et al*. Effect of oral naloxone hydrochloride on gastrointestinal transit in premature infants treated with morphine. *Acta Paediatr* 2009;**98**:442–7.

American Academy of Pediatrics. Committee on Drugs. Naloxone dosage and route of administration for infants and children: addendum to emergency doses for infants and children. *Pediatrics* 1990;**86**:484–5. (See also 1998;**101**:1085.)

Furman WL, Menke JA, Barson WJ, *et al*. Continuous naloxone infusion in two neonates with septic shock. *J Pediatr* 1984;**105**:649–51.

Guinsburg R, Wykoff MH. Naloxone during neonatal resuscitation: acknowledging the unknown. *Clin Perinatol* 2006;**33**:121–32. [SR]

Jordan S, Emery S, Bradshaw C, *et al*. The impact of intrapartum analgesia on infant feeding. *Br J Obstet Gynaecol* 2005;**112**:927–34.

Morland TA, Brice JEH, Walker CHM, *et al*. Naloxone pharmacokinetics in the newborn. *Br J Clin Pharmacol* 1979;**9**:609–12.

Tenenbein M. Continuous naloxone infusion for opiate poisoning in infancy. *J Pediatr* 1984;**105**:645–8.

Werner PC, Hogg MI, Rosen M. Effects of naloxone on pethidine-induced neonatal depression. Part II – intramuscular naloxone. *BMJ* 1977;**2**:229–31.

Use
Neostigmine and edrophonium are used in the diagnosis and treatment of myasthenia.

Myasthenia
Myasthenia gravis is an acquired autoimmune disorder causing progressive muscle fatigue and weakness. About 10–15% of the babies born to myasthenic mothers are affected by transient neonatal myasthenia due to transfer from the maternal circulation of antibodies directed against the acetylcholine receptors of the muscle–nerve junction. Symptoms present within 1–3 days and usually persist for 3–6 weeks. There is no way of knowing before birth whether a baby is going to be affected or not, but most affected babies have mothers with high antibody titres and a history of affected siblings. The presence of hydramnios predicts severe involvement. In contrast, maternal disease is sometimes only recognised when the baby presents with symptoms at birth. Symptoms persist for months in the other congenital, recessively inherited, forms of myasthenia, although they usually become less severe with time. Respiratory and feeding difficulty may cause prolonged apnoea, aspiration and even death. Hypotonia is common, and stridor can be a problem. Some babies have multiple joint contractures (arthrogryposis) at birth. Ptosis (a drooping of the upper eye lid) is usually only seen in babies with maternally acquired autoimmune disease. Aminoglycoside antibiotics are hazardous in patients with any of the myasthenic disorders because they interfere with neuromuscular transmission causing respiratory depression. Some congenital myasthenic syndromes do not respond to neostigmine and pyridostigmine.

Pharmacology
Neostigmine (first developed in 1931) inhibits cholinesterase activity and therapy prolongs and intensifies the muscarinic and nicotinic effects of acetylcholine, causing vasodilatation, increased smooth muscle activity, lacrimation, salivation and improved voluntary muscle tone. It is therefore the drug of choice in the management of both maternal and neonatal myasthenia gravis. Intravenous edrophonium has a similar and much more rapid effect, but the response frequently only lasts 5–10 minutes. For this reason, most clinicians now prefer to use intramuscular neostigmine methylsulphate (with or without atropine to control any side effects), both for diagnostic and for maintenance purposes since this produces a response lasting 2–4 hours after a latent period of 20–30 minutes. Other rarer disorders require more complex diagnostic techniques (see Matthes *et al.* 1991; Newsom-Davis 1998).

Diagnostic use
Always have 15 micrograms/kg of IV atropine on hand to control any undue salivation, and equipment to control any unexpected respiratory arrest.
Edrophonium: Give 20 micrograms/kg IV followed, after 30 seconds, by a further 80 micrograms/kg IV if there is no adverse effect. Watch for bradycardia or arrhythmia. Double this dose has been used.
Neostigmine methylsulphate: Use a 150 microgram/kg IM test dose.

Treatment
Short-term management: 150 micrograms/kg of neostigmine methylsulphate subcutaneously, or IM, once every 6–8 hours is usually used for maintenance, but twice this dose may be necessary once every 4 hours. Oral treatment with neostigmine bromide can be used once control is achieved. An oral dose that is 10–20 times the IM maintenance dose will need to be given every 3 hours.
Long-term management: Oral pyridostigmine (another anticholinesterase) is preferable in the long-term management of myasthenia because it has a slightly longer duration of action. The usual starting dose is 1 mg/kg by mouth every 4 hours (unless the child is asleep). Adjust later as necessary.
Reversing drug-induced muscle paralysis: The effects of non-depolarising muscle relaxants such as pancuronium can be largely reversed by giving a combined IV injection of 10 micrograms/kg of glycopyrronium and 50 micrograms/kg of neostigmine (as outlined in the monograph on glycopyrronium).

Supply and administration
1 ml (2·5 mg) ampoules of neostigmine methylsulphate for IM use cost 58p each. For accurate administration take the contents of the ampoule and dilute to 16·5 ml with glucose or glucose saline immediately before use to give a solution containing approximately 150 micrograms/ml. 1 ml (10 mg) ampoules of edrophonium (costing £4·80) are also available on request. Inexpensive oral suspensions of neostigmine bromide or pyridostigmine in syrup are available on request.

References
Dubowitz V. Myasthenia. In: *Muscle disorders in childhood*, 2nd edn. London: Saunders, 1995: pp. 298–421.
Matthes JWA, Kenna AP, Fawcett PRW. Familial infantile myasthenia: a diagnostic problem. *Dev Med Child Neurol* 1991;**33**:924–9.
Morel E, Eymard B, Vernet de Gatabedian B, *et al*. Neonatal myasthenia gravis: a new clinical and immunological appraisal of 30 cases. *Neurology* 1988;**38**:138–42.
Newsom-Davis J. Autoimmune and genetic disorders at the neuromuscular junction. *Dev Med Child Neurol* 1998;**40**:199–206.
Volpe J. Neuromuscular disorders. In: *Neurology of the newborn*, 4th edn. Philadelphia: Saunders, 2001: pp. 657–70.

NEVIRAPINE

Use

Nevirapine is used to prevent babies of human immunodeficiency virus (HIV) positive women becoming infected during delivery. Use should always follow current guidelines. Combined treatment with zidovudine (q.v.) costs more, but further reduces viral transmission, and may make later drug resistance less likely. In resource-poor countries continued daily prophylaxis (2 mg/kg for 2 weeks and then 4 mg/kg a day) greatly decreases the risk of infection during lactation (see web commentary).

Pharmacology

Nevirapine is a *non*-nucleoside reverse transcriptase inhibitor (NNRTI) that binds to reverse transcriptase, thus inhibiting viral replication. For prophylaxis, use with at least one nucleoside reverse transcriptor inhibitor (NRTI) drug – the most widely studied is zidovudine (q.v.). Nevirapine is well absorbed by mouth, widely distributed ($V_D \sim 1.2$ l/kg), penetrates the CSF well and, because it is lipophilic, is rapidly transferred across the placenta. There is no evidence of teratogenicity. It is extensively metabolised by the cytochrome P450 isoenzyme system in the liver with a half life of 40–60 hours when treatment is first started – a half life that is almost halved by enzyme autoinduction after 1–2 weeks. It is also reduced in patients on rifampicin, but extended in patients taking a range of other drugs including cimetidine, erythromycin and fluconazole. The most important adverse effects with sustained use, commonest in the first months of treatment, are a skin rash (sometimes severe) and liver dysfunction (which may make it necessary to suspend or stop treatment). Hypersensitivity reactions can also be a problem. Enough nevirapine appears in breast milk to inhibit viral replication.

Post-delivery care of babies born to HIV infected mothers

Without treatment at least one-third of babies born to infected mothers will themselves become infected, and half of these will die, or become ill with the acquired immune deficiency syndrome (AIDS) by the age of 6 years. Most will become symptomatic within 5–11 months. The higher the mother's viral load, the greater the risk of transmission. Vertical infection can be assumed if virus or antigen is detected (using a viral DNA PCR probe) in blood samples taken on two separate occasions (excluding any sample taken at birth because of the risk of contamination with maternal blood). One of these samples should be collected at least 4 months after birth. Conversely, freedom from infection can be presumed if two separate blood samples from the baby are antibody negative and no virus or antigen has ever been detected – provided the baby is *not* breastfeeding (transplacentally acquired maternal antigen can persist in the baby for up to 18 months). With appropriate treatment it has recently become possible to reduce the risk of vertical transmission to 1%. However, expert advice **must** be sought. The best advice often involves the use of more than one drug, and is frequently revised. Check for up to date treatment guidelines – USA: www.AIDSinfo.nih.gov, and UK: www.bhiva.org

Simple intrapartum prophylaxis in a resource-poor setting

The following strategies are *only* appropriate in a previously untreated mother in a resource-poor setting.
If started before delivery: Give a 200 mg oral dose of nevirapine at the start of labour to *all* mothers not on any retroviral drug treatment, and one 2 mg/kg dose of nevirapine to the baby 2 days after birth.
If started after delivery: Give the baby one 2 mg/kg dose of nevirapine by mouth as soon as possible after birth, and 4 mg/kg of zidovudine by mouth twice a day for 7 days.

Full intrapartum prophylaxis using several drugs

See the recommendations in the monograph on lamivudine.

Post-delivery multidrug treatment of suspected infection

Neonate: Give 2 mg/kg once a day for 2 weeks and then 5 mg/kg once a day in babies under 2 months old.
Older babies: Start with 4 mg/kg *once* a day for 2 weeks, and than 7 mg/kg *twice* a day unless a rash or other serious side effect develops. Such treatment should only be started where there is at least some provisional evidence that the baby has become infected, as discussed in the monograph on lamivudine.

Supply

200 mg nevirapine tablets cost £2·80 each; 100 ml of a 10 mg/ml suspension in sucrose costs £21.

References

See also the relevant Cochrane reviews

Jackson JB, Musoke P, Fleming T, *et al*. Intrapartum and neonatal single-dose nevirapine compared to zidovudine for prevention of mother-to-child transmission of HIV-1 in Kampala, Uganda: 18 month follow-up of the HIVNET012 randomised trial. *Lancet* 2003;**362**:859–68. [RCT] (See also editorial on pp. 842–3.)

Jourdain G, Ngo-Giang-Huong N, La Coeur S, *et al*. Intrapartum exposure to nevirapine and subsequent maternal responses to nevirapine-based antiretroviral therapy. *N Engl J Med* 2004;**351**:229–40. [RCT] (See also pp. 289–92.)

Kumwenda NI, Hoover DR, Mofenson LM, *et al*. Extended antiretroviral prophylaxis to reduce breast-milk HIV-1 transmission. *N Engl J Med* 2008;**359**:119–29. [RCT] (See also pp. 189–91.)

Shapiro RL, Holland RT, Capparelli E, *et al*. Antiretroviral concentrations in breast-feeding infants of women in Botswana receiving antiretroviral treatment. *J Infect Dis* 2005;**192**:720–7. (See also pp. 709–12.)

Stringer JSA, Rouse DJ, Sinkala M, *et al*. Nevirapine to prevent mother-to-child transmission of HIV-1 among women of unknown serostatus. *Lancet* 2003;**362**:185–3.

Taha TE, Kumwenda NI, Gibbins A, *et al*. Short postexposure prophylaxis in newborn babies to reduce mother-to-child transmission of HIV-1: NVAZ randomised trial. *Lancet* 2003;**362**:1171–7. [RCT]

Volmink J, Marais B. HIV: mother-to-child transmission. *BMJ Clinical evidence handbook*. London: BMJ Books, 2009: pp. 234–6 (and updates). [SR]

Use

Nifedipine is a smooth muscle relaxant used to manage hypertension, cardiomyopathy, angina and Raynaud phenomenon. It seems more effective than β-mimetics and as good as atosiban at delaying preterm birth, and may well be the best drug to use to delay delivery long enough for betametasone (q.v.) to speed the maturation of the fetal lung even if the baby is still born early.

Pharmacology

Nifedipine, first introduced in 1968, is one of a range of oral drugs used to cause a reduction in vascular tone (including coronary artery tone) by reducing slow channel cell membrane calcium uptake. All calcium channel-blocking drugs also reduce cardiac contractility, but the vasodilator effect of nifedipine is more influential than the myocardial effect. Nifedipine also reduces uterine muscle tone. It is quite well absorbed through the buccal mucosa (having some effect within 5 minutes) and is then metabolised by the liver (adult half life 2–3 hours) before being excreted in the urine. Despite widespread use, the manufacturers are not yet prepared to recommend use in childhood, or in pregnancy, although there is no evidence of teratogenicity in man. Breastfeeding is not contraindicated since the baby only receives about 3% of the maternal dose when intake is calculated on a weight-for-weight basis.

Controlling preterm labour

Unexplained spontaneous preterm labour accounts for more than half of all births before 32 weeks' gestation, and obstetric intervention has yet to make any impact on this cause of preterm birth. Indometacin (q.v.), ethanol (alcohol), nifedipine and the betamimetics terbutaline and salbutamol (q.v.) are all capable of delaying delivery for 2–3 days, but nifedipine is the only tocolytic that has yet been shown to inhibit labour for long enough to reduce the number of babies requiring intensive care and use did halve the number delivering within 7 days in one small trial. Atosiban (q.v.), an oxytocin receptor antagonist introduced in 1998, is probably at least as effective (although no very satisfactory head-to-head trial has yet been done) and does not run the risk of causing hypotension, but it is much more expensive and has to be given IV. Antibiotic treatment does nothing to delay delivery in uncomplicated preterm labour, but treatment with erythromycin (q.v.) *did* delay delivery and improve neonatal outcome in women with preterm prelabour rupture of membranes. Progesterone (q.v.) prophylaxis may benefit those women with a past history of unexplained very preterm labour with a very short cervix.

Treatment

Controlling preterm labour: Crush one 10 mg capsule between the teeth to achieve sublingual absorption. Up to three further doses may be given at 15-minute intervals while watching for hypotension if contractions persist. If this stops labour give between 20 and 50 mg of modified-release nifedipine three times a day for 3 days. Some then recommend giving 20 mg three times a day until pregnancy reaches 34 weeks.

Hyperinsulinaemic hypoglycaemia: 100–200 micrograms/kg by mouth once every 6 hours seems to improve glucose control in some patients also taking diazoxide (q.v.). Where there is no response, doubling or tripling the dose may occasionally be helpful. Watch for hypotension.

Hypertension in children: 200–500 micrograms/kg by mouth every 6–8 hours is now increasingly used to control hypertension, and to treat angina in Kawasaki disease. Start with the lowest dose and increase as necessary. Consider managing the initial reduction in pressure in a controlled way using IV labetalol (q.v.), especially where hypertension has existed for a sustained, or unknown, time.

Drug interactions

The simultaneous use of magnesium sulphate sometimes causes sudden profound muscle weakness.

Supply

10 mg nifedipine capsules cost 4p each. A range of modified release tablets and capsules are available, and a sustained release tablet, that only needs to be taken once a day, is also now available for use in adults. A 20 mg/ml (1 mg per drop) dropper bottle formulation is importable on a 'named patient' basis for babies. A suspension containing 1 mg/ml can be prepared on request which is stable for a month if protected from light. No IV or IM formulation is available.

References

See also the relevant Cochrane reviews and UK guideline on tocolysis

Adcock KM, Wilson JT. Nifedipine labelling illustrates the pediatric dilemma for off-patent drugs. *Pediatrics* 2002;**109**:319–21.

Blaszak RT, Savage JA, Ellis EN. The use of short-acting nifedipine in pediatric patients with hypertension. *J Pediatr* 2001;**139**:34–7.

Haas DM. Preterm birth. *BMJ Clinical evidence handbook*. London: BMJ Books, 2007: pp. 435–7 (and updates). [SR]

Jacquemyn Y. Atosiban v nifedipine. [Letter] *BMJ* 2009;**338**:904.

Lamont RF, Khan KS, Beattie B, *et al*. The quality of nifedipine studies used to assess tocolytic efficacy: a systematic review. *J Perinat Med* 2005;**33**:287–95. [SR]

Müller D, Zimmering M, Roehr CC. Should nifedipine be used to counter low blood sugar levels in children with persistent hyperinsulinaemic hypoglycaemia? *Arch Dis Child* 2004;**89**:83–5. [SR]

Papatsonis DNM, Kok JH, van Geijn HP, *et al*. Neonatal effects of nifedipine and ritodrine for preterm labour. *Obstet Gynecol* 2000;**95**:477–81. [RCT]

Simhan HN, Caritis SN. Prevention of preterm birth. [Review] *N Engl J Med* 2007;**357**:477–87.

Tsatsaris V, Papatsonis F, Goffinet D, *et al*. Tocolysis with nifedipine or beta-adrenergic agents: a meta-analysis. *Obstet Gynecol* 2001;**97**:840–7. [SR]

Use

Nitazoxanide is a relatively new drug that can be used to treat a range of parasitic infections including, uniquely, the illness caused by the protozoal parasites *Cryptosporidium parvum* and *C. hominis*.

Pharmacology

Nitazoxanide is a nitrothiazole benzamide that is increasingly recognised as being an effective treatment for a wide range of intestinal protozoal and helminthic infections. It was initially developed in 1975 as a veterinary drug because of its activity against intestinal nematodes, cestodes and liver trematodes, and has been used, as an investigational drug, since 1996 to treat children with debilitating diarrhoea due to a range of protozoal infections, including cryptosporidiosis and giardiasis. It seems more effective than albendazole (q.v.) in the treatment of children with whipworm (infection with *Trichuris trichiura*), and as effective (if more expensive than) albendazole in the treatment of ascariasis (infection with the round worm *Ascariasis lumbricoides*). It is also effective in fascioliasis (infection with *Fasciola hepatica*), amoebiasis (infection with *Entamoeba histolytica* and *E. dispar*) and isosporiasis (infection with *Isospora belli*). More importantly, it is the first drug to be recognised as effective in the management of cryptosporidiosis, and the manufacturers were permitted to recommend its use in North and South America in 2002 for children with this condition who are at least 12 months old. Use to treat giardiasis was also approved, but this is usually as effectively (and more cheaply) treated with metronidazole (q.v.). Early reports suggest it may also be effective in rotavirus diarrhoea. The drug has been in use in Latin America for 10 years, but has not yet been reviewed by UK licensing authorities.

Nitazoxanide is well absorbed when taken by mouth, and absorption is improved when the drug is taken with food. This prodrug is rapidly metabolised by glucuronidation in the liver to the active drug tizoxanide, and then cleared from the blood with a terminal half life of 7 hours. Two-thirds appears in bile and faeces, and one-third in the urine. Children metabolise the drug in much the same way as adults, but drug handling has not yet been studied in children less than a year old. Adverse effects (abdominal pain and vomiting) seem no commoner than with placebo treatment. Animal studies suggest that use during pregnancy is unlikely to be hazardous, and extensive plasma protein binding means that very little active drug appears in breast milk.

Cryptosporidiosis

Cryptosporidium parvum is a spore-forming coccidian protozoal parasite found in a wide range of hosts including mammals, birds and reptiles. Serious waterborne outbreaks are not uncommon and may make it important to boil drinking water (since the parasite is resistant to chlorine). Swimming pools are a common source of cross infection, and child-to-child transmission is also common. The organism is also a common cause of 'traveller's diarrhoea'. The incubation period is usually about 7 days (range 2–14 days). Infection causes frequent, non-bloody, watery diarrhoea. This clears spontaneously in 2–3 weeks in most healthy individuals, but infection often causes severe persistent infection and even death in immunocompromised individuals. Persisting infection can also stunt growth and impair later cognitive function in seriously malnourished young children even when there is no evidence of HIV infection, and, in a severely ill, hospitalised, child, there is currently a 10–20% risk of death. Diagnosis is best made by examining the stool for oocysts, but these are small (4–6 μm in diameter) and easily missed unless a floatation-concentrated stool smear is examined after auramine-phenol staining. Measures to prevent dehydration and to correct any electrolyte imbalance are all that are necessary in a child who was previously well, but the search for an antimicrobial agent that is curative had been unavailing until nitazoxanide first became available.

Treatment

100 mg by mouth twice a day for 3 days was shown to be effective in combating diarrhoea, and in reducing mortality in seriously malnourished 1–3-year-old children with severe cryptosporidiosis in one recent small trial. It also eliminated all parasites from the stool. One study used a dose of 7·5 mg/kg twice a day for 3 days in children less than a year old. Albendazole seems more effective in children with HIV infection.

Supply

Nitazoxanide is made by Romark Laboratories, Tampa, Florida (tel. 813 282 8544). It has FDA approval but no UK licence. 1·2 grams of powder currently costs $60. Reconstitute with 48 ml of tap water to obtain 60 ml of a sucrose-containing, strawberry-flavoured 20 mg/ml suspension. Shake before use, and discard after 7 days.

References

Abaza H, El-Zayadi A, Kabil SM, *et al*. Nitazoxanide in the treatment of patients with intestinal protozoan and helminthic infections: a report on 546 patients in Egypt. *Curr Ther Res* 1998;**59**:116–21.

Amadi B, Mwiya M, Musuku J, *et al*. Effect of nitazoxanide on morbidity and mortality in Zambian children with cryptosporidiosis: a randomised controlled trial. *Lancet* 2002;**360**:1375–80. [RCT]

Bailey JM, Errsmouspe J. Nitazoxanide treatment for giardiasis and cryptosporidiosis in children. *Ann Pharmacother* 2004;**38**:634–40. [SR]

Davies AP, Chalmers RM. Cryptosporidiosis [Review] *BMJ* 2009;**339**:b4168.

Romero-Cabello R, Guerrero LR, Muñóz-Garcia M, *et al*. Nitazoxanide for the treatment of intestinal protozoan and helminthic infections in Mexico. *Trans R Soc Trop Med Hyg* 1997;**91**:701–3.

Rossignol J-F, Abu-Zekry M, Hussein A, *et al*. Effect of nitazoxanide for treatment of severe rotavirus diarrhoea: randomised double-blind placebo-controlled trial. *Lancet* 2006;**368**:124–9. [RCT] (See also pp. 100–1.)

Rossignol JF, Ayoub A, Ayers MS. Treatment of diarrhea caused by *Cryptosporidium parvum*: a prospective randomized, double-blind, placebo-controlled study of nitazoxanide. *J Infect Dis* 2001;**184**:103–6. [RCT]

Use

Nitisinone is used to prevent the accumulation of toxic metabolites in patients with type I tyrosinaemia.

Biochemistry

Tyrosinaemia type I is a rare, recessively inherited disorder that is caused by a deficiency of fumarylacetoacetase, the enzyme involved in the fifth step of tyrosine breakdown. It is seen in about 1:100,000 births. Symptoms result from the accumulation of fumarylacetoacetate and succinylacetone, which are toxic. The condition is of variable severity but can present within weeks of birth with signs of liver failure, including jaundice (which is often misleadingly mild), diarrhoea, vomiting, oedema, ascites, hypoglycaemia and a severe bleeding tendency. Cirrhosis usually develops over time, and there is a significant long-term risk of hepatocellular carcinoma. Milder cases present later in childhood or early adult life with isolated hepatomegaly, liver failure or hypophosphataemic rickets due to renal tubular dysfunction. Plasma tyrosine levels are usually elevated, but diagnosis depends on demonstrating raised urinary levels of succinylacetone. In a few patients succinylacetone levels are only slightly raised, and enzyme assay may be needed to confirm the diagnosis. Acute neurological crises can occur, with abdominal pain, muscle weakness and hypertension, when toxic metabolites trigger other problems similar to those seen in acute intermittent porphyria.

Management was transformed in 1992 by the development of nitisinone (2-(2-nitro-4-trifluoro-methylbenzoyl)-1,3-cyclohexanedione) or NTBC. This inhibits the second enzyme in the pathway of tyrosine metabolism (4-hydroxy-phenylpyruvate dioxygenase). However, while this prevents the formation of fumarylaceto-acetate and succinylacetone, it causes a marked rise in the plasma tyrosine concentration. Very high tyrosine levels can lead to the deposition of crystals in the cornea, causing photophobia and corneal erosions; it is also possible that high tyrosine levels may cause learning difficulties. Because of this, treatment with nitisinone still needs to be combined with a diet low in tyrosine and phenylalanine. Other adverse effects include transient thrombocytopenia and neutropenia. Treatment should be started as soon as the diagnosis is made, and continued indefinitely. Whether management with nitisinone can completely eliminate the need for liver transplantation will only be known once it is shown that such treatment removes the latent risk of liver cancer. Use during pregnancy or lactation is, as yet, unevaluated.

Treatment

Initial care: Infants presenting with liver failure when first diagnosed require intensive support, and should, if possible, be transferred to a liver unit because a few do not respond to nitisinone and require urgent transplantation. Fresh frozen plasma (q.v.) may be required for coagulation failure.
Continuing care: Start regular maintenance with 0·5 mg/kg of nitisinone twice a day by mouth. Slightly more may sometimes be necessary. The intake of natural protein may need to be restricted and the diet supplemented using an amino acid mixture free of tyrosine and phenylalanine. Supplemental oral vitamin K is sometimes required, and rickets may benefit from treatment with additional vitamin D (q.v.).

Monitoring

Patients should be managed in collaboration with a specialist in metabolic disease. Diet needs to allow normal growth while aiming to keep the plasma tyrosine level below 500 µmol/l. The dose of nitisinone is adjusted by assessing the biochemical response. Some centres also monitor the plasma concentration (the therapeutic nitisinone level usually being between 25 and 50 µmol/l). Serum α-fetoprotein levels should be measured serially, and regular liver scans undertaken to watch for early signs of liver cancer.

Supply and administration

2, 5 and 10 mg capsules of nitisinone (costing £9·30, £18·80 and £34 each) are available on a 'named patient' basis from Orphan Europe. Divide the daily dose, where possible, into two (not necessarily equal) parts, given morning and evening. The capsules can be opened and the content suspended, immediately before use, in a little water or milk. An application for a licence to market this product is said to be pending with the European regulatory authorities.

References

Chakrapani A, Holme E. Disorders of tyrosine metabolism. In: Fernandes J, Saudubray J-M, van den Berghe G, et al., eds. *Inborn metabolic diseases. Diagnosis and treatment*, 4th edn. Berlin: Springer-Verlag, 2006: pp. 233–43.
Holme E, Lindstedt S. Tyrosinaemia type 1 and NTBC (2-(2-nitro-4-trifluomethylbenzoyl)-1,3,-cyclohexanedione). *J Inherit Metab Dis* 1998;**21**:507–17.
McKiernan PJ. Nitisinone in the treatment of hereditary tyrosinaemia type 1. *Drugs* 2006;**66**:743–50.
Mitchell GA, Grompe M, Lambert M, et al. Disorders of tyrosine metabolism. In: Scriver CR, Beaudet AL, Sly WS, et al., eds. *The metabolic and molecular bases of inherited disease*, 8th edn. New York: McGraw-Hill, 2001: pp. 1777–806.

Use

Nitric oxide use can reduce the need for extracorporeal membrane oxygenation (ECMO) in babies of ≥34 weeks' gestation with persisting high pulmonary vascular resistance, but survival is not increased. Prior echocardiography must be done to confirm pulmonary hypertension and exclude structural heart disease. No trial has yet shown treatment to be of convincing and sustained benefit in babies less mature than this.

Pharmacology

It has long been realised that one influence on the muscles that surround all blood vessels is a 'relaxing factor' produced in the vessel's endothelial lining cells. That 'factor' was finally shown, in 1987, to be nitric oxide. This small, elusive molecule influences blood flow by affecting vessel tone, and inhibits labour by reducing uterine muscle tone. It also influences macrophage function, and acts as a neurotransmitter. Breathing this highly diffusable colourless gas can reduce the tone of blood vessels in the lung and, because the gas only has a very short half life in the body (2–4 seconds), it can lower pulmonary vascular resistance without lowering systemic blood pressure. Nebulised nitroprusside (q.v.) seems to be an equally effective, and much cheaper, short-term option. Tolazoline (q.v.) has been given as an endotracheal bolus to a few babies, and might be expected to have a more sustained effect. Neubulised epoprostenol (q.v.) has also been tried. 'Rescue' treatment with nitric oxide only seems of transient benefit in babies of <34 weeks' gestation, but further trials are looking for evidence that earlier intervention might be more effective.

Excess nitric oxide enters the blood stream where it is quickly inactivated, combining with haemoglobin to produce methaemoglobin. While this molecule is inert, its existence reduces the oxygen-carrying capacity of the blood. The level should therefore be checked an hour after treatment is started and then once every 12 hours, aiming to keep the level below 2·5%. Try to reduce the dose of nitric oxide if the level exceeds 4%, and give methylene blue (q.v.) if it exceeds 7%. Many trials have limited recruitment to babies with a platelet count of >50 × 10^9/l, INR of <2 and/or partial thromboplastin time (PTT) of <72 seconds because nitric oxide increases the risk of haemorrhage by inhibiting platelet aggregation, but use does not usually seem to cause a bleeding problem. Nitric oxide (NO) reacts with oxygen to form nitrogen dioxide (NO_2), and the level of this needs to be monitored, since some byproducts are toxic. Leakage could put staff at risk unless an alarm system exists, and poorly ventilated areas need a gas scavenging system, but most delivery systems address these issues.

Use in babies with persisting pulmonary hypertension

Starting treatment: Start by adding 20 parts per million (ppm) of nitric oxide to the ventilator gas circuit. If this produces a response (a rise of at least 3 kPa in post-ductal arterial pO_2 within 15 minutes while ventilator settings are held constant) the amount given should be reduced, after 1 hour, to the lowest dose compatible with a sustained response. Wean off treatment promptly if there is no response.

Weaning: Failure to use the lowest effective dose causes dependency. So does prolonged use. Try to reduce the dose needed in 'responders' once every 12 hours. Lower the concentration by 10% once every 3 minutes, but reverse any reduction that causes arterial saturation to drop more than 2–3%. Babies sometimes require a low dose (<0·5 ppm) for several days during weaning, even if no response was seen initially. Increasing the inspired oxygen concentration 20% may facilitate final 'weaning'.

Use in other children

Use can occasionally help to control postoperative pulmonary hypertension in older children after cardiac surgery, but there are *no* clear-cut indications for use. One trial did find that low-dose use started in preterm babies still ventilated at 7–14 days might marginally increase the number alive and not in oxygen (28% *v.* 49%) at 36 weeks. Several other large trials have, however, now shown that, except in the rare baby with overt echocardiographic evidence of pulmonary hypertension, use does *not* improve survival, or reduce the incidence of disability at 2 years in babies born more than about 8 weeks early, even when it does initially make the baby slightly less oxygen dependent. The scope for use in other children with severe respiratory failure remains unclear. Use is not helpful in patients with adult respiratory distress syndrome (ARDS).

Supply and administration

Nitric oxide was, until recently, an ill-defined therapeutic product, but use in term infants with pulmonary hypertension has now been approved by the regulatory authorities in Europe and North America. Now that the gas has received formal recognition as a medicinal product, a single company (INO Therapeutics Inc.) has acquired sole marketing rights, and this company makes uniform delivery and monitoring systems available to hospitals for an hourly fee. Since this arrangement seems to have increased the cost of treatment more than ten-fold, it is going to be important to mount further studies into the cost-effectiveness of this and other strategies for modifying pulmonary vascular tone.

References

See also the relevant Cochrane reviews

Barrington KJ, Finer NN. Inhaled nitric oxide for preterm infants: a systematic review. *Pediatrics* 2007;**120**:1088–99. [SR]

Hibbs AM, Walsh MC, Martin RJ, *et al.* One-year respiratory outcomes of preterm infants enrolled in the Nitric Oxide (to Prevent) Chronic Lung Disease Trial. *J Pediatr* 2008;**153**:525–9. [RCT]

Kinsella JP. Inhaled nitric oxide in the term newborn. [Review] *Early Hum Dev* 2008;**84**:709–16.

Tanaka Y, Hayashi T, Kitajima H, *et al.* Inhaled nitric oxide therapy decreases the risk of cerebral palsy in preterm infants with persistent pulmonary hypertension of the newborn. *Pediatrics* 2007;**119**:1159–64.

Use

Sodium nitroprusside is a direct, very rapid acting, peripheral vasodilator often used to reduce afterload when left ventricular function is impaired. It can be used to control systemic hypertension, and has been used, experimentally, as an alternative to tolazoline (q.v.) to produce selective pulmonary vasodilatation.

Pharmacology

Sodium nitroprusside is a potent vasodilator first developed in 1951 that is now known to cause smooth muscle relaxation by acting as a direct nitric oxide donor. At **low** doses nitroprusside reduces systemic vascular resistance and increases cardiac output. This may be associated with a slight increase in heart rate, but significant tachycardia is unusual. It decreases right atrial pressure, pulmonary capillary wedge pressure and pulmonary vascular resistance. However, a **high** IV dose of nitroprusside can produce serious systemic hypotension and can also exacerbate myocardial ischaemia (a tendency aggravated by volume depletion). When directed specifically at the pulmonary vasculature by nebulisation it can cause very marked pulmonary vasodilatation without having any detectable systemic effect. Indeed one study has suggested that such treatment can be as effective, in the short term, as treatment with nitric oxide (q.v.) in babies with hypoxic respiratory failure. It is also cheaper, and use does not require specialist equipment.

Little is known about the long-term use or safety of nitroprusside when prescribed during pregnancy or lactation, but short-term use to control pregnancy-induced hypertension seems safe even though it causes a 30% reduction in uterine blood flow. Nitroprusside is broken down to cyanide in the body, which is quickly metabolised to thiocyanate in the liver and then slowly excreted by the kidneys (half life 4 days). Tissue levels exceed plasma levels (V_D ~3 l/kg). Prolonged or high-dose infusions of nitroprusside, or the presence of hepatic or renal impairment, can cause a dangerous accumulation of these toxic products. Prolonged use can also lead to hypothyroidism as thiocyanate inhibits iodine uptake into the thyroid gland.

The manufacturers have not yet issued any advice about the use of nitroprusside in children, but toxic side effects have never been described at infusion rates of 2 micrograms/kg per minute, and rates of up to 8 micrograms/kg per minute are generally considered safe. The cerebral vasodilatation caused by nitroprusside may be undesirable in some neonates, but many cardiothoracic centres routinely use this drug in the initial control of the paradoxical hypertension sometimes seen after coarctectomy. The rapidity with which the drug works, and the rapidity with which the drug is degraded, make nitroprusside a relatively safe drug to use with due monitoring in an intensive care setting. Continuous blood pressure monitoring is advisable, and invasive monitoring wise. A single 1 mg/kg dose of phenoxybenzamine, a powerful α blocker, may be better at maintaining organ perfusion during cardiopulmonary bypass surgery, but causes sustained vasodilatation only reversible using vasopressin (q.v.).

Treatment

Intravenous: Give 500 nanograms/kg of nitroprusside per minute. Monitor systemic blood pressure and increase the dose infused cautiously, as necessary, to no more than 8 micrograms/kg per minute.

Nebulised: Giving a nebulised solution containing 25 mg of nitroprusside dissolved in 2 ml 0·9% sodium chloride into the ventilator gas circuit causes very effective, short lasting, selective pulmonary vasodilatation.

Compatibility

Nitroprusside can be added (terminally) to an IV line containing atracurium, dobutamine and/or dopamine, glyceryl trinitrate, midazolam or milrinone.

Antidote

Tachycardia, arrhythmia, sweating and an acidosis suggest cyanide toxicity, especially after sustained treatment despite poor renal function. Correct the acidosis and give 0·3 ml/kg of 3% sodium nitrite IV (unless there is overt cyanosis) followed by 0·8 ml/kg of a 50% solution of IV sodium thiosulphate.

Supply and administration

Nitroprusside: 50 mg vials cost £6·60. Reconstitute for IV use with 2 ml of 5% glucose. Take 0·2 ml (5 mg) of this solution and dilute up to 10 ml with 5% glucose (500 micrograms/ml). Then take 3 ml of this solution for each kg the baby weighs and dilute to 25 ml with 5% glucose (60 micrograms/kg per ml). Infuse this solution at 1 ml/hour to give 1000 nanograms/kg (i.e. 1 microgram/kg) per minute. Prepare a fresh infusion once every 24 hours. Store ampoules in the dark (discarding any that become brownish), and shade the infusate from light, because this causes nitroprusside to break down to cyanide and ferrocyanide.

Phenoxybenzamine hydrochloride: 2 ml (100 mg) vials cost £32 each.

References

Mestan KKL, Carlson AD, White M, *et al*. Cardiopulmonary effects of nebulized sodium nitroprusside in term infants with hypoxic respiratory failure. *J Pediatr* 2003;**143**:640–3.

Motta P, Mossad E, Toscana D, *et al*. Comparison of phenoxybenzamine and sodium nitroprusside in infants undergoing surgery. *J Cardiothorac Vasc Anesth* 2005;**19**:54–9.

Palhares DB, Figueiredo CS, Moura AJM. Endotracheal inhalatory sodium nitroprusside in severely hypoxic newborns. *J Perinat Med* 1998;**26**:219–24.

NITROUS OXIDE

Use

A mixture of 50% nitrous oxide (N_2O) provides very safe conscious analgesia in children (although there are, as yet, few reports of its use in children under 1 year). Higher concentrations bring little extra benefit.

History

Humphry Davy, who first described this gas in 1800, was shrewd enough to see that it might be used 'with great advantage in surgical operations where no great effusion of blood takes place.' Despite this, it was the intoxicating and amnesic effect of 'laughing gas' that was exploited for 44 years before Wells first used the drug during dentistry. Although Queen Victoria used chloroform, it was many years before inhalation analgesia became common in childbirth, partly because the early Minnitt machine could leave a woman breathing as little as 10% oxygen. The 'Lucy Baldwin' machine (named after the UK Prime Minister's wife who did much to champion its use by midwives) made safe pain relief available during home births, but single cylinders containing a 50:50 nitrous oxide:oxygen mixture then came into use in the 1960s.

Pharmacology

Use of a 50% mixture causes conscious analgesia after 3 minutes, and this persists for about 3 minutes after inhalation ceases. Swallowing is depressed but laryngeal reflexes are retained. Use in any patient with an air-containing closed space (such as a pneumothorax or loculated air within a damaged lung) is potentially dangerous because nitrous oxide diffuses into the space causing a significant increase in pressure. Diffusion hypoxia, due to nitrous oxide returning to the alveoli from the blood stream more rapidly than it is replaced by nitrogen at the end of the procedure, can be minimised by giving oxygen.

A recent large French study has shown that nurse-supervised use in children to provide short-term analgesia for a range of investigative and treatment procedures can be extremely safe. The only significant problems encountered during procedures lasting up to 30 minutes were mild hypoxaemia, brief apnoea, bradycardia and oversedation (loss of verbal contact lasting more than 5 minutes), though such problems were only encountered in 0·3% of all procedures. They were, however, slightly commoner in children who had also been given both an opioid and a benzodiazepine sedative, and in children less than 1 year old (where 2% experienced some mild adverse effect). Transient dizziness and nausea can be a problem, but only 1% of procedures had to be cancelled because of inadequate sedation or a side effect.

Safe use in young children

Use must be supervised by someone who has undergone appropriate training, and should be supervised by a qualified anaesthetist in any child who is drowsy or who has also had another sedative (especially any benzodiazapine or opioid). Do nothing for 4 hours after the child last had milk or solid food (2 hours after clear liquids). Do nothing painful for 3 minutes after starting to give the gas, and stop the procedure if pain relief is inadequate, as may inexplicably happen in 5% of all procedures. Always use a pulse oximeter and have oxygen to hand in case brief diffusion hypoxia occurs during recovery. Use always requires the presence of at least two people, because the person undertaking the procedure for which analgesia is being offered must **never** be the person supervising the administration of nitrous oxide. See the website for a review of use in very young children. Very frequent use in a child could lower body cobalamin (B_{12}) stores.

Pain relief

Maternal pain relief in labour: An MRC trial found a 50% mixture in oxygen uniformly safe and helpful. A 70% mixture probably brought added benefit, but rendered a few women briefly unconscious.
Pain relief in infancy: Use must be supervised by appropriately trained staff (see above).

Supply and administration

Premixed supplies of 50% nitrous oxide in oxygen (Entonox® and Equanox®) come in blue cylinders with a blue and white shoulder. Refills cost about £10. Storage at temperatures below −6°C can cause the gases to separate – should this happen the cylinder *must* be laid horizontally in a warm room for 24 hours and briefly inverted before use. School-age children should be encouraged to use a mouth piece or face mask and demand valve, because self-control ensures that use ceases if the patient becomes drowsy. A constant flow system with a blender like the Quantiflex®, which shuts down if the oxygen supply fails, makes safe administration of a variable dose possible. Good room ventilation, or a waste gas scavenging system, must be provided where frequent use occurs, to stop the ambient level exceeding 100 ppm, since chronic exposure could interfere with the action of vitamin B_{12} and cause megaloblastic anaemia. There is one report that chronic exposure (once common during dental surgery) might lower female fertility.

References

See SIGN guidelines on sedation of children for procedures

Babl FE, Oakley E, Seaman C, *et al*. High-concentration nitrous oxide for procedural sedation in children: adverse events and depth of sedation. *Pediatrics* 2008;**121**:e528–32.

Gall O, Annequin D, Benoit G, *et al*. Adverse events of premixed nitrous oxide and oxygen for procedural sedation in children. *Lancet* 2001;**358**:1514–15.

Medical Research Council, Committee on Nitrous Oxide and Oxygen Analgesia in Midwifery. Clinical trials of different concentrations of oxygen and nitrous oxide for obstetric analgesia. *BMJ* 1970;**i**:709–13.

Rosen MA. Nitrous oxide for relief of labour pain; a systemic review. *Am J Obstet Gynecol* 2003;**186**:S110–26. [SR]

Use
Noradrenaline is a potent vasoconstrictor that is sometimes used to treat severe refractory hypotension (as in patients with septic shock) once any hypovolaemia caused by fluid leaking from damaged capillaries into the extravascular tissue space has been corrected. Milrinone (q.v.) may prove more effective if the hypotension is, at least in part, due to a fall in cardiac output.

Pharmacology
Sympathomimetic agents mimic the actions produced by stimulation of the postganglionic sympathetic nerves, preparing the body for 'fight or flight'. Three natural catecholamine agents have been identified: dopamine (primarily a central neurotransmitter), noradrenaline (a sympathetic neurotransmitter) and adrenaline (which has metabolic and hormonal functions). Metabolism is rapid, if variable, so stable concentrations are reached within 10–15 minutes of starting an infusion and clearance is not influenced by renal function. The agents, and their synthetic counterparts, differ in their actions according to the receptors on which they mainly act (though many stimulate most to a varying degree): α_1 smooth muscle receptors, which cause vasoconstriction; α_2 presynaptic nerve receptors, which are thought to inhibit gastrointestinal activity; β_1 receptors, which stimulate cardiac activity; β_2 smooth muscle receptors, which cause vascular and bronchial dilatation; and two CNS dopamine receptors (D_1 and D_2).

Noradrenaline is the main postganglionic neurotransmitter in the sympathetic nervous system. Some is also produced along with adrenaline (q.v.) by the adrenal glands in response to stress. It is inactivated when given by mouth and cannot be given by subcutaneous or IM injection because it is such a powerful vasoconstrictor. The main effects are to increase cardiac contractility, heart rate and myocardial oxygen consumption (via β_1 stimulation), but high-dose infusions also cause intense peripheral vasoconstriction (an α_1 agonist effect) unless vasopressin (q.v.) insufficiency has developed. Such peripheral vasoconstriction can sometimes, by increasing the afterload on the heart, counteract the drug's inotropic effect and cause a decrease in cardiac output. Similarly, the increase in myocardial oxygen consumption can exacerbate any existing cardiac failure and compromise ventricular function. For these reasons the drug should only be used when the need to increase arterial pressure outweighs the risk of lowering cardiac output. Infants with sepsis who are hypotensive but have good cardiac function and adequate vascular volume are the most likely to benefit, though even here the optimum dose calls for careful judgement. Use in babies with persistent pulmonary hypertension may marginally improve oxygenation by changing the balance between pulmonary and systemic artery pressure. Noradrenaline can cause the pregnant uterus to contract.

Drug equivalence
1 mg of noradrenaline acid tartrate contains 500 micrograms of noradrenaline base. The drug is always best prescribed in terms of the amount of **base** to be given, to prevent ambiguity.

Treatment
Start with an infusion of 100 nanograms/kg per minute of noradrenaline base (0·1 ml/hour of a solution made up as described below) and infuse into a *central* vein. Severe complications can be associated with peripheral infusion as outlined in the monograph on dopamine. The rate of infusion can be increased slowly to a maximum of 1·5 micrograms/kg per minute (1·5 ml/hour), as long as limb perfusion and urine output are watched carefully. Monitor central vascular pressures where possible.

Compatibility
Noradrenaline can be added (terminally) into a line containing dobutamine, heparin, milrinone or standard TPN (with or without lipid). The safety of physical mixture with dopamine remains unassessed.

Supply and administration
Noradrenaline is available in 2 and 4 ml ampoules containing 2 mg/ml of noradrenaline acid tartrate (the equivalent of 1 mg/ml of noradrenaline base) costing £1 and £1·50 each. To give an infusion of 100 nanograms/kg per minute of noradrenaline base take 1·5 mg (1·5 ml) of noradrenaline base for each kg the baby weighs, dilute to 25 ml with 10% glucose or glucose saline, and infuse at a rate of 0·1 ml/hour. The drug is stable in solutions with a low pH, such as glucose, but is best prepared afresh every 24 hours unless protected from light. Protect ampoules from light during storage, and discard if discoloured. Tissue extravasation can be dangerous and should be treated as outlined in the monograph on hyaluronidase.

References
Carcillo JA, Fields AI. Clinical practice parameters for hemodynamic support of pediatric and neonatal patients in septic shock. *Crit Care Med* 2002;**30**:1365–78. [SR]
Ceneviva G, Paschall JA, Maffei F, *et al*. Hemodynamic support in fluid refractory septic shock. *Pediatrics* 1998;**102**:e19.
Seri I. Circulatory support of the sick preterm infant. [Review] *Semin Neonatol* 2001;**6**:85–95.
Tourneux P, Rakza T, Bouissou A, *et al*. Pulmonary circulatory effects of norepinephrine in newborn infants with persistent pulmonary hypertension. *J Pediatr* 2008;**153**:345–9.
von Rosensteil N, von Rosensteil I, Adam D. Management of sepsis and septic shock in infants and children. *Paediatr Drugs* 2001;**3**:9–27.

NYSTATIN

Use
Nystatin is used to treat gastrointestinal and topical *Candida albicans* infection and low-dose prophylaxis may stop overt infection developing. Miconazole gel (q.v.) seems better at eliminating oral infection.

Pharmacology
Nystatin was the first naturally occurring antifungal polyene antibiotic to be developed in 1951, and is still the most widely used. It is very insoluble and is usually prescribed as a suspension. Nystatin is particularly active against yeast-like fungi and has long been used in the treatment of topical infection with *C. albicans*. Full purification is impracticable and the drug dosage is therefore usually quoted in 'units'. The drug works by combining with the sterol elements of fungal cell membranes causing cell death by producing increased cell wall permeability. Oral absorption is poor. While there is no evidence to suggest that it is unsafe to use nystatin during pregnancy or lactation, treatment with miconazole seems to be a more effective way of eliminating vaginal candidiasis.

The dose usually recommended for oral infection ('thrush') in a baby is 1 ml of the suspension four times a day, but this is not as effective as treatment with oral miconazole gel. A 4 ml dose of nystatin may be more effective, but this still needs controlled trial confirmation. Oral drops can be used to clear *Candida* from the gastrointestinal tract, and ointment used to treat skin infection. Fluconazole (q.v.) costs more, but is probably more effective, and it should certainly be used if there is tracheal colonisation or systemic infection. Such colonisation can turn into serious overt systemic infection in babies on broad-spectrum antibiotic treatment (because of the resultant change in the normal bacterial flora).

Maternal breast and nipple pain
A tender, lumpy, inflamed breast is best treated for incipient bacterial mastitis with flucloxacillin (q.v.). Local *nipple* pain is usually due to poor positioning (an art that has to be learnt), and this can be rapidly relieved by improved technique. Topical treatments usually do more harm than good, and some mothers are even sensitive to lanolin cream. Keep the skin dry (while allowing any expressed milk to dry on the nipple). *Candida* infection ('thrush') can occasionally be part of the problem, and should be suspected if trouble comes on after lactation has been established, especially if the baby has signs of this infection, or the mother has vaginitis. Recent antibiotic treatment makes this problem more likely. Miconazole cream and oral gel (q.v.), sold 'over the counter' under the trade name Daktarin® may help, but a maternal course of fluconazole is the treatment of choice when there is severe, sustained, stinging or radiating pain, presumably due to duct infection. Give nystatin drops as well to minimise the risk of reinfection if the baby seems to be heavily colonised or more widely infected. Sudden severe pain with marked blanching may be a vasomotor reaction. Anxiety can be one trigger. Local warmth may help; keeping warm may forestall trouble. Some cases seem to be a form of Raynaud phenomenon, and this occasionally merits pharmacological intervention – giving the mother a 30 mg slow release tablet of nifedipine (Adalat® Retard) once a day often brings rapid relief.

Neonatal treatment
Prophylaxis: 1 ml (100,000 units) of the oral suspension every 8 hours can lower the risk of systemic infection in the very low birthweight baby. Fluconazole once a day is also very affective but more expensive.
Oral candidiasis (thrush): It is standard practice to give 1 ml (100,000 units) by mouth four times a day after feeds, but a larger dose may be more effective.
Candida (*Monilia*) **dermatitis:** Dry the skin thoroughly and apply nystatin ointment at least twice a day for a week. Leave the skin exposed if possible. A cream is better if the skin is broken and wet.
General considerations: Continue to treat for 3 days after a response is achieved to minimise the risk of a recurrence. Consider the possibility of undiagnosed genital infection, especially in the mother of an infected but otherwise healthy full term baby. Check that the child is not reinfected by a contaminated bottle or teat. Treat the gastrointestinal tract as well as the skin if there is a stubborn monilial nappy (diaper) rash.

Supply
The 30 gram tubes of nystatin cream (costing £2·20) contain benzyl alcohol, and some formulations also contain propylene glycol, but the 30 gram tubes of ointment (costing £1·80) do not. One 30 ml bottle of the sugar-free oral suspension (100,000 units/ml) costs £2. The 500,000 unit tablets cost 8p each.

References
See also the relevant Cochrane reviews

Anderson JE, Held N, Wright K. Raynaud's phenomenon of the nipple: a treatable cause of painful breastfeeding. *Pediatrics* 2004;**113**:e360–4.
Borderon JC, Therizol FM, Saliba E, *et al*. Prevention of *Candida* colonisation prevents infection in a neonatal unit. *Biol Neonat* 2003;**84**:37–40.
Ganesan K, Harigopal S, Neal T, *et al*. Prophylactic oral nystatin for preterm babies under 33 weeks' gestation decreases fungal colonisation and invasive fungaemia. *Arch Dis Child* 2009;**94**:F275–8.
Goins RA, Ascher D, Waecker N, *et al*. Comparison of fluconazole and nystatin oral suspensions for treatment of oral candidiasis in infants. *Pediatr Infect Dis J* 2002;**21**:1165–7. [RCT]
Ozturk MA, Gunes T, Koklu E, *et al*. Oral nystatin prophylaxis to prevent invasive candidiasis in neonatal intensive care unit. *Mycoses* 2006;**49**:484–92. [RCT]
Sims ME, Too Y, You H, *et al*. Prophylactic oral nystatin and fungal infections in very-low-birthweight infants. *Am J Perinatol* 1988;**5**:33–6. [RCT]
Tanquay KE, McBean MR, Jain E. Nipple candidiasis among breastfeeding mothers. *Can Fam Phys* 1994;**40**:1407–13.

Use

Octreotide is used to treat intractable hypoglycaemia due to persisting neonatal hyperinsulinism when diazoxide (q.v.) fails to abolish all dangerous episodes of hypoglycaemia. It has also found to be useful in the management of persistent pleural effusions caused by lymphatic chyle (chylothorax).

Pharmacology

Octreotide is an analogue of hypothalamic hormone somatostatin, a naturally occurring 14 amino acid peptide that acts to inhibit the release of several pituitary hormones as well as glucagon and insulin from the pancreas. It also seems to have some influence over the secretion of pepsin, gastrin and hydrochloric acid in the stomach and duodenum and to play some poorly understood role in the perception of pain by the brain. Somatostatin was first isolated in the Salk Institute in 1973 and the potent octapeptide, octreotide, was synthesised there in 1982. It is rapidly absorbed following subcutaneous injection and then partly metabolised by the liver and partly excreted unchanged in the urine. While its pharmacokinetic behaviour may be non-linear, the normal half life is about 90 minutes. The drug's main initial use was in the control of acromegaly, in the control of upper intestinal bleeding and in the management of secretory neoplasms. It can help prevent complications during and after pancreatic surgery and has also been found to be of use in the control of both malignant and non-malignant chylous effusions of the chest and abdomen, although the mechanism by which this is achieved is less clear.

Babies who cannot be weaned from IV glucose with diazoxide are likely to require surgical intervention such as subtotal pancreatectomy, but may be stabilised while this step is being contemplated by the use of octreotide. A dose of 5 micrograms/kg given subcutaneously every 6−8 hours is usually sufficient. Rarely, doses of as much as 7 micrograms/kg every 4 hours may be required to maintain a safe blood glucose level of at least 4 mmol/l. It can also be given as an intra-venous or subcutaneous infusion in a dose of 5−25 micrograms/kg per day. Such treatment should only be contemplated under the direct supervision of a consultant paediatric endocrinologist. There is no animal evidence to suggest that octreotide is fetotoxic or teratogenic and, since the drug is ineffective when given by mouth, no likelihood that use during lactation will prove hazardous.

Babies with persistent chylothorax unresponsive to a medium-chain triglyceride diet or parenteral nutrition may respond to octreotide subcutaneously or by continuous intravenous infusion. Dosage is titrated against the volume of pleural drainage and, following satisfactory resolution, octreotide is weaned over 2−4 days.

Necrotising enterocolitis has been reported in a neonate following treatment with octreotide for chylothorax following repair of coarctation of the aorta.

Treatment

Hyperinsulinaemic hypoglycaemia: Start with 5 micrograms/kg by subcutaneous injection 6−8 hourly, increasing incrementally based on response to 7 micrograms/kg 4 hourly if necessary. Alternatively, consider a dose of 5−25 micrograms/kg per day by subcutaneous or IV infusion.
Chylothorax: Start with 5 micrograms/kg subcutaneously 8 hourly increasing slowly to 20 micrograms/kg if needed. Alternatively, give a continuous infusion of octreotide starting at 1 microgram/kg per hour and increasing incrementally as high as 10 micrograms/kg per hour if required.

Supply

1 ml single-dose ampoules containing 50 micrograms of octreotide (costing £3·50 each) are available, as are 5 ml multidose vials containing 200 micrograms/ml (costing £65). Ampoules and vials are best stored at 4−8°C, but are stable at 25°C for 2 weeks. Multidose vials can be kept for 2 weeks once open.

References

Chan S, Lau W, Wong WHS, *et al.* Chylothorax in children after congenital heart surgery. *Ann Thorac Surg* 2006;**82**:1650−7.

Copons FC, Benitez SI, Casillo SF, *et al.* Quilotórax neonatal: etiología, evolución y respuesta al tratamiento. *An Pediatr Barc* 2008;**68**:224−31.

de Lonlay P, Saudubray J-M. Persistent hyperinsulinemic hypoglycemia. In: Fernandes J, Saudubray J-M, van den Berghe G, *et al.*, eds. *Inborn metabolic diseases. Diagnosis and management*, 4th edn. Berlin: Springer, 2006: pp. 143−9.

Helin RD, Angeles STV, Bhat R. Octreotide therapy for chylothorax in infants and children: a brief review. *Pediatr Crit Care Med* 2006;**7**:576−9. [SR]

Hoe FM, Thornton PS, Wanner LA, *et al.* Clinical features and insulin regulation in infants with a syndrome of prolonged neonatal hyper-insulinism. *J Pediatr* 2006;**148**:207−12.

Kapoor RR, Flanagan SE, James C, *et al.* Hyperinsulaemic hypoglycaemia. [Review] *Arch Dis Child* 2009;**94**:450−7.

Lindley KJ, Dunne MJ. Contemporary strategies in the diagnosis and management of neonatal hyperinsulinaemic hypoglycaemia. [Review] *Early Hum Devel* 2005;**81**:61−72.

Roehr CC, Jung A, Proquitté H, *et al.* Somatostatin or octreotide as treatment options for chylothorax in young children: a systematic review. *Intensive Care Med* 2006;**32**:650−7. [SR]

Young S, Dalgleish S, Eccleston A, *et al.* Severe congenital chylothorax treated with octreotide. *J Perinatol* 2004;**24**:2002.

OMEPRAZOLE

Use

Omeprazole is used to suppress gastric acid secretion when endoscopically proven oesophagitis or peptic ulceration persists despite treatment with ranitidine. Use is not of benefit in most young children with reflux.

Pharmacology

Omeprazole, a substituted benzimidazole, was the first gastric acid pump inhibitor (proton pump inhibitor) to come into clinical use (in 1983). Lansoprazole, a closely related drug, came onto the market 10 years later and esomeprazole (the S-isomer of omeprazole) 10 years after that. All three drugs work by inhibiting the last step in the chain of reactions that leads to the secretion of hydrochloric acid by the parietal cells of the stomach. The resultant reduction in gastric acidity, even in the fed state, allows even severe oesophageal erosions to heal. Treatment is only necessary once a day even though the plasma half life in adults is only about 1·5 hours, since a single dose more than halves the secretion of gastric acid for over a day. Side effects are uncommon. Pharmacokinetic studies suggest that children handle the proton pump inhibitor drugs in much the same way as adults, but the few studies that have been done in children of less than a year old suggest that drug accumulation might well occur if a child less than 9 months old is given more than twice the normal starting dose. The plasma half life is particularly short in later childhood, but this does not, on its own, seem to explain the higher treatment dose sometimes found necessary. Manufacturers have not yet endorsed the IV use of omeprazole in children, and only recommend oral use in children over 1 year.

Formal trials have shown that omeprazole and lansoprazole do nothing to reduce the symptoms suffered by most children with gastroesophageal reflux, and one trial has suggested that use may, in some unexplained way, actually increase the risk of lower respiratory tract infection. Studies show that esomeprazole seems to be no more effective than omeprazole. The latter, with two antibiotics (commonly amoxicillin and 7·5 mg/kg of clarithromycin twice a day) is widely used to teat *Helicobacter pylori* gastritis in older children. It does not seem to be teratogenic, but less is known about lansoprazole. There is only one report of use during lactation but, since the drug is rapidly destroyed by acid (the reason why the drug is formulated in enteric-coated granules), use during lactation is unlikely to affect the baby. Oral bioavailability, even with coating, is only about 65%. Prophylactic IV use has been used to minimise the risk of aspiration pneumonitis (Mendelson syndrome) in advance of urgent Caesarean delivery under general anaesthesia, but ranitidine (q.v.) seems an equally effective, and better studied, alternative.

Drug interactions

Omeprazole significantly prolongs the half life of several benzodiazepine drugs.

Treatment

By mouth: Start by giving 0·7 mg/kg by mouth once a day half an hour before breakfast, and double this dose after 7–14 days if this does not inhibit gastric acid production. A few patients may need as much as 2·8 mg/kg a day but progressive drug accumulation might occur if a baby <3 months old is given more than 1·4 mg/kg. Sustained treatment is hard to justify unless there continuing evidence of active oesophagitis.

IV use: Give 0·5 mg/kg once a day over 5 minutes (a dose that can be tripled if acid production persists).

Supply and administration

10 and 20 mg dispersible, film-coated tablets cost 68p and £1 each. Capsules containing enteric-coated granules are also available at the same cost. Small doses can be given by giving half a tablet dissolved in water, or by sprinkling some of the content of a capsule into a small quantity of yoghurt or fruit juice. Powders that can be reconstituted and administered IV are available in 40 mg vials costing £5·20. Similar vials exist for IM use. Because granules can block any nasogastric tube they are forced down, many hospitals now routinely first dilute the granules in bicarbonate solution – a product that has half the bioavailability of the standard product (see Song *et al*. 2001).

References

Bishop J, Furman M, Thomson M. Omeprazole for gastroesophageal reflux disease in the first two years of life: a dose finding study with dual-channel monitoring. *J Pediatr Gastroenterol* 2007;**45**:50–5.

Hoyo VC, Venturelli CR, Gonázlez H, *et al*. Metabolism of omeprazole after two oral doses in children 1 and 9 months old. *Proc West Pharmacol Soc* 2005;**48**:108–9.

Moore DJ, Tao BS-K, Lines DR, *et al*. Double-blind placebo-controlled trial of omperazole in irritable infants with gastroesophageal reflux. *J Pediatr* 2003;**143**:219–23. [RCT]

Nikfar S, Abdollahi M, Moretti ME, *et al*. Use of proton pump inhibitors during pregnancy and rates of major malformations: a meta-analysis. *Dig Dis Sci* 2002;**47**:1526–9.

Omari T, Davidson G, Bondarov P, *et al*. Pharmacokinetics and acid-suppression of esomeprazole in infants 1–24 months old with symptoms of gastroesophageal reflux disease. *J Pediatr Gastroenterol Nutr* 2007;**45**:530–7.

Omari TI, Haslam RR, Lundborrg P, *et al*. Effect of omeprazole on acid gastroesophageal reflux and gastric acidity in preterm infants with pathological acid reflux. *J Pediatr Gastroenterol Nutr* 2007;**44**:41–4.

Omari T, Lundborg P, Sandström M, *et al*. Pharmacodynamics and systemic exposure to esomeprazole in preterm infants and term neonates with gastroesophageal reflux disease. *J Pediatr* 2009;**155**:222–8.

Orenstein SR, Hassall E, Furmaga-Jablonska W, *et al*. Mulitcenter, double-blind, randomized, placebo controlled trial assessing the efficacy and safety of proton pump inhibitor lansoprazole in infants with symptoms of gastroesophageal reflux. *J Pediatr* 2009;**154**;514–20. [RCT] (See also editorial on pp. 475–6 and correspondence on pp. 601–2.)

Song JC, Quercia RA, Fan C, *et al*. Pharmacokinetic comparison of omeprazole capsules and a simplified omeprazole suspension. *Am J Health-Syst Pharm* 2001;**58**:689–94.

Use

Ondansetron is now widely used to control postoperative nausea and vomiting. More recently it has also been shown to be of value in children with gastroenteritis severe enough to merit hospital referral.

Pharmacology

Ondansetron first came on to the market in 1990, having been found by pharmacologists working for Glaxo to be a potent blocker of the receptors for the neurohormone 5-hydroxytryptamine ($5HT_3$) in the gut and central nervous system. Initially it was only used (together with dexamethasone) to control the nausea and vomiting caused by stimulation of the vagus nerve when $5HT_3$ is released from enterochromaffin cells in the gut during chemotherapy and radiotherapy. Studies by cancer specialists found it to be more effective than metoclopramide (q.v.), and it is now also quite widely used to pre-empt postoperative vomiting (even though the manufacturer has not yet endorsed use in children less than 2 years old). More recently it has been shown to be of value in the management of the severe vomiting that occasionally accompanies acute gastroenteritis in young children (and the only drug for which there is objective evidence of efficacy). Only about 60% of the drug reaches the circulation when the drug is given by mouth because of first pass uptake by the liver. The drug is then widely distributed in the body (V_D ~2 kg/l) before being metabolised in a range of different ways in the liver and, because of this, some have argued that a loading dose should probably be considered before starting chemotherapy. Repeat treatment should also be curtailed in patients with severe liver failure. The terminal half life is about 3 hours (and possibly a little less in young children). Metabolism in the first year of life does not seem to have been studied. A serious overdose can cause seizures and make respiratory support necessary, but recovery occurred within 24 hours in the only case reported to date.

Use in pregnancy

Ondansetron (10 mg every 6 hours) has occasionally been given during pregnancy to control severe nausea and vomiting (hyperemesis gravidarum). There is no evidence to suggest that it is teratogenic, and it seems to be less sedating than promethazine (see Part 3). Lesser degrees of nausea are most commonly controlled by meclozine (see Part 3), which is available without prescription. Nothing is known about the use of ondansetron during lactation, and the drug's small molecular size makes some transfer likely.

Use in infancy

Pre-anaesthetic prophylaxis: Give a single preoperative 150 microgram/kg oral or slow IV dose.
Severe gastroenteritis: A single 200–300 microgram/kg oral or slow IV dose is usually used.
During emetogenic chemotherapy: Give 125 micrograms/kg shortly before treatment, and two further doses 4 and 8 hours later. Consider giving dexamethasone as well. Adults are also often given aprepitant.

Drug interactions

The BNF has raised the possibility of an interaction with other drugs that can prolong the QT interval.

Supply and administration

2 ml ampoules containing 4 mg of ondansetron cost £5·40. Take 2 ml and dilute to 20 ml with glucose or glucose saline to obtain a solution containing 200 micrograms/ml. Rapidly dissolving 4 mg tablets cost ~£3 each. A pack that, when reconstituted, provides 50 ml of a sugar-free, strawberry-flavoured syrup containing 0·8 mg/ml of ondansetron costs £36. Zofran® syrup contains sodium benzoate.

References

See also the relevant Cochrane reviews

Bolton CM, Myles PS, Carlin JB, *et al.* Randomized double-blind study comparing the efficacy of moderate-dose metoclopramide and ondansetron for the prophylactic control of postoperative vomiting in children after tonsillectomy. *Br J Anaesth* 2007;**99**:699–703. [RCT]
Culy CR, Bhana N, Plosker GL. Ondansetron: a review of its use as an antiemetic in children *Paediatr Drugs* 2001;**3**:471–9. [SR]
DeCamp LR, Byerley JS, Doshi N, *et al.* Use of antiemetic agents in acute gastroenteritis. A systematic review and meta-analysis. *Arch Pediatr Adolesc Med* 2008;**162**:858–65. [SR] (See also pp. 866–9.)
Einarson A, Maltepe C, Navioz Y, *et al.* The safety of ondansetron for nausea and vomiting of pregnancy: a prospective comparative study. *Br J Obstet Gynaecol* 2004;**111**:940–3.
Freedman SB, Adler M, Seshadri R, *et al.* Oral ondansetron for gastroenteritis in a pediatric emergency department. *N Engl J Med* 2006;**354**:1698–705. [RCT]
Hesketh PJ. Chemotherapy-induced nausea and vomiting. [Review] *N Engl J Med* 2008;**358**:2482–94.
Köseaoğlu V, Kürekçi AE, Sarici Ü, *et al.* Comparison of the efficacy and side-effects of ondansetron and metoclopramide-diphenhydramine administered to control nausea and vomiting in children treated with antineoplastic chemotherapy: a prospective randomised study. *Eur J Pediatr* 1998;**157**:806–10. [RCT]
Kris MG, Hesketh PJ, Somerfield MR, *et al.* American Society for Clinical Oncology guideline for antiemetics in oncology: update 2006. *J Clin Oncol* 2006;**24**:2932–47.
Roslund G, Hepps TS, McQuillen KK. The role of oral ondansetron in children with vomiting as a result of acute gastritis/gastroenteritis who have failed oral rehydration therapy: a randomized controlled trial. *Ann Emerg Med* 2007;**52**:22–9.e6. [RCT]
Stork CM, Brown KM, Reillly TH, *et al.* Emergency department treatment of viral gastritis using intravenous ondansetron or dexamethasone in children. *Acad Emerg Med* 2006;**13**:1027–33. [RCT]
Sullivan CA, Johnson CA, Roach H, *et al.* A pilot study of intravenous ondansetron for hyperemesis gravidarum. *Am J Obstet Gynecol* 1996;**174**:156–58. [RCT]
Szajewska H, Gieruszczak-Bialek D, Dyag M. Meta-analysis: ondansetron for vomiting in acute gastroenteritis in children. *Aliment Pharmacol Ther* 2007;**25**:393–400. [SR]

ORAL REHYDRATION SOLUTION (ORS)

Use

Giving a solution of salts in glucose by mouth, or down a nasogastric tube, is both the simplest and best way to rehydrate a child suffering from diarrhoea. Limited initial IV correction is only needed in the few children who present with particularly severe dehydration (more than 9% acute loss of weight). In all other situations it is inappropriately invasive, complex and expensive. Ondansetron (q.v.) can help with vomiting.

Recognising dehydration

Dehydration due to diarrhoea currently kills several thousand young children in the world every day, and may account for a third of all death in the first year of life. Dehydration has to be recognised clinically – laboratory tests are of no real help. Minor dehydration (less than 3% loss of body weight) is self-correcting, but loss greater than this calls for corrective action. These children seem irritable, restless and thirsty; their eyes and the anterior fontanelle are slightly sunken; the skin and mucous membranes seem dry; and the extremities are cool. However, the three most reliable signs of significant dehydration (≥5% weight loss) are a raised respiratory rate, delayed (>2 second) capillary refill time and increased skin turgor (delayed recoil when a fold of skin is picked up between the thumb and finger). Children who have become lethargic, are reluctant or unable to drink, and have weak pulses or an abnormal heart rate have probably suffered a >9% loss.

Pathophysiology

The management of gastroenteritis has four elements: the correction of any dehydration that has already occurred; the replacement of ongoing fluid and electrolyte loss; the continued provision of basic nutrition; and, more selectively, the provision of oral zinc and, where indicated, antimicrobial therapy. Parents can easily come to believe that treatment 'is not working' if the diarrhoea does not stop promptly – they need to be reassured that almost all infectious gastrointestinal illness is self-limiting, and that the two key aims of care are first to replace lost water and salts, and then to keep the child fed until the illness resolves. Diarrhoea is usually viral, but bloody stools (dysentery) may point to bacterial infection meriting antibiotic treatment once the organism is identified.

Research into the management of cholera in the late 1960s showed how oral rehydration could be achieved in cholera by harnessing the coupled transport of sodium and glucose molecules across the intestinal brush border. The World Health Organisation (WHO) have been extolling the merits of a simple oral rehydration solution (ORS) containing equimolar amounts of sodium and glucose for more than 30 years, and the superiority of this approach is now admitted even in countries addicted to 'high tech' medicine.

Treatment

Severe dehydration: Babies who have suffered more than a 9% loss of weight need urgent revival with 20–30 ml/kg of 0·9% sodium chloride or, where this is available, compound sodium lactate (Hartmann) solution given over an hour IV, followed by a further 70 ml/kg of the same solution over the next 5 hours. Hartmann solution is to be preferred because it provides potassium and also lactate which, metabolised to bicarbonate, corrects acidosis. Nasogastric administration may work if IV access can not be achieved, but ileus can sometimes make intraosseous (or even intraperitoneal) administration the only remaining option.
Less severe dehydration: Rehydrate with 75 ml/kg of ORS over 4 hours. Then resume breastfeeding, or the child's normal diet. Give a further 50–100 ml of ORS for each further episode of diarrhoea or vomiting. Lactose usually remains well tolerated. Avoid carbonated (fizzy) drinks and carbohydrate-enriched juices.
Oral zinc: Adding 40 mg/l of elemental zinc (as gluconate) to the ORS speeds recovery in some communities.

Supply

WHO formulation: The WHO has, since 2004, recommended a powder containing 2·6 g of sodium chloride, 1·5 g of potassium chloride, 2·9 g of sodium citrate and 13·5 g of anhydrous glucose which, when added to enough water to give 1 litre of fluid, provides a solution containing 75 mmol of sodium, 20 mmol of potassium, 65 mmol of chloride, 10 mmol of citrate and 75 mmol of glucose per litre.
UK formulations: Most commercial UK products differ slightly from the WHO solution in that they deliver marginally less sodium (usually 50–60 mmol/l rather than 75 mmol/l). Fruit-flavoured powders suitable for children less than a year old include Dioralyte® Relief, Electrolade® and Rapolyte®. All come in sachets designed for reconstitution just before use with 200 ml of cool, freshly boiled, water. Such sachets typically cost 20–30p each. Any of the solution not used promptly can be kept for 24 hours, if it is stored in a fridge.

References

See also the relevant Cochrane reviews

Bahl R, Bhandari N, Saksena M, *et al.* Efficacy of zinc-fortified oral rehydration solution in 6- to 35-month-old children with acute diarrhea. *J Pediatr* 2002;**141**:677–82. [RCT]
Centres for Disease Control and Prevention. Managing acute gastroenteritis among children: oral rehydration, maintenance, and nutritional therapy. *MMWR* 2003;**52**(RR-16):1–16.
Dalby-Payne J, Elliottt E. Gastroenteritis in children. *BMJ Clinical evidence handbook*. London: BMJ Books, 2009: pp. 86–7 (and updates). [SR]
Fonseca BK, Holdgate A, Craig JC. Enteral vs intravenous rehydration therapy for children with gastroenteritis: a meta-analysis of randomized controlled trials. *Arch Pediatr Adolesc Med* 2004;**158**:483–90. [SR]
Spanorfer PR, Alessandrini EA, Joffe MD, *et al.* Oral versus intravenous rehydration of moderately dehydrated children: a randomised, controlled trial. *Pediatrics* 2005;**115**:295–301. [RCT]
Steiner MJ, DeWalt DA, Byerley JS. Is this child dehydrated? *JAMA* 2004;**291**:2746–54. [SR]

Use

Supplemental oxygen is used to correct hypoxia in babies with pulmonary problems, especially where this is causing a mismatch between the ventilation and the perfusion of the lung.

Pathophysiology

Oxygen deserves its place in any pharmacopoeia because – like almost any other drug – oxygen can do a lot of harm as well as a lot of good. It needs to be used with care; all use should be documented, and the 'dose' recorded. While lack of oxygen can be damaging, the body can manage with blood that is only about 50–60% saturated as long as the *quantity* of oxygen delivered to the tissues is adequate. Were this not true, the fetus would be in substantial trouble before birth, as would the brain of the baby with cyanotic heart disease. Cardiac output and tissue perfusion matter more than blood pressure, and anaemia can undermine oxygen delivery as much as overt cyanosis. While tissue hypoxia can be damaging, it is the combined effect of CO_2 accumulation and oxygen lack (asphyxia) that is most damaging, causing a respiratory (carbonic acid) as well as a metabolic (lactic acid) acidosis.

Too much oxygen can also be damaging, however. Prolonged exposure to more than ~60% oxygen can be toxic to the pulmonary epithelium, and hyperbaric oxygen can cause convulsions. There is also evidence that a relatively high partial pressure of oxygen in the blood is one of a range of factors that can interfere with the normal growth of blood vessels into the retina at the back of the eye in the last 10 weeks of what should have been intrauterine life. In most cases this retinopathy of prematurity (ROP) resolves spontaneously, leaving no damage, but severe change can lead to permanent scarring if it involves more than the outer rim of the retina, and this can sometimes progress to retinal detachment and blindness. Good controlled trial evidence that excess oxygen could cause blindness first appeared in 1952, but we still do not know precisely what constitutes 'excess' oxygen. Even the 'routine' use of 100% oxygen during resuscitation at birth is now being questioned.

The more immature the baby, the greater the risk to the eye, but changes take at least 6 weeks to develop, and most severe disease develops at a postconceptional age of 33–40 weeks. Damage can be reduced by surgery to limit the capillary proliferation that precedes permanent scarring, but the disease can progress quite rapidly. It is essential, therefore, for every baby born before 28 weeks' gestation to be seen by an experienced ophthalmologist when they reach a postmenstrual age of 31 weeks, and then serially every 7–14 days until any acute proliferative change has started to regress. Babies of 28–32 weeks' gestation first merit review when 4 weeks old. Review can be discontinued after 36 weeks if there is still no retinal abnormality because disease appearing for the first time after this is extremely unlikely to progress to permanent scarring. Diode-laser treatment should be offered *immediately* if stage 3 change develops in zone I (the central area of the retina), or if any change develops in this zone accompanied by 'plus' disease (vessel dilatation and tortuosity involving two quadrants (usually 6 or more clock hours)). It is also indicated if stage 2 or 3 change with 'plus' disease develops in zone II. The recent ET-ROP trial showed that there was a 15% risk of the child becoming near blind in that eye if nothing was done once the disease process had become that extensive, and that prompt intervention can probably reduce that risk by a third.

Administration

Oxygen is usually given into an incubator, especially in small babies, but cot nursing using a nasal cannula is a valuable (and economic) alternative that simplifies parental involvement. Some form of humidification is, however, called for if the baby is getting much oxygen this way. Devices delivering a high flow of warm humidified gas for cannula use are becoming increasingly popular, but there is concern that, at flows of more than 2 l/min, the main benefit derived from their use is caused by the fact that they deliver an unmeasured, uncontrolled and potentially dangerously high form of constant positive airway pressure (or CPAP). A humidified head box (see below) is the only satisfactory way of providing more than 50% oxygen to a baby requiring incubator care – oxygen tents are seldom very satisfactory at any age. It is also possible – although not generally recognised – that substantial (but not very precisely controlled) amounts of oxygen can be given directly into any high-sided carry cot or basinette since oxygen, because of its temperature and density, 'layers' immediately above the surface of the mattress; it is not necessary to put a plastic sheet over the top of the basinette.

Measurement in air

The amount of oxygen each baby is breathing (as a percentage) should be recorded regularly. Those given oxygen via a nasal catheter should have the ambient concentration needed to provide an equivalent arterial saturation documented periodically, because the relation between catheter flow and the inspired concentration varies. Equipment needs daily calibration against room air (20·9% oxygen).

Measuring blood levels

What constitutes a safe range for arterial oxygen pressure is not known. It is said that there must be 50 g/l of desaturated haemoglobin for cyanosis to be visible. Cyanosis is certainly difficult to detect by eye until 25% of the blood is desaturated, and in the neonate this often only occurs when the arterial partial pressure (PaO_2) is down to 35 mmHg or 4·7 kPa (the left dashed line in Fig. 1). The use of arterial catheters can reduce the pain and trauma caused by repeated capillary sampling, but there is no evidence that use improves long-term outcome. Transcutaneous pressure and saturation monitors are valuable but not free from error.

A cohort study in 1992 showed an association between the prevalence of acute retinopathy and exposure to transcutaneous oxygen ($TcPO_2$) levels of more than 80 mmHg (~10·7 kPa) and, as a result, many units started to aim for $TcPO_2$ levels of 6–10 kPa, and to withdraw supplemental oxygen from preterm babies with a $TcPO_2$ level higher than this. Pulse

Continued on p. 192

191

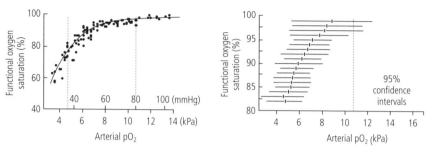

Fig. 1

Fig. 2

oximetry is widely used to replace monitoring of $TcPO_2$ even though the relation between PaO_2 and arterial saturation is quite variable in babies (Fig. 1) because of the differing effects of varying shunt and changes in ventilation:perfusion ratio on the curve relating FiO_2 to SaO_2. A more detailed discussion with a link to an interactive algorithm for determining shunt and V_A/Q can be found in the website commentary. To be certain of keeping $TcPO_2$ (and PaO_2) below 80 mmHg, the *functional* saturation in babies has to be kept from exceeding 95% (Fig. 2) – equivalent to a *fractional* saturation of 93%. Even this may leave preterm babies at a small risk of 'hyperoxia' as oximeter manufacturers only claim an accuracy of ±3%. Five trials are currently trying to identify what range of saturation optimises long-term outcome.

No such restriction needs to limit management in babies in whom retinal vascular development is complete. Here monitoring is only necessary to identify hypoxia, and significant central cyanosis is not difficult to detect (although badly chosen fluorescent lighting can affect assessment). Babies with chronic lung disease are often given oxygen in the belief that this will improve weight gain and reduce emergency hospital readmission, but there was no evidence of this in the first Australian BOOST trial, and babies given enough supplemental oxygen to maintain a *fractional* saturation of 96–99% in the American STOP-ROP trial actually had *more* pulmonary problems than those only given enough to achieve a saturation of 89–94%. Views differ as to how often home use is necessary, and a UK register of such use (CHORD) has recently been set up.

Supply

Piped hospital supplies result in our taking the provision of oxygen for granted; the same is not true in many developing countries. Arrangements for providing oxygen for home use in the UK have recently undergone a major, and initially unsettling, change. The supply of an oxygen concentrator and of lightweight cylinders by one of four commercial companies must now be authorised by a designated official in each Trust hospital.

Humidification

Piped supplies and cylinders are devoid of water vapour, and humidification is essential to avoid excessive drying of the respiratory tract when giving >40% oxygen. A range of commercial equipment (such as the Vapotherm®) has now become available for delivering a flow of warm, well-humidified gas with a variable oxygen content. Bubbling gas through water at room temperature adds 20 grams of water to each cubic metre of gas (equivalent to 50% saturation at body temperature), and this is generally adequate unless flow is high or the nose's humidification system has been partially bypassed. For babies breathing high concentrations of head box oxygen in an incubator, reasonable humidification can be achieved without a heated humidifier by bubbling oxygen through a small bottle situated *inside* the incubator.

References

See also the relevant Cochrane reviews and UK guideline on managing ROP

Askie LM, Henderson-Smark DJ, Irwig L, *et al*. Oxygen saturation targets and outcomes of extremely preterm infants. *N Engl J Med* 2003;**349**:959–67. [RCT]

Balfour-Lynn IM, Primahak RA, Shaw BNJ. Home oxygen for children: who, how and when? *Thorax* 2005;**60**:76–81. (See also the related British Thoracic Society guideline on home oxygen use and its paediatric supplement: www.brit-thoracic.org.uk.)

Castillo A, Sola A, Baquero H, *et al*. Pulse oxygen saturation levels and arterial oxygen tension in newborns receiving oxygen therapy in neonatal intensive care unit: is 85% to 93% an acceptable range? *Pediatrics* 2008;**121**:882–9.

Early Treatment for Retinopathy of Prematurity (ET-ROP) Cooperative Group. Revised indications for the treatment of retinopathy of prematurity. *Arch Ophthalmol* 2003;**121**:1684–96. [RCT] (See also pp. 1697–701 and 1769–71.)

Finer NN. Nasal cannula use in the preterm infant: oxygen or pressure? *Pediatrics* 2005;**116**:1216–17.

Gerstmann D, Berg R, Haskell R, *et al*. Operational evaluation of pulse oximetry in NICU patients with arterial access. *J Perinatol* 2003;**23**:378–83.

Harrison GT, Shaw B. Prescribing home oxygen. *Arch Dis Child* 2007;**92**:F241–3.

Quine D, Stenson BJ. Arterial oxygen tension (PaO₂) values in infants <29 weeks of gestation at currently targeted saturations. *Arch Dis Child* 2009;**94**:F51–3.

Rowe L, Jones JG, Quine D, *et al*. A simplified method for deriving shunt and reduced V_A/Q in infants. *Arch Dis Child* 2010;**95**:F47–52.

Saugstad OD, Ramji S, Soll RE, *et al*. Resuscitation of newborn infants with 21% or 100% oxygen: an updated systematic review and meta-analysis. *Neonatology* 2008;**94**:176–82. [SR]

Tin W, Gupta S. Optimum oxygen therapy in preterm babies. [Review] *Arch Dis Child* 2007;**92**:F143–7.

Use
Oxytocin is used (and misused) to induce or augment labour, and to reduce postpartum haemorrhage.

Pharmacology
Oxytocin is a synthetic octapeptide identical to the naturally occurring hypothalamic hormone. Crude pituitary extracts were first used clinically in 1909, and became commercially available in 1928. Its structure was confirmed by synthesis in 1953. It was long used to initiate and augment labour (given continuously IV because uptake is erratic from mucous membranes and the natural half life is only 3–4 minutes), but prostaglandin (q.v.) induction is now the preferred option unless the membranes have already ruptured spontaneously. A sudden bolus can cause vasodilatation and tachycardia, and secondary hypotension can be dangerous in patients with underlying heart disease. Uterine hyperstimulation can also cause fetal hypoxia, but this can be reversed by stopping the infusion and/or giving a betamimetic drug. There is some risk of uterine rupture, especially in patients with a uterine scar, even in the absence of cephalopelvic disproportion. Doses of more than 15 mU/min have an antidiuretic effect, and the risk of symptomatic fetal and maternal hyponatraemia is compounded if the mother ingests excessive fluid in labour. It helps if IV oxytocin is always given through a separate line using a motor-driven syringe pump, but oral intake is also sometimes excessive. Recent studies have not supported earlier claims that oxytocin nasal spray can augment lactation.

While use in mothers delivering under epidural anaesthesia can speed up the second stage of labour, there is no controlled trial evidence that use (with or without early amniotomy) to 'augment' spontaneous labour is of any significant clinical benefit. On the other hand, such augmentation can certainly cause increased pain and there is a significant risk of uterine hyperstimulation. A 10 unit dose given when the anterior shoulder delivers reduces the risk of postpartum haemorrhage and is commonly given IM (although it is only licensed for IV use), while a continuous infusion can be used if bleeding continues after the placenta is delivered. A combined IM injection of oxytocin and ergometrine maleate (Syntometrine®) is marginally more effective in reducing blood loss, but causes a transient rise in blood pressure and can cause nausea and vomiting. A 100 microgram IV dose of carbetocin (a longer acting synthetic analogue of oxytocin) seems to be equally effective and cause less nausea. Misoprostol (q.v.) is an extremely effective way of containing excessive post-delivery blood when it does occur, especially in a setting where it is difficult to keep supplies of oxytocin refrigerated. The inadvertent administration of Syntometrine to a baby (in mistake for an injection of vitamin K) is known to cause respiratory depression, seizures and severe hyponatraemia, but survivors, luckily, seem to make a complete recovery.

Units used when prescribing oxytocin
Oxytocin is such a potent drug that only a few nanograms are needed. Many staff feel insecure trying to use nanogram units and, for this reason, oxytocin remains (like insulin) one of the few drugs still widely prescribed using the old pharmaceutical unit of potency – the 'unit' – and, because of its short half life, is prescribed in milliunits per minute (often written as mU/min) to avoid writing 'start by giving 0·001 units/min'.

Treatment
Inducing and augmenting labour: Start with 1 or 2 mU/min and increase this by 1 mU/min every 30 minutes as necessary using a motor-driven syringe. If more than 4 mU/min proves necessary increase the dose by 2 mU/min increments once every 30 minutes to a maximum of 20 mU/min.

Postpartum use: Give 10 units of oxytocin (or 1 ml of Syntometrine) IM once the anterior shoulder of the baby is safely delivered. Continuous IV oxytocin will usually limit residual postpartum bleeding.

Supply and administration
Oxytocin comes in 5 or 10 unit (1 ml) ampoules. For accurate, continuous, dose-adjusted IV administration, dilute 3 units of oxytocin to 50 ml with 0·9% sodium chloride (or Hartmann solution). This gives a solution containing 60 mU/ml which, when infused at a rate of 1 ml/hour, gives the patient 1 mU/min of oxytocin. (1 unit = 2·2 micrograms of oxytocin). 1 ml ampoules of Syntometrine contain 5 units of oxytocin and 500 micrograms of ergometrine. UK midwives can use these products on their own authority. They cost about £1 per ampoule. 100 microgram ampoules of carbetocin cost £12. Keep all three products in the dark at 4°C.

References
See also the relevant Cochrane reviews and UK guideline on induction of labour

Chelmow D. Postpartum haemorrhage: prevention. *BMJ Clinical evidence handbook*. London: BMJ Books, 2009: pp. 478–80 (and updates). [SR]

Clark SL, Simpson KR, Knox GE, *et al*. Oxytocin: new perspectives on an old drug. *Am J Obstet Gynecol* 2009;**200**:35.e1–6.

Dargaville PA, Campbell NT. Overdose of ergometrine in the newborn infant: acute symptomatology and long-term outcome. *J Paediatr Child Health* 1998;**34**:83–9.

Fewtrell MS, Loh KL, Blake A, *et al*. Randomised, double blind trial of oxytocin nasal spray in mothers expressing breast milk for preterm infants. *Arch Dis Child* 2006;**91**:F169–74. [RCT]

Hinshaw K, Simpson S, Cummings S, *et al*. A randomised controlled trial of early versus delayed oxytocin augmentatrion to treat dysfunctional labour in nulliparous women. *Br J Obstet Gynaecol* 2008**115**:1289–96.

Leung SW, Ng PS, Wong WY, *et al*. A randomised trial of carbetocin versus syntometrine in the management of the third stage of labour. *Br J Obstet Gynaecol* 2006;**113**:1459–64. [RCT]

Moen V, Brudin L. Rundgren M, *et al*. Hyponatraemia complicating labour – rare or unrecognised? A prospective observational study. *Br J Obstet Gynaecol* 2009;**116**:552–61.

Su LL, Rauff M, Chan YH, *et al*. Carbetocin versus syntometrine for the third stage of labour following vaginal delivery – a double-blind randomised controlled trial. *Br J Obstet Gynaecol* 2009;**116**:1461–6. [RCT]

PALIVIZUMAB

Use
Prophylactic use of this monoclonal antibody can reduce the risk of a baby requiring hospital admission with bronchiolitis as a result of respiratory syncytial virus (RSV) infection. Treatment is of no use in babies with established infection. Neither is treatment with RSV immune globulin (RSV-IVIG).

Respiratory syncytial virus infection
Infection occurs in epidemic form every winter. Adults usually only get a mild cold, but babies can develop a chest infection severe enough to need hospital admission, and a few need ventilation. Infection is rapidly diagnosed from a nasopharyngeal wash specimen using immunofluorescence or an ELISA test (though the latter is not always positive early on). Coryza and/or apnoea may be the only symptoms in a preterm baby, but infants 2–9 months old can become seriously ill, particularly if they have congenital heart disease or chronic lung disease. Much can be done to reduce these risks by making parents more aware of the extent to which handwashing and limiting 'social' family exposure can lessen cross-infection. Barrier nursing reduces the risk of infection spreading to other vulnerable inpatients. Most babies merely need brief help with fluid intake and a little oxygen – support that may not always require hospital admission. Pulse oximetry can help to identify those needing admission, but a concern to keep saturation above 90% risks generating some unnecessary admissions. Antibiotics can usually be reserved for babies with heart disease, and for those who need intensive care or become infected while in hospital. Nebulised adrenaline (q.v.) lowered the number needing hospital admission in one recent trial, and nebulised hypertonic saline (see the monograph on sodium chloride) given every 2–4 hours reduced the length of stay in four small trials. Corticosteroids may benefit a few of those starting to reveal early signs of asthma, but is of no general value. Ribavirin. salbutamol and montelukast are of no proven value.

Pharmacology
Palivizumab is a combined human and murine monoclonal antibody produced by recombinant DNA technology that inhibits RSV replication. It has a 20-day half life. The first large placebo-controlled trials were reported in 1998. A monthly injection during the seasonal winter epidemic reduces the need for hospitalisation due to RSV infection in babies of less than 36 weeks' gestation. However, use does *not* reduce total health service costs, even when treatment is limited to babies who are still oxygen dependent because of chronic lung disease, unless readmission rates are atypically high. The risk of such babies becoming ill is further increased where there are other young school-age children in the house. Side effects, other than pain and swelling at the injection site, are rare. Use does not interfere with the administration of other vaccines. Monthly RSV-IVIG treatment (750 mg/kg IV) might be more appropriate in babies needing immunoglobulin for other reasons, and it offers some protection from other viral illnesses, but it is no longer commercially available and it seemed to do more harm than good in babies with cyanotic heart disease.

Prophylaxis
Some babies who are, or were until recently, oxygen dependent because of post-ventilator lung scarring probably merit treatment. So may a few babies with haemodynamically significant congenital heart disease (see web commentary). Give 15 mg/kg IM once a month for 3–5 months from the start of the winter RSV epidemic. Use the outer thigh (employing two sites where the injection volume exceeds 1 ml).

Supply and administration
The 50 and 100 mg vials of palivizumab (costing £360 and £600) should be stored at 4°C. Do not freeze. The small 50 mg vial actually contains more than 50 mg of palivizumab, but it is not possible to draw all the drug back out of the vial after reconstitution. This is why the manufacturers recommend that the powder should be dissolved by running 0·6 ml (50 mg vials) or 1 ml (100 mg vials) of water for injection slowly down the side of the vial. Rotate gently for 30 seconds without shaking and then leave it at room temperature for at least 20 minutes until the solution clarifies (it will remain opalescent). The resultant 100 mg/ml solution must be used within 6 hours. Cost can be reduced by using the larger vial, and scheduling several babies for treatment on the same day. RSV-IVIG is only licensed in the USA.

References
See also the Cochrane reviews of management of bronchiolitis

American Academy of Pediatrics, Subcommittee on Diagnosis and Management of Bronchiolitis. Diagnosis and management of bronchiolitis. *Pediatrics* 2006;**118**:1774–93. (See also 2007;**120**:890–2 and 893–4.)

Baumer JH. SIGN guideline on bronchiolitis in infants. *Arch Dis Child* 2007;**92**:ep149–51.

Duttweiler L, Nadal D, Frey B. Pulmonary and systematic bacterial co-infection in severe RSV bronchiolitis. *Arch Dis Child* 2004;**89**:1155–7.

Gooding J, Millage A, Rye A-K, *et al.* The cost and safety of multidose use of palivizumab vials. *Clin Pediatr* 2008;**47**:160–3.

Jefferson T, Foxlee R, Del Mar C, *et al.* Physical interventions to interrupt or reduce the spread of respiratory viruses: systematic review. *BMJ* 2008;**336**:77–80. [SR] (See also pp. 55–6.)

King VJ, Viswanathan M, Bordley WC, *et al.* Pharmacologic treatment of bronchiolitis in infants and children. A systematic review. *Arch Pediatr Adolesc Med* 2004;**158**:127–37. [SR] (See also pp. 119–26.)

Kumal-Bahl S, Doshi J, Campbell J. Economic analysis of respiratory syncytial virus immunoprophylaxis in high-risk infants. *Arch Pediatr Adolesc Med* 2002;**156**:1034–41. [SR] (See also pp. 1180–1.)

Kuzik BA, Al Qadhi SA, Kent S, *et al.* Nebulized hypertonic saline in the treatment of viral bronchiolitis in infants. *J Pediatr* 2007;**151**:266–70. [RCT] (See also pp. 235–7.)

Use
Pancreatic supplements are given to aid digestion in patients with cystic fibrosis.

Cystic fibrosis
Cystic fibrosis (CF) is a relatively common, recessively inherited, genetic disorder associated with abnormal mucus production. It seems to be caused by a primary defect of chloride ion secretion. Pancreatic damage causes malabsorption, while the production of viscid sputum renders patients vulnerable to recurrent bacterial infection. Thick meconium may cause intestinal obstruction (meconium ileus) at birth. Other complications include liver disease (due to biliary tract obstruction) and male infertility. The high chloride content of sweat is diagnostic, and a sample of sweat for laboratory analysis can be obtained by pilocarpine iontophoresis in most term babies more than a few weeks old. Most defective mutant genes are identifiable in the laboratory, and prenatal diagnosis is now possible. Lung damage, including bronchiectasis, used to limit the number of patients reaching adult life, but survival has now improved significantly. Diagnosis and treatment should start as soon after birth as possible to minimise lung scarring, and management should be supervised from a specialist clinic. Nutritional support plays an important part in improving survival. Lung transplantation has been offered to a few patients, but progressive liver disease remains an unsolved problem. Gene therapy offers hope for the future. Now that the value of neonatal screening (using an immunoreactive trypsin blood test) is well established, this is starting to become national policy in many countries including the US and UK.

The condition, which affects about 1:2500 of all children born in Europe and North America, was rapidly fatal when first recognised 50 years ago, but the median age of survival is now into the late 20s and still rising. Lower respiratory tract infection needs prompt and vigorous treatment, and there is one small controlled trial to suggest that continuous prophylaxis with 250 mg a day of oral flucloxacillin (q.v.) during the first 2 years of life may reduce the need for frequent hospital admission. Only a few babies need pancreatic supplements at birth, but almost all need supplementation before they are 6 months old. One small study has recently suggested that regular nebulised hypertonic (7%) saline can delay the emergence of pulmonary problems.

Pharmacology
Pancreatin is an extract prepared from pancreatic tissue that is given by mouth to aid digestion in patients with cystic fibrosis and pancreatic insufficiency. It contains protease enzymes that break protein down into peptides and proteases, lipases that hydrolyse fats to glycerol and fatty acids, and amylases that convert starch into dextrins and sugars. It is available as a powder, in capsules containing powder, in capsules containing enteric-coated granules, as free granules, and as tablets. Pancreatin should be taken with food, or immediately before food, in order to speed transit into the small intestine, because the constituent enzymes are progressively inactivated by stomach acid. The extent to which the enteric-coated formulations actually improve intact passage into the duodenum is open to some doubt. Buccal soreness can occur if the powdered product is not swallowed promptly. Perianal soreness can be helped by a zinc oxide barrier ointment, but it may be a sign of excessive supplementation. High-dose enteric-coated formulations have occasionally caused colonic strictures in children 2–12 years old.

Treatment
Sprinkle the powder from one capsule of Pancrex V® '125' into each feed, and increase this dose cautiously as necessary, as judged by the amount of undigested fat in the stool.

Vitamin supplements
The risk of subclinical vitamin A and D deficiency (the main fat-soluble vitamins) can be eliminated by giving Abidec® drops (as outlined in the monograph on multiple vitamins). Marginally low α-tocopherol levels can persist, even in children on a 25 mg daily oral supplement of vitamin E (q.v.), but whether this matters is far from clear. More seriously, suboptimal vitamin K status frequently affects bone metabolism.

Supply
Pancrex V '125' capsules are a convenient first preparation to use in the neonatal period. They contain a minimum of 160 protease units, 2950 lipase units and 3300 amylase units per capsule, and cost 3p each. Enteric-coated microspheres, which deliver a higher proportion of the constituent enzymes intact into the small intestine, have completely replaced powders for older children. Store all products in a cool place.

References
See also the relevant Cochrane reviews of CF care

Balfour-Lynn IM. Newborn screening for cystic fibrosis: evidence for benefit. *Arch Dis Child* 2008;**93**:7–10.

Conway SP, Wolfe SP, Brownlee KG, *et al.* Vitamin K status among children with cystic fibrosis and its relationship to bone mineral density and bone turnover. *Pediatrics* 2005;**115**:1325–31.

Feranchak AP, Sontag MK, Wagener JS, *et al.* Prospective, long-term study of fat-soluble vitamin status in children with cystic fibrosis identified by newborn screen. *J Pediatr* 1999;**135**:601–10.

Littlewood JM, Wolfe SDP. Control of malabsorption in cystic fibrosis. *Paediatr Drugs* 2000;**2**:205–22.

Minasian C, McCullagh A, Bush A. Cystic fibrosis in neonates and infants. [Review] *Early Hum Dev* 2005;**81**:997–1004.

O'Sullivan BP, Freedman SD. Cystic fibrosis. [Seminar] *Lancet* 2009;**373**:1891–904.

Sims EJ, Mugford M, Clark A, *et al.* Economic implications of newborn screening for cystic fibrosis: a cost of illness retrospective cohort study. *Lancet* 2007;**369**:1187–95.

PANCURONIUM BROMIDE

Use

Pancuronium causes sustained muscle paralysis. Ventilated babies should not be paralysed unless they are sedated, and most sedated babies do not need paralysis. Sustained paralysis is usually only offered to babies needing major respiratory support who continue to 'fight' the ventilator despite sedation.

Pharmacology

Pancuronium is a competitive non-depolarising muscle relaxant developed in 1966 as an analogue of curare (tubocurarine), the arrow-tip poison used by South American Indians. Pancuronium competes (like tubocurarine) with acetylcholine for the neuromuscular receptor sites of the motor end plates of voluntary muscles. It is part metabolised by the liver and then excreted in the urine with a half life that is variably prolonged in the neonatal period. Simultaneous treatment with magnesium sulphate or an aminoglycoside will further prolong the period of blockade. Pharmacokinetic information does not seem to have influenced the empirical dose regimens generally used in neonatal practice. Very little crosses the placenta, but doses of 100 micrograms/kg have been given into the fetal circulation to induce fetal paralysis prior to intrauterine fetal transfusion. Larger doses cause paralysis for 2–4 hours.

Sedation or paralysis can reduce lung barotrauma in small babies requiring artificial ventilation, reducing the risk of pneumothorax and prolonged oxygen dependency due to early bronchopulmonary dysplasia, but there are no grounds for sedating or paralysing babies as a *routine*. Paralysis makes it much more difficult to judge whether a baby is in pain, and sedation or paralysis both make it harder to watch for seizures or assess a baby's neurological status. Rocuronium (q.v.) is a related drug largely cleared from the body through the biliary tract rather than the renal tract; it may be a better drug to use where there is renal failure. Atracurium (q.v.) may be the best drug to use in this situation; it is usually given as a continuous infusion because it has a much shorter duration of action. Suxamethonium (q.v.) is the drug to use when paralysis is only required for a few minutes.

Never paralyse a non-ventilated baby without first checking that you can achieve face mask ventilation, and never paralyse a ventilated baby without first checking whether pain, correctable hypoxia, respiratory acidosis, inadequate respiratory support or an inappropriate respiratory rate is the cause of the baby's continued non-compliance. The prophylactic use of pancuronium might theoretically reduce the risk of fluctuations in cerebral blood flow velocity, but only two very small trials have, as yet, looked at this issue. Pancuronium sometimes produces a modest but sustained increase in heart rate and blood pressure, but does not usually have any noticeable effect on gastrointestinal activity or bladder function, and its use does not preclude continued gavage feeding. Joint contractures responsive to gentle physiotherapy have been reported in a few chronically paralysed babies but such problems seem to resolve spontaneously once the infant is no longer paralysed. More importantly, it has recently been suggested that the sustained high-dose use of any neuromuscular blocking drug in the neonate may make serious, progressive, late-onset deafness more likely in any child who is also treated with a loop diuretic such as furosemide (q.v.).

Treatment

First dose: Give 100 micrograms/kg to obtain prompt paralysis. Take a blood gas sample 20–30 minutes later (or use transcutaneous monitoring) to check for CO_2 accumulation. A restless baby who appears to be 'fighting' the ventilator may have been contributing to his own ventilation because of inadequate artificial ventilatory support, in which case paralysis will only exacerbate the problem.

Further doses: Most babies continue to comply with the imposed ventilatory rate as they 'wake' from the first paralysing dose (especially if a moderately fast rate and a relatively short (<0·7 second) inspiratory time is used) but a few require prolonged paralysis. The standard repeat dose is half the initial dose IV (or IM) every 4–6 hours as need arises, but some larger and older babies seem to require a higher maintenance dose.

Antidote

Give a combination of 10 micrograms/kg of glycopyrronium (or 20 micrograms/kg of atropine) and 50 micrograms/kg of neostigmine IV, as outlined in the monograph on glycopyrronium.

Supply and administration

2 ml ampoules containing 4 mg of pancuronium cost 65p each. Dilute 0·5 ml from the ampoule with 0·5 ml of 0·9% sodium chloride in a 1 ml syringe before use to obtain a preparation containing 100 micrograms in 0·1 ml. Pancuronium is stable for up to 6 weeks at 25°C, but is best stored, wherever possible, at 4°C. Open ampoules should not be kept. The US product contains 1% benzyl alcohol.

References

See also the relevant Cochrane reviews

Besunder JB, Reed MD, Blumer JL. Principles of drug biodisposition in the neonate. A critical evaluation of the pharmacokinetic-pharmacodynamic interface (part II). *Clin Pharmacokinet* 1988;**14**:261–86.

Costarino AT, Polin RA. Neuromuscular relaxants in the neonate. *Clin Perinatol* 1987;**14**:965–99.

Fanconi S, Ensner S, Knecht B. Effects of paralysis with pancuronium bromide on joint mobility in premature infants. *J Pediatr* 1995;**127**:134–6.

Robertson CMT, Tyebkhan JM, Peliowski A, *et al.* Ototoxic drugs and sensorineural hearing loss following severe neonatal respiratory failure. *Acta Paediatr* 2006;**95**:214–23.

Use

Papaverine has been used experimentally in a few centres to reduce the risk of vasospasm and prolong the life of peripheral arterial catheters. Glyceryl trinitrate ointment (q.v.) will sometimes correct any vasospasm that does occur.

Pharmacology

Papaverine is an alkaloid present in opium although it is not related, either chemically or pharmacologically, to the other opium alkaloids. It was first isolated in 1848 and was briefly in vogue as a vasodilator and antispasmodic in the 1920s prior to the development of synthetic analogues of atropine. It has a direct relaxant effect on smooth muscle, probably because it inhibits phosphodiesterase, and it was frequently used for a time by intercavernosal injection in the treatment of male impotence. It can, however, cause general vasodilatation, and it was shown, in a randomised controlled trial involving over 200 children in 1993, to extend the functional life of peripheral arterial cannulas. Such lines also lasted 40% longer in a recent neonatal trial. However, since this study only involved 141 babies, more studies will be needed before we can be sure that this form of prophylaxis is not only effective but also safe when used in the preterm baby. Its use in the first few days of life certainly needs to be approached with some caution because vasodilatation could have adverse cerebrovascular consequences. A sustained low-dose intra-arterial infusion of tolazoline (q.v.) has been used for the same purpose, and has also been used to abolish the acute 'white leg' occasionally caused by femoral artery spasm following umbilical artery catheterisation. Low-dose heparin (q.v.) has been shown to extend the 'life' of intravascular lines in adults, but the only neonatal trials done to date have been too small to show similar benefit with any certainty. The need for invasive arterial sampling has been much reduced by recent developments in pulse oximetry, and systolic blood pressure can also be monitored non-invasively using Doppler sphygmomanometry.

Adverse effects of papaverine are uncommon, but include flushing, hypotension and gastrointestinal disturbances. High doses can cause cardiac arrhythmia. The drug is rapidly metabolised by the liver and excreted in the urine, the adult half life being variable, but usually only a little more than 1 hour. Nothing is known about the time course of drug elimination in the neonatal period, or the effect of maternal use during pregnancy or lactation.

Take care not to confuse papaveretum for papaverine. Papaverine can be confused with papaveretum, a preparation containing a mixture of opium alkaloids (including morphine and codeine as well as papaverine hydrochloride), with potentially fatal consequences.

Treatment

A slow syringe-controlled infusion can be used to help sustain catheter patency. 100 micrograms/ml of papaverine made up as described below, and infused at a rate of 1 ml/hour (with or without additional heparin), can prolong the functional life of a peripheral arterial line. This fluid must *not* be used to flush the catheter through after sampling: any such bolus of papaverine could cause marked vasodilatation.

Compatibility

Papaverine was co-infused with heparin at a rate of 1 ml/hour in both the controlled trials referred to above.

Supply and administration

Papaverine is an unlicensed product obtainable by the pharmacy to special order. Ampoules containing 30 mg in 2 ml cost £2·20 each. To obtain a solution containing approximately 100 micrograms/ml take 5 mg (0·3 ml) of papaverine, dilute to 50 ml with glucose, glucose saline or saline, and infuse at a rate of not more than 1 ml/hour using a syringe pump. While 0·9% sodium chloride is the most frequently used infusion fluid, the sodium this delivers to the baby needs to be considered with some care when calculating a preterm baby's total daily sodium intake – glucose or glucose saline may often be a better option.

References

Griffin MP, Kendrick AS. Does papaverine prevent failure of arterial catheters in neonates? [Abstract] *Pediat Res* 1995;**37**:207A.
Griffin MP, Siadaty MS. Papaverine prolongs patency of peripheral arterial catheters in neonates. *J Pediatr* 2005;**146**:62–5. [RCT]
Heulitt MJ, Farrington EA, O'Shea TM, *et al.* Double blind, randomised, controlled trial of papaverine-containing infusions to prevent failure of arterial catheters in pediatric patients. *Crit Care Med* 1993;**21**:825–9. [RCT]

PARACETAMOL = Acetaminophen (USAN)   (web comment)

Use
Paracetamol is a valuable analgesic also sometimes used to control fever. An IV formulation is now available.

Pharmacology
Paracetamol, which has analgesic and antipyretic but no anti-inflammatory properties, was first marketed as an alternative to phenacetin in 1953. Now that aspirin (q.v.) is no longer recommended for children under 16 (except as an antithrombotic and in Kawasaki disease) because of its link to Reye syndrome, paracetamol has become the most widely used analgesic for children (although dosage is often suboptimal). Intermittent (p.r.n.) administration in response to perceived pain seldom provides optimal relief and, while anticipatory use (treatment started 1–2 hours before surgery) certainly helps to control postoperative pain, visceral pain often needs opiate analgesia. Clearance is slightly slower in babies with visible jaundice. Tolerance does not develop with repeated use (as it does with opioid drugs), and respiratory depression is not a problem, but there is an analgesic ceiling that cannot be overcome by using a higher dose.

Paracetamol is rapidly absorbed by mouth, widely distributed in the body (V_D ~1 l/kg) and mostly conjugated in the liver before excretion in the urine. Optimum pain relief only occurs an hour after the blood level peaks. The main metabolite changes during childhood, but elimination in babies over 3 months old (half life ~3 hours) is as rapid as in adults. It is a little slower in term babies at birth (4 hours), and is initially 8 hours in babies born more than 8 weeks early. Rectal absorption is rapid but incomplete, and influenced by the volume given. Luckily, although the manufacturer has not yet endorsed its use in the preterm baby, the development of an IV formulation (see web commentary) is set to render rectal administration unnecessary. Toxicity is uncommon in infancy, possibly because reduced cytochrome P450 activity limits toxic arene metabolite production, but an overdose could still cause late lethal liver failure if not treated promptly. Paracetamol seems the analgesic of choice in pregnancy, and the breastfed baby is only exposed to 5% of the weight-related maternal dose.

Management of fever
While paracetamol can give symptomatic relief to a child who is feverish (just as an adult will sometimes take two aspirins and retire to bed!), its use to control fever per se is usually uncalled for. One oral 30 mg/kg dose often suffices. Prophylactic use for febrile convulsions is of no proven value, and these are only of concern if they are focal, last more than 15 minutes, or recur during the same febrile illness. Most children just need to be unwrapped. Forced cooling does not work. Ibuprofen (q.v.) may be preferable for babies over 3 months old because asthma seems commoner later on in children who experienced early paracetamol exposure.

Treatment in the neonate
Oral pain relief: Give a 24 mg/kg loading dose (1 ml/kg of the 24 mg/ml oral elixir) and a maintenance dose of 12 mg/kg every 4 hours (every 8 hours in babies of less than 32 weeks' postmenstrual age).
IV administration: Give a 20 mg/kg loading dose over about 15 minutes. Then give further maintenance doses once every 6 hours as follows: 10 mg/kg to babies of less than 30 weeks' postmenstrual age, 12·5 mg/kg to babies of 31–36 weeks' postmenstrual age and 15 mg/kg to term babies.
Rectal administration: Give term babies a 36 mg/kg loading dose and then 24 mg/kg once every 8 hours.
Sustained use: These doses are higher than those suggested by the manufacturer, so it is wise to check the trough blood level before giving high-dose treatment by any route for more than 36 hours to a baby less than 3 months old (sooner in the jaundiced or very preterm baby) to check safety and also optimise pain relief.

Treatment in babies over 3 months old
Oral pain relief: Give a 24 mg/kg loading dose and then 18 mg/kg once every 4 hours.
IV pain relief: Give a 20 mg/kg loading dose and then 15 mg/kg once every 4 hours.

Toxicity
Lethal liver damage can occur in adults if the plasma level exceeds 150 mg/l four or more hours after ingestion (1 mg/l = 6·62 mmol/l). The safe threshold after repeated use is much less certain. Give 150 mg/kg of IV acetylcysteine promptly over 30 minutes, in a little 5% glucose, if there is concern. Then give 12 mg/kg per hour for 4 hours, followed by 4 mg/kg per hour for 48 hours. Later doses can be given orally.

Blood levels
Collect at least 50 μl of plasma, and aim to sustain a trough level of 10 mg/l. Patients can be asymptomatic despite toxic blood levels, but relief of pain almost certainly requires a peak plasma level of over 20 mg/l.

Supply
100 ml of the 24 mg/ml sugar-free elixir costs 41p. Parents can get this for a baby over 3 months old without a prescription. Using this elixir rectally (instead of a suppository) speeds absorption. 50 ml (10 mg/ml) IV vials cost £1·50. Use within an hour of dilution. 10 ml ampoules of acetylcysteine (200 mg/ml) cost £2·50.

References
See also the relevant Cochrane reviews

Anderson BJ, Allegaert K. Intravenous neonatal paracetamol dosing: the magic 10 days. [Editorial] Paediatr Anaesth 2009;**19**:289–95.
Duggan ST, Scott LJ. Intravenous paracetamol (acetaminophen). Drugs 2009;**69**:101–13.
Jacqz-Aigrain E, Anderson BJ. Pain control: non-steroidal anti-inflammatory agents. Sem Fetal Neonatal Med 2006;**11**:251–9.
Palmer GM, Atkins M, Anderson BJ, et al. IV acetaminophen pharmacokinetics in neonates after multiple doses. Br J Anaesth 2008;**101**:523–30.

Use

Paraldehyde provides a very effective, and currently underutilised, way of terminating persistent non-hypoglycaemic convulsions especially if there is no response to one of the drugs commonly used first – IV phenobarbital (q.v.) in the neonate, or a benzodiazepine (such as buccal midazolam, intranasal lorazepam or rectal diazepam (q.v.)) in later infancy. The IM route is preferable when the dose involved is less than 1 ml.

Pharmacology

Paraldehyde, a polymer of acetaldehyde, has been used for a century as a sedative-hypnotic and for seizure control. It is a potent anticonvulsant capable of controlling seizures refractory to phenobarbital, phenytoin and the benzodiazepines without causing respiratory depression. It exerts its action rapidly and is then eliminated from the body with a half life that is rather variable, but only a little shorter than that of most other anticonvulsants used in the neonatal period. It crosses the placenta, but there is nothing to suggest that its use is hazardous in pregnancy. There are no reports of use during lactation.

Drug elimination is by oxidation to acetaldehyde and carbon dioxide in the liver and also by direct excretion through the lungs. Dispersal into body tissues is very variable (V_D ~4 l/kg). The half life in babies is also very variable (8–27 hours) but generally rather longer than in children (7·5 hours) and adults (6 hours). The dose given does not need to be modified in babies with kidney failure because renal clearance is negligible, but the drug's variable and prolonged half life probably makes repeated dosing unwise in the first few weeks of life. It has been suggested that high barbiturate levels can retard drug clearance by the liver, probably because of competition for the liver's oxidative pathways, but this remains to be confirmed. It is equally possible that the prolonged half life often seen in the first week of life could be a consequence of the impact of intrapartum asphyxia on liver metabolism. The management of babies in whom EEG evidence of seizure activity persists despite treatment with both phenobarbital and phenytoin (q.v.) is in urgent need of further study. Paraldehyde has fallen out of favour, but might well turn out to be quite effective if a blood level of 100 mg/l can be achieved. Clonazepam (q.v.), lidocaine (q.v.) and valproate (q.v.) are alternatives currently under study.

The IM route was once widely used in babies, but standard texts now generally consider the rectal route safer. Large IM injections are certainly painful, and they can cause an unpleasant sterile abscess with subsequent muscle and/or nerve damage, but such problems are *very* uncommon following the deep IM injection of volumes not exceeding 1 ml (which is all that any neonate should need), and the response to an IM injection is much quicker than the response to rectal administration. Rectal diazepam was once widely used to control seizures in a home setting, but a dose of liquid lorazepam or midazolam (q.v.) given into the nose or mouth is usually equally effective and families often find this approach more acceptable. However, paraldehyde provides a very effective way of stopping prolonged seizure activity in *any* setting if IV access proves difficult.

Treatment

Rectal: Give a single 0·4 ml/kg dose of paraldehyde mixed with an equal volume of olive oil (or mineral oil).
Intramuscular: Give 0·2 ml/kg *deep* IM. A second identical dose can be given if seizures persist or recur, but no further doses should be given to the neonate after that for 36 hours because the half life is unpredictable.
Intravenous: Paraldehyde *can* be given as an IV infusion, but the use of this route is now generally discouraged, and it is not really necessary given the drug's long neonatal half life. To give 0·4 ml/kg of paraldehyde (the maximum safe dose) as an IV infusion, dilute 2·5 ml of paraldehyde to 50 ml with 5% glucose and then give 4 ml/kg of this solution over *just 2 hours* as a slow continuous infusion protected from light.

Supply and administration

Supply: Amber glass bottles that contain 15 ml of paraldehyde already mixed with 15 ml of olive oil are available on special order in the UK for rectal administration. They cost £6. Ampoules of pure paraldehyde (containing 1 g/ml) are still available in some countries, but are no longer marketed in the UK. Never use either product if there is brown discolouration, or if there is a sharp pungent odour of acetic acid when the container is first opened. Keep all products below 25°C during storage.
Administration: Paraldehyde reacts chemically with rubber and with most plastics (polythene and polypropylene syringes being more resistant than those made of polyvinyl chloride (PVC)), but it can be given using any plastic syringe as long as it is injected just as soon as it is drawn up. However, a polypropylene syringe (such as a Plastipak® syringe made by Becton Dickinson) and a polypropylene extension set (such as one of the products marketed by Vygon) **must** be used if a sustained IV infusion is to be given.

References

Ahmad S, Ellis JC, Kamwendo H, *et al.* Efficacy and safety of intranasal lorazepam versus intramuscular paraldehyde for protracted convulsions in children: an open randomised trial. *Lancet* 2006;**367**:1591–7. [RCT]
Armstrong DL, Battin MR. Pervasive seizures caused by hypoxic-ischaemic encephalopathy: treatment with intravenous paraldehyde. *J Child Neurol* 2001;**16**:915–17.
Giacoia GP, Gessner IK, Zaleska MM, *et al.* Pharmacokinetics of paraldehyde disposition in the neonate. *J Pediatr* 1984;**104**:291–6.
Johnson DL, Vigoreaux JA. Compatability of paraldehyde with plastic syringes and needle hubs. *Am J Hosp Pharm* 1984;**41**:306–8.
Koren G, Butt W, Tajchgot P, *et al.* Intravenous paraldehyde for seizure control in newborn infants. *Neurology* 1986;**36**:108–11.
Rowland AG, Gill AM, Stewart AB, *et al.* Review of the efficacy of rectal paraldehyde in the management of acute and prolonged tonic-clonic convulsions. *Arch Dis Child* 2009;**94**:720–3.

Use

Amino acid solutions, together with glucose and other trace nutrients, are used with or without Intralipid® (q.v.), to supplement or replace enteral feeding when milk feeds are contraindicated or poorly tolerated.

Nutritional factors

Intravenous solutions are capable of providing every nutrient necessary for growth, although enteral feeding is always to be preferred where possible. Serious progressive cholestatic jaundice can occur in the preterm baby who is not offered at least a little milk by mouth, and sepsis can exacerbate this problem. Preterm babies not given at least 1 g/kg of protein a day develop a progressive negative nitrogen balance, and an intake of at *least* 2·5 g/kg a day seems necessary to support growth. If parenteral nutrition is given, and some argue that it is given too often, there should be enough protein to minimise the interruption of growth.

The standard neonatal preparation that is most widely used in the north of England contains glucose and a mixture of synthetic L-amino acids (Vaminolact®) with trace minerals (7·5 ml/l of Peditrace®), water-soluble vitamins (seven-tenths of the contents of a vial of Solivito N®) and an extra 30 mg of ascorbic acid per litre, and a basic quantity of sodium (27 mmol/l), potassium (20 mmol/l), calcium (12·5 mmol/l), magnesium (1·3 mmol/l) and phosphate (12·3 mmol/l). This provides either 2·7 or 3·5 g/l of nitrogen (17 or 22 g/l of protein), and is available formulated so that the final glucose concentration is 10%, 12·5% or 15% (providing 400, 500 or 600 kcal/l of energy). It contains no iron. Solutions containing more than 10% glucose rapidly cause thrombophlebitis unless infused into a large vessel. Intralipid with Vitlipid N® infant should be added to augment the calorie intake and provide the baby's other nutritional needs. Amino acid solutions with a profile mimicking that provided by the placenta or breast milk are now generally used. These contain taurine, and do not produce the high plasma tyrosine and phenylalanine levels previously seen with egg protein-based products. The acidosis that develops when the intake of non-metabolisable chloride exceeds 6 mmol/kg per day can be reduced by substituting up to 6 mmol/kg of acetate. Aluminium (present as a contaminant in some ingredients – notably calcium gluconate) can affect bone density and cause permanent neurological damage.

Intake

Babies taking nothing by mouth can usually be started on 5 ml/kg per hour of the standard 10% solution with 2·7 g/l of nitrogen as soon as they are stable (6 ml/kg in babies over 2 days old). Energy intake can then be increased further *either* by using a formulation containing 12·5% or 15% glucose (if a central 'long line' is available), *or* by increasing the infusion rate to 7 or 8 ml/kg per hour. While this policy provides 2·4 g/kg of protein a day from the outset, the product containing 3·5 g/l of nitrogen will come closer to optimising the protein intake needed for sustained growth. More phosphate (q.v.) may also be needed. Some babies of <30 weeks' gestation need another 2–3 mmol/kg of sodium a day to replace loss due to renal immaturity.

Administration

Individually 'customised' infusions are rarely necessary. Their routine use causes much unnecessary blood sampling, the results are no better, and any such policy doubles the total cost. How beneficial it is to add heparin (q.v.) remains inadequately studied. A few other drugs (as noted in the relevant monographs in this compendium) can be co-infused with the formulation specified here if lack of vascular access so demands, but this may increase the risk of sepsis. These should be infused using a Y-connector sited as close to the patient as possible. Add *nothing* to any amino acid solution after it leaves the pharmacy.

Monitoring

Clinically stable children require only marginally more biochemical monitoring than bottle-fed babies when on the standard formulation described here: it is the problem that made parenteral nutrition necessary that usually makes monitoring necessary. Ignore urinary glucose loss unless it exceeds 1%. Liver function should be monitored. Sepsis is the main hazard associated with any reliance on IV nutrition.

Tissue extravasation

'Tissue burns' are much more serious than those caused by a comparable solution of glucose. A strategy for the early treatment is described in the monograph on hyaluronidase.

Supply

Pre-prepared standard nominal half-litre bags cost about £20 to produce and remain safe to use for a month. Bags should be changed aseptically after 48 hours; change the bag, filter *and* giving set every 96 hours.

References

See also the relevant Cochrane reviews

Beecroft C, Martin H, Puntis JWL. How often do parenteral nutrition prescriptions for the newborn need to be individualized? *Clin Nutr* 1999;**18**:83–5.

Clark RH, Chase DH, Spitzer AR. Effects of two different doses of amino acid supplements on growth and blood amino acid levels in premature neonates admitted to a neonatal intensive care unit: a randomized controlled trial. *Pediatrics* 2007;**120**:1286–96. [RCT] (See also **121**:865–6.)

Embleton ND. Optimal protein and energy intakes in preterm infants. *Early Hum Dev* 2007;**83**:831–7.

Lenclen R, Crauste-Manciet S, Narcy P, *et al.* Assessment and implementation of a standardized parenteral formulation for early nutritional support of very preterm infants. *Eur J Pediatr* 2006;**165**:512–18.

Poindexter BB, Langer JC, Dusik AM, *et al.* Early provision of parenteral amino acids in extremely low birth weight infants: relation to growth and neurodevelopmental outcome. *J Pediatr* 2006;**148**:300–5. (See also pp. 291–4.)

Yeung MY, Smyth JP, Maheshwari R, *et al.* Evaluation of standardized versus individualised total parenteral nutrition regime for neonates less than 33 weeks gestation. *J Paediatr Child Health* 2003;**39**:613–17.

Use

Benzylpenicillin is the treatment of choice for pneumococcal, meningococcal, syphilitic, gonococcal and aerobic and anaerobic streptococcal infection. It is also very adequate for *Listeria* infection, although ampicillin or amoxicillin (q.v.) are better. Flucloxacillin (q.v.) is more appropriate for staphylococcal infection because most strains produce penicillinase. Procaine penicillin (q.v.) is sometimes used to treat syphilis.

Pharmacology

Benzylpenicillin is a naturally occurring, bactericidal substance, first used clinically in 1941, that acts by interfering with bacterial cell wall synthesis. Fetal concentrations approach those in maternal serum, but extremely little is ingested in breast milk. Since it is also destroyed by gastric acid and poorly absorbed by the gut, there is no contraindication to its use during lactation. Use phenoxymethylpenicillin (penicillin V), which is acid stable, when giving penicillin by mouth, giving 25 mg/kg doses at similar time intervals as for the IV or IM drug (although oral amoxicillin is a more widely used alternative in this situation). Active excretion by the renal tubules is the most important factor affecting the serum half life, which falls from 4–5 hours at birth to 1·5 hours by 1 month (gestation at birth having only a modest influence on this). Exposure may further stimulate tubular secretion. Very high levels are neurotoxic, making it important to reduce the dose or choose a different drug when there is renal failure. Transient thrombocytopenia can also occur. Allergic reactions are the main hazard in those with a history of prior exposure. The dose regimen recommended here allows for the fact that CSF penetration is poor even when the meninges are inflamed. Intrathecal treatment is not advisable.

Group B streptococcal infection

Death caused by exposure to group B streptococcal (GBS) bacteria during birth is now commoner than death from surfactant deficiency in babies weighing ≥1·5 kg, but prevalence in the UK does not seem to justify the universal screening policy advocated in North America. Intermittent bowel carriage is common in adults and, while it seldom causes symptoms, it can cause urinary infection during pregnancy. However, half the babies born to carriers also become carriers for a time, and 1–2% develop life-threatening infection within hours of birth. Carriage cannot be eliminated by antenatal treatment, and early neonatal infection often spreads too rapidly for post-delivery treatment to be effective, but prophylaxis started at least 4 hours before delivery can reduce the risk of neonatal illness. Current US guidelines recommend that known carriers, and all mothers with intrapartum pyrexia (≥38°C) or whose membranes have been ruptured ≥18 hours, should be given 3 g of benzylpenicillin every 6 hours as a slow IV injection during labour. Women allergic to penicillin should receive IV erythromycin or clindamycin (q.v.). Babies only require further investigation or treatment after delivery if symptomatic or born before 35 weeks' gestation. Some have suggested giving all infected babies and their mothers 4 days of oral rifampicin (q.v.) as well as penicillin, because penicillin on its own does little to eliminate the risk of continued carriage, and 2% of infected babies suffer a second episode of overt infection, but this may not eliminate carriage. An alternative strategy for protecting babies from *all* early-onset bacterial sepsis when membranes rupture before the onset of labour appears in the monograph on ampicillin.

Treatment

Dose: Give 60 mg/kg per dose IM or (slowly) IV when there could be evidence of meningitis (especially GBS meningitis); 30 mg/kg is more than adequate in all other circumstances. Consider giving gentamicin synergistically as well for 48 hours for infection with group B streptococci or *Listeria*.

Timing: Give one dose every 12 hours in the first week of life, one dose every 8 hours in babies 1–3 weeks old, and one dose every 6 hours in babies 4 or more weeks old. The dose should be halved and the dosage interval doubled when there is renal failure. Give treatment for at least 7–10 days in proven pneumonia and septicaemia, and in the management of congenital syphilis. Treat meningitis for 3 weeks and osteitis for 4 weeks. Oral medication is sometimes used to complete a course of treatment.

Supply and administration

A 600 mg (1 million units or one 'mega unit') vial costs 43p. Add 5·6 ml of sterile water for injection to get a solution containing 10 mg in 0·1 ml. Slow IV administration has been advocated, but there is no published evidence to support this advice (see website commentary). A 60 mg/kg dose of the UK product contains 0·17 mmol/kg of sodium (most US products contain the potassium salt). Staff handling penicillin regularly should avoid hand contact as this can cause skin sensitisation. Penicillin V (25 mg/ml) is available as a syrup (£1·70 per 100 ml) which is stable for 2 weeks after reconstitution if stored at 4°C.

References

See the relevant Cochrane reviews of GBS prophylaxis

American Academy of Pediatrics. Committee on Infectious Disease and Committee on Fetus and Newborn. Revised guidelines for prevention of early onset group B streptococcal (GBS) infection. *Pediatrics* 1997;**99**:489–96.

Colbourn TE, Asseburg C, Bojke L, *et al.* Preventive strategies for group B streptococcal and other bacterial infections in early infancy: cost effectiveness and value of information analysis. *BMJ* 2007;**335**:655–8. [SR] (See also pp. 622–3.)

Fernandez M, Rench MA, Albanyan EA, *et al.* Failure of rifampin to eradicate group B streptococcal colonization in infants. *Pediatr Infect Dis J* 2001;**20**:371–6.

Mercer BM, Carr TL, Beazley DD, *et al.* Antibiotic use and drug-resistant infant sepsis. *Am J Obstet Gynecol* 1999;**181**:816–21.

Oddie S, Embleton ND. Risk factors for early onset neonatal group B streptococcal sepsis: case control study. *BMJ* 2002;**325**:308–11.

Royal College of Obstetrics and Gynaecology. *Prevention of early onset neonatal group B streptococcal disease.* Guideline 36. London: RCOG Press, 2003. [SR] (See www.rcog.org.uk.)

Schrag SJ, Zywicki S, Farkey MM, *et al.* Group B streptococcal disease in the era of intrapartum antibiotic prophylaxis. *N Eng J Med* 2000;**342**:15–20.

Use
Pethidine remains widely used to relieve pain during labour, although evidence of efficacy is limited. Use in infancy has received little study, and toxic quantities of the active metabolite, norpethidine, can accumulate with repeated usage. Morphine (q.v.) remains by far the best studied neonatal analgesic.

Pharmacology
Pethidine is a synthetic opioid developed in Germany during a review of the many analogues of atropine in 1939. The dose required to provide analgesia is variable. It is only a tenth as potent as morphine and its analgesic effect is not as well sustained. It was originally hoped that, because it bears no chemical similarity to morphine, it would not be addictive, but this is not so. Oral bioavailability is limited (about 50%) because of rapid first pass clearance by the liver, where the drug undergoes hydrolysis or demethylation and conjugation before excretion. Tissue levels markedly exceed plasma levels ($V_D \sim 7$ l/kg), and clearance in the first 3 months is much slower than later in infancy. The average half life in young babies is about 11 hours and also *very* variable (range 3–60 hours), but in babies 3–18 months old may be even lower than it is in adults ($t^1/_2$ about 3·5 hours). Similar half life changes have been documented for morphine. This variation between patients and over time, and the lack of any clear evidence as to what constitutes an effective analgesic dose, makes it difficult to recommend the use of pethidine in young children. The active metabolite, norpethidine, is renally excreted. It has an extended half life, and neurotoxic quantities can accumulate with repeated usage, particularly if there is renal failure.

Increased scepticism is being voiced about the drug's central place in the management of pain relief in labour but, at the moment, it remains the only parenteral analgesic that midwives in the UK can give on their own authority. It often causes more drowsiness, disorientation and nausea than genuine relief from pain. Morphine is no better. Sclerotic legislation denies midwives and their patients straight access to any other parenteral analgesic while the scope for nitrous oxide (q.v.) analgesia remains undervalued.

Pethidine crosses the placenta rapidly, and cord levels in babies delivered 1–5 hours after the mother had an IM injection during labour are higher than the corresponding maternal levels. Neonatal respiratory depression is most often seen 2–3 hours after such an injection. Feeding may be slow, and some babies show impaired behavioural responses and EEG abnormalities for 2–3 days after birth. Maternal use during lactation only exposes the baby to about 2% of the weight-related maternal dose. There is no evidence of teratogenicity.

Pain relief
Maternal pain relief in labour: A single dose of 100 or 150 mg is usually administered IM. This may be repeated once during labour but rarely, if ever, more often than this. Try to avoid using a total of more than 1·5 mg/kg.
Pain relief in infancy: A dose of 1 mg/kg IM or IV has been used, but usually only in babies receiving ventilatory support. No repeat dose should be given for 10–12 hours in babies less than 2 months old (or for 4–6 hours in infants more than 3 months old) if drug accumulation is to be avoided.

Antidote
Neonatal respiratory depression is readily reversed by naloxone (q.v.), but *serious* depression is very seldom caused by the use of an opiate to relieve pain during labour. Opiate use during labour can, however, cause sustained neonatal drowsiness and interfere with the early initiation of lactation, and there are many who argue that IM naloxone should be used more widely to counter this problem.

Supply and administration
1 and 2 ml ampoules containing 50 mg/ml are available. They cost approximately 50p each. Take 0·2 ml (10 mg) from the ampoule and dilute to 1 ml with glucose, glucose saline or saline to obtain a preparation containing 10 mg/ml for accurate IM or IV administration.

The storage and administration of pethidine is controlled under Schedule 2 of the UK Misuse of Drugs Regulations 1988 (Misuse of Drugs Act 1971). Midwives in the UK have the legal right to prescribe pethidine or pentazocine with or without promazine, oxytocin or Syntometrine®, and naloxone, and to give lidocaine during labour, on their own authority (as outlined in the website commentary). Other analgesics can be given if use is covered by a Patient Group Direction.

References
See also the relevant Cochrane reviews

Armstrong PJ, Bersten A. Normeperidine toxicity. *Anaesth Analg* 1986;**65**:536–8.
Bricker L, Laender T. Parenteral opioids for labour pain relief: a systematic review. *Am J Obstet Gynecol* 2002;**186**:S94–109. [SR]
Hunt S. Pethidine: love it or hate it. *MIDIRS Midwifery Digest* 2002;**12**:363–5.
Pokela M-L, Olkkola KT, Koivisto M, *et al*. Pharmacokinetics and pharmacodynamics of intravenous meperidine in neonates and infants. *Clin Pharmacol Ther* 1992;**52**:342–9.
Pokela M-L. Pain relief can reduce hypoxia in distressed neonates during routine treatment procedures. *Pediatrics* 1994;**93**:379–83. [RCT]
Saneto RP, Fitch JA, Cohen BH. Acute neurotoxicity of meperidine in an infant. *Pediatr Neurol* 1996;**14**:339–41.

Phenobarbitone (former BAN) = **PHENOBARBITAL**

Use

Phenobarbital is widely used in the initial management of neonatal fits. It is seldom the most appropriate drug to use in the longer term management of epilepsy.

Pharmacology

Phenobarbital, first marketed as a hypnotic in 1904, was widely used as an anticonvulsant for many years, but use in children then declined sharply because sustained exposure was thought to have an adverse effect on behaviour (a perception robustly challenged by a recent well-designed trial undertaken in Bangladesh). Other trials have failed to detect the supposed parallel adverse effect on cognition. Many adults certainly still remain well controlled on long-term medication. Oral phenobarbital is only slowly absorbed, and IM absorption can take 2–4 hours, so the drug must be given IV if a rapid response is required. An overdose can cause drowsiness, vasodilatation, hypotension and dangerous respiratory depression. Therapeutic hypothermia (33–34°C) doubles the half life. The drug is largely metabolised by the liver, but a quarter is excreted unchanged in the urine in the neonatal period. The plasma half life is so long in the neonatal period (**2–4 days**) that treatment once a day is perfectly adequate, but the half life decreases with age, and is halved after 1–2 weeks of medication because the drug acts to induce liver enzymes. This enzyme-inducing property has been used to speed the liver's conjugation and excretion of bilirubin. It also influences the metabolism and half life of a number of other drugs. Phenobarbital, phenytoin and carbamazepine all induce hepatic microsomal enzymes, speeding the metabolism of oestrogens and progestogens thus making it unwise for women to rely on low-dose oral contraceptives when taking any of these anticonvulsants.

Maternal use

See the valproate website for a general discussion of anticonvulsant use during pregnancy and lactation.

Fetal consequences: Barbiturates rapidly cross the placenta, the fetal blood level being two-thirds the maternal level. There is little clear evidence of teratogenicity, but minor cardiac anomalies, skeletal defects and palatal clefts are more common in the babies of mothers taking anticonvulsants for epilepsy. Phenytoin has been implicated more than phenobarbital in this regard and some of the reported defects may have more to do with the epilepsy than its treatment. Fetal exposure to phenobarbital may have some impact on later cognitive development. The hazards associated with uncontrolled epilepsy are, however, almost certainly greater than the hazards associated with continued medication.

Neonatal consequences: The babies of mothers taking phenobarbital are occasionally hypoprothrombinaemic at birth, but this bleeding tendency can be easily corrected by giving the baby 100 micrograms/kg of vitamin K (q.v.) IM at birth. (A standard 1 mg dose is widely used.) Giving phenobarbital during labour can cause the baby to be rather sleepy and feed poorly for 2–3 days. Some authorities (including the BNF) feel that breastfeeding may be unwise in mothers taking phenobarbital on a regular basis, and calculations suggest that neonatal blood levels could approach or exceed those seen in the mother. More information is needed, because few problems have been reported in practice. Drowsiness has occasionally been alluded to, however, and there is one report of a baby who appeared to develop severe withdrawal symptoms when breastfeeding was stopped abruptly at 7 months.

Use to prevent intraventricular haemorrhage (IVH): While early reports that giving phenobarbital immediately after birth could reduce the incidence of IVH were not supported by later larger trials, there remained a belief that *antenatal* prophylaxis (typically 10 mg/kg slowly IV to the mother, followed by an oral maintenance dose of 100 mg once or twice a day) might be beneficial. Six trials involving over 1600 women have now been reported and it would seem that, yet again, the benefits suggested by a number of small trials of variable quality have not been confirmed by subsequent larger studies.

Use to prevent neonatal jaundice: Maternal treatment (typically 100 mg a day) reduces the chance that neonatal jaundice will need treatment. Neonatal treatment (typically 5–8 mg/kg a day for 2–7 days) also has a measurable effect, but is not widely used. Phototherapy (q.v.) usually suffices.

Neonatal use

Intrapartum asphyxia: Animal evidence suggests that phenobarbital reduces the amount of damage caused by cerebral anoxia (independent of its anticonvulsant effect) and the evidence from one small trial using a prompt 40 mg/kg loading dose suggests it may also be of clinical value, although another small study, and a small trial of the barbiturate thiopental (q.v.), failed to find evidence of clinical benefit. Further trials are clearly called for. Other possible strategies are discussed in the monograph on hypothermia.

Cholestatic jaundice: Phenobarbital (5 mg/kg per day) will improve bile flow and can sometimes alleviate pruritis, although ursodeoxycholic acid (q.v.) is usually more effective. Additional vitamin K will be required. Vitamins A, D and E (q.v.) may be needed if jaundice is prolonged.

Maternal drug dependency: Babies of mothers who are dependent on other drugs as well as opiates who are suffering *serious* withdrawal symptoms sometimes benefit from a short 4–6-day course of phenobarbital. Start with the same loading as for seizure control (see below).

Seizures: There is no evidence that failure to control *all* seizure activity puts the baby at increased risk of long-term cerebral damage. However, it is now also becoming clear that electroencephalographic (EEG) seizure activity often occurs in the absence of visible motor activity in the newborn baby, and that when such activity is semi-continuous it is potentially damaging. Animal evidence certainly points in that direction. Much remains to be learnt from conventional or amplitude-integrated (aEEG) examination. Although some babies who fail to respond to a standard loading dose of phenobarbital seem to respond clinically to a higher loading dose, it is not yet clear how often this actually stops EEG seizure activity. While high-dose treatment (with a loading dose up to 40 mg/kg) has its advocates, it certainly makes many babies drowsy

Continued on p. 204

enough to render neurological assessment more difficult, if not impossible, and cause some preterm babies to become ventilator dependent. Where a high loading dose *has* been used, no daily maintenance dose should be started for at least 3–4 days (especially if there has been intrapartum asphyxia). Seizures that fail to respond to phenobarbital may respond to phenytoin (q.v.) or high-dose lidocaine (q.v.), although some believe paraldehyde (q.v.) is a more appropriate first option. Clonazepam and midazolam (q.v.) seldom arrest EEG evidence of seizure activity if phenobarbital has not been successful. See the website for a longer discussion of what is known about the available options. Pyridoxine dependency (q.v.), biotin deficiency (q.v.) and folinic acid-responsive seizures **must** be considered if unexplained seizures do not respond to phenobarbital.

The tonic posturing and motor automatisms, repetitive stereotypic mouthing movements, rotatory arm movements, pedalling and stepping activity that is seen in most encephalopathic babies is clearly abnormal. The background (interictal) EEG activity in these babies is also usually very abnormal.

Isolated seizures in a baby who appears alert, awake and normal when not actually fitting are usually well controlled by phenobarbital. These babies usually have a normal interictal EEG, and their long-term prognosis is usually good. If pheno-barbital and phenytoin fail, carbamazepine (q.v.), valproate (q.v.) or vigabatrin (q.v.) may work. It is seldom necessary to use more than one drug. Most babies given an anticonvulsant in the neonatal period can be weaned from all treatment within 14 days, and few need medication at discharge from hospital.

Treatment

Give 20 mg/kg as a slow IV loading dose over 20 minutes to control seizures (once any biochemical disturbance such as hypoglycaemia has been excluded or treated), followed by 4 mg/kg once a day IV, IM or by mouth. Increase this to 5 mg/kg once a day if treatment is needed for more than 2 weeks. While higher loading doses have been used (see above), these can cause respiratory depression in the preterm baby.

Blood levels

The therapeutic level of phenobarbitone in the blood in the neonatal period is 20–40 mg/l (1 mg/l = 4·42 µmol/l), which is higher than the range generally quoted for use in later childhood. Drowsiness is common, especially if levels exceed 50 mg/l, and respiratory depression becomes progressively more likely. Some clinicians aim for a free (unbound) level of ~25 mg/l. Levels can be measured in 50 µl of plasma. Because of the long half life, timing is not critical.

Supply and administration

IV ampoules contain viscid propylene glycol (80–90% w/v). 1 ml (30 mg) ampoules, costing £1·70, are convenient for neonatal use; dilution with an equal quantity of water (giving a 15 mg/ml solution) makes injection through a fine (24 gauge) cannula easier. Greater dilution, though widely recommended, is *not* necessary with slow administration when this strength ampoule is used (and no dilution is necessary when the 15 mg/ml ampoule is used), but slow administration is important to minimise the risk of shock, hypotension or laryngospasm. Extravasation is also damaging because of the solution's high osmolality and high pH (10–11). A 3 mg/ml oral BNF elixir is available, but its alcohol content is potentially toxic. An aqueous, sugar-free, preparation with a 2-week shelf life can be made in various strengths on request (100 ml for about 70p). Use is controlled under Section 3 of the UK Misuse of Drugs Regulations 1985 (Misuse of Drugs Act 1971).

References
See also the relevant Cochrane reviews

Banu SH, Jahan M, Koli UK, *et al*. Side effects of phenobarbital and carbamazepine in childhood epilepsy: randomised controlled trial. *BMJ* 2007;**334**:1207–10. [RCT]

Coyle MG, Ferguson A, Lagasse L, *et al*. Diluted tincture of opium (DTO) and phenobarbital versus DTO alone for neonatal opiate withdrawal in term infants. *J Pediatr* 2002;**140**:561–4. [RCT]

Hall RT, Hall FK, Daily DK. High-dose phenobarbital therapy in term newborn infants with severe perinatal asphyxia: a randomised, prospec-tive study with three-year follow-up. *J Pediatr* 1998;**132**:345–8. [RCT]

Hellstrom-Westas L, Blennow G, Londroth M, *et al*. Low risk of seizure recurrence after withdrawal of antiepileptic treatment in the neonatal period. *Arch Dis Child* 1995;**72**:F97–101.

Murray DM, Boylan GB, Ali I, *et al*. Defining the gap between electrographic seizure burden, clinical expression and staff recognition of neonatal seizures. *Arch Dis Child* 2008;**93**:F187–91.

Painter MJ, Scher MS, Stein AD, *et al*. Phenobarbital compared with phenytoin for the treatment of neonatal seizures. *N Engl J Med* 1999;**341**:485–9.

Silverstein FS, Jensen FE, Inder T, *et al*. Improving the treatment of neonatal seizures: National Institute of Neurological Disorders and Stroke workshop report. *J Pediatr* 2008;**153**:12–15.

Toet MC, van Rooij LGM, de Vries LS. The use of amplitude integrated electroencephalography for assessing neonatal neurologic injury. [Review] *Clin Perinatol* 2008;**35**:665–78.

Use
Phenytoin controls acute neonatal seizures as effectively as phenobarbital (q.v.), but phenytoin is seldom the first anti-convulsant used because of its very unpredictable half life. Giving one or other of these drugs controls about 45% of all neonatal seizures; giving both controls about 60%.

Pharmacology
Phenytoin was first developed and used as an antiepileptic drug in 1936. Cosmetic changes, such as gum hypertrophy, acne, hirsutism and facial coarsening have now reduced the popularity of phenytoin as a drug of first choice in the long-term management of epilepsy. Unwanted psychological changes, such as aggression, sedation, depression and impaired memory, are also common, making carbamazepine (q.v.) and sodium valproate (q.v.) preferable first choice drugs. Phenytoin may control the arrhythmia seen with digoxin toxicity. An overdose can cause restlessness or drowsiness, vomiting, nystagmus and pupilary dilatation, but symptoms resolve without specific intervention when treatment is stopped. The related prodrug fosphenytoin (1·5 mg of fosphenytoin = 1 mg of phenytoin) is less irritant, but neonatal experience is limited and prescribing this drug in 'phenytoin equivalent' units risks causing confusion.

Pharmacology in pregnancy
Phenytoin crosses the placenta freely and there is a slightly increased risk of congenital malformation (especially cleft palate and congenital heart disease) in the babies of mothers with epilepsy, which is thought to be at least partially due to anticonvulsant medication. Fetal exposure can also occasionally affect the child's appearance and measurably retard growth and intelligence. Issues relating to the use of antiepileptic drugs in pregnancy are more fully discussed in a website entry linked to the monograph on valproate. Mothers who need to remain on phenytoin during pregnancy may need to take more of this drug in the third trimester because of pharmacodynamic changes. *In utero* exposure can depress fetal vitamin K-dependent clotting factor levels, but the risk of haemorrhage can be controlled by giving IM vitamin K (q.v.) at birth. Treatment during lactation will result in the baby receiving about a tenth of the mother's dose on a weight-related basis.

Pharmacology in the first year of life
Phenytoin is excreted as a glucuronide by the liver, but the rate of elimination is very variable, especially in the first few weeks and months of life. Co-treatment with quite a few commonly used drugs can significantly alter the half life. The elimination process is also rapidly saturated at plasma levels near the upper end of the therapeutic range. Small changes in the amount prescribed can have a disproportionate effect on the plasma level once clearance exceeds half the maximum rate possible (the Michaelis constant), prolonging the half life ('zero-order' kinetics). An initial IV loading dose of 18 mg/kg and then 2·5–5 mg/kg by mouth twice a day is now generally considered the optimum strategy for children more than 4–6 months old. However, because the volume of distribution is almost twice as high in young babies ($V_D \sim 1·2$ l/kg) as it is in later life, a higher loading dose seems appropriate in babies less than 6 months old. Similarly, because the rate of elimination is so variable, treatment should only be sustained for more than a couple of days if plasma levels can be measured.

Treatment
A loading dose of 20 mg/kg given IV over 10–20 minutes (to prevent hypotension, arrhythmia and pain at the injection site) will usually control acute status epilepticus at any age. The optimum maintenance dose is variable but 2 mg/kg IV every 8–12 hours will usually maintain a therapeutic level in the first week of life, and the same maintenance dose usually works when given by mouth (at least in babies over 2 weeks old). Older babies may require two or three times as much as this. Crystallisation makes the IM route unsatisfactory.

Blood levels
The optimum plasma concentration is usually 10–20 mg/l (1 mg/l = 3·96 µmol/l), but 20% less than this in the first 3 months of life because of reduced protein binding. Levels must be measured if phenytoin is given for more than 2–3 days in babies only a few months old. Collect 50 µl of plasma just before the next dose is due.

Supply and administration
5 ml (250 mg) ampoules of phenytoin cost £3·40. Give IV through a filter **always** preceded and followed by a bolus of 0·9% sodium chloride because crystals form when phenytoin comes into contact with any solution containing glucose. To give IV maintenance treatment, accurately first draw 1 ml of fluid from the ampoule into a syringe and dilute to 10 ml with 0·9% sodium chloride to get a solution containing 5 mg/ml. The fluid is very alkaline (pH 12). UK ampoules contain 2 g propylene glycol; the US product also contains 10% benzyl alcohol. An oral suspension in sucrose contains 6 mg/ml (100 ml costs 85p). 750 mg (10 ml) vials of fosphenytoin (which can be given IV or IM) cost £40.

References
See also the relevant Cochrane reviews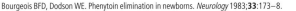

Bourgeois BFD, Dodson WE. Phenytoin elimination in newborns. *Neurology* 1983;**33**:173–8.

Frey OR, von Brenndorff AI, Probst W. Comparison of phenytoin serum concentrations in premature neonates following intravenous and oral administration. *Ann Pharmacother* 1998;**32**:300–3.

Painter MJ, Scher MS, Stein AD, *et al*. Phenobarbital compared with phenytoin for the treatment of neonatal seizures. *N Engl J Med* 1999;**341**:485–9. [RCT]

Takeoka M, Krishnamoorthy KS, Soman TB, *et al*. Fosphenytoin in infants. *J Child Neurol* 1998;**13**:537–40,

PHOSPHATE

Use
Supplemental phosphate (as oral sodium phosphate) can be used prophylactically to prevent neonatal rickets due to phosphate deficiency in the very low birthweight baby.

Nutritional factors
The transplacental fetal uptake of calcium and phosphate is high especially in the second trimester of pregnancy and comparable intakes are hard to achieve after birth in the preterm baby. The mineral content of breast milk is particularly inadequate but ordinary neonatal milk formulas (q.v.) are also deficient. Most preterm formulas and breast milk fortifiers (q.v.) contain additional calcium and phosphate for this reason.

Deficient mineral intake after birth compromises subsequent bone growth. Poor bone mineralisation leads to osteopenia, and pathological fractures can develop once bone growth starts to accelerate after 6–8 weeks; severe deficiency can also cause rickets with fraying and cupping of the bony metaphyses on X-ray. When breast milk is used phosphate deficiency is normally the limiting factor. Low plasma phosphate levels are associated with increased hydroxylation of 25-hydroxycholecalciferol to 1,25-dihydroxycholecalciferol (the metabolically active form of vitamin D), increased phosphate absorption from the gut, maximum renal retention of phosphate, and hypercalciuria (which is corrected by phosphate supplementation). Parenterally fed babies develop similar problems. Formula-fed babies can, on the other hand, sometimes develop a calcipenic type of rickets with marginal hypocalcaemia and no renal calcium spill, but secondary hyperparathyroidism with hyperphosphaturia. There is evidence of a prenatal deficiency of phosphate in some very low birthweight babies possibly as a result of pre-eclampsia and/or placental insufficiency. A controlled trial of oral phosphate supplementation in babies with a low plasma phosphate level and a high initial urinary calcium loss shortly after birth found that early supplementation can prevent the development of osteopenia of prematurity. Post-discharge supplementation does not seem necessary.

Treatment
Oral administration: Very low birthweight babies developing a plasma phosphate level of <1·5 mmol/l in the first few weeks of life should be offered ~500 micromol/kg of extra phosphate twice a day by mouth. Some babies benefit from supplementation three times a day.
IV administration: The low solubility of inorganic calcium and phosphorus can compromise bone growth in low birth-weight babies needing prolonged parenteral nutrition (q.v.). Intake can be increased to 1·5 mmol/kg per day by using the soluble organic salt, sodium glycerophosphate.

Monitoring
Treatment can be reduced or stopped when the plasma phosphate level exceeds 1.8 mmol/l and/or the tubular reabsorption of phosphate in the urine falls below 95% (in the absence of acute tubular necrosis). The renal tubular phosphate resorption (%TPR) can be calculated from the formula:

$$\%TPR = 1 - \frac{\text{Urine phosphate}}{\text{Urine creatinine}} \times \frac{\text{Plasma creatinine}}{\text{Plasma phosphate}} \times 100$$

Supply
An oral solution containing 1 mmol/ml of phosphate (with 1.28 mmol/ml Na, 0.2 mmol/ml K) can be obtained by dissolving a 500 mg Phosphate-Sandoz® tablet (costing 16p) in water, and then making the resultant solution up to 16 ml. Alternatively, the formulation used in the study published in the *Lancet* (Holland *et al.* 1990) containing 500 micromol/ml (50 mg/ml) of phosphate can be prepared by adding 94·5 grams of disodium hydrogen phosphate dodecahydrate and 41 grams of sodium dihydrogen phosphate dihydrate to 1 litre of chloroform water.

10 ml ampoules containing 2·16 grams of anhydrous sodium glycerophosphate suitable for continuous IV infusion are available in the UK from the Queen's Medical Centre Pharmacy, Nottingham. These 'special order' ampoules contain 1 mmol/ml of phosphate and 2 mmol/ml of sodium. They cost £1·10.

References

Catache M, Leone CR. Role of plasma and urinary calcium and phosphorus measurements in early detection of phosphorus deficiency in very low birthweight infants. *Acta Paediatr* 2003;**92**:76–80.
Costello I, Powell C, Williams AF. Sodium glycerophosphate in the treatment of neonatal hypophosphataemia. *Arch Dis Child* 1995;**73**:F44–5.
Harrison CM, Johnson K, McKechnie E. Osteopenia of prematurity: a national survey and review of practice. *Acta Paediatr* 2008;**97**:407–13.
Holland PC, Wilkinson AR, Diaz J, *et al.* Prenatal deficiency of phosphate, phosphate supplementation, and rickets in very-low-birthweight babies. *Lancet* 1990;**335**:697–701. [RCT]
Kurl S, Heinonen K, Lansimies E. Randomized trial: effect of short versus long duration of calcium and phosphate supplementation on bone mineral content of very low birth weight (VLBW) infants born <32 weeks gestation. [Abstract] *Pediatr Res* 2004;**55**:448A.
Pohlandt F. Prevention of postnatal bone demineralisation in very-low-birth-weight infants by individually monitored supplementation with calcium and phosphorus. *Pediatr Res* 1994;**35**:125–9.
Ryan S. Nutritional aspects of metabolic bone disease in the newborn. *Arch Dis Child* 1996;**74**:F145–8.

Use
Effective phototherapy will immediately stop jaundice increasing unless there is abnormal haemolysis.

Physiology
Bilirubin is formed during the breakdown of the iron-containing haem component of the haemoglobin molecule. Biliverdin, the first product formed, is then converted to bilirubin in the reticuloendothelial system. One gram of haemoglobin yields 35 mg of bilirubin, and the newborn baby normally produces 8–10 mg/kg of bilirubin a day. Before birth this then crosses the placenta to be conjugated in the mother's liver and excreted in the bile, a task that the neonatal liver has to take on after birth. Conjugated (direct acting) bilirubin is water soluble and harmless, but excess unconjugated bilirubin is toxic to the brain causing deafness, athetoid cerebral palsy and death from 'kernicterus', so babies go through a vulnerable period until their liver enzymes 'switch on' after birth. Normal bilirubin levels in the healthy fully breastfed term baby are shown in Fig. 1. Levels above the 97th centile at 24–36 hours do not always predict high levels at 4–5 days, but levels

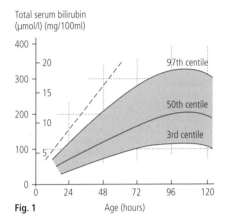

Fig. 1

above the dashed line suggest abnormal red cell breakdown (haemolysis), requiring further diagnostic assessment. Values below 470 µmol/l (~27 mg/dl) seldom damage the healthy term baby if there is no overt haemolysis.

Photochemistry
Phototherapy causes photo-oxidation or bleaching (as recognised by a neonatal nursing sister in 1958), a reversible configurational isomerisation (a change in molecular shape without any change in composition) and a non-reversible structural isomerisation of bilirubin, to a product called lumirubin, which is rapidly excreted in the bile and the urine without prior conjugation in the liver. The natural isomer is toxic and fat soluble, but not very water soluble. The products produced by phototherapy are non-toxic and water soluble. As a result, phototherapy starts to detoxify the bilirubin in the blood stream even before any lumirubin is excreted into the gut, or any decline in the plasma bilirubin is detectable. The bilirubin level will also fall within 2 hours, unless there is excess haemolysis, making early 'just in case' treatment of moderate jaundice quite unnecessary. Skin bronzing can occur if biliary stasis causes a high *conjugated* bilirubin level, from an effect of light on accumulating copper porphyrin.

Treatment
Use phototherapy to prevent the *total* plasma bilirubin (in µmol/l) reaching a value that is equal to ten times the gestational age (in weeks). Lower this ceiling by 50 µmol/l if there is haemolysis, or the baby is ill. Remember that duplicate measurements, even from the same laboratory, may differ by 15% (95% confidence limits). Some allowance can be made for conjugated bilirubin in babies over a week old, but such measurements only have limited accuracy. Exchange transfusion is seldom needed, but does have a role where antibodies have developed in response to feto-maternal red cell incompatibility, not so much to correct anaemia or jaundice, as to remove antibody-coated cells, especially where anaemia (Hb <130 g/l) has developed before birth and no intrauterine transfusion was undertaken. Units need to audit the effectiveness of the strategy of treatment they use to satisfy themselves that it effectively stops the bilirubin level rising further when there is no haemolysis.

Administration
Phototherapy only works when jaundice already exists, so there is little point starting treatment until the plasma bilirubin level approaches 170 µmol/l. The speed of decline is directly related to the amount of light used, until a plateau intensity is reached similar to that achieved outdoors in the shade on a sunny day (an irradiance of about 2 mW/cm²). Unfortunately, much standard treatment is 'homeopathic': a standard light cradle with 4–8 white strip lights placed 50 cm above the baby only provides about one-fifth as much light as this. Halogen lamps and halogen fibreoptic devices like the BiliBlanket® are even less effective. Halving the distance between the cradle and the baby, or placing a second device below the baby, will double the speed with which the bilirubin level falls. Doing both speeds the fall four-fold. Use a white bed sheet and cot-sides. 'Special blue' (F20T12/BB) lights are more effective than white lights, so are blue light-emitting diodes (LEDs). Maximise skin exposure, but cover the eyes to prevent retinal damage. Treatment can be stopped while feeding. Extra fluid is not necessary. Skin colour can not be used to judge jaundice once phototherapy has been started.

References
See also the relevant Cochrane reviews

Hansen TWR. Acute management of extreme neonatal jaundice – the potential benefits of intensified phototherapy and interruption of enterohepatic bilirubin circulation. *Acta Paediatr* 1997;**86**:843–6.

Maisels MJ, Watchko JF. Treatment of jaundice in low birthweight babies. [Review] *Arch Dis Child* 2003;**88**:F459–63. (See also pp. F455–8.)

Newman TB, Liljestrand P, Jeremy RJ, *et al.* Outcomes among newborns with total serum bilirubin levels of 25 mg per deciliter or more. *N Eng J Med* 2006;**354**:1889–900. (See also pp. 1947–9.)

Trikalinos TA, Chung M, Lau J, *et al.* Systematic review of screening for bilirubin encephalopathy in neonates. *Pediatrics* 2009;**124**:1162–71. [SR] (See also pp. 1172–7, 1193–8 and 1199–202.)

Vreman HJ, Wong RJ, Murdock JR, *et al.* Standardised bench method for evaluating the efficacy of phototherapy devices. *Acta Paediatr* 2008;**97**:3081–6.

Use
There are few established indications for using plasma albumin – 0·9% sodium chloride, gelatin (q.v.) or pentastarch, expand plasma volume at lower cost. Fresh frozen plasma (FFP) (q.v.) is more appropriate when there is a bleeding tendency, and hypotension is better managed with an inotrope like dobutamine (q.v.).

Blood levels
Ninety-five per cent of normal babies have a plasma albumin of between 20 and 40 g/l at term, but values of between 10 and 30 g/l are normal at 28 weeks' gestation.

Products
Pooled plasma prepared from donated whole blood contains soluble proteins and a caprylate stabiliser, but no bactericide or clotting factors. It is prepared by cold ethanol fractionation, sterilised by filtration, and heated to 60°C for 10 hours to inactivate any contaminating viruses. An isotonic solution with a similar colloid osmotic pressure to plasma contains 4·5% albumin. A hyperoncotic, isotonic 20% solution is also available. Some products contain significant amounts of aluminium. Albumin cost five times as much as pentastarch, and ten times as much as dextran and gelatin. The Australian SAFE trial, involving 6933 adult intensive care patients, failed to confirm the danger associated with albumin use that the 1998 Cochrane review had identified, but it did show that mortality was higher in those with a serious head injury. Giving albumin did not improve the outcome in any subgroup, but some still think that plasma has a role in treating burns and in severe sepsis.

Indications
Hypovolaemia: The value of plasma infusions in the neonatal period is very imperfectly established. Persisting hypotension immediately after birth, once acidosis has been corrected, can, rarely, be due to acute hypovolaemia, and this is best treated by blood transfusion. Most cases are more appropriately treated with an inotrope such as dopamine and/or dobutamine. Trials in adults with burns or trauma found that crystalloids (like Ringer lactate) reduce mortality more than an albumin infusion. Some artificial colloids, such as gelatin, may nevertheless be of value in selected patients with anaphylaxis, peritonitis or septic shock when there are features suggesting increased capillary permeability (a capillary 'leak' syndrome), although few trials to support such a view have yet been done apart from one small study in children with severe malaria in 2005.

Hypoproteinaemia: Underproduction due to liver failure, or to excess gut or renal loss, can cause oedema and hypovolaemia, triggering a compensatory retention of salt and water. Where this does not respond to a diuretic, 20% albumin may produce a diuresis, although the effect will be relatively short lived because most of the body's albumin is in the extravascular space, intercompartmental exchange is rapid (even when vascular permeability is normal), and plasma protein turnover is high (25% per day). The use of albumin to treat hypoproteinaemia actually *increased* the risk of death in one recent systematic review.

Polycythaemia: A partial (dilutional) exchange transfusion is sometimes done in a symptomatic child if the venous haematocrit is over 75% at birth, but there is no evidence that this improves the long-term outcome, and it can occasionally cause necrotising enterocolitis. Colloid (20–30 ml/kg of 4·5% albumin) is occasionally used, but 0·9% sodium chloride is just as effective. The haematocrit will start to fall within 6–12 hours anyway.

Treatment
20 ml/kg of 4·5% albumin or 5 ml/kg of 20% albumin may be pick-abacked terminally into an existing glucose infusion: stopping the glucose will merely precipitate reactive hypoglycaemia. Infusion (distal to any filter) into a line containing an amino acid solution (TPN) increases the risk of bacterial proliferation, but may have to be accepted. Any 20% albumin **must** be given slowly to prevent vascular overload.

Supply
50 ml bottles of 4·5% human albumin solution cost £6·50, and 50 ml bottles of 20% human albumin solution cost £22·40. Blood grouping is not necessary. Preparations contain 120–150 mmol/l of sodium and small amounts of potassium and are stable for 3 years at room temperature. Do not use if turbid.

References
See also the relevant Cochrane reviews

Cochrane Injuries Group Albumin Reviewers. Human albumin administration in critically ill patients: systematic review of randomised controlled trials. *BMJ* 1998;**317**:235–40. [SR]

Dempsey EM, Barrington K. Short and long term outcomes following partial exchange transfusion in the polycythaemic newborn: a systemic review. *Arch Dis Child* 2006;**91**:F2–6. [SR] (See also the systematic review by de Wall on pp. F7–10.)

Haynes GR, Navickis RJ, Wilkes MM. Albumin administration – what is the evidence of clinical benefit? A systematic review of randomised controlled trials. *Eur J Anaesthesiol* 2003;**20**:771–93. [SR]

Maitland K, Pamba A, English M, *et al*. Randomized trial of volume expansion with albumin or saline in children with severe malaria: preliminary evidence of albumin benefit. *Clin Infect Dis* 2005;**40**:538–45. [RCT]

Morris I, McCallion N, El-Khuffash A, *et al*. Serum albumin and mortality in very low birth weight infants. *Arch Dis Child* 2008;**93**:F210–12. (See also p. F326.)

SAFE Study Investigators. Effect of baseline serum albumin concentration on outcome of resuscitation with albumin or saline in intensive care units: analysis of data from the Saline versus Albumin Fluid Evaluation (SAFE) study. *BMJ* 2006;**333**:1044–6. [RCT] (See also pp. 1029–30.)

SAFE Study Investigators. Saline or albumin for fluid resuscitation in patients with traumatic brain injury. *N Engl J Med* 2007;**357**: 874–84. [RCT]

Sarkar S, Rosenkraantz TS. Neonatal polycythemia and hyperviscosity. [Review] *Semin Fetal Neonat Med* 2008;**13**:248–55.

Use

Platelet concentrates are used in the management of severe thrombocytopenia with bleeding (Fig. 1).

Pathophysiology

The risk of serious internal haemorrhage increases significantly when the platelet count falls below 30×10^9/l, and the risk of intracranial haemorrhage may be particularly high in the preterm baby shortly after birth. Always check first that the 'thrombocytopenia' is not due to clots in the sample!

A number of inherited conditions and syndromes (such as thrombocytopenia absent radius (TAR) syndrome) are associated with thrombocytopenia. These seldom call for active treatment. Ill babies can have sepsis or a consumption coagulopathy (disseminated intravascular coagulation or DIC): the main need here is usually to treat the underlying condition. Platelets can pool in the spleen in conditions causing hypersplenism (such as Rhesus isoimmunisation), and exchange transfusion can further exacerbate thrombocytopenia. A low count may point to focal infection or to thrombus formation on a long line. Marrow disorders will reduce platelet production, but the results of a full blood count and examination of a blood film will usually provide a diagnostic clue in these situations. Heparin therapy (q.v.) occasionally causes a dangerous thrombocytopenia that is made worse if platelets are given.

Platelet antibodies cause most cases of severe *isolated* neonatal thrombocytopenia. Platelet transfusions are of little value in **auto**immune thrombocytopenia because the maternal antiplatelet antibodies also attack any transfused platelets. Most of these mothers will have idiopathic thrombocytopenia (ITP) or systemic lupus erythematosus

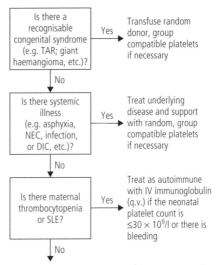

(SLE). **Allo**immune thrombocytopenia is more hazardous. Here, maternal antibodies, produced as a result of transplacental sensitisation, attack fetal platelets (in a process analogous to the red cell destruction that occurs in Rhesus haemolytic disease), treatment with immunoglobulin (q.v.) may be appropriate, and fully compatible platelets are required (i.e. they must lack the antigen against which the antibodies are directed). The transfusion service can usually provide platelets that are both HPA-1a and HPA-5b negative (the antibodies responsible for 95% of all problems). These will almost always be suitable, and can be used if the situation is urgent before platelet grouping and any formal confirmation of the diagnosis is possible. Maternal washed and irradiated platelets can be used on those rare occasions when the blood transfusion service finds itself unable to provide suitable donor platelets.

Administration

10 ml/kg of platelets from a single ABO and Rh compatible CMV-negative donor will usually suffice unless there is alloimmune thrombocytopenia. Here more is given, and a higher minimum count aimed for, because platelet function in poorer. To minimise loss, draw the contents of the pack into a 50 ml syringe through a special platelet or blood transfusion set with a 170–200 μm filter and then infuse over 30 minutes, using a narrow bore extension set linked (near the patient) to an IV line primed with 0.9% sodium chloride. ***Always confirm compatibility by checking that the patient's name is on the pack***.

Supply

Leucodepleted 50 ml single-unit packs containing 60×10^9 platelets are available from hospital blood banks. They cost about £70 to prepare and dispense. Packs for intrauterine use are irradiated and further concentrated before issue. Platelets need to be stored under special conditions, kept at room temperature and used *promptly* on receipt. They quickly loose their therapeutic power if this is not done, and bacterial contamination also becomes increasingly likely. Send 2 ml of blood for grouping.

References

See also the UK website guidelines **DHUK**

Baer VI, Lambert DK, Henry E, *et al*. Severe thrombocytopenia in the NICU. *Pediatrics* 2009;**124**:e1095–100.
Birchall JE, Murphy MF, Kaplan C, *et al*. European Fetomaternal Alloimmune Thrombocytopenia Study Group. European collaborative study of the antenatal management of feto-maternal alloimmune thrombocytopenia. *Br J Haematol* 2003;**122**:275–88.
British Society for Haematology. Guidelines for the use of platelet transfusions. *Br J Haematol* 2003;**122**:10–23.
Chakravorty S, Murray N, Roberts I. Neonatal thrombocytopenia. [Review] *Early Hum Dev* 2005;**81**:35–41.
Killie MK, Kjeldsen-Kragh J, Husebekk A, *et al*. Cost-effectiveness of antenatal screening for neonatal alloimmune thrombocytopenia. *Br J Obstet Gynaecol* 2007;**114**:588–95. (See also **115**:412–14.)
Porcelijn L, Van den Akker ESA, Oepkes D. Fetal thrombocytopenia. [Review] *Semin Fetal Neonat Med* 2008;**13**:223–30.
Roberts I, Murray NA. Neonatal thrombocytopenia: causes and management. *Arch Dis Child* 2003;**88**:F350–64.
Roberts I, Murray NA. Neonatal thrombocytopenia. [Review] *Semin Fetal Neonat Med* 2008;**13**:256–64.
Sola MC, Del Vecchio A, Rimsza LM. Evaluation and treatment of thrombocytopenia in the neonatal intensive care unit. *Clin Perinatol* 2000;**27**:655–79.

PNEUMOCOCCAL VACCINES

Use
Two vaccines are now available offering protection from some, but not all, forms of pneumococcal meningitis, septicaemia, pneumonia and otitis media. Universal availability might prevent over 500,000 deaths a year.

Pneumococcal infection
A range of serious bacterial infections are caused by the encapsulated Gram-positive coccus *Streptococcus pneumoniae*; 84 capsular forms have been identified, but 8–10 of these are responsible for 85% of the cases currently seen in the UK. It often causes community-acquired pneumonia, and is now the commonest cause of lethal or disabling bacterial meningitis. Patients with impaired immunity are at particular risk. Penicillin remains the drug of choice except in areas where the minimum inhibitory concentration for penicillin is now >2 μg/ml.

Infants at *high risk* include those with homozygous sickle cell disease, with no spleen (or a poorly functioning spleen), or with congenital or acquired immunodeficiency (including HIV infection). Such patients should be offered prophylactic antibiotics (see the monograph on immunisation), because the current vaccines only offer protection from *some* of the capsular types of pneumococcal infection. They may also benefit from being given the multivalent plain polysaccharide vaccine when 2 years old, and such immunisation should also be offered to patients 2 weeks ahead of any planned splenectomy or chemotherapy.

Products
Plain polysaccharide vaccine: An unconjugated vaccine, active against 23 of the more commonly encountered capsular types of pneumococcal infection, has been available for some years. Because this vaccine offers relatively little protection when given to children under 2 years old, it has generally only been offered to adults and to older children considered to be at particularly high risk of infection.

New conjugate vaccine: A new 7-valent protein-polysaccharide vaccine (active against the 4, 6A, 6B, 9V, 14, 18C, 19F and 23F strains) was first licensed for use in young children in 2000. Its use caused a 70% decrease in invasive pneumococcal disease in the young in 3 years. Cases due to vaccine-related serotypes fell by almost 80%, but serotypes not covered by the vaccine are now becoming commoner.

Contraindications
Avoid immunisation during an acute infection, and while pregnant. Patients already immunised with the plain 23-valent vaccine (or the earlier 12- or 14-valent vaccines) do not need to be re-immunised with the present 23-valent vaccine for 3–5 years.

Interactions
The conjugate vaccine can be given (into a different limb) at the same time as any other childhood vaccine, but parents who seem unhappy at the thought of their child facing more than one 'needle' at a single clinic visit can, if necessary, be offered a different, staged, plan. The plain vaccine should not be given until at least 8 weeks after the new conjugate vaccine has been given. Anaphylaxis is extremely unlikely – its management is discussed in the monograph on immunisation.

Administration
Conjugate vaccine: Young children who have not yet started their primary course of immunisation should be offered three 0·5 ml doses of the new conjugate 7-valent vaccine. Children in the UK are offered this when 2, 4 and 13 months old, and the WHO has now made use a priority in all countries where mortality is high.

Plain vaccine: High-risk children (see above) who are 2 or more years old should still be offered a single 0·5 ml deep IM injection of the plain 23-valent vaccine because it provides broader protection from pneumococcal infection.

Documentation
Tell the family doctor every time a child is immunised in hospital, and record what was done in the child's own personal health booklet. Community-based registers of vaccine uptake also need to be informed.

Supply
0·5 ml vials of the plain polysaccharide vaccine (Pneumovax® or Pnu-Imune®) cost £10. 0·5 ml vials of the conjugate vaccine (Prevenar®) cost £39 (but are available cheaper on the NHS). Always store at 4°C.

References
See also the relevant Cochrane reviews and UK guidelines

Cardoso MRA, Nascimento-Carvalho CM, Ferrero F, *et al.* Penicillin-resistant pneumococcus and risk of treatment failure in pneumonia. *Arch Dis Child* 2008;**93**:221–5.

Grijalva CG, Nuorti JP, Arbogast PG, *et al.* Decline in pneumonia admissions after routine childhood immunisation with pneumococcal conjugate vaccine in the USA: a time-series analysis. *Lancet* 2007;**369**:1179–86. (See also pp. 1144–5.)

O'Brien KL, Wolfon LJ, Watt JP, *et al.* Burden of disease caused by *Streptococcus pneumoniae* in children younger than 5 years: global estimates. *Lancet* 2009;**374**:893–902. (See also pp. 854–6.)

Pichichero ME, Casey JR. Emergence of a multiresistant serotype 19A pneumococcal strain not included in then 7-valent conjugate vaccine as an otopathogen in children. *JAMA* 2007;**298**:1772–8.

Sinha A, Levine O, Knoll MD, *et al.* Cost-effectiveness of pneumococcal conjugate vaccination in the prevention of child mortality: an international economic analysis. *Lancet* 2007;**369**:389–96. (See www.gavialliance.org.)

Van der Poll T, Opal SM. Pathogenesis, treatment and prevention of pneumococcal pneumonia. [Seminar] *Lancet* 2009;**374**:1543–56.

Whitney CG, Pilishvilli T, Farley MM, *et al.* Effectiveness of seven-valent pneumococcal conjugate vaccine against invasive pneumococcal disease: a matched case-control study. *Lancet* 2006;**368**:149–502. (See also pp. 1469–70.)

Use

Polio vaccine gives lasting immunity to the three polio viruses.

Poliomyelitis

Poliomyelitis is a notifiable infectious illness that has now been eradicated from most of the world, but cases were still being recorded in Afganistan, Chad, Ethiopia, north India, Indonesia, Pakistan, Nigeria and the Yemen in 2005. The World Health Organisation launched a global 15-year plan to rid the world of this disease in 1988 and one country – northern Nigeria – now accounts for almost half of all the new cases being reported across the world each year. Infection may be clinically inapparent, but may also produce aseptic meningitis and severe lasting paralysis. An injectable formaldehyde-inactivated triple strain (Salk) vaccine first became available in 1958, a live attenuated triple strain oral (Sabin) vaccine was introduced in 1962, and a more potent monovalent product was licensed for use in India in 2005. The Salk vaccine is now the only product used in north America, and is being used with increasing frequency in most parts of Europe. Indeed, though the Sabin vaccine was still used in the UK until September 2004, there is now a global move towards greater use of the inactivated Salk vaccine. The two products have, between them, certainly made the eventual global eradication of polio a realistic aim. While polio (and measles) could eventually, with sustained commitment and good management, be eradicated from the world, just as smallpox was in 1980, it is not proving easy.

Indications

Inactivated parenteral vaccine (IPV): With the arrival of a combined, injectable vaccine, which also offers protection from diphtheria, tetanus, whooping cough and *Haemophilus* (Hib) infection, this is now becoming the product of choice worldwide. Give three doses IM at least 4–8 weeks apart, starting at least 6 weeks (and usually 2 months) after birth. Because the live and inactivated products are interchangeable, there is nothing to stop the inactivated vaccine being used to complete a course of treatment started using the live oral vaccine.

Live oral vaccine (OPV): Give three doses by mouth at monthly intervals (as with the inactivated vaccine). Remember, however, that children excrete the live virus in their stools for up to 6 weeks after immunisation, putting other unimmunised and immunocompromised patients and family contacts at risk. This product should never, therefore, be used in a maternity hospital setting. There is also a one in a million chance of the live, attenuated vaccine itself causing paralytic disease.

Contraindications

Early pregnancy, immunodeficiency, immunosuppression, reticuloendothelial malignancy and high-dose corticosteroid treatment (the equivalent of >1 mg/kg prednisolone a day, or 2 mg/kg for more than 1 week in the last 6 weeks) are contraindications to the use of any live vaccine (but *not* for the IPV vaccine). Children should not be immunised while febrile, or given the oral vaccine while suffering from diarrhoea or vomiting. For anaphylaxis (rare even with the IM product), see under immunisation.

Drug interactions

Polio vaccine can be given at the same time as other live and inactivated vaccines. The live vaccine should not, ideally, be given less than 3 weeks before or 3 months after a dose of normal immunoglobulin.

Administration

Inactivated vaccine: Give 0·5 ml by deep IM injection into any limb not simultaneously being used to give some other vaccine using a fresh syringe and a 25 mm, 23 gauge, needle.

Oral live vaccine: The normal dose is 3 drops by mouth. Repeat if regurgitated. Older children have, traditionally, been offered the drops on a sugar cube.

Documentation

Tell the family doctor every time a child is immunised in hospital, and record what was done in the child's own personal health booklet. Community-based registers of vaccine uptake also need to be informed.

Supply

The combined (DTaP/IPV/Hib) vaccine (Pediacel®) made by Aventis Pasteur is the inactivated polio vaccine (IPV) now used in the UK. Always shake each 0·5 ml vial before use. A monovalent inactivated vaccine is also available on request. The live oral polio vaccine (OPV) remains available in some countries in 10-dose containers (which should be discarded at the end of any session), and in 10 × one-dose packs. Store all products in the dark at 2–8°C.

References

See also the full UK website guidelines

Advisory Committee on Immunization Practice. Updated ACIP recommendations regarding routine poliovirus vaccination. *MMWR* 2009;**58**:829–30.

American Academy of Pediatrics Committee on Infectious Diseases. Poliomyelitis prevention: revised recommendations for use of only inactivated poliovirus vaccine for routine immunisation. *Pediatrics* 1999;**104**:1404–6.

Ehrenfeld E, Chumakov K. Monovalent oral poliovirus vaccines – a good tool but not a total solution. [Editorial] *N Engl J Med* 2008;**359**:1726–7.

Ehrenfeld E, Glass RI, Agol VI, *et al.* Immunisation against poliomyelitis: moving forward. *Lancet* 2008;**371**:1385–7.

Grassly NC, Wenger J, Durrani S, *et al.* Protective efficacy of a monovalent oral type 1 poliovirus vaccine: a case-control study. *Lancet* 2007;**369**:1356–62. (See also pp. 1320–2 and 2007;**370**:129–33.)

MacLennan C, MacLennan J. What threat from persistent vaccine-related poliovirus? *Lancet* 2005;**366**:351–3. (See also pp. 359–60 and 394–6.)

Thompson KM, DuintjerTebbens RJ. Eradication versus control for poliomyelitis: an economic analysis. *Lancet* 2007;**369**:1363–71.

Use

Sodium and calcium polystyrene sulphonate are cation-exchange resins administered orally or rectally in the treatment of severe hyperkalaemia (a plasma potassium level of ≥7·5 mmol/l). IV salbutamol (q.v.) seems to provide a more immediate, and an IV glucose infusion with added insulin (q.v.) a more reliable, way of achieving a sustained lowering of the plasma potassium level in the neonatal period by causing influx of potassium into cells. Neither salbutamol nor glucose and insulin will remove potassium from the body.

Pharmacology

Sodium and calcium polystyrene sulphonate are cation-exchange resins used to draw potassium out of the body and into the gut in exchange for sodium or calcium, thus effecting the elimination of potassium from the body in the faeces. Faecal impaction has been reported following rectal administration in children, as have gastrointestinal concretions when the drug is given by mouth in early infancy, especially if there is already some degree of intestinal ileus for any reason.

Because none of the exchange resins are entirely selective for potassium it is best to choose a calcium resin if the plasma calcium level is already low, since a sodium resin will inevitably draw further calcium out of the body. The calcium resin is also to be preferred if the plasma sodium level is already high, because a sodium resin is likely to cause a further rise in the plasma sodium level, and severe hypernatraemia (a plasma sodium level of ≥160 mmol/l) can cause serious neurological damage. Each gram of sodium resin is capable, in practice, of extracting about 1 mmol of potassium from the body (as much as 3 mmol in theory). An equivalent weight of the calcium resin is marginally less effective.

Do not attempt *any* treatment for hyperkalaemia without first checking that the apparently high plasma potassium level is not merely due to potassium leaking from damaged red cells (as a result of haemolysis) into the plasma sample sent for laboratory analysis. Neonates seem to tolerate high plasma potassium levels much better than older patients, but treatment should be considered, as a matter of urgency, if there are significant electrocardiographic changes. Correct any hypocalcaemia with 10% IV calcium gluconate (q.v.) and give 1 mmol/kg of IV sodium bicarbonate (q.v.) to reduce the risk of sudden, potentially life-threatening, cardiac arrhythmia. Intravenous or nebulised salbutamol, and intravenous glucose and insulin, are both capable of lowering plasma potassium levels more rapidly than any cation-exchange resin, but they do not rid the body of excess potassium. An exchange transfusion with *fresh* blood (or washed red cells), although it may take a little time to set up, is probably the best way of achieving a *sustained* fall in the plasma potassium level in the neonatal period, while a cation-exchange resin may be the more appropriate strategy in older children where bowel complications are less likely. Peritoneal dialysis, or haemodialysis, is an even better option in centres with the necessary expertise to do this, although such a strategy is usually only necessary when there is renal failure and/or fluid overload. Consider adrenal failure (usually due to congenital adrenal hyperplasia) if there is hyponatraemia, hypoglycaemia and/or hypotension, and treat as outlined in the monograph on hydrocortisone.

Treatment

Give 500 mg/kg as a retention enema. Ensure evacuation by colonic irrigation after 8–12 hours (preferably with the aid of X-ray image intensification) in order to ensure complete recovery of the resin. Treatment may be repeated after 12 hours if necessary. Double this dose can be employed at least once in severe hyperkalaemia. Do *not* give polystyrene sulphonate resins by the oral route in the neonatal period. Monitor the plasma electrolytes to minimise the risk of overtreatment.

Supply and administration

Sodium polystyrene sulphonate (Resonium A®) can be provided as a powder by the pharmacy on request. Calcium polystyrene sulphonate (Calcium Resonium®) can also be provided where the use of a sodium-containing resin has to be avoided because of latent hypocalcaemia or hypernatraemia. Both resins cost about 15p per gram. The sodium resin contains approximately 4·5 mmol of sodium per gram. It is best to get the pharmacy to prepare the enema in advance using a mixture of water and 9% methylcellulose (which acts as a faecal softener), but the resin can be prepared on the ward immediately prior to use if necessary using 6 ml/kg of water. In the United States polystyrene sulphonate resins are usually made up in a solution of 25% sorbitol rather than in a mixture of water and methylcellulose.

References

Filippi L, Cecchi A, Dani C, *et al*. Hypernatraemia induced by sodium polystyrene sulphonate (Kayexalate®) in two extremely low birth weight newborns. *Paediatr Anaesth* 2004;**14**:271–5.

Hu P-S, Su B-H, Peng C-T, *et al*. Glucose and insulin infusion versus kayexalate for the early treatment of non-oliguric hyperkalaemia in very-low-birth-weight infants. *Acta Paediatr Taiwan* 1999;**40**:314–18.

Malone TA. Glucose and insulin versus cation-exchange resin for the treatment of hyperkalaemia in very low birth weight infants. *J Pediatr* 1991;**118**:121–3.

O'Hare FM, Molloy EJ. What is the best treatment for hyperkalaemia in a preterm infant? *Arch Dis Child* 2008;**93**:174–6. [SR]

Use

Potassium is an essential nutrient and potassium chloride is often used to correct bodily depletion.

Pathophysiology

An intake of 2 mmol/kg of potassium per day is more than enough to meet all the body's normal needs. Breast milk, artificial milk formulas (q.v.) and the standard neonatal parenteral nutrition solution (q.v.) all contain more than enough potassium to meet basic needs, and a low plasma potassium level in the neonatal period (hypokalaemia) is more often the result of potassium redistribution than any true body deficit.

While urinary sodium loss (as summarised in the monograph on sodium chloride) can vary widely in the neonatal period, potassium loss seldom varies very much. Most healthy preterm babies remain in positive potassium balance throughout the neonatal period. Stressed, ventilator-dependent, preterm babies sometimes show a raised renal potassium loss during the first 2 days of life, although this almost always resolves spontaneously within 3–4 days and seldom causes a serious fall in plasma level. Indeed urinary loss is almost always sufficiently small as to make supplementation unnecessary in an unfed baby even if fluid support is limited to the provision of glucose saline for up to a week after birth. There are, however, a few conditions associated with excessive renal potassium loss that can produce severe hypokalaemia. Some diuretics if used for a sustained period can cause significant urinary potassium loss (cf. the monographs on chlorothiazide and furosemide), while chronic diarrhoea can also induce a significant body potassium deficit.

Potassium is the most important intracellular cation in the body, and a cellular deficit causes ileus, retention of urine, neuromuscular weakness and ECG changes (including ST segment depression, a low-voltage T wave and U wave changes). Alkalosis drives extracellular potassium into the cells, making the plasma level a poor marker of whole body depletion. Insulin can have a similar effect. Compartmental shifts are the commonest cause of apparent neonatal hypokalaemia; true depletion requiring replacement is really quite rare. Overtreatment, on the other hand, can easily cause hyperkalaemia (a serious management problem discussed in the monograph on salbutamol). A dose of 3 mmol/kg has been used to cause immediate cardiac asystole in those rare situations where deliberate fetocide is deemed necessary.

Treatment

Oral treatment: This is the preferred route for correcting any potassium deficit. Start with a total of 2 mmol/kg a day given in a series of small divided doses with feeds to minimise gastric irritation. The oral rehydration fluid (q.v.) recommended by the World Health Organisation provides both the simplest and the quickest way of correcting the salt and fluid loss caused by diarrhoea.

Intravenous treatment: Correct any true body deficit slowly over 1–2 days, using a solution that does not contain more than 40 mmol of potassium per litre, given at a rate of no more than 0·2 mmol/kg per hour (a higher rate of up to 0·5 mmol/kg per hour may rarely be justified if there is severe potassium depletion). ECG monitoring is recommended during infusion in some centres. Concentrated solutions can cause thrombophlebitis and pain at the injection site, while extravasation can cause tissue necrosis. ***Always check the dose carefully: an overdose can be rapidly fatal.***

Supply and administration

A sugar-free oral 7·5% solution of potassium chloride containing 1 mmol (75 mg) per ml is available from the pharmacy on request (100 ml costs 70p).

10 ml ampoules of strong 15% potassium chloride (containing 1·5 g, or approximately 20 mmol, of potassium) for IV use are available as stock costing 42p each. Note that ampoules are also available in a range of *other* strengths. Strong potassium chloride must normally be ***diluted at least 50-fold*** with 0·9% sodium chloride (or a mixture of 0·9% sodium chloride in glucose) prior to administration, and the resultant solution mixed with some care in order to make quite sure that the potassium does not separate or 'layer' out prior to administration.

The inadvertent use of potassium chloride instead of sodium chloride during the reconstitution of other IV drugs has caused several deaths. There are strong grounds for insisting that all potassium chloride ampoules should be stored well away from all other routinely used ampoules. Many hospitals keep all such ampoules with the controlled drugs.

References

Brem AS. Electrolyte disorders associated with respiratory distress syndrome and bronchopulmonary dysplasia. *Clin Perinatol* 1992;**19**:223–32.

Engle WD, Arant BS Jr. Urinary potassium excretion in the critically ill neonate. *Pediatrics* 1984;**74**:259–64.

John E, Klavdianou M, Vidyasagar D. Electrolyte problems in neonatal surgical patients. *Clin Perinatol* 1989;**16**:219–32.

Tubman M, Majumdar SR, Lee D, *et al.* Best practices for safe handling of products containing concentrated potassium. *BMJ* 2005;**331**:274–7.

Use

Probiotics can be used to restore a healthy balance of bowel microorganisms in children troubled by diarrhoea. Eleven controlled trials have also shown that use reduces the risk of necrotising enterocolitis (NEC). Maternal use during pregnancy and lactation seems safe and may help to 'normalise' the range of bacteria always present in the vagina, but it has not yet been shown to reduce the risk of preterm birth.

Microbiological issues

Interest in the use of lactic acid-producing bacteria to retain or restore a healthy balance of microorganisms in the gut has grown steadily in the last 20 years, and commercially available live cultures of these organisms are now often called 'probiotics'. *Lactobacillus bulgaricus*, which occurs in naturally soured milk, was the first organism to be widely studied, but this does not grow well in the human gut, and various other lactobacilli including *L. acidophilus*, a normal inhabitant of the gut, and *L. casei* are now more commonly used. Other organism studies include *Saccaromyces boulardi*, *Streptococcus thermophilus* and various *Bifidobacterium* species. Early studies focused on the ability of these microbial supplements to re-establish a more normal bowel flora in children suffering for serious diarrhoea, and other studies looked to see if use could enhance growth in early infancy. Studies in the last 10 years have now, more importantly, looked to see whether early prophylactic use can minimise the risk of excessive and unbalanced early colonisation of the gut by other potentially pathogenic organisms in the vulnerable preterm baby. The few trials done as yet to see whether use can reduce disease severity in babies with severe atopic dermatitis have had inconsistent outcomes.

Sustained close contact with the mother helps the normal baby acquire a balance of healthy gut bacteria at birth, as can breastfeeding. The gut of the unfed, antibiotic-treated, preterm baby is, in contrast, at high risk of being colonised by potential pathogens, and this may be one of the prime factors that renders the baby vulnerable to NEC – a condition in which the gut wall can perforate, causing toxic peritonitis and septicaemia, after it is invaded and killed by pathogenic gas-forming organisms. Reduced gut blood flow in the period immediately before and after birth (which is particularly common in the light-for-dates baby) puts the baby at even greater risk. Serious NEC currently occurs in about 7% of babies born more than 12 weeks early, and is one of the commonest causes of death in those who manage to surmount the respiratory problems seen in the first week of life. Even in survivors, the need for surgery, and for further respiratory support, can have a serious impact on subsequent growth and development, especially if surgery involves the removal of a significant length of gut. The use of breast milk seems to reduce the risk of NEC. So, too, can prophylaxis with an oral antibiotic (as outlined in the monograph on gentamicin), but this strategy is seldom used at present because of continuing concern that such treatment could encourage the proliferation of multiply-resistant organisms. Hope is rising that probiotic priming, and the more consistent use of breast milk, could greatly reduce the current scourge of NEC. Whether selective oral antibiotic prophylaxis could further enhance these two strategies is not yet known.

Prophylactic neonatal use

It is increasingly clear that treatment is beneficial in babies of less than 30 weeks' gestation, but the best product to use is not yet clear. A 125 mg/kg dose of Infloran® (a mixture of *L. acidophilus* and *B. bifidum*) was given twice a day in the two largest trials reported to date. Start prophylaxis as soon as feeds are started, and give for 6 weeks. A further NIHR funded trial (PIPS) using the BBG strain of *Bifidobacerium* was due to start recruiting babies of less than 31 weeks' gestation in the south of England in late 2009.

Supply and administration

Infloran is imported into the UK from Austria by IDIS World Medicines. Twenty 250 mg capsules (which should be stored at 4°C) cost £14. Mix half the content of one capsule with milk immediately before it is given.

References

See also the relevant Cochrane reviews

Bin-Nun A, Bromiker R, Wilschanski M, *et al*. Oral probiotics prevent necrotizing enterocolitis in very low birth weight neonates. *J Pediatr* 2005;**147**:19–26. [RCT]

Deshpande G, Rao S, Patole S. Probiotics for prevention of necrotising enterocolitis in preterm neonates with very low birth weight: a systematic review of randomised controlled trials. *Lancet* 2007;**369**:1614–20. [SR] (See also pp. 1578–80.)

Embleton ND, Yates R. Probiotics and other preventative strategies for necrotising enterocolitis. *Semin Fetal Neonat Med* 2008;**13**:35–43.

Huurre A, Laitinen K, Rautava S, *et al*. Impact of maternal atopy and probiotic supplementation during pregnancy on infant sensitization: a double-blind placebo-controlled study. *Clin Exp Allergy* 2008;**38**:13428. [RCT]

Lee J, Seto D, Bielory L. Meta-analysis of clinical trials of probiotics for prevention and treatment of pediatric atopic dermatitis. *J Allergy Clin Immunol* 2008;**121**:11621.e11. [SR]

Lin H-C, Hsu C-H, Chen H-L, *et al*. Oral probiotics prevent necrotizing enterocolitis in very low birth weight preterm infants: a multicenter, randomized, controlled trial. *Pediatrics* 2008;**122**:693–700. [RCT]

Lin H-C, Su B-H, Chen A-C, *et al*. Oral probiotics reduce the incidence and severity of necrotizing enterocolitis in very low birth weight infants. *Pediatrics* 2005;**115**:1–4. [RCT]

Manzoni P, Mostert M, Leonessa ML, *et al*. Oral supplementation with *Lactobacillus casei* subspecies *rhamnosus* prevents enteric colonization by *Candida* species in preterm neonates: a randomized study. *Clin Infect Dis* 2006;**42**:1735–42. [RCT]

Samanta M, Sarkar M, Ghosh P, *et al*. Prophylactic probiotics for prevention of necrotising enterocolitis in very low birth weight newborns. *J Trop Pediatr* 2009;**55**:128–31. [RCT]

Van Neil CW, Feudtner C, Garrison MM, *et al*. Lactobacillus therapy for acute infectious diarrhea in children: a meta-analysis. *Pediatrics* 2002;**109**:678–84. [SR]

Weston S, Halbert A, Richmond P, *et al*. Effects of probiotics on atopic dermatitis: a randomised controlled trial. *Arch Dis Child* 2005;**90**:892–7. [RCT] (See also pp. 881–3 and 2005;**91**:276.)

Use
Procaine G penicillin was, for many years, the antibiotic normally used to treat congenital syphilis, but benzylpenicillin, or penicillin (q.v.), if given diligently, is now known to be just as effective.

Pharmacology
Procaine benzylpenicillin is a sustained release drug that is slowly hydrolysed to benzylpenicillin after deep IM injection. Its microbiological properties are the same as those of benzylpenicillin. Benzathine penicillin (which is even more slowly hydrolysed to benzylpenicillin over 2–3 weeks) was once widely used to treat syphilis in pregnancy, but it is no longer available in the UK. Luckily, the *Treponema pallidum* organism still remains totally sensitive to benzylpenicillin despite more than 60 years of near-universal use.

Congenital syphilis
Latent untreated maternal syphilis is associated with a 20% risk of fetal loss and a 20% risk of premature delivery, even if maternal infection has only been present for 1–2 years. Intrauterine growth retardation is common. The placenta is often large, and fetal hydrops may develop. Half the liveborn babies will have congenital syphilis at birth. The longer the maternal disease has been left untreated, the greater the risk to the fetus. Florid neonatal disease is now rare, but babies can present with hepatosplenomegaly, anaemia, thrombocytopenia, jaundice and generalised lymphadenopathy. Skin desquamation is a characteristic feature, as is a typical pink maculopapular rash that later turns brown. Osteitis is usually asymptomatic at birth, and rhinitis ('snuffles') only develops after a few weeks.

Syphilis is starting to become more common in the UK, and some women currently escape diagnosis and treatment before delivery. It still remains very common in some countries. A non-treponemal serological test (a Venereal Disease Research Laboratory (VDRL) or rapid plasma-reagin (RPR) test) is usually used to make the diagnosis, and false-positive tests identified, if facilities exist, by undertaking a fluorescent treponemal antibody absorption (FTA-ABS) or *T. pallidum* particle agglutination (TPPA) test. Antenatal treatment was traditionally a single 1·8 gram (2·4 million-unit) IM dose of benzathine penicillin, but long-standing infection requires at least three doses at weekly intervals. A single 2 gram oral dose of azithromycin (q.v.) seems as effective as one IM dose of benzathine penicillin. However, most genitourinary specialists in the UK now give a 3 gram dose of benzylpenicillin IV or IM once every 4 hours for 10–14 days. Check for other venereal disease, including HIV, and review all sexual contacts. Manage penicillin allergy as outlined on the CDC website (see references).

If the mother was fully treated at least 1 month before delivery, as demonstrated by at least a four-titre fall in a serological non-treponemal (VDRL or RPR) test, and the baby seems asymptomatic at birth, neonatal treatment is not called for. Follow up is, however, essential at 3, 6 and 12 months to ensure that all the serological tests eventually become negative. If there is any doubt about the adequacy of treatment, or this was only started in the second half of pregnancy, it is probably wise to X-ray the baby's long bones for osteitis and to do a VDRL test on the CSF (also looking at the cell count and protein level). Treat any possible infection after birth like proven infection. It may also be appropriate to screen siblings for latent syphilis.

Treatment
In babies thought to be infected at birth it was once traditional to give 50 mg/kg of procaine benzylpenicillin IM once a day for 10 days. However, this can easily cause a sterile abscess with subsequent fibrosis and muscle atrophy, and 30 mg/kg of benzylpenicillin IV or IM once every 12 hours for 10 days is equally effective (and penetrates the CSF rather better). If syphilis is only first suspected when the baby is already more than 2 weeks old then, if benzylpenicillin is to be used, it needs to be given once every 6 hours. While *asymptomatic* babies born to mothers with evidence of untreated syphilis are often given a single 100 mg/kg dose of IM procaine benzylpenicillin at birth in many resource-poor countries, further study may show oral azithromycin to be a useful second option as long as the community prevalence of azithromycin-resistant *T. pallidum* is low.

Supply
Procaine benzylpenicillin acts by slowly releasing benzylpenicillin from an intramuscular depot. It should **never** be given IV. It comes in the UK as a suspension in ready-to-use 600,000 unit (1 ml) and 1·2 million-unit (2 ml) cartridges, which need to be stored at 4°C. In many countries it is still provided as a powder, for reconstitution with water, in 1 gram (1 million-unit) vials that are stable at room temperature.

References
See also the Cochrane review of treatment for syphilis

Association for Genitourinary Medicine and the Medical Society for the Study of Venereal Disease. *UK national guidelines on the management of early syphilis*. See www.bashh.org/guidelines/2002/early$final0502.pdf.

Centers for Disease Control and Prevention. Sexually transmitted diseases treatment guidelines – 2002. *MMWR* 2002;**51**(RR-6):1–80. (See the CDC website www.cdc.gov/STD/treatment/.)

Chakraborty R, Luck S. Syphilis is on the increase: the implications for child health. *Arch Dis Child* 2008;**93**:105–9.

Nathan L, Bawdon RE, Sidawi JE, *et al.* Penicillin levels following the administration of benzathine penicillin G in pregnancy. *Obstet Gynecol* 1993;**82**:338–42.

Paryani SG, Vaughn AJ, Crosby M, *et al.* Treatment of asymptomatic congenital syphilis: benzathine versus procaine penicillin G therapy. *J Pediatr* 1994;**125**:471–5. [RCT]

Rieder G, Rusizoka M, Todd J, *et al.* Single-dose azithromycin versus penicillin G benzathine for the treatment of early syphilis. *N Engl J Med* 2005;**353**:1236–44. [RCT] (See also pp. 1291–3.)

PROGESTERONE

Use
Several trials are currently studying the prophylactic use of this natural hormone in women with a previous history of preterm labour, or found, during mid-pregnancy screening, to have an unusually short cervix.

Pharmacology
The chemical structure of progesterone, a natural hormone produced by the ovary's corpus luteum, was first determined in 1934. It was synthesised artificially soon after that and used, intermittently, for many years in the treatment of various menstrual disorders despite very little objective evidence of benefit. It has also been in intermittent use, ever since 1960, to reduce the risk of miscarriage. While there was no evidence that it does manage to reduce the general miscarriage rate in a Cochrane review of 14 small trials in 2003, there did seem to be a case for mounting a further trial in women who had already suffered at least three miscarriages. Indeed a systematic review undertaken in 1990 did suggest that it might also have a role in reducing the risk of preterm labour in women with a strong prior history of this problem, and interest in this approach to the prevention of recurrent preterm labour has increased significantly in the last 10 years.

Considerable interest was generated by some small trials suggesting that use reduced the risk of preterm birth in women who have already experienced preterm birth, but larger trials failed to replicate these findings. However, in a trial that involved the mid-pregnancy screening of an unselected population of women (Fonseca et al., 2007), prophylaxis in the 1·7% with a very short cervix (≤15 mm) almost halved delivery before 34 weeks. Retrospective review in another recent trial (DeFranco et al., 2007) also detected efficacy in the subgroup with a mid-trimester cervical length of less than 28 mm. Treatment does not seem to be effective in twin pregnancy.

Warnings about exposure to any progestogen in early pregnancy were issued in the 1960s after reports appeared saying that this could cause masculinisation of the female fetus, but it seems, in retrospect, that most cases were caused by exposure to norethisterone rather than progesterone. There would seem to be a three-fold increase in the risk of second- or third-degree hypospadias in boys after first trimester use, but later use does not seem to be associated with any general excess of congenital abnormality. The only study of intrauterine use as a contraceptive during breastfeeding found no evidence that this interfered with lactation.

Prophylaxis in a singleton pregnancy
Vaginal capsules: The nightly insertion of a 200 mg progesterone capsule into the vagina from the 24th to 34th week of pregnancy nearly halved the risk of preterm birth in women found to have a short cervix on mid-pregnancy screening in one recent trial. The current OPTIMUM trial is also testing a 200 mg pessary.
IM prophylaxis: 250 mg depot injections of hydroxyprogesterone caproate given IM once a week from the 20th to 36th week of pregnancy reduced the risk of recurrent preterm delivery in one small trial.

Supply and administration
Vaginal capsules: Capsules containing 200 mg of micronised progesterone (Utrogestan®) made by Besins International in Belgium were used in the trial reported by Fonseca et al. in 2007.
Vaginal gel: Vaginal applicators delivering a gel containing 90 mg of progesterone (Prochieve®) made by Columbia Laboratories, NJ, USA were used in the trial reported by O'Brien et al. and DeFranco et al. in 2007.
IM prophylaxis: 17α-hydroxyprogesterone caproate (also known as hydroxyprogesterone hexanoate (BANM)) is the analogue of the natural hormone that was used in the studies by Meis in 2003 and Facchinetti et al. in 2007. 250 mg ampoules made up in castor oil, with benzyl benzoate as a preservative, are manufactured by Schering Health Care Ltd, and can be imported into the UK from Germany on request.

References
See also the relevant Cochrane reviews

Borna S, Sahabi N. Progesterone for maintenance tocolytic therapy after threatened preterm labour: a randomised controlled trial. Aust NZ Obstet Gynaecol 2008;**48**:58–63. [RCT]
Carmichael SL, Shaw GM, Laurent C, et al. Maternal progestin intake and risk of hypospadias. Arch Pediatr Adolesc Med 2005;**159**:957–62.
Daya S. Efficacy of progesterone support for pregnancy in women with recurrent miscarriage: a meta-analysis of controlled trials. Br J Obstet Gynaecol 1989;**96**:275–80. [SR]
DeFranco EA, O'Brien JM, Adair CD, et al. Vaginal progesterone is associated with a decrease in the risk of early preterm birth and improved neonatal outcome in women with a short cervix: a secondary analysis from a randomized, double blind, placebo-controlled trial. Ultrasound Obstet Gynecol 2007;**30**:697–705. [RCT]
Facchinetti F, Paganelli S, Comitini G, et al. Cervical length changes during preterm cervical ripening: effects of 17-alpha-hyproprogesterone caproate. Am J Obstet Gynecol 2007;**196**:453–54. [RCT]
Fonseca EB, Celik E, Parra M, et al. Progesterone and the risk of preterm birth among women with a short cervix. N Engl J Med 2007;**357**:462–9. [RCT] (See also pp. 498–501 and the supplementary appendix on the web at www.nejm.org.)
Lamont RF, Jayasooriya GS. Progesteroral agents for the prevention of preterm burth. [Short review] J Perinatat Med 2009;37:12–14.
Norman JE, Mackenzie F, Owen P, et al. Progesterone for the prevention of preterm birth in twin pregnancy (STOPPIT): a randomised, double blind, placebo-controlled study and meta-analysis. Lancet 2009;**373**:2034–40. [RCT] (See also pp. 2000–2.)
O'Brien JM, Adair CD, Lewis DF, et al. Progesterone vaginal gel for the reduction of recurrent preterm birth: primary results from a randomized, double-blind, placebo-controlled trial. Ultrasound Obstet Gynecol 2007;**30**:687–96. [RCT]
Romero R. Prevention of spontaneous preterm birth: the role of sonographic cervical length in identifying patients who may benefit from progesterone treatment. [Commentary] Ultrasound Obstet Gynecol 2007;**30**:675–86.
Rouse DJ, Caritis SN, Peaceman AM, et al. A trial of 17 alpha-hydroxyprogesterone caproate to prevent prematurity in twins. N Engl J Med 2007;**357**:454–61. [RCT]

Use

A dose of chloroquine (q.v.) once a week was for many years the most widely used strategy for preventing malaria, but a combination of weekly chloroquine and daily proguanil is now the more widely recommended option. Proguanil with atovaquone, or mefloquine (q.v.), is now the strategy that has to be used for prophylaxis in the many parts of the world where most parasites have now become resistant to chloroquine.

Pharmacology

Proguanil is a biguanide, first developed in the UK during the Second World War as the result of a collaboration instigated by the MRC's Joint Chemotherapy Committee, that is rapidly absorbed when taken by mouth and quickly turned in the liver into the active metabolite cycloguanil. Both are then excreted largely in the urine (the somewhat variable half life in adults being about 20 hours).

Atovaquone is an antiprotozoal developed in the early 1990s that is sometimes used to prevent or treat *Pneumocystis* infection in patients unable to tolerate co-trimoxazole (q.v.) and, along with proguanil, in the prevention and treatment of malaria. It has a plasma half life of 2–3 days (probably because of enterohepatic recycling) before it is excreted largely unchanged in the stools. Almost nothing is yet known about the use of atovaquone during pregnancy or lactation.

Malarone® is a widely used fixed combination tablet of proguanil hydrochloride with atovaquone.

Other prophylactic strategies

Nets impregnated with permethrin offer substantial night-time protection. Diethyltoluamide (DEET) sprays and lotions are effective for 5–10 hours. Use a formulation with <30% DEET to minimise the risk of toxicity. Long sleeves and trousers lessen the risk after dusk.

Drug resistance

See the monograph on mefloquine for how to access advice on how drug resistance varies in different parts of the world. Proguanil with atovaquone is the drug now most widely recommended for use by visitors to those parts of sub-Saharan Africa, Southeast Asia (including India and China), the Pacific Islands and South America where there is substantial risk of infection.

Prophylaxis

In pregnancy: Malaria can be a devastating disease during pregnancy and prophylaxis with proguanil is known to be of considerable value in areas where infection is endemic. Side effects are minimal with the standard prophylactic dose (200 mg once a day) and there is no evidence of teratogenicity. Consider giving a daily folate supplement as well. More needs to be learnt about maternal use during lactation, but use certainly exposes the baby to much less drug than would result from standard prophylactic treatment (5 mg/kg once a day). Less is known about combined use with atovaquone, and most would argue that the combination should only be employed if no other alternative is available. No authority has yet recommended the use of Malarone during lactation.

In infancy: Start giving Malarone once a day 1–2 days before entering any area where malaria is prevalent and continue treatment for 1 week after leaving. It is probably safe to give children weighing at least 6 kg half of one paediatric tablet (i.e. 12·5 mg of proguanil and ~41 mg of atovaquone) if the risk of infection is high, but it is better to use other strategies to avoid exposure and treat any signs of infection promptly if these do occur. Children weighing over 10 kg can certainly take one crushed tablet once a day.

Treatment

One option is to give any small child with overt signs of infection two crushed tablets of the paediatric strength Malarone once a day for 3 days. There is little experience of treating babies weighing less than 5 kg as yet. See the monograph on quinine for a review of all the treatment options in early infancy.

Supply

Proguanil: Scored 100 mg tablets (which only cost 8p) can be quartered, crushed and administered on a spoon or down a nasogastric tube. A suspension could be prepared, but its 'shelf life' is not yet certain, and there is no evidence that the greater precision this might offer is important.

Proguanil with atovaquone: Malarone provides an alternative approach to prophylaxis and treatment, but the manufacturers have not yet recommended prophylactic use in early infancy. The standard paediatric tablet contains 25 mg of proguanil hydrochloride and 62·5 mg of atovaquone. No suspension exists.

References

Croft A. Malaria: prevention in travellers. *Clin Evid* 2005;**14**:954–72 (and updates). [SR]

Gilveray G, Looareesuwan S, White NJ, *et al*. The pharmacokinetics of atovaquone and proguanil in pregnancy in women with acute falciparum malaria. *Eur J Clin Pharmacol* 2003;**59**:545–52.

Lell B, Luckner D, Ndjavé M, *et al*. Randomised placebo-controlled study of atovaquone plus proguanil for malaria prophylaxis in children. *Lancet* 1998;**351**:709–13. [RCT]

Marra F, Salzman JR, Ensom MH, *et al*. Atovaquone-proguanil for prophylaxis and trestment of malaria. *Ann Pharmacother* 2003;**37**:1266–75.

Nakato H, Vivancos R, Hunter PR. A systematic review and meta-analysis of the effectiveness and safety of atovaquone-proguanil (Malarone) for chemoprophylaxis against malaria. *J Antimicrob Chemother* 2007;**60**:929–36. [SR]

Taylor WRJ, White NJ. Antimalarial drug toxicity: a review. *Drug Saf* 2004;**27**:25–61.

Use

Propofol is a rapid-acting intravenous anaesthetic. Adults needing intensive care are often sedated with a continuous infusion, but serious (sometimes lethal) metabolic complications were encountered when this strategy was used in children. Pain control requires an opiate, such as remifentanil (q.v.), as well.

Pharmacology

Propofol is a clear, colourless, insoluble phenolic compound supplied in an isotonic, oil-in-water, Intralipid® emulsion that came into use as a useful, short-acting IV anaesthetic in 1984. It is unrelated, chemically, to any other anaesthetic agent, but behaves rather like ketamine (q.v.). Recovery from propofol is, however, rather more rapid, and 'hangovers' are less common. The drug is rapidly redistributed into fat and other body tissues and more than half leaves the circulation within 10 minutes, even after neonatal IV administration (V_D ~4 l/kg). It is then conjugated and metabolised in the liver, the elimination half life being 5−10 hours although, with sustained use, elimination from deep stores may take 2−3 days. Propofol is not teratogenic or fetotoxic in animals but crosses the placenta readily, and the manufacturers do not recommend use during pregnancy or delivery, although no problems have been encountered with use for Caesarean delivery. Neither has the main manufacturer yet recommended the use of propofol to induce anaesthesia in the neonate, to sustain anaesthesia in patients less than 3 years old, or to provide continuous sedation in patients under 17. Substantial quantities appear in breast milk, but a baby taking milk from the breast 12 hours after the mother's delivery under propofol anaesthesia would ingest less than 1% of the weight-related maternal dose.

The drug was used as a sedative in paediatric intensive care for 15 years before any controlled trials were undertaken, and it was several years before reports of unexpected metabolic acidosis, and rhabdomyolysis, with sudden life-threatening cardiac and renal failure started to appear. In one still unpublished control trial, in which 222 children received a sustained 1% or 2% propofol infusion and 105 some other sedative, all but 4 of the 25 deaths occurred in children given propofol. It is now clear that prolonged infusion can sometimes cause a myopathy due to impaired fatty acid oxidation in patients of *any* age which is only reversible by stopping treatment at once and offering prompt haemoperfusion. Maintaining a generous glucose infusion may make this hazard less likely by limiting the tendency of the body to mobilise energy stores from fat.

Use during neonatal intubation

2·5 mg/kg of propofol given IV over 10 seconds will usually cause relaxation without apnoea, and render the baby oblivious to the stress of intubation, but some babies need a second dose. The addition of a 3 microgram/kg bolus of remifentanil can be used to provide pain-free working conditions within 90 seconds, but this can cause brief apnoea, and intubation on its own should cause relatively little pain.

Use for continuous IV sedation or anaesthesia

Maintenance anaesthesia: Anaesthesia for any procedure lasting more than 10−15 minutes requires a maintenance infusion of propofol. Evidence suggests that this should ***never*** be given to any young child at a rate exceeding 4 mg/kg per hour. Where (as is often the case) this fails to provide adequate pain relief, an opiate, such as remifentanil, should be given as well − the dose of propofol should not be increased.

Prolonged sedation: Propofol is now widely used to provide sustained sedation for patients requiring intensive care, but it should ***not*** be used in this way, especially in children less than 3 years old because there is a small, but currently unpredictable, risk of sudden 'propofol infusion syndrome' collapse.

Precautions

Propofol use must be supervised by an experienced intensivist, and recovery monitored until it is complete.

Supply and administration

20 ml ampoules of an IV emulsion containing 10 mg/ml cost £2·30. Store ampoules at room temperature, shake before use and do not freeze. The lipid content makes it important to protect any line used for sustained infusion from microbial contamination. Do not infuse through a <1·2 μm filter. IV injection can cause transient pain, but this can be relieved by adding 50 micrograms of lidocaine to each mg of propofol.

References

Allegaert K, de Hoon J, Verbesselt R, et al. Maturational pharmacokinetics of single intravenous bolus of propofol. Pediatr Anesth 2007;**17**:1028−34.

Allegaert K, Peeters MY, Verbesselt R, et al. Inter-individual variability in propofol pharmacokinetics in preterm and term neonates. Br J Anaesth 2007;**99**:864−70.

Cornfield DN, Tegtmeyer K, Nelson MD, et al. Continuous propofol infusion in 142 critically ill children. Pediatrics 2002;**110**:1177−81.

Duncan HP, Zurick NJ, Wolf AR. Should we consider awake neonatal intubation? A review of the evidence and treatment strategies. Paediatr Anaesth 2001;**11**:135−45.

Ghanta S, Abdel-Latif ME, Lui K, et al. Propofol compared with the morphine, atropine, and suxamethonium regimen as induction agents for neonatal endotracheal intubation: a randomized, controlled trial. Pediatrics 2007;**119**:e1248−55. [RCT] (See also 2007;**120**:932−3.)

Kam PCA, Cardone D. Propofol infusion syndrome. [Review] Anaesthesia 2007;**62**:690−701. [SR]

Meyer S, Grundmann U, Gottschling S, et al. Sedation and analgesia for brief diagnostic and therapeutic procedures in children. Eur J Pediatr 2007;**166**:291−302.

Reeves ST, Havidich JE, Tobin DP. Conscious sedation of children with propofol is anything but conscious. Pediatrics 2004;**114**:e74−6.

Tsui BCH, Wagner A, Usher AG, et al. Combined propofol and remifentanil anesthesia for pediatric patients undergoing magnetic resonance imaging. Pediatr Anesth 2005;**15**:397−401.

Use

Oral propranolol is used to manage hypercyanotic spells in Fallot tetralogy, in neonatal thyrotoxicosis, and (with hydralazine) in the control of dangerous hypertension. It is sometimes used to control arrhythmia, to manage the long QT syndromes and, experimentally, in the management of severe infantile haemangiomas.

Pharmacology

Propranolol hydrochloride was the first non-selective ß-adrenoreceptor blocking agent. It reduces the rate and force of contraction of the heart and slows cardiac conduction. The hypotension and bradycardia seen with an overdose are best treated with glucagon (q.v.). Respiratory depression and fits can also occur. Propranolol, together with a vasodilator such as hydralazine, is of value in the management of severe hypertension although its mode of action remains unclear. Caution is essential when the drug is used in the presence of heart failure. The half life in children and adults is 3–6 hours; the neonatal half life is not known. It is not teratogenic, but maternal use can cause transient neonatal bradycardia and hypoglycaemia and may also retard fetal growth. It is excreted in breast milk, but use only exposes the baby to 1% of the maternal dose on a weight-for-weight basis. It can be given IV in the initial management of arrhythmia and cyanotic 'spells', but a 600 microgram/kg bolus of IV esmolol over 1–2 minutes (followed, if necessary, by a continuous infusion of 300–900 micrograms/kg per minute) may be a safer alternative, because esmolol has a very short half life. Patients started on IV propranolol will need significantly more once oral treatment is started because of high first pass liver metabolism. Oral nadolol may be preferable for long-term management because most babies only need 1 mg/kg once a day.

Neonatal thyrotoxicosis

This rare but potentially fatal disorder, seen in 1–2% of the offspring of mothers with Graves disease, results from the transplacental passage of thyrotropin receptor antibody. Neonatal problems are most frequently seen in babies of mothers with a high antibody titre. This can occur even after the mother has been rendered medically or surgically euthyroid. Propylthiouracil (5 mg/kg every 12 hours) should be given to symptomatic babies. Propranolol is a further mainstay of treatment in severe cases. It may need to be continued for 3–12 weeks after delivery. Lugol iodine (which contains 130 mg/ml of iodine) provides the most easily obtained source of iodine for inhibiting thyroid function. Digoxin (q.v.) and a diuretic may be required if there is heart failure. Sedation is occasionally called for. Always seek the advice of an experienced paediatric endocrinologist if symptoms are severe.

Treatment

Neonatal thyrotoxicosis: Give 250–750 micrograms/kg every 8 hours by mouth to control symptoms, with one drop of Lugol iodine every 8 hours to control the transient neonatal thyrotoxicosis.
Arrhythmia: Try 20 micrograms/kg IV over 10 minutes with ECG monitoring and increase this, in steps, to a cumulative total of 100 micrograms/kg if necessary. Give the effective dose IV once every 8 hours for maintenance. The same strategy may also work for the 'spells' sometimes seen in severe Fallot tetralogy (with oxygen, morphine and, if necessary, sodium bicarbonate, to correct serious acidosis). For sustained oral maintenance try 1 mg/kg (never more than 2 mg/kg) once every 8 hours.
Long QT syndromes: Start by giving 1 mg/kg by mouth once every 8 hours. Oral nadolol once a day (see above) may be a more convenient long-term option.
Neonatal hypertension: Start with 250 micrograms/kg every 8 hours by mouth together with hydralazine (q.v.) and increase as necessary to a maximum of 2 mg/kg per dose.

Blood levels

The therapeutic blood level in adults is said to be 20–100 mg/l (1 mg/l = 3·9 µmol/l), but it is best to judge the amount of drug to give by reference to the patient's blood pressure and response to treatment.

Supply and administration

1 mg (1 ml) ampoules of propranolol cost 21p. For accurate IV use dilute to 10 ml with 10% glucose to get a 100 microgram/ml solution. It is also available as a 1 mg/ml oral solution (100 ml for £8·30). 100 mg (10 ml) vials of esmolol cost £7·80. Nadolol is available as a 6 mg/ml oral suspension with a 30-day 'shelf life' (100 ml costs £45), and an inexpensive suspension of propylthiouracil can be supplied on request.

References

Gardner LI. Is propranolol alone really effective in neonatal thyrotoxicosis? *Arch Dis Child* 1980;**134**:707–8. (See also pp. 819–20.)
Hussain T, Greenhalgh K, McLeod KA. Hypoglycaemia syncope in children secondary to beta-blockers. *Arch Dis Child* 2009;**94**:968–9.
Mehta AV, Chidambraram B. Efficacy and safety of intravenous and oral nadolol for supraventricular tachycardia. *J Am Coll Cardiol* 1992;**19**:630–5.
Moss AJ, Zareba W, Hall WJ, *et al.* Effectiveness and limitations of beta-blocker therapy in congenital long-QT syndromes. *Circulation* 2000;**101**:616–23.
Ogilvy-Stuart AL. Neonatal thyroid disorders. [Review] *Arch Dis Child* 2002;**87**:F165–71.
Sans V, Dumas de la Roque E, Berge J, *et al.* Propranolol for severe infantile hemangiomas: follow-up report. *Pediatrics* 2009;**124**:e423–31.
Villain E, Denjoy I, Lupoglazoff JM. Low incidence of cardiac events with β-blocking therapy in children with long QT syndrome. *Eur Heart J* 2005;**25**:1405–11.

PROSTAGLANDIN E$_2$ = Dinoprostone (rINN)

Use
Prostaglandin E$_2$ gels and vaginal tablets are now widely used to initiate and augment labour. Prostaglandin E$_1$ and E$_2$ are both widely used to maintain patency of the ductus arteriosus pending surgery in babies with a duct-dependent congenital heart defect, but they can take several hours to become fully effective.

Pharmacology
Prostaglandin E$_1$ (alprostadil) and E$_2$ (dinoprostone) are potent vasodilators originally isolated from prostate gland secretions that inhibit platelet coagulation and stimulate uterine contractility. Prostaglandin E$_2$ was first synthesised in 1970 and is still occasionally used to terminate pregnancy by extra-amniotic administration, while tablets, gels and pessaries are now very widely used to ripen the cervix and/or initiate labour at term. Misoprostol (q.v.), an analogue of prostaglandin E$_1$, is also sometimes used to initiate labour, and is more widely used to control postpartum bleeding, although the manufacturers have not yet sought permission to market the drug for use in this way. Caution must be employed before using prostaglandins and oxytocin simultaneously because each drug potentiates the effect of the other.

Prostaglandins were first used experimentally to sustain ductal patency in 1975, and continuous IV infusions are now frequently employed in the early preoperative management of babies with duct-dependent congenital heart disease. While prostaglandin E$_1$ is the licensed preparation, a similar dose of prostaglandin E$_2$ is equally effective and eight times as cheap. Because of rapid inactivation during passage through the lung, the half life during IV infusion is less than a minute, and no loading dose is necessary. Monitor oxygen saturation. Respiratory depression and apnoea are common with high-dose treatment (some texts still recommend a dose that is much higher than necessary) and may occur, even with the dose recommended here, especially in the cyanosed or preterm baby. High-dose treatment causes vasodilatation and hypotension, and has rarely caused diarrhoea, irritability, seizures, tachycardia, pyrexia and metabolic acidosis. Watch for hypoglycaemia. Continued IV use for more than 5 days can cause gastric outlet obstruction due to reversible antral hyperplasia, and long-term use can cause hyperostosis of cortical bone.

Sustained oral administration is still sometimes used in a few centres, but it is rarely employed in the UK now because delay is not thought to render surgery any less technically difficult. Start with 25 micrograms/kg by mouth once an hour and double this if necessary. Some babies manage with treatment every 3–4 hours, but many need a dose every 2 hours to remain stable. Watch for rising renal electrolyte loss.

Treatment
Maternal: 1 mg of vaginal gel (2 mg if the cervix is unfavourable) inserted high into the posterior fornix, or a 3 mg vaginal tablet similarly positioned, is now the most widely used method of inducing labour. A second dose of either can be given, if necessary, after 6–8 hours. An infusion of 0·25–1 micrograms per minute is now only rarely used to initiate labour, but is still occasionally employed to induce labour after fetal death.

Neonatal: Start with a 10 nanogram/kg per minute IV infusion through a secure line (0·6 ml/kg per hour of a solution made up as described below) and leave this dose running for a few hours before using oxygen saturation to adjust this dose up, or down, as necessary. Always aim to use the lowest effective dose – a dose as high as 40 nanograms/kg per minute is very rarely necessary.

Preventing neonatal apnoea
Use the minimum effective dose of prostaglandin. If high-dose treatment *is* necessary the risk of apnoea can be reduced by giving IV aminophylline (see the monograph on theophylline). Caffeine (q.v.) would probably be equally effective.

Compatibility
Prostaglandin E$_2$ (dinoprostone) is very unstable in solution, and should never be infused with any other drug. In contrast it *may* be acceptable to add prostaglandin E$_1$ (alprostadil) (terminally) when absolutely necessary, into a line containing adrenaline, dopamine, glyceryl trinitrate, heparin, lidocaine, midazolam, morphine or nitroprusside, although the manufacturers remain reluctant to endorse this advice.

Supply and administration
One 0·75 ml IV ampoule of prostaglandin E$_2$ (containing 1 mg/ml) costs £8·50. Note that *10 mg/ml* ampoules are sometimes stocked for use in termination of pregnancy. To give an infusion of 10 nanograms/kg per minute, add 0·5 ml of dinoprostone from a 1 mg/ml ampoule to 500 ml of 10% glucose or glucose saline to produce a solution containing 1 microgram of dinoprostone per ml, and infuse this at a rate of 0·6 ml/kg per hour. A less concentrated solution of dextrose or dextrose saline can be used where necessary. Store ampoules at 4°C, and prepare a fresh IV solution daily. A sugar-free oral solution with a 1-week shelf life can be prepared on request. Vaginal gels and tablets are widely used to induce labour; the two are *not* strictly bioequivalent, but a 3 mg tablet is cheaper than 2 mg of gel (£10 *v.* £18).

References
See also the Cochrane reviews of obstetric use

Brodie M, Chaudari M, Hasan A. Prostaglandin therapy for ductal patency: how long is too long? *Acta Paediatr* 2008;**97**:1303–4.
Kaufman MB, El-Chaar GM. Bone and tissue changes following prostaglandin therapy in neonates. *Ann Pharmacother* 1996;**30**:269–77.
Lálosi G, Katona M, Túri S. Side-effects of long-term prostaglandin E$_1$ treatment in neonates. *Pediatr Int* 2007;**47**:335–40.
Madar RJ, Donaldson T, Hunter S. Prostaglandins in congenital heart disease. *Cardiol Young* 1995;**5**:202–3.
Meckler GD, Lowe C. To intubate or not to intubate? Transporting infants on prostaglandin E$_1$. *Pediatrics* 2009;**123**:e25–30.

Use

Pyrazinamide is used in the first phase treatment of tuberculosis (TB). To minimise the risk of drug resistance developing, the management of this notifiable disease should always be overseen by a clinician with substantial experience of this dangerous, and frequently contagious, condition.

Pharmacology

Pyrazinamide, like isoniazid (q.v.), to which it is chemically related, is bacteriostatic or bactericidal against *Mycobacterium tuberculosis* depending on the dose used. Other mycobacteria, including *M. bovis*, are resistant. Fifty years after its discovery in 1952 its mode of action is still unknown, but its metabolite, pyrazinoic acid, seems to prevent intracellular bacterial replication. Resistance develops rapidly if other drugs are not taken at the same time. It is well absorbed by mouth and should always be used when TB meningitis is a possibility because it rapidly penetrates all body tissues. The half life in adults is 9–10 hours, but it does not seem to have been studied in children. Excretion is impaired in severe renal failure, but drug accumulation does not occur during peritoneal dialysis. Liver toxicity is the main hazard, so liver function should be checked before treatment is started, and repeated at intervals if there is pre-existing liver disease. Review treatment at once if any sign of liver toxicity (such as nausea, vomiting, drowsiness or jaundice) develops during treatment. Manufacturers in the US have endorsed use in children, but no such move has been made in the UK.

While the continued lack of published information has left authorities in the US reluctant to recommend use during pregnancy or lactation, such use has been endorsed by the International Union against Tuberculosis and Lung Disease and by the British Thoracic Society. The breastfed baby almost certainly gets less than 1% of the maternal dose on a weight-for-weight basis, but this estimate is based on a single case report.

Infants exposed to a case of infectious TB

Babies born to mothers with TB: See the monograph on isoniazid for maternal treatment. Give the baby 5 mg/kg of isoniazid as chemoprophylaxis once a day for 3 months, and then do a Mantoux test. If this test is negative and the mother is no longer infectious, BCG can be given and treatment stopped; if it is positive give 10 mg/kg of isoniazid for a further 3 months. Do not discourage breastfeeding. Congenitally acquired infection usually becomes symptomatic in 2–3 weeks. Treat evidence of active disease as summarised below.

Babies not previously given BCG: Give 10 mg/kg of isoniazid for 6 weeks and then do a Mantoux test. Give a further 20 weeks of isoniazid if this proves positive or the interferon gamma test proves positive (where facilities exist for performing this test). Offer full active treatment (see below) if there are X-ray changes.

Babies previously given BCG: Offer isoniazid for 6 months if the Mantoux test is strongly positive, or if it becomes strongly positive on retesting 6 weeks later. Offer full treatment if there is evidence of active disease.

Treating overt TB in infancy

TB can progress rapidly in young children. Generalised (or miliary) TB is a real possibility if treatment is not started promptly, infecting bone or the meninges round the brain. Treatment is a two stage process – an initial 2-month phase using three (or even four) drugs designed to reduce bacterial load to a minimum and minimise the risk of drug resistance developing, and a 4-month maintenance phase using just two drugs.

Pyrazinamide: Give 35 mg/kg of pyrazinamide by mouth once a day for the first 2 months of treatment. It is critically important to ensure that the dose is correct, and that treatment is taken every day as prescribed. There is a very real risk that dangerous drug-resistant bacteria will evolve and put both the patient, and the community, at risk if this is not done.

Other drugs: Give 10 mg/kg of isoniazid and 10 mg/kg of rifampicin (q.v.) as well by mouth once a day for at least 6 months. Any possible meningeal involvement calls for at least a year's expert treatment and the use of a fourth drug for the first 2 months. A 15 mg/kg dose of ethambutol given once a day for 2 months is the most commonly employed option. While this drug can occasionally cause serious visual loss, which can become permanent if not recognised promptly, there are no well attested reports of this occurring in a young child with the dose recommended here. A 20–30 mg/kg IM dose of streptomycin once a day for 2 months may be the most acceptable alternative (checking periodically that the trough level does not exceed 5 mg/l).

Supply

500 mg tablets of pyrazinamide cost 7p, and 100 mg tablets of ethambutol cost 20p each. Sugar-free oral suspensions can be provided with a 4-week shelf life. 1 gram vials of streptomycin cost £8 each in the UK.

References

Joint Tuberculosis Committee of the British Thoracic Society. Chemotherapy and management of tuberculosis in the United Kingdom: recommendations 1998. *Thorax* 1999;**53**:536–48.

Joint Tuberculosis Committee of the British Thoracic Society. Control and prevention of tuberculosis in the United Kingdom: code of practice 2000. *Thorax* 2000;**55**:887–901.

Marais BJ, Pai M. Recent advances in the diagnosis of childhood tuberculosis. *Arch Dis Child* 2007;**92**:446–52.

Raju B, Schluger NW. Tuberculosis and pregnancy. *Semin Respir Crit Care Med* 1998;**19**:295–306.

Skevaki CL, Kafetzis DA. Tuberculosis in neonates and infants: epidemiology, pathogenesis, clinical manifestations, diagnosis, and management issues. *Pediatr Drugs* 2005;**7**:219–34.

Teo SSS, Riordan A, Alfaham M, *et al.* Tuberculosis in the United Kingdom and Republic of Ireland. *Arch Dis Child* 2009;**94**:263–7.

Vallejo JG, Ong LT, Starke JR. Clinical features, diagnosis, and treatment of tuberculosis in infants. *Pediatrics* 1994;**94**:1–7.

PYRIDOXINE (Vitamin B$_6$) and PYRIDOXAL PHOSPHATE

Use

Pyridoxine, and its active metabolite, pyridoxal phoshate, are used to treat two inborn errors of metabolism that cause convulsions in early infancy. Pyridoxine is also used in the management of homocystinuria.

Biochemistry

Pyridoxine is widely available in most foodstuffs and nutritional deficiency is extremely rare. Pyridoxine is converted in the body to pyridoxal phosphate, which is a cofactor for a number of enzymes. Pyridoxine dependency is an autosomal recessive condition associated with mutations in the antiquitin (ALDH7A1) gene. This defect leads to the accumulation of piperideine-6-carboxylate, which binds and inactivates pyridoxal phosphate. Pyridoxine dependency should be considered in any baby with severe seizures even if they seem to have a clear cause (e.g. asphyxia). Most cases present soon after birth, and seizures have even been sensed *in utero*. Development may still be delayed even though pyridoxine controls the fits. The diagnosis can be confirmed by measuring CSF plasma or urine α-aminoadipic semialdehyde (α-AASA).

Pyridoxine is converted to pyridoxal phosphate by pyridox(am)ine phosphate oxidase, and patients with the rare recessive defect of *this* enzyme present with neonatal seizures that respond to pyridoxal phosphate, but *not* to pyridoxine. It should be noted that pyridoxine and pyridoxal phosphate also display anticonvulsant activity in some patients who do not have either of these conditions for reasons that are not yet understood.

Homocystinuria most commonly results from cystathionine β-synthase deficiency. Pyridoxal phosphate is the cofactor for this enzyme, and many patients improve biochemically and clinically with pharmacological doses of pyridoxine. Cases of homocystinuria detected by neonatal screening programmes, however, tend not to be pyridoxine responsive. Other patients present with developmental delay, or subsequently with dislocated lenses, skeletal abnormalities or thromboembolic disease.

Diagnostic use

Defects of pyridoxine metabolism: One 100 mg IV dose of pyridoxine stops most fits within minutes. Watch for apnoea. The test is best conducted while the EEG is being monitored (although visible seizure activity may cease some hours or even days before the EEG trace returns to normal), but this test should not be delayed if monitoring proves hard to organise. If the response is negative, or equivocal, and pyridoxine dependency is a likely diagnosis, then oral pyridoxine should be given for 2 weeks. Finally, a trial of pyridoxal phosphate (see below) should be considered in patients who do not respond to pyridoxine.

Fits later in infancy: Some patients with pyridoxine dependency present when more than 4 weeks old. All infants with infantile spasms or drug-resistant seizures merit a trial of pyridoxine or pyridoxinal phosphate (50 mg/kg of either drug by mouth once a day for a minimum of 2 weeks).

Homocystinuria: Pyridoxine responsiveness should be assessed by measuring plasma methionine and homocysteine under basal conditions, and during a 2–3 weeks trial of pyridoxine, while ensuring a constant protein intake. Start by giving 100 mg a day (although a dose of up to 250 mg/day may deliver added benefit). Give 5 mg folic acid a day to be sure the response is not impaired by folate deficiency.

Treatment

Fits: Infants with fits that respond to pyridoxine should then receive 50–100 mg indefinitely once a day if tests show excess α-AASA in the urine. The prognosis for siblings may be improved if mothers with a pyridoxine-dependent child take 100 mg of pyridoxine daily in any subsequent pregnancy.

Homocystinuria: Pyridoxine-responsive infants are usually given 50 mg twice a day; older patients are usually given 50–250 mg twice a day, depending on their response. Most patients take 5 mg of folic acid once a day. If this does not completely correct the abnormality, treatment can be combined with a low methionine diet, betaine (q.v.) and/or vitamin B$_{12}$ (q.v.). These forms of treatment can also be used in patients unresponsive to pyridoxine.

Adverse effects

The first dose of pyridoxine or pyridoxal phosphate in a neonate can cause hypotonia or apnoea requiring support. High doses in adults have caused a sensory neuropathy (and might be neurotoxic in children), so long-term management should be overseen by a paediatric neurologist or metabolic physician.

Supply

Pyridoxine: All units should have access to a stock of 2 ml (50 mg/ml) IV ampoules. They cost about £1 each. A sugar-free oral suspension is available, as are 10, 20 and 50 mg tablets (costing 2p each).

Pyridoxal phosphate: 50 mg tablets cost 12p each; a sugar-free suspension is also available.

References

See also the relevant Cochrane reviews

Clayton PT, Surtees RAH, DeVile C, *et al.* Neonatal epileptic encephalopathy. *Lancet* 2003;**361**:1614.

Mills PB, Struys E, Jakobs C, *et al.* Mutations in antiquitin in individuals with pyridoxine-dependent seizures. *Nat Med* 2006;**12**:307–9.

Rankin PM, Harrison S, Chong WK, *et al.* Pyridoxine-dependent seizures: a family phenotype that leads to severe cognitive deficits, regardless of treatment regime. *Dev Med Child Neurol* 2007;**49**:300–5.

Wang H-S, Kuo M-F, Chou M-L, *et al.* Pyridoxal phosphate is better than pyridoxine for controlling idiopathic intractable epilepsy. *Arch Dis Child* 2005;**90**:512–5. (See also pp. 441–2.)

Use
Pyrimethamine is used, with sulfadiazine (q.v.), to treat toxoplasmosis and, with sulfadoxine, to treat malaria (as an alternative to co-trimoxazole (q.v.)) in areas where resistance has not yet developed.

Pharmacology
Pyrimethamine is a di-aminopyrimidine that blocks nucleic acid synthesis in the malaria parasite. It also interferes with folate metabolism. It was developed in 1951 and is still widely used in the treatment of toxoplasmosis (the natural history of which is briefly summarised in the monograph on spiramycin) although the only proof of efficacy comes from trials in patients where toxoplasmosis was a complication of HIV infection. Prolonged administration can depress haemopoiesis. Other side effects are rare, but skin rashes may occur and high doses can cause atrophic glossitis and megaloblastic anaemia. Folinic acid (the 5-formyl derivative of folic acid) is used to prevent this during pregnancy because folinic acid does not interfere with the impact of pyrimethamine on malaria and *Toxoplasma* parasites. Pyrimethamine is well absorbed by mouth and slowly excreted by the kidney, the average plasma half life being about 4 days. Tissue levels exceed plasma levels (V_D ~3 l/kg). The efficacy of pyrimethamine in treating toxoplasmosis is increased eight-fold by sulfadiazine. Other sulphonamides are not as effective. Efficacy in treating malaria is also improved by giving sulfadoxine. For this reason a sulphonamide should *always* be prescribed when pyrimethamine is used to treat a baby for malaria or toxoplasmosis unless there is significant neonatal jaundice, even though the manufacturer only endorses such use in children over 5 years old. Long-term administration can sometimes cause problems (as outlined in the monograph on sulfadiazine). Lactation can continue during treatment, even though the baby receives about a third of the maternal dose on a weight-for-weight basis.

Intermittent prophylactic use where malaria is endemic
Insecticide-treated bed nets are an effective and underused strategy for preventing infection. See the web commentary on pre-emptive drug use to control subclinical infection during pregnancy and in early infancy.

Treatment of malaria
During pregnancy: A single 3-tablet dose of Fansidar® (a total of 75 mg of pyrimethamine and 1·5 g of sulfadoxine) and a 3-day course of amodiaquine (q.v.) effectively eliminates tissue parasites. Some think this unwise in the first trimester, but the teratogenicity seen in animals seems absent in man.
In infancy: Uncomplicated malaria was once commonly treated with one dose of a synergistic mixture of 1·25 mg/kg of pyrimethamine and 25 mg/kg of sulfadoxine (i.e. Fansidar), but resistance to these two drugs has now rendered this strategy ineffective in many parts of the world, and an artemether-based approach (q.v.) has now been adopted in many countries. Quinine (q.v.) remains the best studied way of treating children with *severe* malaria, although an artemether-based approach may be equally effective.

Treatment of *Toxoplasma* infection
During pregnancy: Spiramycin (q.v.) is often used to try and prevent transplacental spread. If fetal infection is thought to have occurred, sustained maternal treatment with 50 mg of pyrimethamine once a day and 1 g of sulfadiazine three times a day by mouth may possibly lessen disease severity.
In infancy: Give an oral loading dose of 1 mg/kg of pyrimethamine twice a day for 2 days followed by maintenance treatment with 1 mg/kg once a day for 8 weeks if there is evidence of congenital infection. Treatment with 50 mg/kg of oral sulfadiazine once every 12 hours should be started at the same time. Check weekly for possible thrombocytopenia, leukopenia and megaloblastic anaemia.
Older children: It is not known whether a year's sustained treatment improves the outcome. Dormant cysts, which often give rise to ocular disease in later life, can not be eradicated by such an approach. Some centres intersperse continued treatment as outlined above with 4–6-week courses of spiramycin.
Ocular disease: Clindamycin (q.v.) is sometimes given in babies with ocular disease. Consider photocoagulation for choroidal scars. Prednisolone (2 mg/kg once a day) remains of uncertain value.

Prophylaxis with calcium folinate (= leucovorin (USAN))
Give 15 mg by mouth twice a week during pregnancy to prevent pyrimethamine causing bone marrow depression. Exactly the same dose is often given to infants on long-term pyrimethamine treatment.

Supply and administration
Pyrimethamine: 25 mg tablets cost 7p, and 25 mg tablets compounded with sulfadoxine as Fansidar (see above) cost 25p each. Suspensions can be provided on request, but dosage is not critical and it is often good enough to give small babies a quarter or half tablet.
Calcium folinate: 15 mg tablets and 15 mg (2 ml) ampoules cost £4·80 and £7·80, respectively.

References
See also the relevant Cochrane reviews

Fegan GW, Noor AM, Akhwale WS, *et al*. Effect of expanded insecticide-treated bednet coverage on child survival in rural Kenya: a longitudinal study. *Lancet* 2007;**370**:1035–9. (See also pp. 1009–10.)
Omari A, Garner P. Severe life threatening malaria in endemic areas. *BMJ* 2004;**328**:154. [SR] (See also p. 155.)
Plowe CV, Kublin JG, Dzinjalamala FK, *et al*. Sustained clinical efficacy of sulphadoxine-pyrimethamine for uncomplicated falciparum malaria in Malawi after 10 years of first line treatment: five year prospective study. *BMJ* 2004;**328**:545–8. (See also pp. 534–5.)

Use

Quinine remains the best studied drug for treating severe malaria in the very young child but, in a child well enough to take treatment by mouth, treatment with an artemisinin (see the monographs on artemether with lumefantrine or amodiaquine with artesuate) may – where affordable – prove an even more reliable strategy.

Pharmacology

Four hundred years ago Jesuit priests noted that an extract from the bark of the cinchona tree had long been valued in Peru as a specific cure for marsh or 'four day' (quaternary) fever. It contains the alkaloid quinine, which kills malarial schizonts when they enter the blood stream. G6PD deficiency is not a contraindication. High-dose quinine is a recognised abortificant, but use to treat maternal malaria in pregnancy does not seem hazardous, and use during lactation would only expose the baby to ~5% of the weight-adjusted maternal dose.

Managing severe malaria

Malaria can be rapidly fatal, especially in children less than a year old, and symptoms may be non-specific. There may be vomiting, diarrhoea and weakness or drowsiness as well as fever, and speedy intervention can make the difference between life and death. Many severely ill children are hypovolaemic and benefit from an immediate transfusion of 20 ml/kg of plasma albumin (q.v.) or, if this is not available, 0·9% sodium chloride. Then correct severe anaemia (haematocrit <15%) with blood (q.v.) or, if the anaemia is gross, or more than 10% of the red cells are parasitised, by exchange transfusion. Monitor, prevent and treat hypoglycaemia with sublingual or, if necessary, IV glucose (q.v.). Give lorazepam (q.v.) for seizures and, if this fails, paraldehyde (q.v.). IV mannitol is not helpful, but shock may suggest there is both malaria and septicaemia (with or without meningitis) – start treatment for both if the situation is unclear and review later. Transplacentally acquired infection may only manifest itself 2–8 weeks later with fever, jaundice, anaemia, respiratory symptoms and a large spleen.

Initial treatment

By mouth: See that those well enough to take quinine sulphate (or dihydrochloride) by mouth take 10 mg/kg once every 8 hours for a full 7 days (repeating the dose if vomiting occurs within an hour).
As an IV infusion: Give a loading dose of 20 mg/kg of quinine dihydrochloride (2 ml/kg of a solution made up as specified below) over 4 hours – followed 12 hourly by 10 mg/kg infused over 2–4 hours. Always use a pump or in-line infusion chamber to avoid cardiotoxicity from rapid administration. Follow with a full course of oral treatment with quinine or any artemisinin combination, e.g. artemether and lumefantrine (q.v.).
IM administration: 10 mg/kg once every 12 hours for 3 days (or until oral treatment is possible).
Rectal administration: Give 20 mg/kg of quinine, as outlined below, once every 12 hours for 3 days (or until the 7-day course can be completed by mouth). IV artesunate is now becoming the treatment of choice but an early rectal dose of quinine or artemether can be lifesaving when skilled care is hours away.

Secondary treatment

Complete treatment as soon as oral medication is possible by giving doxycycline or clindamycin or, alternatively, in those areas where the parasites are still sensitive, pyrimethamine and sulfadoxine.
Doxycycline: Give 2·5 mg/kg of this tetracycline by mouth once every 12 hours for 7 days.
Clindamycin: A 10 mg/kg dose of clindamycin (q.v.) given by mouth once every 8 hours for 7 days is an alternative that avoids the risk of dental staining caused by tetracycline use.
Pyrimethamine and sulfadoxine: Give a quarter tablet of Fansidar® on the last day of treatment. Babies 3 or more months old can have half a tablet. For more information see the monograph on pyrimethamine.

Supply and administration

Quinine: Quinine sulphate is available as dividable 200 mg (7p) tablets, and as an IV product (quinine dihydrochloride) from Martindale Pharmaceuticals, Romford, UK in 1 and 2 ml ampoules containing 300 mg/ml that cost £2·60 and £3·50 respectively. Take 1 ml of this preparation and dilute it to 30 ml with 5% or 10% glucose saline to get an IV solution containing 10 mg/ml. IM injection is painful, but quinine can also be given into the rectum – just draw up the dose required, dilute to 4 ml with water, and give using a syringe. A less painful buffered product containing four cinchona alkaloids (Quinimax®) is widely used in Africa.
Doxycycline: 50 mg capsules cost 6p each. Scored 100 mg dispersible tablets cost 60p. A 5 mg/ml suspension and a 10 mg/ml syrup (Vibramycin®) are available in America.

References

See also the relevant Cochrane reviews

Achan J, Tibenderana JK, Kyabayinze D, *et al.* Effectiveness of quinine versus artemether-lumefantrine for treating uncomplicated falciparum malaria in Ugandan children: randomised trial. *BMJ* 2009;**339**:b2763. [RCT]
Barennes H, Balima-Koussoubé T, Nagot N, *et al.* Safety and efficacy of rectal compared with intramuscular quinine for the early treatment of moderately severe malaria in children: randomised clinical trial. *BMJ* 2006;**332**:1055–7. [RCT] (See also p. 1216.)
Maitland K, Nadel S, Ollard AJ, *et al.* Management of severe malaria in children: proposed guidelines for the United Kingdom. *BMJ* 2005;**331**:337–41.
Maitland K, Pamba A, English M, *et al.* Randomized trial of volume expansion with albumin or saline in children with severe malaria: preliminary evidence of albumin benefit. *Clin Infect Dis* 2005;**40**:538–45. [RCT]
Omari A, Garner P. Malaria: severe, life threatening. *BMJ Clinical evidence handbook.* London: BMJ Books, 2009: pp. 274–5 (and updates). [SR] (See also pp. 276–7.)
Phillips RE, Looareesuwan S, White NJ, *et al.* Quinine pharmacokinetics and toxicity in pregnant and lactating women with falciparum malaria. *Br J Clin Pharmacol* 1986;**21**:677–83.
van der Torn M, Thuma PE, Mabeza GF, *et al.* Loading dose of quinine in African children with cerebral malaria. *Trans R Soc Trop Med Hyg* 1998;**92**:325–31.

Use

Ranitidine is used to treat symptomatic oesophagitis, gastritis and peptic ulceration. Omeprazole (q.v.) may sometimes be more effective. Use the gastric pH to judge the best dose to give in early infancy.

Pharmacology

Ranitidine (first developed in 1979) reduces stomach acidity by blocking the H_2-histamine receptors in the stomach that control the release of gastric acid. A low-dose 75 mg tablet is now available without prescription for the short-term treatment of heartburn and indigestion in adults. A higher dose is used to treat peptic ulceration, but does little for stress-related upper gastrointestinal bleeding. No measurable benefit has yet been seen in trials of prophylaxis in children or adults requiring intensive care.

The pharmacology of ranitidine is very similar to that of cimetidine (q.v.), but ranitidine does not interact with the metabolism of other drugs in the same way as cimetidine, and it has no anti-androgenic properties. Higher doses have to be used when the drug is given by mouth because of rapid first pass metabolism in the liver (oral bioavailability being about 50% but rather variable in the neonate). Tissue levels exceed plasma levels (neonatal $V_D \sim 1.8$ l/kg). Most of the drug is excreted in the urine, the half life being 3·5 hours a birth but closer to 2 hours (as in adults) by 6 months. It is even longer, at first, in the preterm baby. Most neonatal reports of the use of ranitidine relate to IV administration (a route the manufacturers are not yet ready to recommend in children less than 6 months old). Necrotising enterocolitis may be commoner in babies given an H_2 blocker, and one report has suggested that neonatal use is associated with a higher risk of late-onset sepsis.

There is no evidence that ranitidine is teratogenic and, although high concentrations are found in breast milk, the baby will only get about a tenth of the normal therapeutic dose, and there have been no adverse reports following use by mothers during lactation. Ranitidine is widely used, with or without an antacid, to minimise the risk of potentially life-threatening pneumonitis that can result from the maternal aspiration of gastric fluid into the lung during birth (Mendelson syndrome). The standard maternal dose for this is 150 mg by mouth, repeatable after 6 hours. A liquid non-particulate antacid, such as 30 ml of 0·3 M sodium citrate, is often given as well if a general anaesthetic becomes necessary. Such a strategy has been shown to reduce gastric acidity, and seems safe for the baby, but, because the complication is so uncommon, it is difficult to prove that this reduces the threat of serious pneumonitis, and aspiration can still occur despite prophylaxis.

Treatment

By mouth: Variable first pass metabolism affects uptake in the term baby. Try 2 mg/kg every 8 hours.

IV administration: Use gastric pH to titrate the right dose: 500 micrograms/kg given slowly IV twice a day will usually keep the gastric pH above 4 in babies of less than 32 weeks' gestation in the first week of life, but term babies may need 1 or 1·5 mg/kg every 8 hours. Rapid administration can (rarely) cause an arrhythmia.

Continuous IV infusion: Give a 1·5 mg/kg loading dose, followed by a maintenance infusion of 50 micrograms/kg per hour. Half this dose is more than adequate in the very preterm baby soon after birth.

Renal failure: Double the dosage interval if there is renal failure and during ECMO treatment.

Compatibility

Ranitidine can be added (terminally), when necessary, into a line containing adrenaline, atracurium, dobutamine, dopamine, fentanyl, glyceryl trinitrate, heparin, insulin, isoprenaline, midazolam, milrinone, morphine, nitroprusside, noradrenaline or vancomycin or with standard TPN (with or without lipid).

Supply and administration

2 ml ampoules containing 25 mg/ml of ranitidine hydrochloride for IV or IM use are available costing 60p. For accurate IV administration take 1 ml (25 mg) from this ampoule and dilute to 50 ml with 5% glucose to get a preparation containing 500 micrograms/ml. To give a continuous infusion of 50 micrograms/kg per hour take 1 ml (25 mg) of drug from the ampoule and dilute to 10 ml with 5% glucose. Then take 1 ml of this diluted solution for each kg the baby weighs, make this up to 50 ml with 5% glucose and infuse at a rate of 1 ml/hour. The drug is stable in solution, so a fresh infusion is not needed every day. A 15 mg/ml sugar-free syrup (which should not be diluted further) containing 96% alcohol is also available (100 ml costs £6·70).

References

Bianconi S, Gudavalli M, Sutija VG, et al. Ranitidine and late onset sepsis in the neonatal intensive care unit. J Perinat Med 2007;**35**:147–50.

Fontana M, Massironi E, Rossi A, et al. Ranitidine pharmacokinetics in newborn infants. Arch Dis Child 1993;**68**:602–3.

Garbis H, Elefant E, Diav CO, et al. Pregnancy outcome after exposure to ranitidine and other H_2 blockers. A collaborative study of the European Network of Teratology Information Services. Reprod Toxicol 2005;**19**:453–8.

Guillet R, Stoll BJ, Cotten M, et al. Association of H_2-blocker therapy and higher incidence of necrotizing enterocolitis in very low birth weight infants. Pediatrics 2006;**117**:e137–42. (See also pp. 531–2.)

Kuusela A-L. Long term gastric pH monitoring for determining optimal dose or ranitidine for critically ill preterm and term neonates. Arch Dis Child 1998;**78**:F151–3.

Messori A, Trippoli S, Vaiani M, et al. Bleeding and pneumonia in intensive care patients given ranitidine and sucraflate for prevention of stress ulcer: metanalysis of randomised controlled trials. BMJ 2000;**321**:1103–6. [SR]

Salvatore S, Hauser B, Salvatoni A, et al. Oral ranitidine and duration of gastric pH >4·0 in infants with persisting reflux symptoms. Acta Paediatr 2006;**95**:176–81.

Tighe MP, Afzal NA, Bevan A, et al. Current pharmacological management of gastro-esophagitis in children: an evidence-based systematic review. Pediatr Drugs 2009;**11**:185–202. [SR]

Use

Remifentanil is an ultra short-acting opiate related to fentanyl (q.v.) that can be used to titrate pain relief during surgery without causing troublesome postoperative respiratory depression. It is always given IV. A single dose is now starting to be used to reduce pain and relax the muscles during neonatal intubation.

Pharmacology

Remifentanil hydrochloride is a short-acting, μ-receptor opioid agonist that was first developed in 1991. It achieves its peak analgesic effect within a minute of administration (three or four times faster than fentanyl, and very much faster than morphine). Unlike the other opioid drugs currently in clinical use it is rapidly hydrolysed by non-specific blood and tissue esterases within minutes into a carboxylic acid metabolite that has almost no biological activity, 95% of which is then excreted in the urine. Indeed, it was specifically designed with these properties in mind. The half life, both in infancy and in later life, is just 5 minutes. Clinical recovery is therefore rapid and it is thought that, because of this, many of the problems of drug dependence and progressive drug accumulation often seen with other opioid drugs can be avoided. Sustained use does, however, seem to cause tolerance to develop. A single IV dose provides pain relief within 1 minute which normally only lasts for 5–10 minutes irrespective of the magnitude of the dose given. As a result, sustained analgesia for longer operative procedures requires the administration of a continuous infusion. The commonest side effects of such use are nausea, vomiting and headache. While these problems are less often seen when midazolam (q.v.) is given as well, dual treatment significantly increases the risk of respiratory depression. High-dose treatment may cause muscle rigidity of the type sometimes seen with fentanyl. Brief bradycardia is also not uncommon. The manufacturers have not yet recommended use in children less than a year old.

Little is yet known about the potential effect on the baby of maternal use during pregnancy or lactation but, given the drug's short biological half life, adverse effects seem unlikely. There is evidence, however, that use during operative delivery could cause brief neonatal respiratory depression.

Treatment

Short-term pain relief: 1 microgram/kg IV provides 5–10 minutes of pain relief after 60 seconds, but some brief respiratory depression. Giving 2 micrograms/kg provides as much muscle relaxation as suxamethonium.

Sustained pain relief: Start by giving 1 microgram/kg per minute IV, after taking control of the child's respiratory needs, and double this if necessary for a while to give 'real time' control over operative pain of variable intensity. Even higher doses have been used. Remember that pain relief will only last a few minutes once the infusion is stopped or interrupted, and that most other analgesics take time to become effective.

Sedation during ventilation: A tenth this dose (0·1 microgram/kg per minute) sedates the preterm baby.

Antidote

Naloxone (q.v.) is an effective antidote, but remifentanil's short half life should render use unnecessary.

Compatibility

Remifentanil can be added (terminally) to a line containing fentanyl, midazolam or morphine.

Supply and administration

Use is controlled under Schedule 2 of the UK Misuse of Drug Regulations (Misuse of Drugs Act 1971).

Reconstitution: Prescribing conventionally refers to the amount of remifentanil base, and the product is supplied in vials of varying strength. A vial containing 1 mg of remifentanil base (or approximately 1·1 mg of remifentanil hydrochloride) costs £5·50. Reconstitute the lyophilised powder in this with 1 ml of sterile water.

Dilution for single-dose use: Take 0·1 ml of the reconstituted powder and dilute to 10 ml with 0·9% sodium chloride to get a solution containing 10 micrograms/ml.

Preparing to give a sustained infusion: Take 0·2 ml (200 micrograms) of the reconstituted powder for each kg the baby weighs, and dilute to 10 ml with 0·9% sodium chloride to get a solution that delivers 1 microgram/kg per minute when infused at a rate of 3 ml/hour (for sustained pain relief), or 0·1 microgram/kg per minute when infused at a rate of 0·3 ml/hour (for sedation).

References

Crawford MW, Hayes J, Tan JM. Dose-response of remifentanil for tracheal intubation in infants. *Anesth Analg* 2005;**100**:1599–604.

e Silva YP, Gomez RS, Marcatte J de O, *et al.* Morphine versus reminfentanil for intubating preterm neonates. *Arch Dis Child* 2007;**92**:F293–4. [RCT]

e Silva YP, Gomez RS, Marcatto J de O, *et al.* Early awakening and extubation with remifentanil in ventilated premature neonates. *Pediatr Anesth* 2008;**18**:17683. [RCT]

Giannantonio C, Sammartino M, Valente E, *et al.* Remifentanil analgosedation in preterm newborns during mechanical ventilation. *Acta Paediatr* 2009;**98**:1111–15.

Van de Velde M, Keunkens A, Kuypers M, *et al.* General anaesthesia with target controlled infusion of propofol for planned caesarean section: maternal and neonatal effects of a remifentanil-based technique. *Int J Obstet Anesth* 2004;**13**:153–8.

Weale NK, Rogers CA, Cooper R, *et al.* Effect of remifentanil infusion rate on stress response to the by-pass phase of paediatric cardiac surgery. *Br J Anaesth* 2004;**92**:187–94.

Welzing L, Kribs A, Huenseler C, *et al.* Remifentanil for INSURE in preterm infants: a pilot study for evaluation of efficacy and safety, *Acta Paediatr* 2009;**98**:1426–20.

Welzing L, Roth B. Experience with remifentanil in neonates and infants. *Drugs* 2006;**66**:1339–50. [SR]

Use
An immunoglobulin used to prevent rhesus isoimmunisation.

Product
A human immune globulin (currently collected by apheresis from the plasma of donors with high levels of anti-D antibody in the US) has been used since 1970 to prevent Rhesus-negative mothers developing antibodies to transplacentally acquired RhD-positive fetal red cells during childbirth. It is also used after miscarriage, threatened miscarriage and abortion after 12 weeks' gestation or any other obstetric manoeuvre such as chorion villus biopsy, amniocentesis, fetal blood sampling and external cephalic version that could be associated with feto-maternal bleeding. Other events such as ectopic pregnancy, antepartum haemorrhage and blunt abdominal trauma (from, for example, seat belt injury) should also be covered. The product works by eliminating fetal red cells from the circulation before they can stimulate active maternal antibody production. It should be given within 72 hours, if possible, with a view to preventing Rhesus isoimmunisation compromising any future pregnancy, but still offers some protection if given within 12 days. A monoclonal IgG_3 antibody is still under development.

Approximately 1% of Rhesus-negative mothers develop Rhesus antibodies late in their first pregnancy but before delivery in the absence of any recognisable sensitising event. Furthermore, these 'hypersensitive' mothers seem to be at risk of having a baby with disease of atypical severity in any subsequent pregnancy. Antenatal treatment at 28 and 34 weeks' more than halves this risk, but there may be better ways to use the money this would cost in communities where such problems are rare.

Indications
The amount of anti-D (Rh_0) immunoglobulin actually required is proportional to the size of the feto-maternal bleed. For events occurring before 20 weeks' gestation, it has been traditional to give 250 units (50 micrograms) of anti-D immunoglobulin. Later in pregnancy and after delivery the usual dose is 500 units (100 micrograms), but this should be increased if a Kleihauer test on the mother's blood shows more than one fetal cell per 500 adult red cells (equivalent to 4–5 ml of packed fetal red cells). Such bleeds should be quantified by flow cytometry and an additional 150 units of anti-D immunoglobulin given for each millilitre by which the transplacental bleed exceeds 4 ml of packed fetal red cells.

Contraindications
There are no known contraindications. Use of the UK product has never caused the acquisition of any blood product-transmitted infection such as hepatitis B or HIV, and current supplies come from America where there is minimal risk of the donor having latent variant Creutzfeldt–Jakob disease. Simultaneous rubella (or MMR) vaccination is acceptable as long as separate syringes are used and the products injected into different limbs. Treat any reaction as outlined in the monograph on immunisation.

Administration
During pregnancy: All Rhesus (D) negative women should be offered an IM injection at 28 and 34 weeks' gestation (500 units seems adequate, but a 1250 unit dose is widely used) to stop the baby becoming immunised before birth unless (i) antenatal tests have shown that the fetus is Rhesus negative, *or* (ii) the mother knows this is going to be her last pregnancy, *or* (iii) she knows that the child's father is Rhesus negative. Injections are usually given into the deltoid muscle.
After delivery: Give at least 500 units IM to Rhesus-negative mothers whose babies are Rhesus positive (or whose blood group is unknown). It is pointless to treat mothers who have already started to produce antibodies to the D antigen, but important to remember that mothers with *other* antibodies (anti-c, anti-Kell, etc.) may still require protection from the D antigen if they are Rhesus (D) negative.

Supply and administration
A range of commercial and volunteer donor products are now available in vials and prefilled syringes containing from 250 to 1500 units of anti-D immunoglobulin. 500 units of a non-proprietary product cost £20. Most need to be stored at 4°C, but lyophilised powders (which should be reconstituted with 0·9% sodium chloride) are safe for a month at room temperature. The products need prescribing, but maternity units in the UK have now developed Patient Group Directions, because these give midwives a more proactive role in ensuring that all Rhesus-negative mothers have easy access to prophylaxis.

References
See also the relevant Cochrane reviews and UK guidelines

Chilcott J, Lloyd Jones M, Wight J, *et al.* A review of the clinical effectiveness and cost-effectiveness of routine anti-D prophylaxis for pregnant women who are rhesus-negative. *Health Technol Assess* 2003;**7**(4).
Finning K, Martin P, Summers J, *et al.* Effect of high throughput *RHD* typing of fetal DNA in maternal plasma on use of anti-RhD immunoglobulin in RhD negative pregnant women: prospective feasibility study. *BMJ* 2008;**336**:816–18.
Kumar S, Regan F. Management of pregnancies with RhD alloimmunisation. [Clinical review] *BMJ* 2006;**330**:1255–8 and 1485.
Roberts IAG. The changing face of haemolytic disease of the newborn. *Early Hum Dev* 2008;**84**:515–24.
Smits-Wintjens VEHJ, Walther FJ, Lopiore E. Rhesus haemolytic disease of the newborn: postnatal management, associated morbidity and long-term outcome. *Semin Fetal Neonat Med* 2008;**13**:265–71.

Use

Treatment with ribavirin may reduce the severity of bronchiolitis due to respiratory tract viral infection if started within 3 days of the onset of lower respiratory tract symptoms. Combined treatment with interferon alfa (q.v.) controls viraemia and slows disease progression in children with chronic hepatitis C infection.

Pharmacology

Ribavirin (first synthesised in 1972) is a stable, white, synthetic nucleoside with *in vitro* antiviral properties against the respiratory syncytial virus, and some adenoviruses as well as the influenza, parainfluenza and measles viruses. A significant amount of drug is absorbed systemically after aerosol administration and the concentration in respiratory secretions is particularly high. Ribavirin is teratogenic and embryo-lethal and should never be given to pregnant patients; the manufacturers even advise against it being administered by staff who are pregnant. There is some evidence that it can be mutagenic in cell culture, and may (with chronic exposure), induce benign glandular tumours. Its clinical use is therefore currently limited to high-risk children (children with congenital heart disease, existing bronchopulmonary dysplasia or immunodeficiency) with proven lower respiratory tract viral infection. There is only one study suggesting that use speeds recovery in ventilator-dependent infants and little evidence that it reduces the time it takes for patients to stop shedding live virus particles. The only common adverse effect in children with standard treatment is conjunctivitis, but little is known about possible long-term morbidity or toxicity. While widespread American experience suggests that ribavirin is safe used in this way, most clinicians in Europe believe that further evidence of efficacy is needed. Nine small controlled studies have now been done, but the total number of children studied (291 in all) remains inadequate to establish the utility of this form of treatment.

Perinatal hepatitis C infection

When viral RNA can be detected in the mother's blood on PCR testing during pregnancy, there is about a 5% risk of the baby becoming infected, and this increases if the woman also has HIV. There is, however, no reason to undertake Caesarean delivery or advise the woman not to breastfeed unless there is HIV. One study suggests that delaying membrane rupture as long as possible once the woman goes into labour may minimise the risk of transmission. If the woman is anti-HCV positive but viral RNA is not detectable it is very rare for the baby to become infected. When infection occurs during rather than before birth, viral RNA may take 2–3 months to become detectable in the baby but, if it does appear, this indicates active infection and merits referral to a supra-regional liver centre. Other babies should be watched until they become anti-HCV negative. The prognosis for those babies who do become actively infected is variable. It looks as though complete viral elimination occurs in a quarter, but a minority develop progressive disease meriting treatment with ribavirin and interferon alfa to stop liver fibrosis eventually progressing to frank cirrhosis.

Treatment

Nebulised administration: Administer 60 mg/ml of ribavirin for 2 hours three times a day using a small particle aerosol generator (SPAG) for 3–7 days, preferably using a modified Easy Vent® CPAP device. Early treatment *may* be appropriate in high-risk children with a proven viral lower respiratory tract infection to try and reduce the chance of their needing ventilator support. There is no good evidence that use shortens the duration of treatment in children already ill enough to be receiving respiratory support, and such use can easily cause the ventilator to become clogged.

Oral administration: Children with progressive chronic hepatitis C infection have been treated with 15 mg/kg of ribavirin by mouth once a day for 6 or even 12 months. While such treatment is of little benefit on its own, combined treatment with subcutaneous interferon alfa-2b frequently abolishes all detectable evidence of viraemia during treatment and for at least 6 months after treatment stops, especially in patients with genotype 2 or 3 infection. The dose of interferon used has usually been 3 million-units/m^2 of the standard preparation given three times a week, or 15 micrograms/kg of the pegylated (polyethylene glycol conjugated) product once a week. Such treatment has **not** yet been attempted in children less than a year old.

Supply and administration

Ribavirin comes in 100 ml vials containing 6 grams of lyophilised drug costing £116 per vial. For nebulised administration dissolve the powder with 100 ml of sterile water for injection free of all preservatives. Any of the reconstituted solution not used within 24 hours of preparation should be discarded.

References

See also the relevant Cochrane reviews

Davison SM, Mieli-Vergani G, Sira J, *et al*. Perinatal hepatitis C virus infection: diagnosis and management. *Arch Dis Child* 2006;**91**:781–5.
Fischler B. Hepatitis C virus infection. *Semin Fetal Neonat Med* 2007;**12**:168–73.
Gonzalez-Peralta R, Kelly DA, Haber B, *et al*. Interferon alfa 2b in combination with ribavirin for the treatment of chronic hepatitis C in children: efficacy, safety and pharmacokinetics. *Hepatology* 2005;**42**:1010–18.
Guerguerian A-M, Gauthier M, Lebel M *et al*. Ribavarin in ventilated respiratory syncytial virus bronchiolitis. *Am J Respir Crit Care Med* 1999;**160**:829–31. [RCT]
Mohsen A, Norris S. Hepatitis C (chronic). *BMJ Clinical evidence handbook*. London: BMJ Books, 2009: pp. 259–62 (and updates). [SR]
Smedsaas-Löfvenberg A, Nilsson K, Moa G, *et al*. Nebulisation of drugs in a CPAP system. *Acta Paediatr* 1999;**88**:89–92.
Wirth S, Pieper-Boustani H, Lang T, *et al*. Peginterferon alfa-2b plus ribavirin treatment in children and adolescents with chronic hepatitis C. *Hepatology* 2005;**41**:1013–18.

Use

Rifampicin is used with isoniazid (q.v.) to treat tuberculosis and, with vancomycin or teicoplanin (q.v.), to treat severe staphylococcal infection. It is also given prophylactically to the contacts of patients with meningococcal or *Haemophilus* infection, and has a role in the treatment of cholestatic pruritis.

Pharmacology

This bactericidal antibiotic, first developed in 1966, interferes with DNA-dependent RNA polymerase. It has activity against many mycobacteria, *Neisseria meningitidis* and *N. gonorrhoeae*, and is the most active antistaphylococcal agent known. However, since resistant strains of *Mycobacterium* or *Staphylococcus* emerge quickly if rifampicin is used alone, it is recommended that rifampicin should always be used in combination with a second antibiotic except when the drug is used prophylactically to eliminate bacterial carriage and reduce the risk of meningitis. Rifampicin is readily absorbed when given by mouth. It is highly protein bound and undergoes enterohepatic recirculation. Up to 30% may be excreted unchanged, but the metabolites are excreted in urine and bile. Dose intervals do not need to be modified in the presence of renal failure. Rifampicin colours urine and other secretions red. The half life is 3–4 hours, but twice this in the first month of life. Transient jaundice can be ignored, but treatment must be stopped at once if thrombocytopenia, nausea and vomiting or other signs of more serious liver toxicity develop. Such adverse effects are rare in children unless there is prior liver disease. Rifampicin crosses the placenta, but its use is not contraindicated in pregnancy, although use in the third trimester is said to be associated with an increased risk of neonatal bleeding meriting routine IM vitamin K (q.v.) prophylaxis. Very little of the drug appears in breast milk.

Drug interactions

Rifampicin induces microsomal liver enzymes and therefore affects the metabolism of a wide range of other drugs. Chloramphenicol, corticosteroids, most benzodiazepines, digoxin, fluconazole, nifedipine, phenobarbital, phenytoin, theophylline, warfarin and zidovudine are all metabolised more rapidly, and dosage levels may need adjustment. Rifampicin also induces its own metabolism and, as a result, clearance increases markedly during the first 2 weeks of use. Treatment of HIV infection with the protease inhibitors nelfinavir or ritonavir greatly increases the clearance of rifampicin, making co-treatment more complex.

Treatment

Synergistic use with teicoplanin or vancomycin: Experience remains limited. Give 10 mg/kg IV (1 ml/kg of dilute solution made up as described below) slowly once every 12 hours pick-abacked onto an existing IV infusion of glucose or glucose saline for 10 days, or 20 mg/kg once a day by mouth.

Treatment of tuberculosis: Seek expert advice. Give 10 mg/kg once a day by mouth (20 mg/kg if meningitis is suspected), together with isoniazid (q.v.). Warn parents that the urine may turn red. Give 1 mg of IM vitamin K if the child is <3 months old to minimise the risk of vitamin K deficiency bleeding.

Prophylaxis against meningococcal and *Haemophilus* infection: Give a 5 mg/kg dose to children less than 1 month old, and a 10 mg/kg dose to older children. Give four such doses, once every 12 hours to eliminate meningococcal carriage, but once a day to any unvaccinated child under 4 years old exposed to known *H. influenzae* infection.

Preventing continued group B streptococcal carriage: 20 mg/kg once a day by mouth for 7 days will reduce, but not eliminate, the risk of continued carriage. Give carrier mothers 600 mg twice a day as well.

Pruritis due to cholestasis: Give 5 (or 10) mg/kg twice a day. Monitor liver function for the first month.

Supply and administration

Rifampicin is available as a powder for IV use in 600 mg vials (costing £8) normally dispensed with 10 ml of solvent. Reconstitute the 600 mg vial with 9·6 ml of the solvent and shake well. Take 60 mg of rifampicin (1 ml of the fluid from a 600 mg vial), dilute to 10 ml with 5% or 10% dextrose to obtain a solution containing 6 mg/ml of rifampicin, and use within 6 hours. Slow infusion over 30–60 minutes is recommended in adults because of the volume involved, and because there is some slight risk of hypotension and phlebitis. Do not co-infuse with any alkaline solution. Rifampicin should not be given IM. A 20 mg/ml syrup is also available with an undiluted shelf life of 3 years (100 ml costs £3·70).

References

See also the relevant Cochrane reviews

Acocella G. Clinical pharmacokinetics of rifampicin. *Clin Pharmacokinet* 1978;**3**:108–27.

American Academy of Pediatrics, Committee on Infectious Diseases. Chemotherapy for tuberculosis in infants and children. *Pediatrics* 1992;**69**:161–5.

Fernandez M, Rench MA, Albanyan EA, *et al.* Failure of rifampin to eradicate group B streptococcal colonisation in infants. *Pediatr Infect Dis J* 2001;**20**:371–6.

Gregorio GV, Ball CS, Mowat AP, *et al.* Effect of rifampin in the treatment of pruritus in hepatic cholestasis. *Arch Dis Child* 1993;**69**:141–3.

Pullen J, Stolk LML, Degaeuwe PLJ, *et al.* Pharmacokinetics of intravenous rifampicin (rifampin) in neonates. *Ther Drug Monit* 2006;**28**:654–61.

Rosenfeld EA, Hageman JR, Yogev R. Tuberculosis in infancy in the 1990s. *Pediatr Clin North Am* 1993;**40**:1087–103.

Shama A, Patole SK, Whitehall JS. Intravenous rifampicin in neonates with persistent staphylococcal bacteraemia. *Acta Paediatr* 2002;**91**:670–3.

Tan TQ, Mason EO, Ou C-N, *et al.* Use of intravenous rifampicin in neonates with persistent staphylococcal bacteremia. *Antimicrob Agents Chemother* 1993;**37**:2401–6.

ROCURONIUM

Use

Rocuronium can be used instead of suxamethonium (q.v.) to provide rapid muscle paralysis during tracheal intubation, but recovery is much slower. Atracurium and mivacurium (q.v.) are useful (but slower acting) alternatives when short-term paralysis is all that is required, but are more likely to trigger histamine release.

Pharmacology

Rocuronium is a mono-quaternary amino-steroidal muscle relaxant of relatively low potency that first came into clinical use in 1994. It works, like the other non-depolarising muscle relaxants, by competitively attaching itself to the cholinergic receptors on the 'end plates' responsible for transmitting nerve signals to the body's voluntary muscles. Conditions for undertaking laryngeal intubation are achieved almost as quickly with IV rocuronium as they are with IV suxamethonium but recovery takes much longer, rendering use hazardous if unexpected difficulties are encountered in securing the airway. However, if the drug has to be given IM, effective muscle relaxation takes much longer to achieve with rocuronium than with suxamethonium (5–10 v. 3–4 minutes). Rocuronium is mostly eliminated by the liver and the biliary system, but up to a quarter is excreted unchanged in the urine. The half life in infancy (mean 1·3 hours) is marginally longer than it is in older children and not greatly affected by renal dysfunction. The manufacturer has not yet endorsed the use of rocuronium in babies less than a month old.

Vecuronium is another muscle relaxant with a similar chemical structure to rocuronium that first came onto the market in 1980. A 100 microgram/kg IV dose produces paralysis for about as long as rocuronium but, because it takes 2–4 times as long to cause paralysis, it is now less commonly used. The normal plasma elimination half life of vecuronium in adults is 30–60 minutes, but considerably (and unpredictably) longer than this in infancy, especially with high-dose treatment. Renal failure seems has little effect on the duration of neuromuscular blockade, but some of the drug (and of its metabolically active metabolites) is renally excreted, and atracurium may be a better drug to use in a baby with severe renal failure requiring paralysis.

Manufacturers have been reluctant to recommend the use of either rocuronium or vecuronium during pregnancy or lactation, and nothing is known about use during the first trimester, but neuromuscular blocking agents do not, as a group, seem to pose a significant risk to the embryo, fetus or breastfed baby. Placental transfer is limited, and doses of up to 600 micrograms/kg of rocuronium (or 100 micrograms/kg of vecuronium) given to mothers requiring Caesarean delivery have no significant clinical effect on the baby.

Treatment

Brief use to effect intubation: 450 micrograms/kg of rocuronium provides the muscle relaxation needed to effect easy laryngeal intubation within a minute in babies less than a year old, but recovery may take an hour. A larger dose does not speed the onset of paralysis, and may double recovery time in a young baby.

Use to provide sustained paralysis: Start by giving 600 micrograms/kg of rocuronium IV. Most babies continue to comply with the imposed ventilator rate as they wake from this first paralysing dose (especially if a moderately fast rate and a relatively short inspiratory time (<0·7 seconds) is used) but a few require prolonged paralysis. The standard repeat dose is half the initial dose IV (or IM) every 2–4 hours as necessary, but some older babies seem to require a higher maintenance dose. Paralysed babies should always be sedated.

Antidote

Give a combination of 10 micrograms/kg of glycopyrronium (or 20 micrograms/kg of atropine) and 50 micrograms/kg of neostigmine IV, as outlined in the monograph on glycopyrronium.

Supply and administration

Rocuronium: This comes in 5 ml vials containing 10 mg/ml of rocuronium bromide. They cost £3 each. Take 0·1 ml and dilute to 1 ml with 0·9% sodium chloride or 5% glucose to obtain a solution containing 100 micrograms in 0·1 ml for accurate neonatal administration.

Vecuronium: This comes as a powder in 10 mg vials, with water for reconstitution. They cost £4 each. Dissolve the powder with 5 ml of sterile water (as supplied) to give a solution containing 2 mg/ml. Further dilute 0·5 ml of this solution with 0·5 ml of 0·9% sodium chloride or 5% glucose in a 1 ml syringe to obtain a preparation containing 100 micrograms in 0·1 ml for accurate neonatal administration.

References

Atherton DP, Hunter DM. Clinical pharmacokinetics of the newer neuromuscular blocking drugs. *Clin Pharmacokinet* 1999;**36**:169–89.
Kaplan RF, Uejima T, Lobel G, *et al*. Intramuscular rocuronium in infants and children: a multicenter study to evaluate tracheal intubating conditions, onset, and duration of action. *Anesthesiology* 1999;**91**:633–8.
Playfor S. Neuromuscular blocking agents in critically ill children. *Paediat Perinat Drug Ther* 2002;**5**:35–46.
Rapp H-J, Altenmueller CA, Waschke C. Neuromuscular recovery following rocuronium bromide single dose in infants. *Pediatr Anaesth* 2004;**14**:329–35.
Zelicof-Paul A, Smith-Lockridge A, Schnadower D, *et al*. Controversies in rapid sequence intubation in children. *Curr Opin Pediatr* 2005;**17**:355–62.

Use

Rotavirus infection is a ubiquitous, worldwide, cause of diarrhoea, killing many Third World children. Two very effective oral vaccines came onto the market in 2006. Neither seems to cause intussusception in the way the first licensed vaccine (Rotashield®) was found to do in 2001. Unfortunately the communities most in need of the protection that these new vaccines can provide are the communities least able to afford their cost.

Rotavirus diarrhoea

Rotaviruses were first discovered, using the newly invented electron microscope, in 1973, and it soon became clear that almost every child becomes infected with this virus at least once in the first 5 years of life. The peak age for infection is 3–30 months, and most infection is caused by the oral intake of faecal contaminants, although respiratory (aerosol) spread is not that uncommon. Young and malnourished children are always the most seriously affected, and half a million children are currently thought to die in the world each year from rotavirus infection. Although a wide range of serotypes exist there is good evidence that children who have had one infection are much less likely to become ill when later exposed to a different strain, suggesting that natural infection triggers strong cross-immunity.

Rotavirus infection currently kills half a million children in the world every year, and seems to be responsible for more than a third of all hospital admissions caused by diarrhoea. Take care not to overlook a surgical cause if there is abdominal pain, distension, a mass or bilious vomiting. Suspect bacterial rather than viral infection if there is high fever, and a Shiga toxin producing *Escherichia coli* or *Shigella dysenteriae* infection if there is bloody diarrhoea. Children unable to take an oral rehydration solution (q.v.) need hospital care.

An attenuated monovalent live human rotavirus vaccine (Rotarix®), when tested in a trial involving 20,000 children in Latin America and Finland, reduced serious rotavirus gastroenteritis by 85% and 'all cause' gastroenteritis by 40%. A pentavalent bovine–human vaccine (RotaTeq®) proved at least as effective when tested on 68,000 American and European children, and in no study to date has there been any excess of small bowel intussusception. It is not possible to say whether one vaccine is better than the other because no direct head-to-head comparison has yet been done. The pentavalent vaccine is more consistently excreted in the stool and may, therefore, confer greater 'herd' immunity. Neither vaccine has yet been tested in a community where the G2(P4) strain is prevalent, so it is not yet certain how either product will perform in this situation. Studies in Asia, where this strain is more commonly seen, may help to resolve this uncertainty.

Indications

Because infection is particularly dangerous in a very young child, the logical time to start immunisation is 6–8 weeks after birth. Because of lingering concern that intussusception might still be a problem, the American vaccine is currently only licensed for use children less than 8 months old. There is no evidence that administration has to be delayed or avoided because of preterm birth.

Contraindications

Give thought to the balance of risk before giving either vaccine to a child with gastrointestinal symptoms, or to a child who is in close contact with an immunodeficient person. There is not yet enough information to recommend administration to a child with symptomatic or asymptomatic HIV infection.

Interactions

Other intramuscular paediatric vaccines can be given safely and effectively at the same time as an oral rotavirus vaccine. Giving this vaccine within 2 weeks of the oral polio vaccine has not yet been studied.

Administration

Rotarix: Give two doses by mouth at least 4 weeks apart. The first dose can be given 6 weeks after birth.
RotaTeq: Give three doses by mouth (at 2, 4 and 6 months). The first dose should be given 6–12 weeks after birth, and other two doses should then be given 4–10 weeks apart. Do not repeat if spat out.

Supply

Rotarix: This product from GSK, which has so far been licensed for use in Europe and 33 countries in Latin America, Africa and Asia, comes as a lyophilised powder that need to be stored at 2–8°C and reconstituted with buffered diluent. Vials (with a syringe containing 1 ml of the necessary diluent) cost £41 each.
RotaTeq: This American product from Merck comes as a buffered pale yellow liquid in 2 ml ready-to-use, squeezable, plastic dosing tubes that cost $55 each. Store and transport at 2–8°C and protect from light.

References

American Academy of Pediatrics, Committee on Infectious Diseases. Prevention of rotavirus disease: guidelines for rotavirus vaccine. *Pediatrics* 2007;**119**:171–81.

American Academy of Pediatrics, Committee on Infectious Diseases. Prevention of rotavirus disease: updated guidelines for use of rotavirus vaccine. *Pediatrics* 2009;**123**:1412–20.

Chokshi DA, Kesselheim AS. Rethinking global access to vaccines. *BMJ* 2008;**336**:750–3.

Dennehy PH, Bretrand HR, Silas PE, *et al.* Coadministration of RIX4414 oral human rotavirus vaccine does not impact on immune response to antigens contained in routine infant vaccine in the United States. *Pediatrics* 2008;**122**:e1062–6.

Elliott EJ. Acute gastroenteritis in children. *BMJ* 2007;**334**:35–40. [SR]

Linhares AC, Velázquez FR, Pérez-Schael I, *et al.* Efficacy and safety of an oral life attenuated human rotavirus vaccine against rotavirus gastroenteritis during the first 2 years of life in Latin American infants: a randomised, double-blind, placebo-controlled phase IIII trial. *Lancet* 2008;**371**:1181–9. [RCT] (See also pp. 1144–5.)

Use

A live attenuated rubella virus vaccine was introduced in 1970 to provide active immunity against rubella in children, and in seronegative women of child-bearing age. A trivalent vaccine offering protection against measles, and mumps as well as rubella (MMR vaccine) is the product now used in the UK.

Rubella

Rubella (or German measles) is a mild notifiable illness with an incubation period of 14–21 days. Patients are infectious from a week before the rash appears for a period of about 10 days. Symptoms may be minimal, and the rash is often not diagnostic (see www.phls.org.uk/topics_az/rashes/rash/pdf). Diagnosis currently depends on testing paired sera taken 2–3 and 8–9 days after the first appearance of the rash for rubella antibody, or a single sample taken 1–6 weeks after the rash first appears tested for the presence of rubella-specific IgM antibody. An alternative is identification of specific IgM in saliva – a test that can be made available by the Public Health Laboratory Service. Natural infection usually causes lasting immunity. Maternal infection in early pregnancy or just prior to conception can cause serious fetal damage, as first recognised by Gregg during the Australian epidemic in 1941, although the multifaceted nature of this damage only became clear 25 years later. Infection at 8–10 weeks damages up to 90% of babies. The risk of damage is about 10–20% by week 16. It is negligible after this. A 750 mg dose of normal immunoglobulin IM (q.v.) is sometimes given to reduce the chance of clinical infection in pregnant seronegative mothers, but there is no good evidence that it does much good.

Problems associated with congenital infection include cataract, glaucoma, pneumonia, meningoencephalitis, hepatitis, purpuric skin lesions and fetal growth retardation. Cardiac lesions include patent ductus, septal defects and pulmonary artery stenosis. Progressive deafness may develop even in babies who seem normal at birth. Infection in pregnancy is now rare in countries with a policy of universal vaccination in infancy, but such a policy has yet to be instituted in most of Africa, much of South East Asia and some parts of eastern Europe, and it has been estimated that about 100,000 children are probably still born with congenital rubella in the world every year (and even more die of measles). Without a policy of universal immunisation, these viruses will continue to circulate putting young children and the babies of unimmunised mothers at continued risk.

Product

A vaccine made from an attenuated live virus first came into use in the UK in 1970. One dose of the vaccine promotes an antibody response in over 95% of recipients, and a second dose has been recommended since 1996. The antibody response is well maintained for at least 20 years, and protection against clinical rubella seems to persist even after antibody levels decline. Nevertheless, natural infection does occasionally occur after immunisation (due, presumably, to primary vaccination failure or subsequent loss of immunity), as it can after natural infection, and such infection can cause fetal damage if it occurs in early pregnancy.

Indications in adult life

All women of child-bearing age should be made aware of their rubella status and told the outcome of any serological test. Any found to be seronegative during pregnancy should also be offered vaccination before discharge from the maternity unit after delivery. It is perfectly acceptable to give a rubella-containing vaccine and anti-D (Rh_0) immunoglobulin at the same time as long as different syringes and different sites are employed. Blood transfusions during delivery blunt the response to vaccination, however. In such cases a test for seroconversion should be undertaken 8 weeks later and revaccination offered if necessary. Short-term contraceptive cover can, if necessary, be offered in the interim using medroxyprogesterone acetate (Depo-Provera®) as long as the mother is counselled appropriately and shown the manufacturer's leaflet first. Give 150 mg in 1 ml once by deep IM injection.

Vaccination should be avoided in early pregnancy (and patients advised not to become pregnant within a month of vaccination), but there has been no recorded case of fetal damage in the USA, Canada, Costa Rica, Sweden, Germany or the UK among the significant number of mothers inadvertently immunised with the attenuated virus in early pregnancy. Seronegative male and female health service staff in maternity units should also be vaccinated to prevent their transmitting rubella to pregnant patients. A mild reaction with fever, rash and arthralgia may occur 1–3 weeks after vaccination.

Indications in childhood

All children should be offered one dose of the MMR vaccine when 12 months old unless there is a specific contraindication (see below) and a second dose as part of the preschool programme. Children not immunised at this time should be immunised before they start school (or nursery school), and again 3 months later. Measles, mumps and rubella are all notifiable illnesses. All became very uncommon in the UK after the MMR vaccine was introduced in 1988, but epidemics of measles and congenital rubella are sure to recur unless the current fall in uptake is soon reversed. Recurring media-fuelled fears that the vaccine could be causing autism or a non-specific colitis still persist even though no study to date has shown any such link. Term babies mount a poor response to the MMR vaccine before they are 9 months old, but, in communities where measles is still prevalent, a case can be made for giving the most vulnerable preterm babies two doses of the MMR vaccine 3 months apart once they are at least 6 months old.

Interactions

More than one live vaccine can be given at different sites on the same day, but an interval of 3 weeks should be allowed if vaccination is not simultaneous. If a booster injection of the diphtheria and tetanus vaccine is to be given at the same time as primary MMR immunisation, the two products should be given into a different limb. Do not give within 4 weeks of BCG administration.

Continued

Contraindications

Pregnancy, immunodeficiency, immunosuppression, reticuloendothelial malignancy and high-dose corticosteroid treatment (the equivalent of more than 1 mg/kg of prednisolone a day, or 2 mg/kg for more than 1 week, in the last 6 weeks) are generally considered contraindications to vaccination, as is known hypersensitivity to gelatin or neomycin. HIV infection is not, however, a contraindication (unless the CD4 count is below 500 cells/µl); nor is egg allergy, as was at one time feared. A history of fits is not a contraindication to either the monovalent or the trivalent vaccine, but advice should be given on how to manage any febrile response to immunisation as outlined in the monograph on paracetamol. Vaccination should be delayed if there is any febrile illness and postponed after immunoglobulin injection (other than Rhesus anti-D) for 3 months. For the latest advice on the safety of the combined MMR vaccine see the UK Government's website, www.doh.gov.uk/mmr/index.html.

Administration

Over 95% of patients achieve immunity with a single 0·5 ml deep IM injection of the monovalent or trivalent vaccine with a 25 mm 23 gauge needle, but a two dose regimen is now generally recommended.

Anaphylaxis

The management of anaphylaxis (which is very rare) is outlined in the monograph on immunisation.

Documentation

Tell the family doctor every time a child is immunised in hospital, and record what was done in the child's own personal health booklet. Community-based registers of vaccine uptake also need to be informed.

Case notification

All cases of suspected congenital rubella (with or without symptoms) in the UK should continue to be notified to the National Congenital Rubella Surveillance Programme. This can be done directly (tel: Pat Tookey on 020 7905 2604; e-mail: ptookey@ich.ucl.ac.uk) or via the British Paediatric Surveillance Unit (tel: 020 7323 7911; fax: 020 7905 2604). Women inadvertently vaccinated during pregnancy, or less than a month before becoming pregnant, should also be notified direct to this register.

Supply

Single-dose vials of the freeze-dried live trivalent (MMR) vaccine are available in the UK and distributed free, in England, by Farillon. In resource-poor countries immunisation against measles is the main priority, and this is offered as a mono-valent vaccine at 6 and 9 months. Although a simple monovalent rubella vaccine is available in some of these countries, this particular vaccine is no longer obtainable in the UK. Store vaccines at 2−8°C and use within an hour of reconstitution with the diluent provided. Do not freeze.

References

See also the relevant Cochrane reviews and UK guidelines

Badilla X, Morice A, Avila-Aguero ML, *et al.* Fetal risk associated with rubella vaccination during pregnancy. *Pediatr Infect Dis J* 2007;**26**:830−5.

Banatvala JE, Brown DWG. Rubella. [Seminar] *Lancet* 2004;**363**:1127−37.

Best J. Rubella. *Semin Fetal Neonat Med* 2007;**12**:182−92.

Best JM, O'Shea S, Tipples G, *et al.* Interpretations of rubella serology in pregnancy – pitfalls and problems. *BMJ* 2002;**325**:147−8.

Bloom S, Rguig A, Berrahp A, *et al.* Congenital rubella syndrome burden in Morocco: a rapid retrospective assessment. *Lancet* 2005;**365**:135−41.

Centers for Disease Control and Prevention. Measles on the upswing. *MMWR* 2008;**57**:893−6.

Cooper LZ, Alford CA. Rubella. In: Remington JS, Klein JO, eds. *Infectious diseases of the fetus and newborn infant*, 5th edn. Philadelphia: WB Saunders, 2001: pp. 347−88.

Ellman D, Sengupta N, Bashir H, *et al.* Measles, mumps, and rubella: prevention. *BMJ Clinical evidence handbook*. London: BMJ Books, 2009: pp. 98−101 (and updates). [SR]

Hinman AR, Irons B, Lewis M, *et al.* Economic analyses of rubella and rubella vaccines: a global review. *Bull World Health Organ* 2002;**80**:264−70.

Mehta NM, Thomas RM. Antenatal screening for rubella – infection or immunity? *BMJ* 2002;**325**:90−1. (See also pp. 596−7.)

Miller E, Cradock-Watson JE, Pollock TM. Consequences of confirmed maternal rubella at different stages of pregnancy. *Lancet* 1982;**ii**:781−4.

Muscat M, Bang H, Wohlfahrt J, *et al.* Measles in Europe: an epidemiological assessment. *Lancet* 2009;**373**:383−9. (See also pp. 356−8.)

Sheridan E, Aitken C, Jeffries D, *et al.* Congenital rubella syndrome: a risk in immigrant populations. *Lancet* 2002;**359**:674−5. (See also **360**:803−4.)

Tookey P. Pregnancy is contraindication for rubella vaccination still. *BMJ* 2001;**322**:1489.

Tookey PA, Cortina-Borja M, Peckham CS. Rubella susceptibility among pregnant women in North London 1996−1999. *J Public Health Med* 2002;**24**:211−16.

Tookey PA, Peckham CS. Surveillance of congenital rubella in Great Britain 1971−96. *BMJ* 1999;**318**:769−70.

Vestergaard M, Hviid A, Meldgaard Madsen K, *et al.* MMR vaccination and febrile seizures: evaluation of susceptible subgroups and long-term prognosis. *JAMA* 2004;**292**:351−7.

SALBUTAMOL = Albuterol (USAN)

Use
Salbutamol, ritodrine and terbutaline are β-adrenergic stimulants (betamimetics) widely used by asthmatics for their bronchodilator activity. Given IV they have been used in an attempt to inhibit preterm labour. Use can also temporarily control a sudden rise in plasma potassium by causing influx of potassium into cells.

Pharmacology
Salbutamol is a synthetic sympathomimetic first developed in 1967 which, like noradrenaline and isoprenaline (q.v.), has its main effect on bronchial muscle β₂ receptors. Excessive doses cause tachycardia, tremor and agitation. Headache and nausea have also been reported. Nebulised salbutamol is of short-term benefit in a minority of babies with chronic lung damage, but no trial has shown sustained use to be helpful. Nor is use of much benefit in the majority of 'wheezy' babies in the first 2 years of life. Drug binding to liver and muscle adrenergic receptors stimulates cyclic AMP production causing a rise in intracellular potassium uptake and a fall in plasma potassium.

Use in pregnancy
None of the inhaled steroid or β-adrenergic drugs commonly used to treat asthma during pregnancy or lactation seem to pose a threat to the baby. Undertreatment is the commonest problem. The safety of chromoglycate is less clearly established. Betamimetics can help make external cephalic version easier.

Use in early labour
Atosiban (q.v.), nifedipine (q.v.) and the betamimetics ritodrine, terbutaline and salbutamol all seem capable of inhibiting uterine contractions (so-called 'tocolysis') to a comparable degree, but use has not yet been shown to impact on perinatal morbidity or mortality. All can usefully be used to delay delivery for 2–3 days and 'buy time' to effect transfer and/or offer antenatal steroid prophylaxis (cf. the monograph on betamethasone). However, while IV betamimetic use seems safe provided the risk of pulmonary oedema from IV fluid overload is recognised, use can cause palpitations and an unpleasant tachycardia, particularly in mothers with cardiac disease, hyperthyroidism or diabetes. Mothers with impaired renal function or a multiple pregnancy may also be at increased risk. Atosiban or nifedipine are, for these reasons, generally considered better alternatives. Betamimetics cross the placenta and, while tachycardia is rare, transient neonatal hypoglycaemia and hyperinsulinaemia have been noted after birth.

Neonatal hyperkalaemia
Potassium toxicity (hyperkalaemia) is relatively common in low birthweight babies in the first 3 days of life, and seems to correlate with low early postdelivery systemic blood flow. Plasma levels >6·5 mmol/l are quite common. Most babies remain asymptomatic, but cardiac arrhythmia can occur when potassium levels exceed 7·5 mmol/l. Give IV calcium gluconate (q.v.) to stabilise the myocardium, and correct any acidosis with IV sodium bicarbonate (q.v.). An infusion of glucose and insulin (q.v.) will also reduce plasma potassium levels, and the consequential risk of arrhythmia, by encouraging influx into cells, but IV salbutamol offers a simpler and more rapid way of controlling *anuric* hyperkalaemia, *temporarily* lowering the plasma potassium by at least 1 mmol/l. Nebulised salbutamol can be used if the IV drug is unavailable, and seems, in older children, to produce a more sustained response. Dialysis, exchange transfusion or polystyrene sulphonate resins (q.v.) are required to remove potassium from the body.

Treatment
Hyperkalaemia: Give an infusion of 4 micrograms/kg IV over 5–10 minutes. Sustained benefit may sometimes require one repeat infusion after a minimum of 2 hours.
Chronic lung disease: A minority of babies show an unequivocal short-term response to nebulised salbutamol. A 1 mg dose is more than enough, but a standard 2·5 mg Nebule® can be used once every 6–8 hours, irrespective of age or body weight, because little of the drug enters the blood stream.

Supply and administration
Salbutamol is available in 5 ml IV ampoules containing 1 mg/ml (costing £2·60 each). To give a 4 microgram/kg infusion take 0·2 ml of this product for each kg the baby weighs, dilute to 50 ml with 10% glucose saline, and infuse at a rate of 6 ml/hour for just 10 minutes. A less concentrated solution of glucose or glucose saline can be used if necessary. 2·5 mg (2·5 ml) Ventolin® nebules (costing 31p) are available for nebuliser use, and ipratropium (see the monograph on atropine) can be added to this fluid.

References
See also the relevant Cochrane reviews and UK guidelines on tocolytic use

Barrington KJ, Finer NN. Treatment of bronchopulmonary dysplasia. *Clin Perinatol* 1998;**25**:177–202.

de Heus R, Mol BW, Erwich J-JHM, *et al*. Adverse drug reactions to tocolytic treatment for preterm labour: prospective cohort study. *BMJ* 2009;**338**:b744. (See also pp. 727–8.)

Helfrich E, de Vries TW, van Roon EN. Salbutamol for hyperkalaemia in children. *Acta Paediatr* 2001;**90**:1213–16.

Impey L, Pandit M. Tocolysis for repeat external cephalic version in breech presentation at term: a randomised, double-blind, placebo-controlled trial. *Br J Obstet Gynaecol* 2005;**112**:627–31. [RCT]

Kluckow M, Evans N. Low systemic blood flow and hyperkalemia in preterm infants. *J Pediatr* 2001;**139**:227–32.

Royal College of Obstetricians and Gynaecologists. *Tocolytic drugs for women in preterm labour*. Clinical Guideline No. 1(B). London: RCOG, 2002.

Singh BS, Sadiq HF, Noguchi A, *et al*. Efficacy of albuterol inhalation in treatment of hyperkalaemia in premature neonates. *J Pediatr* 2002;**141**:16–20.

Tata LJ, Lewis SA, McKeever TM, *et al*. Effect of maternal asthma, exacerbations and asthma medication use on congenital malformations in offspring; a UK population-based study. *Thorax* 2008;**63**:981–7. (See also pp. 939–40.)

Use

Sildenafil is now widely used as a pulmonary artery vasodilator in children with primary and postsurgical pulmonary hypertension. It is also being used to treat persistent pulmonary hypertension of the newborn, and to wean them from inhaled nitric oxide (q.v.) treatment. Efficacy in the preterm baby is not yet established.

Pharmacology

Sildenafil citrate, a phosphodiesterase-5 inhibitor, first came onto the market in 1998 as an oral treatment for male erectile dysfunction. There is a lot of this enzyme present in the lung, so it is not surprising that sildenafil was soon shown to relax the pulmonary arteries by slowing down the resultant degradation of cyclic guanosine monophosphate in a dose that did not cause troublesome systemic vasodilatation. As a result the drug was soon put to use in the management of pulmonary hypertension in adults, and in the management of postoperative pulmonary hypertension in children with congenital heart disease. Oral treatment is now also starting to be used experimentally in the management of babies with severe persisting pulmonary hypertension of the newborn, especially where there is also a diaphragmatic hernia. The drug is quite rapidly absorbed when given by mouth and then metabolised to the inactive N-desmethyl metabolite in the liver before excretion in the faeces and, to a lesser extent, in the urine (the terminal half life in adults being 4 hours). Only about half the ingested dose gets into the systemic circulation because of 'first pass' metabolism in the liver. Drug elimination rises rapidly in the neonate in the first week of life, and the volume of distribution (V_D 1–4 l/kg) is higher than in adult life, making it important to give an initial loading dose.

While an increasing number of case reports of neonatal use have now started to appear, cases where treatment was successful will be more likely to have found their way into print, and there are, as yet, almost no published reports of the successful use of sildenafil in the preterm baby. High-dose treatment could certainly do more harm than good, and combined use with other vasodilators has sometimes increased ventilation–perfusion mismatch in animal studies. There have, however, now been several small structured studies of the drug's neonatal use, first to wean term babies off the need for further treatment with inhaled nitric oxide and also, more recently, to see if use may sometimes make the need for such expensive treatment unnecessary. Clinical reports also suggest that judicious use can improve cardiac output and cerebral blood flow. Obstetric use is now undergoing assessment. The effect of maternal use during pregnancy or lactation on the baby is unknown, but its high molecular weight makes significant transfer unlikely.

Treatment

Oral treatment: Start by giving 300 micrograms/kg once every 6 hours and increase, as required, to no more than 2 mg/kg once every 4 hours. Start with a low dose if there is hepatic or renal impairment. There are a few reports of babies who respond benefiting from sustained oral treatment for some weeks or months.

IV treatment: Start by giving a 200 microgram/kg loading dose over 2 minutes and then, if there is a response, a continuing infusion of 100 micrograms/kg per hour.

Supply

While tablets are available on prescription, the IV preparation is only available for research purposes on direct application from the manufacturers. A liquid for oral use containing 1 mg/ml can be made by dissolving one 25 mg tablet (which costs £4·10) in 25 ml of water (and used for a month if kept refrigerated).

References

See also the relevant Cochrane reviews

Baquero H, Soliz A, Neira F, *et al*. Oral sildenafil in infants with persistent pulmonary hypertension of the newborn: a pilot randomized blinded study. *Pediatrics* 2006;**117**:1077–83. [RCT] (See also **119**:215–16.)

Chaudhari M, Vogel M, Wright C, *et al*. Sildenafil in neonatal pulmonary hypertension due to impaired alveolisation and plexiform pulmonary arteriopathy. *Arch Dis Child* 2005;**90**:F527–8.

Croom KF, Curran MP. Sildenafil. A review of its use in pulmonary arterial hypertension. *Drugs* 2008;**68**:383–97. [SR]

Fernánandez González N, Rodríguez Fernández A, Jerez Rojas J, *et al*. Oral sildenafil: a promising drug for persistent neonatal pulmonary hypertension. [In Spanish] *An Pediatr (Barc)* 2004;**61**:563–8.

Hon K-I E, Cheung K-I, Siu K-I, *et al*. Oral sildenafil for treatment of severe pulmonary hypertension in an infant. *Biol Neonate* 2005;**88**:109–12.

Juliana AE, Abbad FCB. Severe persistent pulmonary hypertension of the newborn in a setting where limited resources exclude the use of inhaled nitric oxide: successful treatment with sildenafil. *Eur J Pediatr* 2005;**164**:626–9.

Lee JE, Hillier SC, Knoderer CA. Use of sildenafil to facilitate weaning from inhaled nitric oxide in children with pulmonary hypertension following surgery for congenital heart disease. *J Intensive Care Med* 2008;**23**:329–34.

Mukherjee A, Dombi T, Wittke B, *et al*. Population pharmacokinetics of sildenafil in term neonates: evidence of rapid maturation of metabolic clearance in the early neonatal period. *Clin Pharmacol Ther* 2009;**85**:56–63.

Nagdyman N, Fleck T, Bitterling B, *et al*. Influence of intravenous sildenafil on cerebral oxygenation measured by near-infrared spectroscopy in infants after cardiac surgery *Pediatr Res* 2006;**59**:46–25.

Noori S, Friedlich P, Wong P, *et al*. Cardiovascular effects of sildenafil in neonates and infants with congenital diaphragmatic hernia and pulmonary hypertension. *Neonatology* 2007;**91**:92–100.

Schulze-Neick I, Hartenstein P, Stiller B, *et al*. Intravenous sildenafil is a potent pulmonary vasodilator in children with congenital heart disease. *Circulation* 2003;**108**(suppl II):II-167–II-173.

Shekerdemain LS, Ravn HB, Penny DJ. Interaction between inhaled nitric oxide and intravenous sildenafil in a porcine model of meconium aspiration syndrome. *Pediatr Res* 2004;**55**:413–18. (See also pp. 370–1.)

Stocker C, Penny DJ, Brizard CP, *et al*. Intravenous sildenafil and inhaled nitric oxide: a randomised trial in infants after cardiac surgery. *Intensive Care Med* 2003;**29**:591–611. [RCT]

Villanueva-García D, Mota-Rojas D, Hernández-González R, *et al*. A systematic review of experimental and clinical studies of sidenafil for intrauterine growth restriction and pre-term labour. *J Obstet Gynaecol* 2007;**27**:255–9. [SR]

Use

Gentle twice daily oiling can improve the appearance and the integrity of the skin in babies of 28–32 weeks' gestation, and reduce the risk that skin bacteria will cause an invasive septicaemia. Simply wiping with a cloth impregnated with 0·25% chlorhexidine can reduce sepsis and neonatal death in a Third World setting.

Physiology

The skin of the very preterm baby is extremely delicate and very easily damaged. That of a baby born more than about 8 weeks early is not even waterproof and, in a baby born more than 12 weeks early, a *lot* of water leaks 'insensibly' out of the body in this way in the first few days of life. (Extra incubator humidity can halve insensible water loss during this time.) However, maturation occurs quite rapidly over a period of 10–14 days after birth as long as the skin is protected from damage during that time, as long as the air is only moderately (~50%) humid. As a result, the skin of a 2-week old baby born at 24 weeks' gestation is much more waterproof than that of a 2-day old baby of 27 weeks' gestation. Prevention is the key ingredient of good nursing care. Even minor trauma (such as the brisk removal of adhesive tape) can easily strip the skin of all its surface sheet of keratinised cells, leaving the baby with the equivalent of a third degree 'skin burn'. Infection can also seriously damage the outer 'waterproofing' layer of the preterm baby's skin.

Pharmacology

Skin thin enough to let water out is also thin enough to let drugs in, and the widely used skin disinfectant, hexachlorophene, had to be withdrawn in 1972 when its use was found to have caused brain damage. Alcoholic lotions not only penetrate the skin of the preterm baby but also damage the outer layer causing haemorrhagic surface necrosis. The risk is highest when the skin is left lying in liquid alcohol for several minutes. Absorption of iodine, or povidone iodine, can make the preterm baby hypothyroid (as can the IV use of X-ray contrast media containing iodine). Analine dyes can cause methaemoglobinaemia by penetrating the skin even in the full term baby. Hydrocortisone, oestrogens, propylene glycol, urea and lindane have all caused toxicity after absorption through the skin, and absorption of the neomycin in Polybactrin® (a triple antibiotic spray) has been incriminated as a possible cause of profound deafness in the very preterm baby. Regular oil massage is common in many cultural groups; trials have shown that the use of a bland product such as olive oil can be beneficial, but some mustard oil products seem toxic.

Routine skin care

The term baby: Towel the baby dry after birth to prevent hypothermia, but do no bathe until body temperature has stabilised (12–24 hours after birth). Washing with 0·25% aqueous chlorhexidine markedly reduces infection in a Third World setting, but soap and water suffices in other settings. Most babies only need to be 'topped and tailed' each day after that. Acetone will remove small areas of vernix if monitoring leads need to be applied. Pre-treatment with 'tinc benz' (compound benzoin tincture BPC) can limit the damage caused by adhesive tape, etc. A pledge of collodion-hardened cotton wool will stabilise a scalp drip better than tape or plaster. A pectin-based barrier (Hollister® skin barrier, or the like) limits the skin damage caused by the tapes used to secure oral and nasal tubing. Zinc ointment BP is a useful barrier agent.

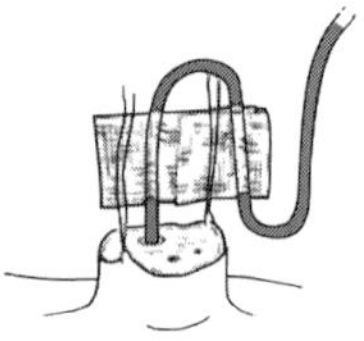

The preterm baby: A transparent plastic wrap will do more than a blanket to prevent the stressful evaporative heat loss that occurs immediately after birth. A waterproof but water vapour permeable, transparent polyurethane dressing or spray (Opsite® or Tegaderm®) can also provide a useful protective barrier over the skin during the first week of life. It does not reduce water loss. Electrodes and transcutaneous blood gas monitoring devices can still be used on areas of skin covered by one such layer (and this dressing can be safely left in place a full week). The use of a stay suture to fix every drain and catheter removes the need to stick *any* tape on the skin (Fig. 1). Applying about 4 g/kg of an emollient cream (aqueous cream BP) or a simple oil (such as sunflower seed oil) twice a day can reduce dermatitis and other signs of minor skin trauma, and reduce the risk of skin commensals causing an invasive blood-borne infection in babies of 28–32 weeks' gestation, but repeated use in the *very* preterm baby may actually be harmful.

Fig. 1

Supply

100 g of the emulsifying ointment Epaderm® costs £3, 100 g of zinc ointment 64p, and 100 g of aqueous cream 21p. A 10 cm² Opsite or Tegaderm dressing costs £1·20, and 10 cm² of Hollister skin barrier £2.

References

See also the relevant Cochrane reviews

Dollison EJ, Beckstrand J. Adhesive tape vs pectin-based barrier use in preterm infants. *Neonatal Network* 1995;**14**:35–39. [RCT]

Donahue ML, Phelps DL, Richter SE, *et al.* A semipermeable skin dressing for extremely low birthweight infants. *J Perinatol* 1996;**16**:20–4. [RCT]

Edwards WH, Conner JM, Soll RF, for the Vermont Oxford Network Neonatal Skin Care Study Group. The effect of prophylactic ointment therapy on nosocomial sepsis rates and skin integrity in infants with birthweights 501 to 1000 g. *Pediatrics* 2004;**113**:1195–203. [RCT]

Mullany LC, Darmstadt GL, Tielsch JM. Safety and impact of chlorhexidine antisepsis interventions for improving neonatal health in developing countries. *Pediatr Infect Dis J* 2006;**25**:665–75. [SR] (See also pp. 676–9.)

Rutter N. Percutaneous drug absorption in the newborn: hazards and uses. *Clin Perinatol* 1987;**14**:911–30.

Smederley P, Lim A, Boyages SC, *et al.* Topical iodine-containing antiseptics and neonatal hypothyroidism in very-low-birthweight infants. *Lancet* 1989;**ii**:661–4.

Use

Skin cleansing is critically important before any invasive procedure. Clean hands are just as important, and supplementing a 30-second hand wash with an alcoholic hand rinse greatly reduces the risk of potential pathogens being passed from one patient to another, especially in a hospital setting. Attempts to keep the healing umbilical stump sterile are misplaced, but heavy bacterial colonisation does need to be controlled.

Pharmacology

Chlorhexidine is a bisguanide antiseptic used to cleanse skin and wounds, and to disinfect working surfaces and instruments. It is sometimes combined with cetrimide (a quaternary ammonium antiseptic). Both can cause skin hypersensitivity. Hexachlorophene (a chlorinated biphenol) is used on skin. All are rapidly bactericidal, and particularly effective against Gram-positive bacteria. Avoid contact with the eyes. Alcohol is a bactericidal antiseptic but use as a cord dressing merely delays its separation. Povidone-iodine (a loose complex of iodine and carrier polymers) also has a slowly lethal effect on bacteria, fungi, viruses and spores.

Neonatal management routines

General skin care: Hexachlorophene dusting powder (Ster-Zac®) can be used to control the heavy staphyloccocal colonisation that usually underpins the development of skin pustules in the neonate. Whole body bathing with hexachlorophene was introduced in the 1950s to deal with the more serious staphylococcal infections often seen when hospital-born babies were regularly nursed in cots only inches apart – a prophylactic ritual that was discontinued very rapidly once it was found to be causing toxic brain damage.

Intravascular access: Cleansing with 0·5% chlorhexidine is better at reducing the risk of catheter-related sepsis in adults than alcohol or povidone-iodine (and an aqueous solution is probably as good as an alcoholic one). The latter two products also pose hazards when used on immature skin (see skin care entry). Employ two different swabs, applying each for 10 seconds, and then leave the skin to dry for 30 seconds. A surgical 'keyhole' drape and no-touch technique will reduce the risk of re-contamination. A transparent polyurethane dressing can help to secure the line, reduce gross soiling and minimise skin damage while allowing regular site inspection. Concern that moisture build up under the dressing could cause catheter colonisation by skin bacteria can be further addressed by placing a chlorhexidine-impregnated disc under the dressing.

Intramuscular injections: While it is sensible to make the skin socially clean, the 'swabaholics' who insist on trying to achieve sterility with spirit or a 'mediswab' are indulging in a pointless ritual. Indeed where a live vaccine is to be given it is said that alcohol should *not* be used.

Umbilical care: Where delivery occurs in hospital, a policy of only treating those stumps that look inflamed reduces true sepsis just as effectively as universal prophylaxis (flucloxacillin (q.v.) being the antibiotic most commonly used for overt infection). In the developing world, however, the situation is very different. Here some traditional ways of dressing the cord risks causing clostridial infection and lethal neonatal tetanus. In any such setting it is now known that the routine use of 4% aqueous chlorhexidine to clean the umbilical stump soon after birth, and then daily for the next few days, greatly reduces the incidence of serious periumbilical infection, and may even reduce neonatal mortality (see website commentary).

Hand washing

Hand washing seldom gets the attention it needs. To be effective, it ***must*** be sustained for at least 30 seconds, sleeves must be rolled up, and all rings and watches removed, but active scrubbing is counterproductive, because of the skin damage that eventually builds up. A medicated soap, such as Hibiscrub®, should be used when starting work and after the hands become soiled, and an alcoholic hand rinse, such as Hibisol®, used before touching any new baby. The importance of all of this was brought vividly home to all the staff on one nursery when five babies in five different rooms developed *Salmonella* infection on a single day from an unwell baby born to an unrecognised maternal carrier. The busy medical resident collected serum bilirubin specimens from all five babies one Christmas morning without washing his hands each time!

Supply

100 ml of 0·5% chlorhexidine in water can be made from a 20% or 25% concentrate for less than 3p. 100 ml of 4% chlorhexidine gluconate liquid hand soap (Hibiscrub) costs 30p; 100 ml of the alcoholic hand rinse (Hibisol) costs 34p; and 30 g of hexachlorophene dusting powder (Ster-Zac) costs 83p.

References

See also the Cochrane review of umbilical cord care

Garland JS, Alex CP, Mueller CD, *et al*. A randomized trial comparing povidone-iodine to a chlorhexidine gluconate-impregnated dressing for prevention of central venous catheter infections in neonates. *Pediatrics* 2001;**107**:1431–6. [RCT]

Girou E, Loyeau S, Legrand P, *et al*. Efficacy of handrubbing with alcohol based solution versus standard handwashing with antiseptic soap: randomsed clinical trial. *BMJ* 2002;**325**:362–5. [RCT]

Kramer A, Rudolph P, Kampf G, *et al*. Limited efficacy of alcohol-based hand gels. *Lancet* 2002;**359**:1489–90. (See also **360**:1509–11.)

Larson EL. APIC guideline for handwashing and hand antisepsis in health care settings. *Am J Infect Control* 1996;**23**:251–69. [SR]

Mullany LC, Darmstadt GL, Khantry SK, *et al*. Topical applications of chlorhexidine to the umbilical stump for prevention of omphalitis and neonatal mortality in southern Nepal: a community-based, cluster-randomised trial. *Lancet* 2006;**367**:910–18. [RCT]

O'Grady NP, Alexander M, Dellinger EP, *et al*. Guidelines for the prevention of intravascular catheter-related infections. *Pediatrics* 2002;**110**:e51. [SR]

Pessoa-Silva CL, Hugonnet S, Pfister R, *et al*. Reductions of health care-associated infection risk in neonates by successful hand hygiene promotion. *Pediatrics* 2007;**120**:e382–90. [RCT]

Timsit J-F, Schwebel C, Bouadma L, *et al*. Chlorhexidine-impregnated sponges and less frequent dressing changes for prevention of catheter-related infections in critically ill adults. *JAMA* 2009;**301**:1231–41. [RCT] (See also pp. 1285–7.)

SODIUM BENZOATE and SODIUM PHENYLBUTYRATE

Use

Sodium benzoate and sodium phenylbutyrate are used to control the hyperammonaemia seen in children with urea cycle defects. A plasma ammonia level above 200 µmol/l needs urgent referral and investigation.

Pharmacology

Sodium benzoate is excreted in the urine as hippurate after conjugation with glycine. As each glycine molecule contains a nitrogen atom, one mole of nitrogen is cleared for each mole of benzoate given, if there is complete conjugation. Phenylbutyrate is oxidised to phenylacetate and also excreted after conjugation with glutamine. Phenylacetate is the intravenous product normally used in North America. Since phenylacetylglutamine contains two nitrogen atoms, two moles of nitrogen are cleared, if there is complete conjugation, for each mole of phenylbutyrate given. All three drugs can lower plasma ammonia levels in patients with urea cycle disorders. Sodium phenylbutyrate is more effective than sodium benzoate but less palatable.

Hyperammonaemia

Plasma ammonia should be measured in any patient with unexplained encephalopathy (vomiting, irritability or drowsiness, etc.), particularly in term neonates who deteriorate after an initial period of good health. Inform the laboratory in advance and send the specimen urgently on ice. Ammonia levels above 200 µmol/l suggest an inborn error of metabolism, but a repeat sample should be sent to check that the result is not artefactual. Severe hyperammonaemia (>500 µmol/l) causes serious neurological damage, and urea cycle defects presenting in the neonatal period have a poor prognosis. Circulating ammonia levels should be lowered as quickly as possible, if treatment is considered appropriate, using haemodialysis (peritoneal dialysis is too slow), and sodium benzoate and sodium phenylbutyrate should also be given while organising dialysis. The main use of these drugs is, however, in the long-term management of urea cycle disorders, including patients with milder defects presenting after the neonatal period. The drugs need to be combined with a low protein diet and other treatment, such as arginine (q.v.), appropriate to each disorder.

Treatment

Acute hyperammonaemia: Brusilow and Horwich (2001) recommend an IV loading dose of 250 mg/kg of each drug, given over 90 minutes, followed by a continuing maintenance infusion of each drug at 10 mg/kg per hour. Co-infusion is safe. Note that an overdose can cause metabolic acidosis and a potentially fatal encephalopathy. There is a theoretical risk that benzoate could displace bilirubin from albumin, so consider treating any severe jaundice. Arginine should generally be given as well.

Look at the website maintained by the British Inherited Metabolic Disease Group (www.bimdg.org.uk) for further advice. Consider haemodialysis if ammonia levels are very high.

Long-term management: Give up to 250 mg/kg per day of sodium benzoate by mouth in 3–4 divided doses. Sodium phenylbutyrate can also be given as well in doses of up to 600 mg/kg a day, also in 3–4 divided doses if necessary. It is, however, possible to achieve very adequate control in some patients using sodium benzoate without phenylbutyrate. The nausea and vomiting caused by the unpleasant taste of the raw products can be minimised by the use of a savoury or fruit-flavoured solution.

Sodium overload

Note that 500 mg of sodium benzoate contains 3·5 mmol of sodium, and 500 mg of sodium phenylbutyrate contains 2·7 mmol of sodium, and take care to avoid sodium overload.

Monitoring

Drug dosages and diet should be adjusted to keep the plasma ammonia concentration below 60 µmol/l, and the plasma glutamine level below 800 µmol/l, while maintaining a normal essential amino acid profile.

Supply

Sodium benzoate: This is available for 'named' patients as a 100 mg/ml sugar-free blackcurrant-flavoured oral liquid from Special Products Ltd (100 ml costs £5). 500 mg tablets are also available. 10 ml (200 mg/ml) ampoules for IV use cost £4·10; dilute the contents with 40 ml of 5% or 10% glucose to obtain a solution containing 50 mg/ml, and give as a continuous infusion.

Sodium phenylbutyrate: This is available from Orphan Europe; 100 g of the EU licensed granules cost £380. It is also available for 'named' patients as a 250 mg/ml strawberry-flavoured liquid from Special Products (100 ml costs £50). Reconstitute the powder with 80 ml of purified water and use within 28 days. 10 ml (200 mg/ml) ampoules for IV use cost £7; dilute the contents with 40 ml of 5% or 10% glucose to obtain a 50 mg/ml solution, and give this as a continuous infusion. It can be put in the same syringe as sodium benzoate.

Ammonul®: This is a commercial formulation of sodium benzoate and phenylacetate widely used in North America.

References

Brusilow SW, Horwich AL. Urea cycle enzymes. In: Scriver CR, Beaudet AL, Sly WS, et al., eds. The metabolic and molecular bases of inherited disease, 8th edn. McGraw-Hill: New York, 2001: pp. 1909–64.

Das AM, Illsinger S, Hartmann H, et al. Prenatal benzoate treatment in urea cycle defects. Arch Dis Child 2009;**94**:F216–17.

Enns GM, Berry SA, Berry GT, et al. Survival after treatment with phenylacetate and benzoate for urea-cycle disorders. N Engl J Med 2007;**356**:2282–92. (See also pp. 2321–2.)

Leonard JV. Disorders of the urea cycle and related syndromes. In: Fernandes J, Saudubray J-M, van den Berghe G, et al., eds. Inborn metabolic diseases. Diagnosis and treatment, 4th edn. Berlin: Springer-Verlag, 2006: pp. 263–72.

Use

Sodium bicarbonate can be used to correct severe metabolic acidosis. Significant respiratory acidosis is almost always more appropriately managed by providing adequate respiratory support.

Pharmacology

Sodium bicarbonate is one of the most important natural buffers of the hydrogen ion (acid) content of the blood, and the body responds to a build up of metabolic acids by increasing the amount of buffering bicarbonate. The process is controlled by the kidney and is very slow to operate. The neonatal kidney also has a limited ability to excrete acid. The infusion of small doses of sodium bicarbonate is a way of maintaining the acid-base balance of the blood by speeding these processes up.

Controversy rages about the role of sodium bicarbonate therapy in neonatal medicine. It was used very liberally for a number of years but is now used less extensively with the recognition that its use can cause sudden osmolar shifts that could be damaging to the brain, and that its excessive use can also cause hypernatraemia. There is also some largely anecdotal evidence to suggest that it can cause intraventricular haemorrhage especially in the preterm baby if administered rapidly. The drug still has a valuable role, however, because there is no doubt that serious acidosis (pH <7·2) compromises cardiac output and surfactant production as well as causing gastrointestinal ileus. THAM (q.v.) is probably a better alternative where there is CO_2 retention or a risk of hypernatraemia (as, for example, when a continuous alkaline infusion is employed in the management of persistent pulmonary hypertension).

Managing severe asphyxia

Term babies normally recover unaided from any episode of severe intrapartum asphyxia within 4 hours, and giving bicarbonate does not seem to speed this recovery or have any impact on the immediate outcome. There may be a stronger case for intervention in a surfactant-deficient preterm baby. The situation is different where asphyxia has been severe enough to bring cardiac output to a complete standstill. Here there is strong (unpublished) evidence that a 1–2 mmol/kg IV bolus of sodium bicarbonate, diluted, if possible, with an equal quantity of 10% glucose, will often restart the circulation when all else fails, as long as it reaches the heart and coronary circulation (which means catheterising the umbilical vein, or performing direct cardiac puncture). Unfortunately only half the babies asphyxiated enough to require any such intervention survive to discharge, and most of those that do later develop severe spastic quadriplegia – the only babies to survive unscathed seem to be those in whom the asphyxial episode was not only severe but of very abrupt onset. Be alert for the rare non-asphyxiated baby in whom acute blood loss has caused hypovolaemic circulatory arrest.

Treatment

Correcting acidosis: Give 0·5 mmol/kg IV for each unit (mmol) by which it is hoped to reduce the measured blood gas base deficit. Do not inject this at a rate of more than 0·5 mmol/kg per minute or allow it to mix with any other IV drug. Partial correction is normally quite adequate, unless pulmonary vasospasm serious enough to cause severe pulmonary hypertension seems to be developing (a condition sometimes called 'persistence of the fetal circulation') in which case it may be necessary to raise the pH above 7·5.

Exchange transfusion: Add 4 mmol of sodium bicarbonate to the first unit and 2 mmol to any second unit of citrate phosphate dextrose (CPD) blood used in any exchange transfusion undertaken in the first day of life to buffer the citrate load. This advice constitutes the one exception to the rule that no drug should ever be added to blood or any blood product.

Symptomatic hyperkalaemia: Maintain mild alkalosis by giving 1 mmol/kg of IV sodium bicarbonate.

Late metabolic acidosis: Preterm babies sometimes develop a late metabolic acidosis because the kidney has only a limited ability to excrete acid, and this can inhibit weight gain. Give 2 mmol/kg of sodium bicarbonate with feeds once a day for 7 days to any baby with a urinary pH that is consistently less than 5·4.

Tissue extravasation

Tissue extravasation due to IV administration can be managed with hyaluronidase (q.v.). The use of a dilute preparation reduces the risk of serious tissue damage.

Supply

Stock ampoules of 8·4% sodium bicarbonate contain 1 mmol of sodium and 1 mmol of bicarbonate per ml. The 10 ml ampoules cost £2. Some units prefer to stock a less concentrated ampoule containing 4·2% sodium bicarbonate (costing £3·50 each). Prior dilution is not necessary as long as any infusion is given slowly (as indicated above). Polyfusor bags containing 200 ml of 8·4% sodium bicarbonate are also available costing £3·50 each. Sachets of powder for oral use that can be used for 24 hours after reconstitution (with instructions on their use) are available on request.

References

See also the relevant Cochrane reviews

Ascher JL, Poland RL. Sodium bicarbonate: basically useless therapy. [Commentary] *Pediatrics* 2008;**122**:831–5.

Kalhoff H, Diekmann L, Stick GJ, *et al*. Alkali therapy versus sodium chloride supplement in low birth weight infants with incipient late metabolic acidosis. *Acta Paediatr* 1997;**86**:96–101. [RCT]

Lokesh L, Kumar P, Murki S, *et al*. A randomized controlled trial of sodium bicarbonate in neonatal resuscitation – effect on immediate outcome. *Resuscitation* 2004;**60**:219–23. [RCT]

Shah PS, Raju NV, Beyene J, *et al*. Recovery of metabolic acidosis in term infants with postasphyxial hypoxic-ischaemic encephalopathy. *Acta Paediatr* 2003;**92**:941–7.

SODIUM CHLORIDE

Use
Sodium is an essential nutrient and, to balance renal loss, orally fed preterm babies benefit from supplements for the first few weeks. Isotonic (0·9%) sodium chloride is often used to correct hypovolaemia, but compound sodium lactate (Hartmann) solution is a better option because it does not cause hyperchloraemic acidosis.

Pathophysiology
The kidney of the term newborn infant rapidly develops an ability to conserve salt, and the fractional excretion of sodium falls ten-fold in the first few days of life, but the preterm infant has a high persisting obligatory salt loss. As a result, the sodium requirement of most healthy infants of less than 34 weeks' gestation is at least 3 mmol/kg per day, while many babies of less than 30 weeks' gestation benefit from getting 6 mmol/kg per day during the first 2 weeks of life. This is more than the sodium intake provided by any of the standard preterm milk formulas (q.v.). Losses may be even higher after renal tubular damage due to severe hypoxia or hypotension.

While **hypo**natraemia is often caused by excessive renal sodium loss, it can also be dilutional, and limitation of water intake is then appropriate. However, if the serum sodium is less than 120 mmol/l, water deprivation alone is unlikely to correct the hyponatraemia, and supplementation to increase the serum sodium to above 120 mmol/l may be necessary. Calculation assumes that sodium is distributed through almost all the extracellular space (i.e. through 60% of the body in the very preterm baby, and 40% of the term baby). Regular weighing and calculation of fractional sodium excretion (as outlined in the introductory section on renal failure (p. 25)) will help to define the disordered electrolyte and fluid balance.

Hypernatraemia is also a risk, however, because the neonatal kidney's ability to excrete excess sodium is also limited, and its maximum ability uncertain. While the apathy and hypotonia caused by serious hyponatraemia (<120 mmol/l) may on occasion render a small baby ventilator dependent, the permanent brain damage caused by severe hypernatraemia (>160 mmol/l) is a disaster of an entirely different magnitude, and this *must* be corrected slowly, by dialysis if necessary. 'Normal' (0·9%) saline and Hepsal® (see the monograph on heparin) both contain 0·15 mmol of sodium (9 mg of sodium chloride) per millilitre. Use during the reconstitution or infusion of a drug, to maintain line patency, or to 'flush' a drug through, can deliver quite a lot of sodium. A baby given a constant infusion of 1 ml of 0·9% sodium chloride an hour gets 3·6 mmol of sodium a day. Aim for a serum sodium of 130–145 mmol/l. Never believe any report based on a sample from a line containing sodium unless the 'dead space' was first cleared by the temporary removal of 5 ml of blood.

Management
IV Intake: A daily IV intake of 150–200 ml/kg of 'fifth-normal' (0·18%) sodium chloride provides between 4·5 and 6 mmol of sodium per kg per day (a safe basic minimum intake for the very preterm baby without being a dangerously high intake for the full term baby). Babies of ≤30 weeks' gestation, especially if they are on a lower total fluid intake than this in the first 2 weeks, may require further oral or IV sodium, particularly if renal function is compromised. It is better not to start supplementation, if the baby requires ventilation, until the physiological adjustment of extracellular fluid volume (and weight loss) that normally occurs in the first few days of life has occurred. Giving large bolus volumes during neonatal resuscitation to correct perceived hypovolaemia serves little purpose and may not be risk free.

Oral Intake: Preterm milk formulas contain enough sodium for most babies of more than 30 weeks' gestation. Babies more immature than this seem to need a further 2 mmol of sodium once a day by mouth for each 100 ml of milk they are given for at least the first couple of weeks of life to optimise both their early growth and their later motor and neuro-psychological development. Those fed breast milk should receive a supplement of 3–4 mmol per 100 ml of milk and this is probably best given, to prevent confusion, once a day at a fixed time. While such dietary supplements do not need a medical prescription it is wise to record the existence of any such supplement in the drug prescription chart.

Nebulised use: Hypertonic (3%) saline (4 ml every 2–4 hours) may speed recovery in babies with bronchiolitis, and a solution twice as strong may help to sustained lung health in infants with cystic fibrosis.

Supply
The 2 ml ampoules of 0·9% sodium chloride frequently used to flush IV lines cost 24p each. 5 ml ampoules of 18% sodium chloride (3 mmol/ml) cost 33p. Take care not to confuse the two. A 1 mmol/ml oral solution can be provided on request. A range of ampoules and packs are available also containing glucose (q.v.), as are 500 ml packs of 0·9% sodium chloride and of Hartmann solution (which also contains 0·25% sodium lactate).

References
See also the relevant Cochrane reviews

Al-Dahhan J, Jannoun L, Haycock GB. Effect of sodium salt supplementation of newborn premature infants on neurodevelopmental outcome at 10–13 years of age. *Arch Dis Child* 2002;**86**:F120–3.

Coulthard MG. Will changing maintenance intravenous fluid from 0·18% to 0·45% saline do more harm than good? *Arch Dis Child* 2008;**93**:335–40. (But see correction on p. 1079 and letters on pp. 285–7 and 1001.)

Elkins MR, Robinson M, Rose BR, *et al.* National Hypertonic Saline in Cystic Fibrosis (NHSCF) Study Group. A controlled trial of long-term inhaled hypertonic saline in patients with cystic fibrosis. *N Engl J Med* 2006;**354**:229–40.

Ewer AK, Tyler W, Francis A, *et al.* Excessive volume expansion and neonatal death in preterm infants born at 27–28 weeks gestation. *Paediatr Perinat Epidemiol* 2003;**17**:180–6.

Kuzik BA, Al Qadhi SA, Kent S, *et al.* Nebulized hypertonic saline in the treatment of viral bronchiolitis in infants. *J Pediatr* 2007;**151**:266–70. [RCT] (See also pp. 235–7.)

Use

Sodium fusidate is a powerful antistaphylococcal antibiotic primarily of value in the treatment of penicillin-resistant osteomyelitis. Only limited information is available on its use in the neonatal period.

Pharmacology

Sodium fusidate is a powerful narrow-spectrum antistaphylococcal antibiotic first isolated in 1960. Virtually all staphylococci are sensitive, including meticillin-resistant and coagulase-negative strains. The antibiotic is also active against *Neisseria* and *Clostridium* species. However, concurrent treatment with a second antistaphylococcal antibiotic (such as flucloxacillin or vancomycin) is advisable, especially if treatment is prolonged, despite a few reports of antagonism *in vitro* because, if this is not done, there is a serious risk of drug resistance developing. Treatment with two antibiotics is generally considered particularly important when treating meticillin-resistant staphylococci. Co-treatment with rifampicin (q.v.) may well be appropriate in this situation in countries like the UK where resistance to rifampicin is still currently uncommon, but co-treatment with a glycopeptide such as vancomycin will be more appropriate in many settings. The frequent use of Fucidin® in the topical management of skin conditions may be one factor in the recent rise in the proportion of all *Staphyococcus aureus* isolates that are resistant to this antibiotic in the UK.

Sodium fusidate is relatively well absorbed from the gastrointestinal tract and widely distributed in most body tissues, but it does not penetrate CSF well. Some crosses the placenta and appears in breast milk, but there is no evidence of teratogenicity, and no evidence to suggest that breastfeeding is contraindicated. Caution is advised, however, in the use of sodium fusidate in any baby with jaundice, because the drug is highly bound to plasma proteins, and there may be competitive binding with bilirubin. Reported toxic effects included skin rashes and jaundice (which can be reversed by stopping treatment). The half life in adults is 10–15 hours; the half life in neonates is less certain. The drug is largely excreted in the bile (making combined treatment with rifampicin unwise). Very little is excreted by the kidney.

Intravenous treatment can cause vasospasm or thrombophlebitis unless the drug is given slowly after suitable dilution into a large vein. Rapid infusion can also cause a high concentration of sodium fusidate to develop locally causing red cell haemolysis and jaundice. Bacterial conjunctivitis responds as rapidly to fucidic acid eye drops as it does to chloramphenicol eye drops, and such treatment has the advantage of only requiring administration twice a day, but such a product is not generally available outside Europe.

Treatment

Oral administration: The only available liquid formulation (fusidic acid) is not as well absorbed as sodium fusidate. Offer 15 mg/kg of fusidic acid once every 8 hours.

IV administration: Infuse 10 mg/kg of sodium fusidate, after reconstitution as described below, once every 12 hours. It should be given slowly over 6 hours (2 hours may be adequate when a central venous line is employed). Doses twice as high as this have been given with apparent safety on occasion.

Long-term administration: High blood levels are often encountered when adult patients are given a standard dose (1·5 grams a day) for more than 4–5 days. In the absence of any reliable pharmacokinetic information it may be advisable to monitor liver function to watch for any rapid rise in liver enzyme levels and/or to reduce the dose used in the neonatal period if treatment is continued for more than 5 days.

Supply and administration

Note that different formulations are used for oral and IV use. A sugar-free oral suspension containing 50 mg/ml of fusidic acid (equivalent to 35 mg/ml of sodium fusidate) is available which should not be diluted prior to administration (50 ml bottles cost £7·20). Vials with 500 mg of sodium fusidate that can be reconstituted with 10 ml of specially provided phosphate/citrate buffer are available for £8 each. Take 0·4 ml of the freshly reconstituted 50 mg/ml concentrate for each kg the baby weighs, dilute to 24 ml with 0·9% sodium chloride, prime the giving set, and infuse at a rate of 2 ml/hour for 6 hours. (Note that this should leave about 10 ml of fluid still in the syringe when the infusion is complete.) The drug is not compatible with acidic solutions, but can be terminally co-infused with 5% or 10% glucose or glucose saline when necessary. While the drug can be kept for up to 24 hours after reconstitution, the vial should not be kept after it has been opened. There is no suitable intramuscular formulation. Sodium fusidate is not currently available in North America.

References

Bergdahl S, Elinder G, Eriksson M. Treatment of neonatal osteomyelitis with cloxacillin in combination with fusidic acid. *Scand J Infect Dis* 1981;**13**:281–2.

Dobie D, Gray J. Fusdic acid resistance in *Staphylococcus aureus*. [Review] *Arch Dis Child* 2004;**89**:74–7.

Normann EK, Bakken O, Peltola J, *et al*. Treatment of acute neonatal bacterial conjunctivitis: a comparison of fucidic acid and chloramphenical eye drops. *Acta Ophthalmol Scand* 2002;**80**:183–7. [RCT]

Reeves DS. The pharmacokinetics of fusidic acid. *J Antimicrob Chemother* 1987;**20**:467–76.

Turnidge J, Collignon P. Resistance to fusdic acid. *Int J Antimicrob Agents* 1999;**12**:S35–44.

SOTALOL

Use

Sotalol can control atrial flutter. It is also being used, under expert supervision, instead of amiodarone (q.v.) or, together with flecainide (q.v.), in the control of ventricular and supraventricular arrhythmia.

Pharmacology

Many β-adrenoreceptor blocking drugs now exist. Such drugs have been widely used, over many years, to control hypertension, manage angina and treat myocardial infarction, arrhythmia, heart failure and thyrotoxicosis, and it is now clear that some are better at some things than others. Some, like propranolol (q.v.), the first β blocker to be developed, are essentially non-selective, and act indiscriminately on receptors in the heart, peripheral blood vessels, liver, pancreas and bronchi (making use in asthmatics hazardous). Others like labetalol (q.v.), which affect receptors more selectively, are used to control hypertension because of their effect on arteriolar tone. Non-cardioselective β blockers like sotalol, which are water rather than lipid soluble, are less likely to enter the brain and disturb sleep, and are excreted largely unchanged in the urine. All β blockers slow the heart and can depress the myocardium. Sotalol, in particular, can prolong the QT interval and cause a life-threatening ventricular arrhythmia, especially if there is hypokalaemia. Because of this sotalol is now *only* used to manage pre-existing arrhythmia. In this sotalol functions both as a class II antiarrhythmic to decrease heart rate and AV nodal conduction as a result of non-selective β-blockade, and as a class III antiarrhythmic by prolonging the atrial and ventricular action potential and the heart muscle's subsequent refractory period. Esmolol is an alternative short-acting cardioselective β blocker.

Sotalol, which was first synthesised in 1964, is well and rapidly absorbed when given by mouth (although food, including milk, decreases absorption). The terminal half life (7–9 hours) remains much the same throughout childhood, but is seriously prolonged in renal failure. The manufacturers have not done the studies needed to be able to recommend use in children. Furthermore, because the drug can provoke as well as control cardiac arrhythmia, patients should be subject to continuous ECG monitoring when treatment is started, and treatment only initiated by a consultant well versed in the management of cardiac rhythm disorders. Sotalol may be the drug of choice for fetal atrial flutter. Lack of controlled trial evidence makes it impossible to say what drug regimen is best for other fetal arrhythmias.

There is no evidence that β blockers are teratogenic, but they can cause intermittent mild fetal bradycardia (90–110 bpm). Sustained high-dose use in the second and third trimester can also be associated with reduced fetal growth. While there is no evidence that this is harmful, the long-term effect of sustained maternal use has not been studied, and warrants evaluation. β blocker use in pregnancy can also cause transient bradycardia and hypoglycaemia in the baby at delivery. Sotalol appears in breast milk in high concentrations (milk:plasma ratio 2·8–5·5). Babies so fed have, to date, been asymptomatic, but it has been shown that they are ingesting 20–40% of the weight-adjusted maternal dose. Propranolol is the β blocker associated with lowest drug exposure during lactation.

Treatment

Mothers: The dose given when trying to control a fetal arrhythmia has usually been between 60 and 160 mg by mouth 2–3 times a day. Watch the mother's ECG carefully for QT changes.

Children: Start cautiously with 1 mg/kg by mouth once every 12 hours and increase the dose as necessary once every 3–4 days to no more than 4 mg/kg. Withdraw treatment gradually.

Toxicity

Absorption is reduced in milk-fed children and, if diarrhoea causes sudden withdrawal, this may cause toxicity. Extend the dosage interval if renal function is poor, and stop treatment if the QT_c interval exceeds 550 milliseconds. An overdose of *any* β blocker can cause bradycardia and/or hypotension. Give 40 micrograms/kg of IV atropine, and treat unresponsive cardiogenic shock with IV glucagons (q.v.) and glucose. Monitor the blood glucose level and control ventilation. Isoprenaline (q.v.) may help. Cardiac pacing is occasionally needed.

Supply

80 mg tablets of sotalol cost 6p each, and a 5 mg/ml oral suspension, stable for up to 3 months at room temperature, can be prepared on request. 4 ml (10 mg/ml) IV ampoules cost £1·70.

References

Beaufort-Krol GCM, Bink-Boelkens MThE. Effectiveness of sotalol for atrial flutter in children after surgery for congenital heart disease. *Am J Cardiol* 1997;**79**:92–4.

Läer S, Elshoff JP, Meibohm B, *et al*. Development of a safe and effective pediatric dosing regimen for sotalol based on population pharmacokinetics and pharmacodynamics in children with supraventricular tachycardia. *J Am Coll Cardiol* 2005;**46**:1322–30.

Lisowski LA, Verheijen PM, Benatar AA, *et al*. Atrial flutter in the perinatal age group: diagnosis, management and outcome. *J Am Coll Cardiol* 2002;**35**:771–7.

Price JF, Kertesz NJ, Snyder CS, *et al*. Flecainide and sotalol: a new combination therapy for refractory supraventricular tachycardia in children <1 year of age. *J Am Coll Cardiol* 2002;**39**:717–20.

Russell GA, Martin AP. Flecainide toxicity. *Arch Dis Child* 1989;**64**:860–2.

Wagner X, Jouglard J, Moulin M, *et al*. Coadministration of flecainide acetate and sotalol during pregnancy: lack of teratogenic effects, passage across the placenta, and excretion in human breast milk. *Am Heart J* 1990;**119**:700–2.

Use

Spiramycin is now widely used to protect the fetus from infection when a woman develops *Toxoplasma* infection during pregnancy. However, since parasitic transmission becomes increasingly unlikely as the mother's immune response builds up, most infection probably occurs before diagnosis is possible.

Pharmacology

Spiramycin is a macrolide antibiotic, first isolated in 1954, that is related to erythromycin. It is well absorbed when taken by mouth, and mostly metabolised in the liver, although biliary excretion is also high. The serum half life in adults is about 8 hours. Spiramycin crosses the placenta, where it is also concentrated, and there is a belief that early treatment can prevent the transplacental passage of the *Toxoplasma* parasite. Treatment with pyrimethamine (q.v.) and sulfadiazine (q.v.) may be a more effective way of limiting damage once fetal infection has occurred, but termination is often offered if there is ultrasound evidence of cerebral damage even though many children with antenatally detected cerebral calcification or ventriculomegaly seem to develop normally. Spiramycin appears in therapeutic quantities in breast milk but it is not the treatment of choice after delivery. It can also prolong the QT interval and has occasionally caused a dangerous neonatal arrhythmia. CSF penetration is poor.

Toxoplasmosis

Toxoplasma gondii is a common worldwide protozoan parasite that infects many warm-blooded animals. Cats are the main host, replication occurring in the small intestine, but sheep, pigs and cattle become infected if they ingest faecally contaminated material, and infected cysts within the muscles and brain then remain viable almost indefinitely. Humans usually only become infected by ingesting cysts from contaminated soil or by eating undercooked or poorly cured meat (although transplant recipients are at risk of cross-infection). Infection normally goes unrecognised but fever, muscle pain, sore throat and a lymphadenopathy may manifest themselves after 4–21 days. Hepatosplenomegaly and a maculopapular rash are sometimes seen. Although the illness is usually benign and self-limiting, chronically infected immunodeficient patients can (like the fetus) experience reactivated central nervous system disease. Screening can not be advocated until the benefit of treatment becomes less uncertain.

The risk of a susceptible woman becoming infected during pregnancy is quite low (~0·5%), and congenital infection is uncommon (1:1000 to 1:10,000 births). The fetus is more likely to become infected if the mother is infected late in pregnancy, but more likely to show *signs* of that infection within 3 years of birth if infected early. Overt signs of infection develop in less than 5% of babies born to mothers infected in the first 16 weeks of pregnancy. Reliable early recognition requires serial testing of all antibody-negative women, since IgM and IgG tests cannot be used to time infection accurately, and often results in mothers receiving unnecessary antenatal treatment even when the baby is not at risk. Fetal infection can be diagnosed by PCR detection of *T. gondii* DNA in amniotic fluid or by mouse inoculation. Persistence of circulating IgG antibodies for a year confirms that the baby was congenitally infected. Most, but not all, have IgM antibodies at birth. Many show no overt sign of illness at birth, but a quarter develop retinochoroiditis, intracranial calcification and/or ventriculomegaly within 3 years. Only a few (<5%) develop severe neurological impairment, but how many develop minor disability is not known. Half of those with retinal lesions eventually develop some visual loss.

Treatment

Mothers: It is common practice to give 1 gram of spiramycin prophylactically once every 8 hours as soon as maternal infection is first suspected to minimise the risk of placental transmission, and this is often continued for the duration of pregnancy. Pyrimethamine and sulfadiazine are often given as well if there is evidence of fetal infection. No controlled trial evidence exists to support this strategy.

Babies: Use pyrimethamine and sulfadiazine to initiate treatment (as outlined in the pyrimethamine monograph). Some clinicians alternate this with 3–4-week courses of spiramycin (50 mg/kg twice a day).

Supply

Spiramycin has a licence for use in Europe (where it has been used for nearly 20 years), but has not yet been licensed for general use in America or the UK. It can, however, be obtained by the pharmacy from Rhône-Poulenc Rorer Ltd for use on a 'named patient' basis on request. The 250 mg (750,000 unit) tablets cost 69p each; 100 ml of the sugar-free suspension (25 mg/ml) costs £10·40.

References

See also the relevant Cochrane reviews

Gras L, Wallon M, Pollak A, *et al*. Association between prenatal treatment and clinical manifestations of congenital toxoplasmosis in infancy: a cohort study in 13 European centres. *Acta Paediatr* 2005;**94**:1721–31.

Kravetz J. Congenital toxoplasmosis. *BMJ Clinical evidence handbook*. London: BMJ Books, 2009: pp. 247–8 (and updates). [SR]

McLoyd R, Boyer K, Karrison T, *et al*. Outcome of treatment for congenital toxoplasmosis. 1981–2004: The National Collaborative Chicago-based Congenital Toxoplasmosis Study. *Clin Infect Dis* 2006;**42**:1383–94.

Montoya JG, Leisenfeld, O. Toxoplasmosis. [Seminar] *Lancet* 2004;**262**:1965–76.

Petersen E. Toxoplasmosis. *Sem Fetal Neonat Med* 2007;**12**:214–23.

SYROCOT (Systematic Review on Congenital Toxoplasmosis) Study Group. Effectiveness of prenatal treatment for congenital toxoplasmosis: a meta-analysis of individual patients' data. *Lancet* 2007;**369**:115–22. [SR]

SPIRONOLACTONE

Use

Sustained treatment with spironolactone is of value in patients with congestive heart failure, in the diagnosis and management of primary hyperaldosteronism, and in the management of ascites due to liver disease. Whether the use of spironolactone, as well as a thiazide diuretic such as chlorothiazide, is of value in babies with bronchopulmonary dysplasia is much less clearly established.

Pharmacology

Spironolactone is a potassium-sparing diuretic developed in 1959 which acts by competitively inhibiting the action of aldosterone (a natural adrenocortical hormone) on the distal part of the renal tubule. It is well absorbed by mouth and mainly excreted (partly metabolised) in the urine. The half life in adults is 1–2 hours, but several of the metabolic products (including canrenone) that also have diuretic properties have a 12–24-hour half life. It is not known whether metabolism and excretion differ in early infancy. Benefits may not become apparent for up to 48 hours after treatment is started and may continue for a similar period after the treatment has stopped. Use declined after sustained high-dose use was shown to cause tumours in rats. However, a large multinational trial in 1999 (the RALES trial) showed that sustained low-dose use in adults with severe heart failure relieves symptoms and reduces the risk of death by as much as 30%. These findings will certainly encourage wider use in infancy even though no comparable evaluation has yet been attempted in children. Fluid retention develops in heart failure when the kidney responds inappropriately to underperfusion, in the same way as it does to volume depletion, by conserving sodium and retaining water. While angiotensin-converting enzyme (ACE) inhibitors such as captopril (q.v.) work by countering this response, at least temporarily, it is now clear that spironolactone use confers additional benefit.

A loop diuretic such as furosemide (q.v.) can improve pulmonary compliance in babies with ventilator-induced chronic lung disease. A thiazide, such as chlorothiazide (q.v.), is better for long-term treatment, and it is common practice to give both a thiazide and spironolactone, although the value of this practice has, as yet, only been assessed in one small trial (that found no evidence of benefit). Spironolactone can be of use in the long-term management of Bartter syndrome while high-dose treatment can also help to control ascites in babies with chronic neonatal hepatitis. Treatment should always be stopped if there is renal failure because of the risk of hyperkalaemia. Spironolactone crosses the placenta and use during pregnancy has produced feminisation in male rat fetuses, but there is no other evidence to suggest that use during pregnancy is dangerous. Some of the metabolites appear in breast milk, but use during lactation has not caused problems and only results in the baby ingesting 1–2% of the maternal dose (when this is calculated on a weight-for-weight basis).

Treatment

Use as a diuretic: Give 1 mg/kg of spironolactone together with 10 mg/kg of chlorothiazide twice a day by mouth in the management of chronic congestive cardiac failure. Congestive failure that fails to respond to this standard dose may sometimes respond if the dose of both drugs is doubled.
Use in hepatic ascites: A dose of up to 3·5 mg/kg by mouth twice a day is sometimes used in ascites secondary to liver disease, although patients need monitoring for possible hyperkalaemia.

Supply

Spironolactone is available as a 2 mg/ml sugar-free oral suspension (costing £10 per 100 ml) although this is a special formulation for which no formal product licence currently exists. Other strength suspensions also exist. It is also widely available in tablet form from a number of pharmaceutical companies.

References

Hobbins SM, Fower RC, Row RD, *et al*. Spironolactone therapy in infants with congestive heart failure secondary to congenital heart disease. *Arch Dis Child* 1981;**56**:934–8. [RCT]

Hoffman DJ, Gerdes JS, Abbasi S. Pulmonary function and electrolyte balance following spironolactone treatment in preterm infants with chronic lung disease: a double-blind, placebo-controlled, randomized trial. *J Perinatol* 2000;**1**:41–5. [RCT]

Kao LC, Durand DJ, Philliops BL, *et al*. Randomized trial of long-term diuretic therapy for infants with oxygen dependent bronchopulmonary dysplasia. *J Pediatr* 1994;**124**:772–81. [RCT]

Pérez-Ayuso RM, Arroyo V, Planas R, *et al*. Randomized comparative study of efficacy of furosemide versus spironolactone in nonazotemic cirrhosis with ascites. *Gastroenterology* 1983;**84**:961–8. [RCT]

Pitt B, Zannad F, Remme WJ, *et al*. The effect of spironolactone on morbidity and mortality in patients with severe heart failure. *N Engl J Med* 1999;**341**:709–17. [RCT] (See also pp. 753–5.)

Shah PS. Current perspectives on the prevention and management of chronic lung disease in preterm babies. *Pediatr Drugs* 2003;**5**:463–80. [SR]

Use

Streptokinase can be used to lyse arterial thrombi when there is symptomatic vascular occlusion. Take the advice of a vascular surgeon where this is available. See the website commentary for a more detailed discussion of the available options.

Pharmacology

Streptokinase is a protein obtained from certain strains of the group C haemolytic *Streptococcus*. It was first purified in 1962, and its amino acid sequence established in 1982. The half life on infusion is about 25 minutes. It activates human plasminogen to form plasmin, a proteolytic enzyme with fibrinolytic effects used to dissolve intravascular blood clots. The plasminogen activator alteplase (q.v.) is a more expensive alternative. Start treatment as soon as there is evidence of an obstructive intravascular thrombus and seek confirmation either by ultrasound or, preferably, by angiography. The relative merits of embolectomy, anticoagulation with heparin and treatment with streptokinase remain undetermined, but embolectomy is often impracticable, and treatment with heparin (q.v.) is of more use as a prophylactic measure than as a therapeutic strategy. Documentary evidence of the value of lytic therapy does not exist, and treatment is not risk free, but treatment is probably merited for arterial lesions that look set to cause tissue necrosis (gangrene). There is no good evidence that thrombosed renal veins benefit from active treatment and even less information on the wisdom of treating other venous thrombi. A collaborative controlled trial might shed some light on these issues. Streptokinase antibodies develop and persist for 6–12 months after treatment making repeat treatment less effective and adverse reactions more likely. Instillation into the pleural cavity has sometimes been used to speed recovery where there is a particularly severe thoracic empyema in older children, but urokinase (q.v.) has been the lytic agent more widely used in published studies of this condition in children. Use during pregnancy to treat maternal thromboembolism does not seem to have caused any direct or indirect threat to the fetus to date, and the teratogenic risk must be minimal because the drug does not cross the placenta. Its use in the intrapartum period might be more problematic. Use during lactation seems unlikely, on theoretical grounds, to pose a serious problem.

Treatment

Arterial thrombi: Give a loading dose of 3000 units/kg of streptokinase slowly IV as soon as the diagnosis is made, followed by a continuous infusion of 1000 units/kg per hour (1 ml/hour of a solution made up as described below). Higher doses have been used with apparent impunity, but there is no evidence, as yet, that they are more effective. Treatment should continue until vascular flow returns, which may only take 4 hours but may be delayed 24–36 hours. Avoid IM injections during treatment and treat any bleeding from puncture sites with local pressure.

Blocked shunts and catheters: Dilute 10,000 units with enough 0·9% sodium chloride to fill the catheter dead space. Instil and leave for 1 hour before aspirating. Flush with heparinised saline.

Dose monitoring

Monitor the fibrinogen level if treatment is necessary for more than 6 hours, aiming for a level of between 1 and 1·4 g/l. Slow or stop the infusion temporarily if the level falls below 1 g/l.

Antidote

Tranexamic acid can control bleeding by inhibiting the activation of plasminogen to plasmin. Try an IV infusion of 10 mg/kg over 10 minutes and repeat if necessary after 8–12 hours.

Supply and administration

Vials of streptokinase as a powder for reconstitution in 5 ml of water for injection are available from the pharmacy (250,000 unit vials cost £14). Take care to prevent the production of foam. Vials kept at 4°C can be used for 12 hours after reconstitution. For IV use take 0·4 ml of reconstituted solution for each kg the baby weighs, dilute to 20 ml with 10% glucose or glucose saline, and infuse at a rate of 1 ml/hour. This provides 1000 units/kg of streptokinase per hour. (A less concentrated solution of glucose or glucose saline can be used if necessary.) Prepare a fresh solution every 12 hours. 5 ml (500 mg) ampoules of tranexamic acid cost £1·50.

References

See also the relevant Cochrane reviews

Cheah F-C, Boo N-Y, Rohana J, *et al*. Successful clot lysis using low dose of streptokinase in 22 neonates with aortic thromboses. *J Paediatr Child Health* 2001;**37**:479–82.

Monagle P, Michelson AD, Bovill E, *et al*. Antithrombotic therapy in children. *Chest* 2001;**119**:344S–370S. [SR]

Nowak-Göttl U, von Kries R, Göbel U. Neonatal symptomatic thromboembolism in Germany: two year survey. *Arch Dis Child* 1997;**76**:F163–7.

Schmidt B, Andrew M. Neonatal thrombosis: report of a prospective Canadian and international registry. *Pediatrics* 1995;**96**:939–43.

Singh M, Mathew JL, Chandra S, *et al*. Randomized controlled trial of intrapleural streptokinase in empyema thoracis in children. *Acta Paediatr* 2004;**93**:1443–5. [RCT]

Turrentine MA, Braems G, Ramirez MM. Use of thrombolytics for the treatment of thromboembolic disease during pregnancy. *Obstet Gynecol Surv* 1995;**50**:534–41.

Use

Giving a newborn baby something sweet to suck reduces the physical response to blood letting. Nevertheless, while such distraction significantly reduces the physical response to pain, it has yet to be shown that sucrose reduces stress, or that it works because it has some pharmaceutical property.

Pharmacology

The potential analgesic effect of sucrose has only been poorly studied. There has been some suggestion that a concentrated sugar solution may affect the endogenous opioid system in young rats if given shortly before pain is inflicted. However, babies pre-exposed to the opioid antagonist naloxone (q.v) actually cried for a shorter, rather than a longer, time in one recent nurse-initiated trial.

Managing brief pain

Fourteen randomised controlled trials included in the Cochrane Review provide unequivocal evidence that babies cry less when given sucrose to suck 2 minutes before being subjected to a painful procedure. However, it has no effect on the rise in heart rate or in oxygen consumption. Blood letting was the cause of pain investigated in all these studies. A wide range of doses have been used (0·01–1 gram), and higher doses do seem to produce a greater effect. Rather fewer studies have yet looked at the efficacy of this strategy in babies more than a month old. Three recent studies suggest that breastfeeding on its own can be just as effective. Efficacy is also enhanced if the baby is held close (cuddled) throughout the procedure or, more impersonally, given a dummy or pacifier to suck. The artificial sweetener aspartame seems as effective as sucrose. So is glucose, but formula milk is not. Sucrose only works when given orally – it is ineffective when given direct into the stomach. Preterm babies show less of a reduction in their 'pain score' than term babies.

Sucrose seems as effective in babies as lidocaine-prilocaine (EMLA) cream. However, other studies have shown that while the latter significantly reduces the pain associated with venepuncture in older children it has relatively little impact on the way babies respond to this procedure (as discussed in the monograph on lidocaine). No comparison with tetracaine (q.v.) has yet been published. Sweets possess a magical ability to keep a child of *any* age quiet, but this does not mean

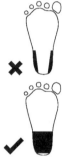

that other strategies do not need to be pursued in parallel (see web commentary). The best way to avoid both heel prick pain and iatrogenic anaemia is, of course, not to take the sample at all. When sampling is necessary, much can be done to ensure that all necessary specimens are collected at one and the same time.

Minimising heel prick pain

Diabetics know that the pain associated with collecting blood is minimised by using a spring-loaded lance. A 2·4 mm Autolet® is ideal for collecting up to 1 ml of blood and seems to cause no more pain than venepuncture. The Tenderfoot®, which has a blade rather than a lance, is more expensive but more effective when a larger sample is required. A wide range of manual devices also exist. Some that are very easy to use (such as the Becton Dickson Microtainer Safety Flow®) look as though they are automated but are not. Prior warming is of negligible value, and ultrasound studies have shown that there is no risk of hitting bone with a 2·4 mm lance irrespective of where you take blood. It is not, therefore, necessary to restrict sampling to the sides of the heel as once recommended. That just leaves the heel of any baby who has had a lot of blood taken hypersensitive and very scarred. The whole dark-shaded area is safe (Fig. 1). Just avoid the area at the back (where you get a blister if your shoes are too tight).

Fig. 1

Care strategy

The optimum approach is probably to drop 2 ml of a 25% solution of sucrose onto the swaddled baby's tongue 2 minutes before starting to take blood, and then give the baby a dummy or comforter to suck.

Supply

Any pharmacy can easily make up a safe, stable 25% solution of sucrose at negligible cost (dissolve 25 g of sucrose in water and make up to 100 ml). The Autolet is manufactured by Owen Mumford Ltd, Woodstock, Oxford, UK, and the Tenderfoot by International Technidyne Corporation, Edison, NJ, USA.

References

See also the Cochrane reviews of pain relief

Anand KJS, and the International Evidence-Based Group for Neonatal Pain. Consensus statement for the prevention and management of pain in the newborn. *Arch Pediatr Adolesc Med* 2001;**155**:173–80.

Bauer K, Ketteler J, Hellwig M, *et al*. Oral glucose before venepuncture relieves neonates of pain, but stress is still evidenced by increase in oxygen consumption, energy expenditure, and heart rate. *Pediatr Res* 2004;**55**:695–700.

Boyle EM, Freer Y, Khan-Orakzai Z, *et al*. Sucrose and non-nutritive sucking for the relief of pain in screening for retinopathy of prematurity: a randomised controlled trial. *Arch Dis Child* 2006;**91**:F166–8. [RCT]

Chermont AG, Falcão LFM, de Souza Silva EH, *et al*. Skin-to-skin contact and/or 25% dextrose for procedural pain relief for term newborn infants. *Pediatrics* 2009;**124**:e1101–7. [RCT]

Codipietro L, Ceccarelli M, Ponzone A. Breastfeeding or oral sucrose solution in term neonates receiving heel lance: a randomized controlled trial. *Pediatrics* 2008;**122**:e71621. [RCT]

Gradin M, Schollin J. The role of endogenous opioids in mediating pain reduction by orally administered glucose among newborns. *Pediatrics* 2005;**115**:1004–7. [RCT]

Jain A, Rutter N. Ultrasound study of heel to calcaneum depth in neonates. *Arch Dis Child* 1999;**80**:F243–5.

Use
Sulfadiazine is used with pyrimethamine (q.v.) in the treatment of toxoplasmosis.

History
The story of how penicillin was discovered has often eclipsed any memory of how the study of a simple chemical dye by Bayer (Prontosil®) led to the discovery of the first effective antibacterial drug in 1932. The German discovery soon led the French to show that the smaller molecule *p*-aminobenzenesulphonamide (or sulphanilamide) was as effective as Prontosil itself, and that Prontosil dye only worked after it was broken down to sulphanilamide within the body. Within 4 years clinical trials backed by the MRC at Queen Charlotte's Hospital in London had established that both drugs could save women from almost certain death from streptococcal infection in childbirth. Alexander Gordon in Aberdeen had been the first to show that it was the birth attendant who transmitted this 'puerperal fever' from mother to mother in 1792, but it took a century, and the work of Louis Pasteur and Joseph Lister, for this to be generally accepted. No other single discovery has ever done so much to make childbirth safe.

Other sulphonamides soon followed, including sulphapyridine by May and Baker (M&B 693), which was effective in pneumococcal pneumonia. Soon all the sulphonamides were shown to work by blocking bacterial folic acid synthesis. The drug was lethal to bacteria and not to man because man acquired folic acid in his diet instead of metabolising it himself. Recognition of this underlying principle was later to help shape the discovery of a wide range of other antimicrobial drugs. While the importance of the sulphonamides has dwindled as many previously susceptible organisms have developed resistance, sulphadimidine is still occasionally used to treat urinary infection, silver sulfadiazine cream was used in several neonatal trials of skin care and is still used in the management of burns, sulfasalazine is used in ulcerative colitis, and sulfamethoxazole is used as a component of co-trimoxazole (q.v.).

Evidence that the prophylactic use of sulfafurazole in preterm babies to prevent infection actually caused an *increase* in death and kernicterus eventually led to a recognition that sulphonamides could displace bilirubin from albumin and cause free bilirubin to enter the brain causing toxic brain damage. The trial by Silverman that brought this problem to light in 1956 did much to convince neonatologists that a trial with random allocation is the only way of establishing both the possible benefits and possible hazards associated with every new form of treatment (as the web commentary describes).

Pharmacology
Most sulphonamides are well absorbed when given by mouth, are widely distributed in the body, and are excreted after partial conjugation by a combination of renal filtration and tubular secretion. Hypersensitivity reactions usually first present with a rash and a fever after about 9 days; treatment should be stopped before more serious symptoms develop. Blood dyscrasias have been reported. Exfoliative dermatitis, epidermal necrolysis (Lyell syndrome) and a severe, potentially lethal, form of erythema multiforme (Stevens–Johnson syndrome) have occurred in children and adults. Haemolysis is a hazard in patients with G6PD deficiency. The adult half life of sulfadiazine is 10 hours, but double this in the first week of life. Sulfadiazine is not very soluble in urine, so damaging crystal formation in the renal tract (with haematuria) is possible if fluid intake is low. Manufacturers remain reluctant to endorse the use of *any* sulphonamide in a child less than 6–8 weeks old because of the risk of kernicteric brain damage, but such a generalisation shows disproportionate caution because sulfadiazine does not displace bilirubin from albumin nearly as strongly as sulfafurazole. There is no evidence that any sulphonamide is teratogenic, but maternal use is probably best avoided in the period immediately before delivery. Only small quantities appear in breast milk, so breastfeeding only needs to be avoided in babies who are jaundiced, or both premature and ill.

Treatment
Maternal disease: Give 1 gram of sulfadiazine every 8 hours by mouth together with 50 mg of pyrimethamine once a day if *Toxoplasma* infection seems to have spread to the fetus. Spiramycin (q.v.) is probably a more appropriate alternative if transplacental spread is not thought to have occurred.
Neonatal disease: Treatment of toxoplasmal infection with pyrimethamine should be augmented by giving 50 mg/kg of sulfadiazine by mouth once every 12 hours.

Supply
500 mg tablets of sulfadiazine cost 31p each. A sugar-free suspension can be prepared from these with a 1 week shelf life stored at 4°C.

References
Fichter EG, Curtis JA. Sulfonamide administration in newborn and premature infants. *Pediatrics* 1956;**18**:50−8.
Loudon I. *Death in childbirth: an international study of maternal care and maternal mortality 1800–1950*. Oxford: Oxford University Press, 1992.
Odell GB. Studies in kernicterus. I. The protein binding of bilirubin. *J Clin Invest* 1959;**38**:823−33.
Silverman WA, Anderson TH, Blanc WA, *et al*. A difference in mortality rate and incidence of kernicterus among premature infants allotted to two prophylactic antibacterial regimens. *Pediatrics* 1956;**18**:614−25. [RCT]

Use

Lack of surfactant is the commonest cause of death in the preterm baby. Synthetic products and products of animal origin both have the ability to reduce mortality by 40% in babies of less than 30 weeks' gestation. Antenatal treatment with betamethasone (q.v.) is an even more cost-effective way of reducing mortality.

Physiology

Although rare inherited congenital defects may render a few term babies permanently unable to make surfactant, the main use for surfactant replacement is in the preterm baby with respiratory distress syndrome (RDS). The lung of the very preterm baby may contain as little as 10 mg/kg of surfactant at birth (a tenth of the amount found at term). Whilst labour and/or birth trigger a surge of production, this takes 48 hours to become effective. Care needs to be exercised during this time; both acidosis and hypothermia interfere with this process, while alveolar collapse increases surfactant consumption. The development of artificial and natural products to bridge this time gap, and their rigorous evaluation, has been one of the major achievements of neonatal medicine in the last 20 years. Endogenous surfactant has a half life of about 12 hours, after which some is recycled and some is degraded. The baby who is deficient at birth, therefore, needs to be given 100 mg/kg as soon as possible to prevent atelectasis (alveolar collapse) developing and, if destruction initially exceeds production, one (and occasionally two) further doses 12 and 24 hours later. Inactivation seems to occur more rapidly when there is infection or meconium aspiration, rendering a larger dose appropriate.

It is now widely accepted that if non-invasive respiratory support can be provided for babies who are surfactant deficient at birth this will reduce the numbers of babies with chronic oxygen dependency. The *first* critical step is to aerate the lung as gently as possible at birth using pressure sustained for several seconds to achieve initial lung expansion before even thinking to 'ventilate' the baby. The *second* critical step is to prevent atelectasis by using CPAP or even non-invasive positive pressure ventilation (NIPPV). The more vulnerable babies may also benefit from early surfactant, but everything should be done to minimise the need to provide ongoing respiratory support using a tube through the larynx.

There is a naïve belief that because all births at 37–41 weeks' gestation are referred to as 'term' births, there is no risk of these babies being surfactant deficient at birth. Unfortunately this is not true – babies delivered electively at 37 weeks' gestation can still be surfactant deficient.

Range of products currently available

Although surfactant deficiency was first recognised to be the cause of RDS in preterm babies in 1959 it was 20 years before the first two **synthetic** products first became available. Only one of these, colfoceril palmitate (Exosurf Neonatal®), which contains 108 mg of phosphatidylcholine, 12 mg of hexadecanol and 8 mg of tyloxapol per vial, is still being produced, and it is now only marketed in a few countries. Many expected that lucinactant (Surfaxin®), which contains a 21 amino acid analogue of part of the surfactant protein B molecule, would become commercially available in 2009. It has been the subject of several large clinical trials, but it has not yet received final clearance from the FDA in America. If competitively priced it might become a well supported option in some countries.

Products of **animal** origin first became widely available in 1990. Poractant alfa (Curosurf®) is an extract of minced porcine lung, with phospholipids and surfactant proteins B and C, while beractant (Survanta®) is a minced bovine lung extract containing phospholipids, neutral lipids, fatty acids and surfactant-associated proteins with added phosphatidylcholine, palmitic acid and tripalmitin. Another product of bovine origin, BLES® (bovine lung extract surfactant), is available in Canada. Two products obtained by bovine lung lavage are also in use: calfactant (Infasurf®) marketed in America, and bovactant (Alveofact®) in Europe.

Natural surfactants have a more rapid onset of action. Head-to-head trials of a natural surfactant (beractant or calfactant) and an artificial surfactant (colfoceril) in 2500 preterm babies with established respiratory distress have shown that survival is marginally, but unequivocally, better with beractant. Using beractant instead of colfoceril produced two more survivors for every 100 babies studied. However, the different natural surfactants may not have identical properties either – poractant alfa seems to act more rapidly than beractant, and survival may be better (although direct comparison is made difficult by differing dosage regimens). New synthetic products currently under development and which contain surfactant proteins and peptides may eventually replace the present natural products.

Indications for use

Babies less than 30 weeks' gestation merit a first dose as soon as possible after birth, more so if they are intubated at that time. The cost of treating babies more mature than this is harder to justify until it is clear that they need more than 40% oxygen to sustain an arterial pO_2 above 7 kPa (90% SaO_2). Babies needing ventilation for pneumonia or meconium aspiration merit consideration for treatment with a product containing surfactant proteins (see website commentary).

Treatment

Poractant alfa: Give 100 mg/kg (1·25 ml/kg) into the trachea as soon after birth as possible if surfactant deficiency seems likely, but be selective over the need for further doses. Some give a second dose after 12 hours if the base deficit at birth was greater than 10 mmol/l, if the baby continues to need ventilation with a mean airway pressure of above 7 cmH₂O in ≥40% oxygen, or if there are signs of pneumonia. Consider giving a larger first dose if there is severe meconium aspiration, or if treatment is started late.

Beractant: Give 100 mg/kg (4 ml/kg) in the same way as for poractant alfa but in 2–3 aliquots. (The manufacturers say up to three further doses can be given, at least 6 hours apart, within the next 48 hours.)

Continued

Optimising usage

Surfactant treatment can be very cost-effective but remains expensive and a lot can be done to limit redundant and unnecessary treatment. If the lung disease is more severe there is much to recommend giving subsequent doses of surfactant earlier than the manufacturers recommend. Likewise there is little to be gained by giving surfactant to a ventilated baby needing ≤30% oxygen when the mean airway pressure is less than 7 cmH$_2$O. One small study has explored giving intratracheal liquid budesonide (q.v.) with surfactant in an attempt to reduce chronic lung disease in very preterm infants.

Administration

It is traditional to instil the prescribed dose down an endotracheal tube using a fine catheter with the baby supine after clearing any mucus and pre-oxygenating the lungs to minimise cyanosis during administration.

For many years it was assumed that if surfactant was required then the baby would need both intubation and sustained respiratory support – neither of these assumptions is necessarily correct. Surfactant can be given using the INSURE procedure (*in*tubation *sur*factant *e*xtubation (Victorin *et al.* 1990)) or even via a fine catheter passed 1·5 cm through the larynx of the unintubated, spontaneously breathing infant (Kribs *et al.* 2009).

A 1–2 mg/kg IV dose of the ultra short-acting opiate remifentanil (q.v.) given 60 seconds before attempting intubation will blunt any pain and cause muscle relaxation, but the 2 mg/kg dose will often depress respiration enough to make it wise to delay extubation for 10–20 minutes. It is widely thought that giving the appropriate dose of surfactant in a small volume of fluid will cause fewer cardiovascular disturbances, but a larger volume leads to a more even dispersal within the lung. Surfactant can be given in less than a minute (rather than 4 minutes, as manufacturers often recommend) without causing bradycardia or cyanosis. Ignore any that subsequently reappears in the tracheal tube. Hand ventilate or reintubate if the tube seems to have become blocked. Natural surfactants increase lung compliance and oxygenation rapidly – you should be prepared to reduce the ventilator settings and, more especially, the amount of oxygen quite soon after they are given.

Supply

Poractant alfa comes in 1·5 and 3 ml ready-to-use vials containing 120 and 240 mg of phospholipid costing £380 and £760 each. Beractant comes in 8 ml vials containing 200 mg of phospholipids, which cost £310; 4 ml (100 mg) vials are also available in some countries. Store vials at 4°C, but warm to room temperature before use, and invert gently without shaking to resuspend the material. Do not use, or return vials to the refrigerator, more than 8 hours after they reach room temperature.

References

See also the relevant Cochrane reviews

Broadbent R, Fok T-F, Dolovich M, *et al*. Chest position and pulmonary disposition of surfactant in surfactant depleted rabbits. *Arch Dis Child Fetal Neonatal Ed* 1995;**72**:F84–9.

Buckmaster AG, Arnolda G, Wright IMR, *et al*. Continuous positive airway pressure therapy for infants with respiratory distress in non-tertiary care centers: a randomized controlled trial. *Pediatrics* 2007;**120**:509–18. [RCT]

Engle WA, and the Committee on Fetus and Newborn. Surfactant-replacement therapy for respiratory distress in the preterm and term neonate. *Pediatrics* 2008;**121**:419–32. [SR]

Kattwinkel J, Bloom BT, Delmore P, *et al*. High- versus low-threshold surfactant retreatment for neonatal respiratory distress syndrome. *Pediatrics* 2000;**106**:282–8. [RCT]

Kribs A, Vierzig A, Hünseler C, *et al*. Early surfactant in spontaneously breathing with nCPAP in ELBW infants – a single centre four year experience. *Acta Paediatr* 2009;**97**:293–8.

Moya M, Maturana A. Animal-derived surfactants versus past and current synthetic surfactants: current status. *Clin Perinatol* 2007;**34**:145–77.

Schaschini M, Nogee LM, Sassi I, *et al*. Unexplained neonatal respiratory distress caused by congenital surfactant deficiency. *J Pediatr* 2007;**15**:649–53.

Sweet D, Bevilacqua G, Carnielli V, *et al*. European consensus guidelines on the management of neonatal respiratory distress syndrome. *J Perinat Med* 2007;**35**:175–86. [SR]

Sweet DG, Halliday HL. The use of surfactants 2009. [Review] *Arch Dis Child Ed Pract* 2009;**94**:78–93.

te Pas AB, Walther FJ. A randomized, controlled trial of delivery-room respiratory management in very preterm infants. *Pediatrics* 2007;**120**:322–9. [RCT]

Verder H, Bohlin K, Kamper J, *et al*. Nasal CPAP and surfactant for treatment of respiratory distress syndrome and prevention of bronchopulmonary dysplasia. [Review] *Acta Paediatr* 2009;**98**:1400–8.

Victorin LH, Deverajan LV, Curstedt T, *et al*. Surfactant replacement in spontaneously breathing babies with hyaline membrane disease – a pilot study. *Biol Neonat* 1990;**58**:121–6.

Welzing L, Kribs A, Huenseler C, *et al*. Remifentanil for INSURE in preterm infants: a pilot study for evaluation of efficacy and safety aspects. *Acta Paediatr* 2009;**98**:1416–20.

Yeh T, Lin HC, Chang CH, *et al*. Early intratracheal instillation of budesonide using surfactant as a vehicle to prevent chronic lung disease in preterm infants: a pilot study. *Pediatrics* 2008;**121**:e1311. [RCT]

SUXAMETHONIUM = Succinylcholine

Use
Suxamethonium was long used to ease endotracheal intubation by providing short-term muscle paralysis.

Pharmacology
Suxamethonium was first developed in 1906, but only came into clinical use in 1951. It acts by mimicking acetycholine, the chemical that normally transmits all nerve impulses to voluntary muscle. However, because suxamethonium is more slowly hydrolysed by plasma and liver cholinesterases (the adult half life being 2−3 minutes), the nerve terminal becomes blocked for a time to all further stimuli. As a result suxamethonium produces rapid and complete muscle paralysis. An effect (phase I block) is seen within 30 seconds after IV injection, but usually only lasts 3−6 minutes. Recovery is spontaneous, but somewhat delayed in patients taking magnesium sulphate. Unlike the *non*-depolarising muscle relaxants, such as pancuronium and rocuronium (q.v.), the action of suxamethonium cannot be reversed.

Large doses cause excessive quantities of suxamethonium to accumulate at the nerve−muscle junction producing prolonged, competitive (phase II) block. Suxamethonium causes a 0·5 mmol rise in plasma potassium, making its use unwise in babies with existing hyperkalaemia. It also causes prolonged paralysis in patients who have inherited one of the abnormal genes associated with deficient cholinesterase production (about 0·04% of the population). While this seldom complicates neonatal care to a serious degree, it can cause prolonged respiratory depression after Caesarean delivery when both mother and baby have such a defect. Children with a parental history of cholinesterase deficiency should probably have their genetic status determined when they are 6 or more months old because the pseudocholinesterase level and type are easily determined from a 2 ml serum sample. Breastfeeding is not contraindicated.

Use to facilitate tracheal intubation
Trials have shown that prior paralysis can prevent the rise in intracranial pressure and reduce the fall in arterial pO_2 usually seen during neonatal intubation, even though it does not prevent some rise in blood pressure. However, paralysis does nothing to reduce the pain and distress associated with intubation while suxamethonium, because it mimics acetylcholine, often causes an initial transient period of painful muscle fasciculation. Indeed the rise in blood pressure rather suggests that the babies in these studies were still under stress. Mivacurium (q.v.) does not cause the muscle spasm seen with suxamethonium, but does leave the baby paralysed for 10−20 minutes. Anaesthetists nearly always administer nitrous oxide, or give a second drug IV, before inducing neuromuscular blockade, to minimise pain. Midazolam, thiopental, methohexital and propofol (q.v.) have all been used for this purpose, but none of these products abolishes pain as effectively as an opiate. Unfortunately morphine takes 5−10 minutes to become fully effective even though it produces a detectable effect within 1 minute. In contrast, the new opiate remifentanil (q.v.) is effective within 90 seconds, and a 3 microgram/kg dose usually causes enough muscle relaxation to make formal muscle paralysis unnecessary in children less than a year old. It now looks as though propofol may be equally effective, rendering the use of even a short-acting opioid like remifentanil unnecessary.

Premedication
A 15 microgram/kg dose of atropine (q.v.) is traditionally given prior to suxamethonium administration, to reduce any reactive bradycardia and increased salivation. However, problems are so uncommon with neonatal *single* dose use that this step can be omitted as long the drug is readily 'to hand'.

Treatment
A 2 mg/kg dose of suxamethonium IV provides 5−10 minutes of muscle paralysis. A 3 mg/kg IV dose provides maximum neuromuscular blockade. A 4 mg/kg dose IM can be used to provide 10−30 minutes of paralysis after a latent period of 2−3 minutes. Staff should **never** paralyse a baby unless they are confident that they can keep the airway open and hand ventilate the baby when necessary.

Supply and administration
2 ml ampoules containing 100 mg of suxamethonium chloride costs 71p. Take 0·2 ml and dilute to 1 ml with 5% glucose or glucose saline in a 1 ml syringe to obtain a preparation containing 10 mg/ml for accurate neonatal administration.

References

Byrne E, MacKinnon R. Should premedication be used for semi-urgent or elective intubation in neonates. *Arch Dis Child* 2006;**91**:79−83. [SR]

Chaudhary R, Chonat S, Gowra H, *et al*. Use of premedication for intubation in tertiary neonatal units in the United Kingdom. *Pediatr Anesth* 2009;**19**:653−8.

Cook DR, Windhard LB, Taylor FH. Pharmacokinetics of succinylcholine in infants, children and adults. *Clin Pharmacol Ther* 1976;**20**:493−8.

Lemyre B, Cheng R, Gaboury I. Atropine, fentanyl and succinylcholine for non-urgent intubation in newborns. *Arch Dis Child* 2009;**94**:F439−42.

Meakin G, McKiernan EP, Baker RD. Dose−response curves for suxamethonium in neonates, infants and children. *Br J Anaesth* 1989; **62**:655−8.

Morton NS. Tracheal intubation without neuromuscular blocking drugs in children. [Editorial] *Pediatr Anesth* 2009;**19**:199−20.

Wyllie JP. Neonatal endotracheal intubation. [Review] *Arch Dis Child Educ Pract Ed* 2008;**93**:44−9.

Use

Teicoplanin is a useful antibiotic that is currently more expensive vial for vial than vancomycin (q.v.), but it only needs to be given once a day, does not need to be given as slowly as vancomycin, and can (when necessary) be given IM. Vancomycin-resistant organisms are sometimes sensitive to teicoplanin.

Pharmacology

Teicoplanin is a complex of five closely related glycopeptide antibiotics with similar antibacterial properties to vancomycin that were first isolated in 1976. Teicoplanin is active against many Gram-positive anaerobes and is particularly potent against *Clostridium* species. It is also active against most *Listeria*, enterococci and staphylococci (including meticillin-resistant strains), although it may work more as a bacteriostatic drug than as a bactericidal drug. Rifampicin (q.v.) can be synergistic in the management of staphylococcal infection. Some coagulase-negative staphylococci are now resistant, requiring treatment with linezolid (q.v.) and rifampicin, and acquired vancomycin cross-resistance is also starting to be reported.

Teicoplanin cannot be given by mouth, but can be given intramuscularly (unlike vancomycin), and does not usually need to be infused slowly to avoid thrombophlebitis when given intravenously (as vancomycin does). Very few children seem to develop adverse effects, and no reports of ototoxicity or nephrotoxicity have yet appeared. Watch for possible leucopenia, thrombocytopenia and disturbances of liver function. Teicoplanin has been used prophylactically in vulnerable babies with a long line in place, but this, like the prophylactic use of vancomycin, remains controversial. Teicoplanin has a high volume of distribution (making an initial loading dose advisable), and penetrates most tissue fluids well, but penetration into the CSF is unsatisfactory and often unpredictable. Almost all the drug is excreted unchanged in the urine, the half life in adults being between 3 and 4 days (many times longer than the half life of vancomycin). Teicoplanin crosses the placenta, and little is yet known about the safety of using teicoplanin during human pregnancy. Use during lactation is unlikely to be hazardous because uptake from the intestinal tract is very limited.

Prophylaxis against bacterial endocarditis

Consider giving babies with structural heart disease 6 mg/kg of teicoplanin and 2 mg/kg of gentamicin IV or IM 30–60 minutes before any invasive operation involving a site where infection is suspected. Amoxicillin (q.v.) or azithromycin (q.v.) are the alternatives more commonly employed.

Treatment

Babies less than 1 month old: Give a 16 mg/kg loading dose IV followed by 8 mg/kg IV or IM once every 24 hours. Treat proven septicaemia for at least 7 days. Double the dosage interval in renal failure.
Older infants: Little has been published on optimising treatment in later infancy (see web commentary). Give three 10 mg/kg IV doses 12 hours apart, and then 10 mg/kg once every 24 hours.

Blood levels

Monitoring is not necessary to avoid toxicity, but may sometimes be appropriate to check that the trough level is at least 10 mg/l (and preferably nearer 20 mg/l) in ill babies with overt, deep-seated infection. The trough level should also be checked where possible after 3 days treatment in babies in renal failure.

Supply

Stock 200 mg vials (costing £18) come with an ampoule of sterile water. Reconstitute by adding the whole of the ampoule of water (3·2 ml) slowly to the vial, and roll the vial gently between the hands until all the powder has dissolved without foaming. If foam does develop let the vial stand for 15 minutes until the foam subsides. Then remove some air and add a further 2 ml of 0·9% sodium chloride. The solution so prepared contains 40 mg/ml of teicoplanin. Administer using a 1 ml syringe. The solution can, if economic pressures so dictate, be kept for up to 24 hours if stored at 4°C, but it contains no preservative. Slow infusion over 30 minutes has sometimes been recommended, especially if the baby is less than a month old, but is not necessary if the administrative procedures outlined in the introduction to this compendium are followed.

References

Degraeuwe PLJ, Beuman GH, van Tiel FH, *et al*. Use of teicoplanin in preterm neonates with staphylococcal late-onset sepsis. *Biol Neonat* 1998;**73**:287–94.
Fanos V, Kacet N, Mosconi G. A review of teicoplanin in the treatment of serious neonatal infections. *Eur J Pediatr* 1997;**156**:423–7.
Kacet N, Dubos JP, Roussel-Delvallez M, *et al*. Teicoplanin and amikacin in neonates with staphylococcal infection. *Pediatr Infect Dis J* 1993;**12**:S10–13.
Lukas JC, Karikas G, Gazouli M, *et al*. Pharmacokinetics of teicoplanin in an ICU population of children and infants. *Pharm Res* 2004;**21**:2064–71.
Möller JC, Nelskamp I, Jensen R, *et al*. Teicoplanin pharmacology in prophylaxis for coagulase-negative staphylococcal sepsis in very low birthweight infants. *Acta Paediatr* 1996;**85**:638–40.
Neumeister B, Kastner S, Conrad S, *et al*. Characterisation of coagulase-negative staphylococci causing nosocomial infections in preterm infants. *Eur J Clin Microb Infect Dis* 1995;**14**:856–63.
Reed MD, Yamashita TS, Myers CM, *et al*. The pharmacokinetics of teicoplanin in infants and children. *J Antimicrob Chemother* 1997;**39**:789–96.
Wilson APR, Clinical parmacokinetics of teicoplanin. *Clin Pharmacokinet* 2000;**39**:167–83.

TETRACAINE = Amethocaine (former BAN)

Use

Tetracaine is a useful, well absorbed, topical anaesthetic.

Pharmacology

Tetracaine is an ester-type local anaesthetic related to *para*-aminobenzoic acid that first came into clinical use in 1932. It acts to block nerve conduction by inhibiting nerve depolarisation, and is destroyed by hydrolysis once it enters the blood stream. Some hydrolysis also occurs in the liver. Systemic absorption can lead to myocardial depression complicated by arrhythmia, while restlessness, tremor and convulsions can be followed by drowsiness, respiratory depression and coma. However, absorption is minimal when the product is only applied to unbroken skin as described here. The elimination half life in adults is about 70 minutes; the neonatal rate of elimination is not known. Methaemoglobinaemia has been reported, but such a problem is much more common with the topical anaesthetic prilocaine. Surface application may cause slight oedema and mild itching, possible due to local histamine release. Some mild erythema is often seen – enough on occasion to delineate the treated area. The manufacturers have not yet endorsed the use of tetracaine gel in preterm babies, or babies less than 1 month old. The product is, however, available 'over the counter' without a doctor's prescription. There is no evidence that its use in pregnancy is hazardous.

Strategies for surface anaesthesia

Several local anaesthetics have been utilised to anaesthetise the skin of the newborn baby. Lidocaine (q.v.) and bupivacaine (q.v.) work best if injected into the skin, but can also be used to infiltrate deep tissues. Lidocaine is more rapidly effective, but bupivacaine provides more sustained pain relief. Lidocaine is less cardiotoxic than bupivacaine if accidentally injected into a blood vessel. Lidocaine gel can be used to anaesthetise the urethra, and has also been used during nasal intubation. A eutectic mixture of 2·5% lidocaine and 2·5% prilocaine (EMLA®) can be used to anaesthetise the skin if applied under an occlusive dressing for at least 1 hour before venepuncture (as outlined in the monograph on lidocaine), but tetracaine gel may be rather more effective. Tetracaine certainly works more quickly (producing anaesthesia after 30–45 minutes that lasts 4–6 hours), and this is probably because it is more lipophilic and therefore better at penetrating the stratum corneum of the skin. It causes some mild vasodilatation, whereas lidocaine causes mild blanching and vasoconstriction. Further comparative study may well show topical tetracaine to be the better product to use before neonatal venepuncture or lumbar puncture, although the greater toxicity of systemic tetracaine needs to be noted. Some treatment failures seem to occur whichever product is used. Unfortunately EMLA cream does not seem to reduce the behavioural response to neonatal heel lancing, and tetracaine gel is of little value either.

Pain relief

To achieve local anaesthesia apply the whole of a 1·5 gram tube of the 4% gel to the skin and cover with an occlusive dressing such as Opsite® (or one of a range of other, rather cheaper, products). Remove the dressing after 30 minutes (1 hour at most) and *wipe away all the remaining gel* before attempting venepuncture. Never apply the gel to mucous membranes, or to damaged or broken skin. Tetracaine gel cannot be recommended as a way to significantly reduce the pain caused by heel prick blood sampling.

Toxicity

Wipe the cream off promptly if signs of blistering develop. The effects of systemic toxicity are reviewed in the monograph on bupivacaine.

Supply

Tetracaine is available as a 4% (40 mg/g) gel in 1·5 gram tubes costing £1·10 each designed to deliver about 1 gram of gel when squeezed. Although this is enough to anaesthetise a 5 × 5 cm area of skin, the gel should never be applied to a larger area of skin than is actually necessary. Use does not require a doctor's prescription, but hospital use in the UK does have to be covered by a Patient Group Direction.

References

See also the relevant Cochrane reviews

Arrowsmith J, Campbell C. A comparison of local anaesthetics for venepuncture. *Arch Dis Child* 2000;**82**:309–10. [RCT]

Jain A, Rutter N. Does topical amethocaine gel reduce the pain of venepuncture in newborn infants? A randomised double blind controlled trial. *Arch Dis Child* 2000;**83**:F207–10. [RCT]

Jain A, Rutter N, Ratnayaka M. Topical amethocaine gel for pain relief of heel prick blood sampling: a randomised double blind controlled trial. *Arch Dis Child* 2001;**84**:F56–9. [RCT]

Lawson RA, Smart NG, Gudgeon AC, *et al*. Evaluation of an amethocaine gel preparation for percutaneous analgesia before venous cannulation in children. *Br J Anaesth* 1995;**75**:282–5.

Long CP, McCafferty DF, Sittlington NM, *et al*. Randomized trial of novel tetracaine patch to provide local anaesthesia in neonates undergoing venepuncture. *Br J Anaesth* 2003;**91**:514–18. [RCT]

O'Brien L, Taddio A, Lyszkiewicz DA, *et al*. A critical review of the topical local anesthetifc amethocaine (Ametop™) for pediatric pain. *Pediatr Drugs* 2005;**7**:41–54. [SR]

Taddio A, Lee C, Yip A, *et al*. Intravenous morphine and topical tetracaine for treatment of pain in preterm neonates undergoing central line placement. *JAMA* 2006;**295**:793–800. [RCT]

Use

Tetracosactide is mainly used diagnostically in the evaluation of adrenal cortex hormone deficiency.

Pharmacology

Serum cortisol levels may be low in the newborn, particularly in babies born before term, and show no detectable diurnal variation for 8–12 weeks, but stimulation tests can be used to test the functional integrity of the adrenal gland. Treatment with dexamethasone (q.v.) and other steroid drugs can suppress cortisol secretion, and the normal reactivity of the adrenal gland can remain depressed for several weeks after treatment stops. Preterm babies with a low cortisol level despite stress in the first few days of life who require ventilation seem to be at greater risk of developing chronic lung damage.

Tetracosactide (Synacthen®) is a polypeptide with properties similar to corticotrophin (or ACTH), the hormone produced by the anterior lobe of the pituitary gland, which stimulates the secretion of several adrenal gland hormones, including cortisol (hydrocortisone) and corticosterone. It was first synthesised in 1961. Corticotrophin secretion is, itself, controlled by corticorelin (CRH) release from the hypothalamus in the brain, and influenced by circulating glucocorticoid hormone levels. Stress can stimulate corticotrophin release. Tetracosactide can be used to test the adequacy of the adrenocortical response to stress (colloquially known as a 'Synacthen test' because that is the trade name of the product). A 1 microgram/kg IV test dose of corticorelin provides a better test of pituitary function. Both hormones are rapidly metabolised to a range of inactive oligopeptides within an hour or two of administration. While it is difficult to see how administration could cause any harm, these hormones should only be given to a pregnant or lactating mother for good reason.

Adverse reactions

Anaphylactic and hypersensitivity reactions can occur, so tetracosactide should only be administered under the direct supervision of an experienced and senior hospital specialist. Most severe reactions occur within 30 minutes. See the monograph on immunisation for the management of anaphylaxis. Intramuscular adrenaline always needs to be followed by a prompt infusion of hydrocortisone.

Test procedure

Standard test: It has been traditional to measure the plasma cortisol level immediately before and exactly 30 minutes after giving a 36 microgram/kg test injection of tetracosactide IV. Some advise the collection of a second specimen 60 minutes after the test injection. Tetracosactide administration normally causes a 70 microgram/l (200 nmol/l) rise in the plasma cortisol concentration unless there is primary adrenal failure, but equivocal results are sometimes obtained, especially in the first month of life. The help and advice of a paediatric endocrinologist should always be sought before undertaking any such test in the neonatal period.

Low-dose tests: The procedure described above involves a supramaximal test dose. Very much smaller doses have been used to assess the response of the adrenal gland to a more physiological stimulus (doses as low as 500 nanograms have sometimes been used in adults). What constitutes a 'normal' response to such a low stimulus in the preterm baby is not yet clear. A 1 microgram/kg dose causes a 2–3-fold rise in the baseline cortisol level within 60 minutes in most, but not all, healthy babies of less than 30 weeks' gestation in the second week of life (mean peak value 500–700 nmol/l).

Initial control of 'infantile spasms'

The simplest way to stop infantile spasms is to give 10 mg of prednisolone four times a day for 2 weeks, and then tail treatment off over the next 2 weeks. Give 20 mg three times a day if fits have not stopped after a week. A few clinicians still prefer to start treatment using 0·5 mg (40 IU) of the Synacthen Depot® preparation on alternate days for the first 2 weeks, but it is still necessary to wean the child off steroids with oral prednisolone (as above) after that. Use vigabatrin (q.v.) instead for babies with tuberous sclerosis or Down syndrome.

Supply

1 ml ampoules containing 250 micrograms of tetracosactide (as acetate) for IV or IM use (made by CIBA and marketed under the trade name Synacthen) cost £2·90 each. Note that a 1 mg depot preparation (using a zinc phosphate complex) for IM use is also available in 1 ml ampoules costing £4·20 each. The depot preparation should **not** be used when conducting the standard diagnostic test described above. All ampoules should be protected from light and stored at 4°C. 5 mg soluble prednisolone phosphate tablets cost 8p each.

References

Bolt RJ, van Weissenbruch MM, Popp-Snijders C, *et al*. Maturity of the adrenal cortex in very preterm infants is related to gestational age. *Pediatr Res* 2002;**52**:405–10.

Hingre RV, Gross SJ, Hingre KS, *et al*. Adrenal steroidogenesis in very low birth weight preterm babies. *J Clin Endocrinol Metab* 1994;**78**:266–70.

Karlsson R, Kalllio J, Irjala K, *et al*. Adrenocorticotropin and corticotropin-releasing hormone tests in preterm infants. *J Clin Endocrinol Metab* 2000;**85**:4592–5.

Korte C, Styne D, Merritt TA, *et al*. Link between early adrenal function and respiratory outcome in preterm infants: airway inflammation and patent ductus arteriosus. *Pediatrics* 2000;**105**:320–24.

Lux AL, Edwards SW, Hancock E, *et al*. The United Kingdom Infantile Spasms Study comparing vigabatrin with prednisolone or tetracosactide at 14 days: a multicentre, randomized controlled trial. *Lancet* 2004;**364**:1773–8. [RCT]

TETRACYCLINE

Use

While there are few reasons for using this antibiotic during childhood, it remains the treatment of choice for brucellosis and rickettsial infection, and the most effective treatment for some uncommon erythromycin-resistant mycoplasmal infections. Malaria is sometimes treated with quinine (q.v.) followed by a tetracycline.

Pharmacology

Tetracycline is a naturally occurring antibiotic produced by a *Streptomyces* fungus. It was first isolated in 1952. Tetracycline is bacteriostatic, inhibiting bacterial protein synthesis and cell growth. It is only partially absorbed from the gastrointestinal tract, absorption being further affected by the formation of insoluble complexes in milk. Oral administration can also cause adverse gastrointestinal symptoms, probably as a result of mucosal irritation. CSF penetration is very poor. Most of the drug is excreted in the urine, but substantial amounts appear in bile and faeces. The half life (8 hours) does not seem to vary with age. Tetracycline can exacerbate any existing renal impairment, and IV treatment should also be avoided where there is hepatic impairment. Tetracycline was once widely used in the management of many Gram-positive and -negative infections but the emergence of drug-resistant strains, and the development of alternative agents, have led to a decline in the use of this once popular antibiotic. Doxycycline (a semisynthetic derivative) is sometimes used along with quinine to treat malaria because of its longer half life.

Systemic tetracycline should normally be avoided during childhood because sustained use causes an unsightly green discolouration of the permanent teeth. It remains of value, however, in the treatment of malaria and brucellosis, and of chlamydial, rickettsial, mycoplasmal and protozoal infection, and there are situations where efficacy, availability and low cost still make short-term treatment a logical option. Tetracycline is also active against most spirochetes including *Borrelia*, the cause of Lyme disease. Treatment can occasionally provoked a dangerous rise in CSF pressure (so-called benign intracranial hypertension). While there is no evidence of teratogenicity, tetracycline should not normally be used during late pregnancy because the drug is avidly taken up by developing fetal teeth and bone. More seriously, use in pregnancy has occasionally been associated with fatal maternal hepatotoxicity. Treatment during lactation probably carries little risk: the amount ingested by the baby in breast milk represents less than 5% of the usual therapeutic dose, and absorption seems to be limited by chelation to calcium. Tetracycline has been shown to retard bone growth in the preterm baby, probably because of its absorption by the epiphyseal plate.

Mycoplasmal infection

The mycoplasmas are the smallest free-living microorganisms. They seem to have evolved from Gram-positive bacterial ancestors but lack a cell wall, making them resistant to most antibiotics (which work by attacking these walls). Special techniques are necessary for laboratory isolation. *Mycoplasma hominis* and *Ureaplasma urealyticum* are potential perinatal pathogens that colonise the female genital tract. *M. pneumoniae* only seems to cause infection in older children. Ureaplasmal infection seems to be an important cause of ascending chorioamnionitis, preterm labour and prelabour rupture of membranes. Overt maternal infection has been documented. Such organisms can cause congenital pneumonia, are suspected of being a cause of postnatal pneumonia, and may be a factor in the pathogenesis of chronic lung disease. Two weeks of erythromycin usually suffices. Tetracycline or chloramphenicol (q.v.) may be necessary to eliminate CNS infection, but isolation of the organism from the trachea, urine or CSF, in the absence of any evidence of inflammation (radiological evidence of pneumonia or a raised white cell count), is not in itself evidence of systemic infection. *M. hominis* infections are resistant to erythromycin and require treatment with tetracycline. Polymerase chain reaction (PCR) tests are now becoming available.

Treatment

Systemic treatment: Treat malaria and erythromycin-resistant *Mycoplasma* infection with 5 mg/kg IV once every 12 hours (or 7·5 mg/kg by mouth once every 8 hours) for at least 7 days.
Eye ointment: Topical chlortetracycline ointment has been used to prevent, or (with oral erythromycin) to treat, *Chlamydia* conjunctivitis, as discussed in the monograph on eye drops, but is not available in the UK.

Supply and administration

500 mg vials are only available in the UK on a 'named patient' basis. They cost £5. Reconstitute the powder with 25 ml of water for injection to obtain a solution containing 20 mg/ml. Take 2·5 ml of this solution, dilute immediately before use to 10 ml with 10% glucose to give a solution containing 5 mg/ml for accurate administration, and give through an IV line that contains a terminal 0·22 µm filter. The IV preparation can also be given by mouth (a fresh vial should be opened daily). A 25 mg/ml suspension is available in the US. Intramuscular injection is painful, and absorption erratic. 250 mg tablets cost 4p each.

References

Hammerschlag MR. Pneumonia due to Chlamydia pneumonia in children: epidemiology, diagnosis and treatment. *Pediatr Pulmonol* 2003;**36**:384−90.

Salsky K, Yahav D, Bishara J, *et al*. Treatment of human brucellosis: systematic review and meta-analysis of randomised controlled trials. *BMJ* 2008;**336**:701−4. [SR] (See also pp. 678−9.)

Theilen U, Lyon AJ, Fitzgerald T, *et al*. Infection with *Ureaplasma urealyticum*: is there a specific clinical and radiological course in the preterm infant? *Arch Dis Child* 2004;**89**:F163−7.

Waites KB, Schelonka RL, Xiao L, *et al*. Congenital and opportunistic infections: *Ureaplasma* species and *Mycoplasma hominis*. *Sem Fetal Neonat Med* 2009;**14**:190−9.

Use
THAM is an organic buffer of occasional value in the management of metabolic acidosis where poor renal function and/or the risk of hypernatraemia make it unwise to use sodium bicarbonate.

Pharmacology
THAM (or *tris-hydroxymethyl amino-methane*) is an organic buffer that was used widely at one time in the management of severe ***metabolic*** acidosis (the appropriate management of ***respiratory*** acidosis being, almost without exception, ventilatory support). It is sometimes known as TRIS (from the first four letters of the drug's full chemical name). The drug has to be given intravenously and is normally fairly rapidly excreted by the kidney; some caution needs to be exercised when the drug is used in a baby with impaired renal function. Infusion has also occasionally been reported to cause apnoea, respiratory depression and hypoglycaemia. Extravasation can cause tissue necrosis after IV infusion (see below).

Metabolic acidosis nearly always corrects itself quite quickly once tissue oxygenation improves. Respiratory acidosis is usually corrected by initiating more vigorous respiratory support. Attempts to keep pH above 7·2 can, however, traumatise the lung. There are, in addition, situations where using THAM or sodium bicarbonate (q.v.) to induce an alkalosis can do much to combat persisting pulmonary hypertension. Such strategies were, for many years, probably overused, but they are now probably underused. THAM should always be used in preference to sodium bicarbonate in patients where CO_2 retention is a problem. Bicarbonate is largely ineffective in such a 'closed' system because the additional CO_2 produced by bicarbonate administration causes respiratory acidosis if it is not eliminated promptly through the lungs. However, because THAM is only 80% ionised when pH is in the physiological range, it is not as therapeutically effective as an equivalent molar volume of sodium bicarbonate.

A mixture of THAM and glucose appeared, in a small number of experiments undertaken nearly 50 years ago, to speed the recovery of an effective cardiac output in animals asphyxiated at birth to the point where they were known to be in terminal apnoea. The strategy has never been subjected to further rigorous study, and the long-term outcome for most of the few babies ill enough to really require this sort of intervention at birth is quite bleak. Nevertheless, if the preceding episode of asphyxia has been hyperacute it is sometime worth giving 1·5 ml/kg of 0·6 M THAM (or some sodium bicarbonate) directly into one of the cavities of the heart mixed, if time allows, with a small amount of 10% glucose, if bradycardia persists despite 0·5 minutes of effective cardiac compression after the lung has been aerated at birth. There is, in contrast, *no* evidence that the short- or long-term outcome is improved if the severe acidosis (pH ≤6·8) present in all these babies at birth is corrected *after* the circulation has been restored.

Treatment
Give 0·6 mmol/kg for each unit (mmol/l) by which it is hoped to lower the base deficit, giving the infusion slowly at a rate never exceeding 0·5 mmol/kg per minute. Because of the risk of respiratory depression the drug is usually only given to babies already receiving respiratory support. Partial correction is usually adequate. It is not usually necessary to give more than 5 mmol/kg, but twice as much as this can be given on demand in a real emergency. Birth-related acidosis in the term baby does not merit any such intervention.

Tissue extravasation
Extravasation following IV infusion can cause tissue necrosis; a strategy for the early management of this complication is described in the monograph on hyaluronidase. Accidental intra-arterial injection of THAM is reported to have produced severe haemorrhagic necrosis in some newborn infants (probably because there was circulatory stasis at the time the drug was injected). Localised liver necrosis has also been reported when THAM is given blind and undiluted into the umbilical vein, but most published reports relate to the use of concentrated solutions containing more than 0·6 mmol/ml.

Supply
A commercial preparation is available from Abbott in the USA, and sterile 5 and 10 ml ampoules containing 3·6% (0·3 M) or 7·2% (0·6 M) THAM costing about £6 each are prepared by a number of NHS manufacturing units in the UK using the Addenbrooke's Hospital formula. The isosmotic 3·6% solution, contains 0·3 mmol/ml; the hyperosmolar 7·2% solution, contains 0·6 mmol/ml (conversion factor: 1 mmol = 120 mg).

References
See also the relevant Cochrane reviews

Adamsons K, Behrman R, Dawes GS, *et al.* Resuscitation by positive pressure ventilation and TRIS-hydroxymethyl-aminomethane of rhesus monkeys asphyxiated at birth. *J Pediatr* 1964;**65**:807–18.

Blench HL, Schwartz WB. TRIS buffer (THAM): an appraisal of its physiological effect and clinical usefulness. *N Engl J Med* 1966;**274**:782–6.

Daniel SS, Dawes GS, James LS, *et al.* Analeptics and the resuscitation of asphyxiated monkeys. *BMJ* 1996;**2**:562–3.

Holmdahl MH, Wiklund L, Wetterberg T, *et al.* The place of THAM in the management of acidemia in clinical practice. *Acta Anaesthesiol Scand* 2000;**44**:524–7.

Hoste EA, Colpaert K, Vanholder RC, *et al.* Sodium bicarbonate versus THAM in ICU patients with mild metabolic acidosis. *J Nephrol* 2005;**18**:303–7.

Nahas GG, Sutin KM, Fermon C, *et al.* Guidelines for the treatment of academia with THAM. *Drugs* 1998;**55**:191–224 and 517.

Wyllie J, Niermeyer S. The role of resuscitation drugs and placental transfusion in the delivery room management of newborn infants. *Semi Fetal Neonat Med* 2008;**13**:416–23.

THEOPHYLLINE

Use

Theophylline (given IV as aminophylline) is a useful bronchodilator. Caffeine (q.v.) has a wider safe therapeutic range when used as a respiratory stimulant. A single dose has been shown to improve renal function in the asphyxiated term baby.

Pharmacology

Theophylline, a naturally occurring alkaloid present in tea and coffee, was widely used in the treatment of asthma for more than 50 years. The optimum bronchodilator effect is only seen with a plasma level of 10–20 mg/l, but toxic symptoms are sometimes seen in the newborn when the level exceeds 14 mg/l, and gastro-oesophageal reflux may be made worse. Sustained use increases urinary calcium loss. Very high blood levels cause hyperactivity, tachycardia and fits that seem to respond to the oral administration of activated charcoal even when the drug has been given IV. Correct any hypokalaemia or metabolic acidosis. Arrhythmias that fail to respond to adenosine (q.v.) may respond to propranolol (q.v.). A single prophylactic 8 mg/kg IV dose seems to reduce some of the adverse renal consequences of perinatal asphyxia. Theophylline is moderately well absorbed in the neonate when given by mouth, but is slowly metabolised by a series of parallel liver pathways, some of which are saturable. The neonatal half life (15–50 hours) is five times as long as in adults. There is no evidence that moderate maternal use during pregnancy or lactation is hazardous to the baby, although calculations suggest that a breastfed baby might receive (on a weight-for-weight basis) about an eighth of the maternal dose.

Caffeine has many advantages over theophylline in the management of neonatal apnoea. The gap between the optimum therapeutic blood level and the blood level at which toxic symptoms first appear is much wider with caffeine than it is with theophylline, and caffeine usually only needs to be given once a day. Theophylline is, in any case, partly metabolised to caffeine in the liver in the neonatal period.

Drug interactions

Toxicity can occur in patients also taking cimetidine, ciprofloxacin, erythromycin or isoniazid unless a lower dose of theophylline is used. Conversely a higher dose may be needed in patients on carbamazepine, phenobarbital, phenytoin or rifampicin because of enhanced drug clearance. Treatment with theophylline, in turn, may make it necessary to increase the dose of phenytoin.

Drug equivalence

Aminophylline (which includes ethylenediamine in order to improve solubility) is only 85% theophylline but there is a suggestion that neonatal bioavailability is reduced by first pass liver metabolism, and that the dose of theophylline used for oral treatment can be the same as the dose of aminophylline given IV.

Treatment

IV treatment for the preterm baby: Try 8 mg/kg of aminophylline as a loading dose over not less than 10 minutes followed by 2·5 mg/kg (or, if necessary, 3·5 mg/kg) once every 12 hours. Because of the long half life, a continuous infusion is not necessary. A rapid IV bolus can cause arrhythmia.

Oral treatment for the preterm baby: Try an initial loading dose of 6 mg/kg of theophylline (if the patient is not already on IV treatment) followed by 2·5 mg/kg every 12 hours.

Term babies suffering intrapartum asphyxia: A single 8 mg/kg dose of IV aminophylline reduces the severity of any consequential renal failure.

Use in older children: To start oral treatment in babies aged 1–11 months calculate the **total** daily dose of theophylline required per kg body weight as 5 mg plus 0·2 times the child's postnatal age in weeks.

Blood levels

The optimum plasma level in neonates is probably 9–14 mg/l (1 mg/l = 5·55 μmol/l). Significant side effects can appear when the level exceeds 15 mg/l in the newborn baby (see p. 9), and when the level exceeds 20 mg/l (100 μmol/l) in older children, the difference probably being due to differences in protein binding. Theophylline can be measured in 0·1 ml of plasma. Timing is not crucial because of the long neonatal half life, but specimens are best collected an hour after the drug has been given.

Supply

One 10 ml ampoule containing 250 mg of aminophylline costs 69p, and 100 ml of an oral syrup containing 12 mg/ml of theophylline hydrate (as sodium glycinate) costs £1. The US product contains 2% benzyl alcohol.

References

See also the relevant Cochrane reviews

Aranda JV, Lopes JM, Blanchard P, *et al*. Treatment of neonatal apnoea. In: Rylance G, Harvey D, Aranda JV, eds. *Neonatal clinical pharmacology and therapeutics*. Oxford: Butterworths, 1991: pp. 95–115.

Bakr AF. Prophylactic theophylline to prevent renal dysfunction in newborns exposed to perinatal asphyxia – a study in a developing country. *Pediatr Nephrol* 2005;**20**:1249–52.

Bhat MA, Shah ZA, Makhdoomi MS, *et al*. Theophylline for renal function in term neonates with perinatal asphyxia: a randomized, placebo-controlled trial. *J Pediatr* 2006;**149**:180–4. [RCT]

Hogue SL, Phelps SJ. Evaluation of three theophylline dosing equations for use in infants up to one year of age. *J Pediatr* 1993;**123**:651–6.

Lowry JA, Jarrett RV, Wasserman G, *et al*. Theophylline toxicokinetics in premature newborns. *Arch Pediatr Adolesc Med* 2001;**155**:934–9.

Use

Thiopental is most widely used during induction of anaesthesia, but it can also be used to control seizures that do not respond to other anticonvulsants as long as ventilation is supported artificially.

Pharmacology

Thiopental sodium is a hypnotic and anticonvulsant barbiturate, but it does not relieve pain. It was first used in 1934. Because it causes marked respiratory depression it should only be used in situations where immediate respiratory support can be provided. Large doses also cause a fall in peripheral vascular resistance and cardiac output. It quickly reaches the central nervous system and is then redistributed away from the brain into body fat stores. The terminal half life is variable but about 10–12 hours in most adults, but shorter than this in children; the neonatal half life is not known for certainty. Drug accumulation (neonatal V_D ~4 l/kg) after a high dose or a continuing infusion has been given is known to result in slow, delayed, triexponential, elimination by the liver. Thiopental crosses the placenta rapidly, but the effect of a single maternal injection is small because the drug only remains briefly in the blood stream. A continuous infusion could, however, cause fetal accumulation. Only a trace appears in breast milk after use during routine operative anaesthesia.

Thiopental can be very effective in controlling seizures that prove resistant to more conventional treatment, but, because the drug acts as a general anaesthetic, its ability to abolish continuing and potentially damaging cerebral discharges can only be reliably confirmed by monitoring the EEG. A cerebral function monitor (aEEG) will suffice for most purposes, but multichannel EEG recordings will usually be necessary – particularly for important management decisions. Most babies whose immediate post-delivery seizures are only controlled by thiopental anaesthesia die before discharge home or become severely disabled in later infancy. However, while thiopental cannot be expected to reverse the cerebral damage already done to a baby with hypoxic-ischaemic encephalopathy, use could well minimise the potential for continuing cortical seizure activity to further compound that damage. Given the frequency with which phenobarbital (q.v.) on its own fails to control such seizure activity, treatment with thiopental almost certainly merits further study.

Thiopental can also be used to provide sedation and analgesia during brief but painful neonatal procedures, and has been shown to halve the time it takes to intubate the trachea. Methohexital sodium is an alternative ultra-short-acting barbiturate with similar anaesthetic but no anticonvulsant properties. A 2 mg/kg bolus dose IV produces anaesthesia after less than a minute. Induction may not be quite as smooth as with thiopental, but recovery starts sooner (usually after 2–5 minutes) and is usually complete within 10 minutes. A single dose or propofol (q.v.) may, however, be as good a choice as either of these barbiturates.

Treatment

To achieve brief anaesthesia: 5 mg/kg IV, flushed in with saline, produces sleep after about 45 seconds. Recovery begins 5–10 minutes later.

To stop seizures resistant to phenobarbital: In the only formal study published to date, a single 10 mg/kg IV dose abolished all abnormal EEG activity in babies receiving respiratory support. The drug's long elimination half life makes continuous infusion unnecessary and inappropriate, but a further dose can be given if seizure activity reappears. Blood levels are not helpful in monitoring treatment.

Tissue extravasation

Extravasation can cause severe tissue necrosis because the undiluted product has very high pH (11·5). Intra-arterial injection should be avoided for the same reason. A strategy for the immediate management of suspected tissue damage is outlined in the monograph on hyaluronidase.

Supply and administration

500 mg vials of thiopental cost £3·10. Reconstitute the vial with 20 ml of preservative-free water for injection; take 125 mg (5 ml) of this solution and dilute to 50 ml with 5% glucose to give a solution containing 2·5 mg/ml for accurate, trouble-free, administration. Methohexital (originally known in the UK as methohexitone) is available in Europe and the United States but not, at present, in the UK.

References

Bhutada A, Sahni R, Rastogi E, *et al.* Randomised controlled trial of thiopental for intubation in neonates. *Arch Dis Child* 2000;**82**:F34–7. [RCT]

Bonati M, Marraro G, Celardo A, *et al.* Thiopental efficacy in phenobarbital-resistant neonatal seizures. *Dev Pharmacol Ther* 1990;**15**:16–20.

Goldberg PN, Moscoso P, Bauer CR, *et al.* Use of barbiturate therapy on severe perinatal asphyxia: a randomised controlled trial. *J Pediatr* 1986;**109**:851–6. [RCT]

Hussain N, Appleton R, Thorburn K. Aetiology, course and outcome of children admitted to paediatric intensive care with convulsive status epilepticus: a retrospective 5-year review. *Seizure* 2007;**16**:305–12.

Naulaers G, Deloof E, Vanhole C, *et al.* Use of methohexital for elective intubation in neonates. *Arch Dis Child* 1997;**77**:F61–4.

Norman E, Malmqvist U, Westrin P, *et al.* Thiopental pharmacokinetics in newborn infants: a case report of overdose. *Acta Paediatr* 2009;**98**:1680–2.

Russo H, Bressolle F. Pharmacodynamics and pharmacokinetics of thiopental. *Clin Pharmacokinet* 1998;**35**:95–134. [SR]

Schrum SF, Hannallah RS, Verghese PM, *et al.* Comparison of propofol and thiopental for rapid anesthesia induction in infants. *Anesth Analg* 1994;**78**:482–5.

Sedik H. Use of intravenous methohexital as a sedative in pediatric emergency departments. *Arch Pediatr Adolesc Med* 2001;**155**:663–8.

Tasker RC, Boyd SG, Harden A, *et al.* EEG monitoring of prolonged thiopentone administration for intractable seizures and status epilepticus in infants and young children. *Neuropediatrics* 1989;**20**:147–53.

Use

Tobramycin is an alternative to gentamicin in the management of Gram-negative bacterial infections.

Pharmacology

Tobramycin is a bactericidal antibiotic related to kanamycin which is handled by the body in much the same way as netilmicin (q.v.). It first came into clinical use in 1968. All the aminoglycoside antibiotics have a relatively low therapeutic:toxic ratio; there is little to choose between amikacin (q.v.), gentamicin (q.v.), netilmicin and tobramycin in this regard. Tobramycin crosses the placenta moderately well, but it has not been found to cause as much ototoxic damage to the fetus as is sometimes seen with streptomycin. It penetrates the CSF and the bronchial lumen rather poorly. Some is also excreted in breast milk but this is of little consequence as oral absorption is negligible.

Tobramycin has certain theoretical advantages over gentamicin in the management of *Pseudomonas* infection because of greater *in vitro* sensitivity, and aggressive high-dose treatment (10 mg/kg once a day in children over 6 months old) is often used when this pathogen colonises the lungs of children with cystic fibrosis. Twice daily inhalation (300 mg in 2–5 ml of 0·9% sodium chloride) for 4 weeks is an alternative strategy that has also been used in this condition, eliminating both lung infection and pseudomonas carriage. Repeat this, if necessary, after 4 weeks off treatment. Gentamicin is more normally used when treating an undiagnosed Gram-negative infection, while a combination of gentamicin and ceftazidime (or gentamicin and azlocillin) is often thought to be the optimum treatment for neonatal *Pseudomonas* infection. The dose regimen recommended in this compendium mirrors the one outlined in the monograph on gentamicin, although very few of the studies of once versus thrice daily aminoglycoside treatment in neonates have actually involved the use of tobromycin. Check that blood levels can be checked by the local laboratory before starting treatment if monitoring is considered important.

Interaction with other antibiotics

Aminoglycosides are capable of combining chemically with equimolar amounts of most penicillins. Such inactivation has been well documented *in vitro*, and is the basis for the advice that these antibiotics should never be mixed together. Problems with combined use have, however, only been encountered in clinical practice when both drugs are given simultaneously to patients with severe renal failure and sustained high plasma antibiotic levels. Leaving a 2–4-hour gap between aminoglycoside and β-lactam antibiotic administration has been shown to enhance bactericidal potency *in vitro* by an unrelated mechanism, but the clinical relevance of this observation remains far from clear.

Treatment

Dose: Give 5 mg/kg IV or IM to babies less than 4 weeks old, and 6 mg/kg to babies older than this (rising to 8 mg/kg at a year). A slow 30-minute infusion is not necessary when this drug is given IV.

Timing: Give a dose once every 36 hours in babies of less than 32 weeks' gestation in the first week of life. Give all other babies a dose once every 24 hours unless renal function is poor. Check the trough level (as below) and increase the dosage interval if the trough level is more than 2 mg/l.

Blood levels

The trough level is all that usually needs to be monitored in babies on intermittent high-dose treatment, and even this is probably only necessary as a *routine* in babies in possible renal failure or less than 10 days old. Aim for a trough level of about 1 mg/l (1 mg/l = 2·14 μmol/l). The 1-hour peak level, when measured, should be 8–12 mg/l. Collect and handle specimens in the same way as for gentamicin.

Supply and administration

1 and 2 ml vials containing 20 mg/ml cost £2·70 and £4·20, respectively. 5 ml (300 mg) nebuliser vials cost £27 each.

References

Barclay ML, Begg EJ, Chambers ST, *et al*. Improved efficacy with nonsimultaneous administration of first doses of gentamicin and ceftazidime in vitro. *Antimicrob Agents Chemother* 1995;**39**:132–6.

Daly JS, Dodge RA, Glew RH, *et al*. Effect of time and temperature on inactivation of aminoglycosides by ampicillin at neonatal dosages. *J Perinatol* 1997;**17**:42–5.

de Hoog M, Schoemaker RC, Mouton JW, *et al*. Tobramycin population pharmacokinetics in neonates. *Clin Pharmacol Ther* 1997;**62**:392–9.

de Hoog M, van Zanten BA, Hop WC, *et al*. Newborn hearing screening: tobramycin and vancomycin are not risk factors for hearing loss. *J Pediatr* 2003;**142**:41–6.

Massie J, Cranswick N. Pharmacokinetic profile of once daily intravenous tobramycin in children with cystic fibrosis. *J Paediatr Child Health* 2006;**42**:601–5.

Ratjen F, Dring G, Nikolaizik WH. Effect of inhaled tobramycin on early pseudomonas aeruginosa colonisation in patients with cystic fibrosis. *Lancet* 2001;**358**:983–4.

Rosenfeld M, Gibson R, McNamara S, *et al*. Serum and lower respiratory tract drug concentrations after tobramycin inhalation in young children with cystic fibrosis. *J Pediatr* 2001;**139**:572–7.

Skopnick H, Heimann G. Once daily aminoglycoside dosing in full term neonates. *Pediatr Infect Dis J* 1995;**14**:71–2.

Smyth A, Tan KH-V, Mulheran M, *et al*. Once versus three-times daily regimens of tobramycin treatment for pulmonary exacerbations of cystic fibrosis – the TOPIC study: a randomised controlled trial. *Lancet* 2005;**365**:473–8. [RCT]

Use

A single dose of tolazoline will often correct pulmonary artery vasospasm when this causes severe right-to-left shunting soon after birth, and the dose recommended here seldom causes systemic hypotension.

Pharmacology

Tolazoline is an α-adrenergic antagonist that produces both pulmonary and systemic vasodilatation. The first paper to describe neonatal use appeared in 1979. Several papers now attest to the drug's ability to improve systemic arterial oxygen tension in some critically ill babies with a transitional circulation, especially where there is clear evidence of pulmonary hypertension. Anecdotal evidence suggests that the drug works best once serious acidosis (pH <7·2) is corrected. Continuous infusion is not nearly as necessary as was once thought, because the half life exceeds 6 hours. Babies given a continuous tolazoline infusion must have their blood pressure measured periodically, but systemic hypotension should be rare with the dose recommended here. Many texts have recommended higher doses and sustained treatment, but this can be cardiotoxic, and, since tolazoline is actively excreted by the kidney but not otherwise metabolised by the baby, such problems will be exacerbated by renal failure. Other side effects of tolazoline include sympathomimetic cardiac stimulation, parasympathomimetic gastrointestinal symptoms and increased gastric secretion due to a histamine-like action. The skin may take on an alarmingly blotchy appearance. Transient oliguria and gastric bleeding have been reported.

Management of pulmonary artery vasospasm

A single bolus dose of tolazoline is quite often all that is required to stop a 'vicious circle' developing, with hypoxia and acidosis fuelling a further increase in pulmonary vascular tone, especially in the period immediately after birth, although the first priority must always be to optimise ventilator management. Raising the pH above 7·5 by a combination of mild hyperventilation (pCO$_2$ 3·5−4·5 kPa) and IV sodium bicarbonate or THAM is often the most potent and physiological way of influencing pulmonary vascular tone. Nitric oxide (q.v.) is frequently effective in babies of ≥34 weeks' gestation, but it is complex treatment strategy to deliver, and many only use it if tolazoline fails. Epoprostenol (q.v.) may be tried if tolazoline is ineffective, but it is seldom of lasting benefit. Systemic hypotension and/or a high right atrial pressure causing right-to-left ductal, or interatrial, shunting, may be a more important factor than a high pulmonary vascular tone in some babies with a 'transitional' circulation. In such circumstances dobutamine (q.v.) with or without adrenaline (q.v.) may be more effective. Magnesium sulphate (q.v.) is still used by some, but seldom has any rapid impact.

Drug interactions

The use of an H$_2$ blocker such as cimetidine or ranitidine (q.v.) prophylactically to minimise the risk of gastric bleeding renders tolazoline ineffective as a vasodilator.

Treatment

IV correction of pulmonary vasospasm: Give 1 mg/kg IV over 2−4 minutes while watching for systemic hypotension. It is just occasionally necessary to sustain this by giving 200 micrograms/kg per hour IV diluted in a little saline or 10% glucose. Prepare a fresh solution daily.
Endotracheal administration: While bolus administration by this route is still under evaluation, there are now several reports that this strategy can be successful. It certainly makes systemic side effects less likely. Try 200 micrograms/kg diluted in 0·5−1 ml of 0·9% sodium chloride.
Use to correct arterial vasospasm: Low-dose infusion (even as little as 20, but more usually 100, micrograms/kg per hour) will often correct the local vasospasm triggered by an indwelling arterial line.

Compatibility

Tolazoline can be added (terminally) into a line containing dobutamine and/or dopamine or vancomycin. One book has an unreferenced claim that it can be added to TPN. Do not add to a line containing lipid.

Supply

1 ml ampoules containing 25 mg of tolazoline are available on special order from Cardinal Health (formerly Martindale) in the UK. Ampoules cost £3 each.

References

Bush A, Busst CM, Knight WB, *et al*. Cardiovascular effects of tolazoline and ranitidine. *Arch Dis Child* 1987;**62**:241−6.
Lemke RP, al Saedi SA, Belik J, *et al*. Use of tolazoline to counteract vasospasm in peripheral arterial catheters in neonates. *Acta Paediatr* 1996;**85**:1497−8.
Nuntnarumit P, Korones SB, Yang W, *et al*. Efficacy and safety of tolazoline for treatment of severe hypoxemia in extremely preterm infants. *Pediatrics* 2002;**109**:852−6.
Parida SK, Baker S, Kuhn R, *et al*. Endotracheal tolazoline administration in neonates with persistent pulmonary hypertension. *J Perinatol* 1997;**17**:461−4.
Ward RM. Pharmacology of tolazoline. *Clin Perinatol* 1984;**11**:703−13.
Ward RM, Daniel CH, Kendig JW. Oliguria and tolazoline pharmacokinetics in the newborn. *Pediatrics* 1986;**77**:307−15.

TRIMETHOPRIM

Use
Trimethoprim is widely used to limit the risk of urinary infection in babies with ureteric reflux or a structural renal tract abnormality. It is also a useful oral antibiotic in the management of many aerobic Gram-positive and -negative infections.

Pharmacology
While trimethoprim is only licensed for neonatal use 'under careful medical supervision', the drug is now very widely used both to prevent and to treat urinary tract infection in infancy and throughout childhood (although there is little control trial evidence to support prophylaxis). Trimethoprim works by inhibiting steps in the synthesis of tetrahydrofolic acid, an essential metabolic cofactor in the synthesis of DNA by bacteria. Adverse effects are rare. Prolonged treatment in adults can rarely cause bone marrow changes, but extensive experience confirms that there is no need to subject young children on sustained low-dose prophylaxis to routine blood testing. A combined preparation with sulfamethoxazole (called co-trimoxazole (q.v.)) has occasionally proved of value in the management of pneumonia and meningitis. Both drugs are known to penetrate the lung, kidney and CSF extremely well. There is, however, no evidence that co-trimoxazole is better than trimethoprim in the prevention, or treatment, of renal tract infection, and trimethoprim has been marketed for use on its own since 1979.

Trimethoprim is well absorbed by mouth, widely distributed (V_D >1 l/kg) and excreted, largely unmetabolised, in the urine, especially in the neonatal period. Dosage should be halved after 2 days treatment, therefore, in the presence of severe renal failure. The half life in the neonate is very variable but averages 18 hours at birth, falling rapidly to only 4 hours within 2 months, before increasing once more to about 11 hours in adults. Since trimethoprim crosses the placenta it should be avoided where possible in the first trimester of pregnancy, because of its teratogenic potential as a folate antagonist. When taken during lactation the baby receives about a tenth of the weight-related maternal dose.

Urinary tract infection
Neonatal infection is uncommon but easily missed. Bag specimens are very misleading, but urine obtained from a collection pad can make bladder tap unnecessary; while bladder tap, even when a eutectic lidocaine cream (q.v.) is used to anaesthetise the suprapublic skin, does not seem to be as pain free as transurethral catheterisation. Immediate direct examination under a phase-contrast microscope, looking for bacteria rather than cells, can provide a prompt working diagnosis, and eliminate many of the 'false-positive' diagnoses generated by routine laboratory culture. Infants with a proven infection need investigation with renal ultrasound, a micturating cystogram and a delayed succimer (dimercaptosuccinic acid or DMSA) radioisotope scan to look for reflux or structural urinary tract abnormality. Consider prophylaxis until structural abnormality is confirmed or disproved.

Prophylaxis
Give 2 mg/kg once a day. Evening administration in older children will generate a peak drug level at the time when infrequent nocturnal bladder emptying makes infection more likely.

Treatment
A loading dose of 3 mg/kg, either IV or by mouth, followed by 1 mg/kg twice a day is widely used to treat urinary infection in the neonatal period. One week's treatment is usually enough. By 6 weeks of age babies require 3 mg/kg twice a day (three times a day for non-renal infection).

Supply
A sugar-free oral preparation (Monotrim®) containing 10 mg/ml, which can be stored at room temperature (5–25°C), is available costing £1·80 for 100 ml. It remains stable for a fortnight if further diluted with water or sorbitol. The only commercial IV preparation has recently been withdrawn, but a formulation also containing sulfamethoxazole is still available, as outlined in the monograph on co-trimoxazole.

References
See also the relevant Cochrane reviews

Anon. The management of urinary tract infection in children. *Drug Ther Bull* 1997;**35**:65–9.

Hoppu K. Age differences in trimethoprim pharmacokinetics: need for revised dosing in children? *Clin Pharmacol Ther* 1987;**41**:336–43.

Hoppu K. Changes in trimethoprim pharmacokinetics after the newborn period. *Arch Dis Child* 1989;**64**:343–5.

Kozer E, Rosenbloom E, Goldman D, *et al*. Pain in infants who are younger than 2 months during suprapubic aspiration and transurethral catheterization: a randomized controlled study. *Pediatrics* 2006;**118**:e51–6. [RCT]

Lambert H, Coulthard M. The child with urinary tract infection. In: Webb N, Postlethwaite R, eds. *Clinical paediatric nephrology*, 3rd edn. Oxford: Oxford University Press, 2003: pp. 197–225.

Larcome J. UTI in children. *BMJ Clinical evidence handbook*. London: BMJ Books, 2009; pp. 120–3 (and updates). [SR]

Rao S, Bhatt J, Houghton C, *et al*. An improved urine collection pad method: a randomised clinical trial. *Arch Dis Child* 2004;**89**:773–5. [RCT]

Smellie JM, Gruneberg RN, Bantock HM, *et al*. Prophylactic co-trimoxazole and trimethoprim in the management of urinary tract infection in children. *Pediatr Nephrol* 1988;**2**:12–17.

Use
Urokinase can clear clotted catheters and shunts, and speed the drainage of a pleural empyema. Streptokinase (q.v.) or alteplase (q.v.) are more frequently used to lyse intravascular thrombi.

Pharmacology
Urokinase is an enzyme derived from human urine that directly converts plasminogen to the proteolytic enzyme plasmin. This then, in turn, converts the fibrin within any clot of blood or plasma into a range of soluble break-down products. It was first isolated in 1947 and crystallised in 1965. Urokinase is rapidly metabolised by the liver (the circulating half life being about 15 minutes). It is often used to clear occluded intravascular catheters, and to lyse intraocular thrombi. Streptokinase has been more commonly used to treat intravascular thrombi, even though there is some suggestion that the risk of a hypersensitivity reaction may be higher. Continuous urokinase infusions are relatively expensive and, because plasminogen levels are relatively low in the neonatal period, high-dose treatment may be necessary. A fresh frozen plasma (q.v.) infusion may help by providing additional plasminogen. The manufacturers do not recommend the use of urokinase during pregnancy or the puerperium because of the possible risk of haemorrhage, but no problems have actually been reported in clinical practice.

A prompt infusion of urokinase-activated plasmin, or a concentrate of plasminogen obtained by fractionating human plasma, both seem to reduce morbidity and mortality from respiratory distress (hyaline membrane disease) in babies of less than 32 weeks' gestation. However, despite evidence from a trial involving 500 babies in its favour in 1977, the strategy was never adopted in clinical practice, nor further evaluated. Concern for a possible increase in the risk of intracerebral haemorrhage may be one reason. How the specially prepared product works remains unclear: it has been suggested that the provision of additional plasminogen may speed the resorption of fibrin from the lungs of babies with surfactant deficiency (the 'hyaline membranes' found in the alveoli at postmortem).

Other strategies for blocked catheters
Instilling enough sterile 0·1 M hydrochloric acid to fill the catheter dead space will usually clear any block caused by calcium or phosphate deposition. A similar quantity of 70% ethanol will often clear a block due to lipid. Alteplase can be used to unblock thrombosed central venous catheters.

Treatment
Blocked catheters: 5000 or 10,000 units of urokinase made up in 2 ml of 0·9% sodium chloride can be used to try to unblock a thrombosed intravascular catheter or shunt. The usual procedure is to instil and leave the urokinase in the catheter for 2 hours. Aspirate the urokinase before then attempting to flush the catheter with heparinised saline with a view to resuming the original infusion.
Vascular thrombi: Try a dose of 5000 units/kg an hour, and consider increasing the dose 2- or even 4-fold if blood flow does not improve within 8 hours.
Pleural empyema: Inject 10,000 units in 10 ml saline and drain after 4 hours. Repeat twice daily for 3 days. Open or thoroscopic surgery may be a better option in selected cases where facilities exist.

Antidote
Tranexamic acid can control bleeding by inhibiting the activation of plasminogen to plasmin. Try an IV infusion of 10 mg/kg over 10 minutes and repeat if necessary after 8–12 hours.

Supply and administration
25,000 unit vials of urokinase (costing £29) can be made available in the UK on a 'named patient' basis. They are also available in America, but the only licensed indication in the USA is pulmonary embolism. Reconstitute with 1 ml of water for injection and then dilute to 5 ml with 0·9% sodium chloride to obtain a solution containing 5000 units/ml. The solution is only fully stable for 12 hours after reconstitution. 100,000 unit vials are also available; they should be reconstituted with 2 ml of water for injection. To give 5000 units/kg per hour place 1 ml of the reconstituted solution from a 100,000 unit vial for each kg the baby weighs in a syringe, dilute to 10 ml with 0·9% sodium chloride, and infuse at a rate of 1 ml/hour. 500 mg (5 ml) ampoules of tranexamic acid are available for £1·30.

References
Ambrus CM, Choi TS, Cunnanan E, et al. Prevention of hyaline membrane disease with plasminogen. JAMA 1977;**237**:1837–41. [RCT]
Avansino GR, Goldman B, Sawin RS, et al. Primary operative versus nonoperative therapy for pediatric empyema: a meta-analysis. Pediatrics 2005;**115**:1652–9. [SR]
Balfour-Lynn IM, Abrahamson E, Cohen G, et al. BTS guidelines for the management of pleural infection in children. Thorax 2005;**60**(suppl 1):i1–21. (For a copy of this British Thoracic Society guideline see www.brit-thoracic.org,uk.)
Rimensberger PC, Humbert JR, Beghetti M. Management of preterm infants with intracardiac thrombi. Paediatr Drugs 2001;**3**:883–98.
Shah SS, DiChristima CM, Bell LM, et al. Primary early thoracoscopy and reduction in length of hospital stay and additional procedures among children with complicated pneumonia: results of a multicenter retrospective cohort study. Arch Pediatr Adolesc Med 2008;**162**:675–81.
Werlin SL, Lausten T, Jessen S et al. Treatment of central venous catheter occlusions with ethanol and hydrochloric acid. J Parent Ent Nutr 1995;**19**:416–18.

URSODEOXYCHOLIC ACID = Ursodiol (USAN)

Use

Ursodeoxycholic acid is used to improve bile acid-dependent bile flow in babies with cholestasis due to biliary atresia and cystic fibrosis, and can relieve the severe itching (pruritus) that can occur when cholestasis occurs as a complication of pregnancy even when it does not retard disease progression. It is less effective in dealing with the cholestasis sometimes caused by parenteral nutrition.

Pharmacology

Ursodeoxycholic acid is a naturally occurring bile acid first isolated by Shoda in Japan in 1927. Small quantities are excreted in human bile and then reabsorbed from the gastrointestinal tract (enterohepatic recirculation). It suppresses the synthesis and secretion of cholesterol by the liver and the intestinal absorption of cholesterol, and a trial in 1980 showed that it could be used to effect the slow dissolution of symptomatic cholesterol-rich gallstones in patients reluctant to undergo surgery or lithotripsy.

Ursodeoxycholic acid has been used in a number of other conditions, although such use is not endorsed by the manufacturers. They do not recommend use during pregnancy, although treatment with 1 gram a day is increasingly being used in patients with intrahepatic cholestasis. Several reports now attest to the drug's ability to reduce the intense itching and to reverse the laboratory signs of liver damage, although control trial evidence that it improves perinatal outcome is still limited. Safe use has also been reported in a patient with primary biliary cirrhosis who took the drug throughout pregnancy. Nothing is known about use during lactation, but it seems unlikely to cause a problem. Reports suggest that the drug is of benefit in some babies with cholestasis due to biliary atresia, α_1-antitripsin deficiency, cystic fibrosis and Alagille syndrome, although it is less clear whether it delays the development of cirrhotic liver damage. Although it may sometimes reduce the serum bilirubin in babies developing cholestasis complicating prolonged parenteral nutrition, liver enzyme levels usually remain high. Side effects are uncommon, although intestinal discomfort may occur initially, and diarrhoea has occasionally been reported. A recent historical cohort review of use in neonatal cholestatic disease has suggested that the drug may not only be ineffective but harmful.

Neonatal hepatitis

A range of individually uncommon conditions cause inflammatory liver disease in infancy interfering with bile flow ('cholestatic' liver disease). Though often referred to as 'hepatitis', few are infectious in origin. Breastfed babies often have prolonged mild jaundice (10% are still clinically jaundiced at a month), but even mild jaundice merits review if the stools become grey or putty coloured rather than yellow or green. Further urgent review is merited if more than 20% of all the plasma bilirubin is conjugated and this component exceeds 18 µmol/l. Survival in biliary atresia (a rare, poorly understood, condition causing perinatal bile duct obliteration affecting one baby in every 15,000) can approach 90% if diagnosed within 8 weeks of birth. No specific treatment is available for most other conditions but it is important to prevent fat-soluble vitamin deficiency. Vitamin K deficiency, in particular, can cause potentially lethal intracranial bleeding. Phenobarbital, and rifampicin (q.v.) are useful, widely used, alternatives to ursodeoxycholic acid for controlling pruritus.

Treatment

In pregnancy: 1 gram a day has not yet been shown to slow disease progression but may help itching.
In infancy: Give 15 mg/kg once a day by mouth. Double this dose has sometimes been given.

Supply

Ursodeoxycholic acid is available as a sugar-free suspension containing 50 mg/ml; 100 ml costs £12·10. 150 mg tablets (costing 30p) and 250 mg capsules (costing 50p) are also available.

References

See also the relevant Cochrane reviews and UK guideline on cholestasis in pregnancy

Arslanoglu S, Moro GF, Tauschel HD, *et al*. Ursodeoxycholic acid treatment in preterm infants: a pilot study for the prevention of cholestasis associated with total parenteral nutrition. *J Pediatr Gastroenterol Nutr* 2008;**46**:228–31.

Chen C-Y, Tsao P-N, Chen H-L, *et al*. Ursodeoxycholic acid (UDCA) therapy in very-low-birth-weight infants with parenteral nutrition-associated cholestasis. *J Pediatr* 2004;**145**:317–21.

Crofts DJ, Michel VJ-M, Rigby AS, *et al*. Assessment of stool colour in community management of prolonged jaundice in infancy. *Acta Paediatr* 1999;**88**:869–74.

Hartley JL, Davenport M, Kelly DA. Biliary atresia. [Seminar] *Lancet* 2009;**374**:1704–13.

Jenkins JK, Boothby LA. Treatment of itching associated with intrahepatic cholestasis of pregnancy. *Ann Pharmacother* 2002;**36**:1462–5. [SR]

Kelly DA, Davenport M. Current management of biliary atresia. *Arch Dis Child* 2007;**92**:1132–5.

Kotb MA. Review of historical cohort: usodeoxycholic acid in extrahepatic biliary atresia. *J Pediatr Surg* 2008;**42**:1321–17.

Kotb MA. Ursodeoxycholic acid in neonatal hepatitis and infantile paucity of intrahepatic bile ducts: review of a historical cohort. *Dig Dis Sci* 2009;**54**:2231–41.

Palma J, Reyes H, Ribalta J, *et al*. Ursodeoxycholic acid in the treatment of cholestasis of pregnancy: a randomised double-blind study controlled with placebo. *J Hepatol* 1997;**27**:1022–8. [RCT]

Powell JE, Keffler S, Kelly DA, *et al*. Population screening for neonatal liver disease: potential for a community-based programme. *J Med Screen* 2003;**10**:112–16.

Saleh MM, Abdo KA. Consensus on the management of obstetric cholestasis: national UK survey. *Br J Obstet Gynaecol* 2007;**114**:99–103.

Scher H, Bishop WP, McCray PB Jr. Ursodeoxycholic acid improves cholestasis in infants with cystic fibrosis. *Ann Pharmacother* 1997;**31**:1003–5.

Tyler W, McKiernan PJ. Prolonged jaundice in the preterm infant – what to do, when and why. *Curr Paediatr* 2006;**16**:43–50.

Willot S, Uhlen S, Michhaud L, *et al*. Effect of ursodeoxycholic acid on liver function in children after successful surgery for biliary atresia. *Pediatrics* 2008;**122**:e1236–41.

Use

Sodium valproate has been widely used in the treatment of several epilepsies since 1974, but the risk of liver toxicity due to an unrecognised metabolic disorder has long served to limit use in early infancy.

Pharmacology

Sodium valproate has a unique chemical structure, and its mode of action is not fully understood although it may involve the modification of gamma amino butyric acid behaviour in the brain. It is slowly but completely absorbed by mouth although peak levels are not reached for 3–8 hours in the newborn. It is highly protein bound and undergoes hepatic metabolism. Sodium valproate has a long half life (10–67 hours) at birth which falls to 7–13 hours by 2 months. It is of particular value in the management of generalised seizures, and the IV preparation is now increasingly used to control status epilepticus in older children and adults. Pancreatitis and severe liver toxicity have been reported in infants and young children, and valproate should only be used with great caution in children less than 2 years old. Nausea, vomiting, lethargy and coma can occur, as can reversible neutropenia and thrombocytopenia. Such problems usually develop soon after treatment is started, but sometimes develop after 3–6 months. Hyperglycinaemia may occur, and has been reported in an infant whose mother was treated during pregnancy. Treatment with 100 mg/kg a day of L-carnitine IV improves survival. Respiratory support may be needed in severe cases.

Sodium valproate crosses the placenta and a constellation of dysmorphic features has been ascribed to valproate exposure in pregnancy, and 1–2% of babies have a neural tube defect. In consequence, where valproate has been used during early pregnancy, it is important to undertake serum α-fetoprotein screening for spina bifida and also to arrange for expert ultrasound screening of the fetal spine at 18 weeks' gestation. Amniocentesis may be necessary in addition if obesity or fetal posture makes detailed examination difficult. High-dose folate prophylaxis may be appropriate (5 mg per day), but this needs to be started before conception. Maternal use does not seem to cause hypoprothrombinaemia requiring neonatal vitamin K prophylaxis at birth in the same way as most other 'first line' anticonvulsant drugs, but afibrinogenaemia has been described. Feeding problems and irritability seem to be common immediately after birth, and hypoglycaemia has been reported. Some of these problems may be dose related. It is also now becoming clear that longer term developmental problems can occur and that, where this has been documented, subsequent siblings may be at increased risk. There is certainly an increased dose-related risk of significant language delay. Readers should check the regularly updated web commentary for the most up-to-date information available on anticonvulsant use during pregnancy. Breastfeeding is not contraindicated in mothers talking valproate, because the baby will only receive 5% of the weight-adjusted maternal dose.

Drug interactions

Treatment with valproate substantially increases the half life of lamotrigine and Phenobarbital.

Treatment

Experience with neonatal use remains *extremely* limited. A 20 mg/kg loading dose (given either by mouth or IV) followed by 10 mg/kg every 12 hours has been suggested. Watch for hyperammonaemia during the first week of administration and suspend treatment at least temporarily if the serum ammonia level exceeds 350 µmol/l. Use blood levels to guide dosage because clearance changes over time.

Blood levels

The immediate pre-dose serum concentration will usually be between 40 and 100 mg/l (1 mg/l = 6·93 µmol/l). However, while monitoring may help to identify non-compliance, it seldom helps to optimise treatment. Levels can be measured in 50 µl of plasma (~150 µl of heparinised whole blood).

Supply

Sodium valproate is available as a red, sugar-free liquid (£2·10 for 100 ml) containing 40 mg/ml. The pharmacy could provide a diluted syrup but the shelf life is only 2 weeks. An IV preparation in powder form (a 400 mg vial with 4 ml of diluent costing £9·60) is also available. The reconstituted solution (containing 100 mg/ml) is compatible with IV glucose and glucose saline but it should not be mixed with any other drug. The oral liquid can be given rectally diluted with an equal volume of tap water.

References

See also the relevant Cochrane reviews

Adab N, Kini U, Vinten J, *et al*. The longer term outcome of children born to mothers with epilepsy. *J Neurol Neurosurg Psychiatr* 2004;**75**:1575–83.

Artama M, Auvinen A, Raudaskoski T, *et al*. Antiepileptic drug use of women with epilepsy and congenital malformations in offspring. *Neurology* 2005;**64**:1874–8. (See also pp. 938–9.)

Bohan TP, Helton E, König S, *et al*. Effect of L-carnitine treatment for valproate-induced hepatotoxicity, *Neurology* 2001;**56**:1405–9.

Meador KJ, Baker GA, Browning N, *et al*. Cognitive function at 3 years of age after fetal exposure to antiepileptic drugs. *N Engl J Med* 2009;**360**:1597–605. (See also pp. 1667–9.)

Smith S, Sharkey I, Cambell D. Guidelines for rectal administration of anticonvulsant medication in children. *Paediatr Perinatal Drug Ther* 2001;**4**:140–7.

Thomas SV, Ajakumar B, Sindu M, *et al*. Motor and mental development of infants exposed to antiepileptic drugs in utero. *Epilepsy Behav* 2008;**13**:229–36.

Williams G, King J, Cunningham M, *et al*. Fetal valproate syndrome and autism: additional evidence of as association. *Devel Med Child Neurol* 2001;**43**:202–6. (See also p. 847.)

VANCOMYCIN

Use

Vancomycin is widely used when staphylococcal infection is caused by an organism resistant to flucloxacillin and/or gentamicin. One alternative is teicoplanin (q.v.). Consider giving rifampicin (q.v.) as well. Empirical use is common when postnatally acquired infection is suspected and the organism is not yet known, but flucloxacillin (q.v.) has the bacterostatic potential needed to keep most 'resistant' coagulase-negative infection in check.

Pharmacology

The glycopeptide antibiotic vancomycin, first isolated in 1956, is bactericidal to most Gram-positive organisms, but is inactive against Gram-negative organisms. It crosses the placenta and penetrates most body fluids reasonably well, but only enters the CSF to any extent when the meninges are inflamed. It is very poorly absorbed by mouth, and causes pain and tissue necrosis when given intramuscularly. Vancomycin is excreted virtually unchanged in the urine, and has to be given with caution in patients with poor renal function. The serum half life is 4–10 hours at birth, later falling to 2–4 hours (6–8 hours in adults). Rapid IV infusion causes erythema and intense pruritis due to histamine release (the so-called 'red man syndrome'), and may cause a dangerous arrhythmia, but there is no evidence that continuous infusion is better than intermittent dosing (except possibly for CNS infection). There is no evidence of toxicity in animals, nephrotoxicity has not been seen with the product currently used, and most patients developing ototoxicity were also taking an aminoglycoside or diuretic (suggesting that damage was wrongly attributed, or that combined use increases the risk). Neutropenia is a rare complication of sustained use. Use during pregnancy or lactation does not seem hazardous to the baby. Giving both vancomycin and rifampicin minimises the risk of initially sensitive organisms becoming resistant, and is particularly useful in catheter and shunt-related coagulase-negative staphylococcal infection.

Prophylaxis

Oral: Giving 15 mg/kg by mouth once every 8 hours for 7 days can reduce the risk of necrotising enterocolitis (as can an oral aminoglycoside), but might encourage the proliferation of multiresistant bacteria.
IV: Adding 25 micrograms of vancomycin to each millilitre of TPN makes catheter-related staphylococcal infection less likely, but such use may not be risk free. Teicoplanin has been used in the same way.

Treatment

Dose: Give 15 mg/kg (3 ml/kg of the dilute solution made up as described below) IV over 1 hour pick-abacked onto an existing IV infusion of glucose or glucose saline.
Timing: Give every 24 hours in babies of less than 29 weeks' gestation in the first week of life, every 12 hours in all other babies of less than 36 weeks' postmenstrual age, every 8 hours in babies of 36–44 weeks, and every 6 hours in babies of over 44 weeks' postmenstrual age. Treat proven CNS infection for 2 weeks.
Monitoring: Monitor the trough blood level if treatment needs to be started in the first week of life, if there is renal failure or if treatment does not seem to be working, and adjust the dosage interval as necessary.
Continuous IV use: 30 mg/kg a day (50 mg/kg in babies over 3 months old) can be given as a continuous infusion, but a prompt therapeutic level will *only* be achieved if a first 10 mg/kg loading dose is given over 1 hour.
Intrathecal use: Give 2 mg/kg of the normal IV preparation once a day, or once every other day, into the ventricles if the CSF is not sterile within 48 hours. Two to four doses will usually suffice. Adjust the initial dose as necessary to achieve a trough CSF level of about 20 mg/l. Consider giving rifampicin as well.

Blood levels

A plasma trough level of 5–10 mg/l (1 mg/l = 0·67 μmol/l) usually suffices, but aim for 15–20 mg/l if endocarditis, a CNS or a meticillin-resistant staphylococcal infection is suspected. Submit 0·5 ml of blood.

Compatibility

Vancomycin may be added (terminally) to TPN with or without lipid, and mixed (terminally) with caffeine, insulin, midazolam, milrinone, morphine, remifentanil or ≤1 unit/ml heparin. Do not mix vancomycin with IV gelatin.

Supply

Stock 500 mg vials cost £8·70 each. Add 9.7 ml of sterile water for injection to the dry powder to get a solution containing 50 mg/ml. Because concentrated solutions cause thrombophlebitis, individual doses for IV or oral use are prepared by drawing 1 ml of this reconstituted (50 mg/ml) solution into a syringe and diluting to 10 ml with 10% glucose or glucose saline to provide a solution containing 5 mg/ml. The fluid has a pH of 2·8–4·5.

References

See also the relevant Cochrane reviews

Arnell K, Enblad P, Wester T, *et al.* Treatment of cerebrospinal fluid shunt infections in children using systemic and intraventricular antibiotic therapy in combination with externalisation of the ventricular catheter: efficacy in 34 consecutively treated infections. *J Neurosurg* 2007;**107**(suppl 3):213–19.

de Hoog M, van den Anker JN, Mouton JW. Vancomycin: pharmacokinetics and administration regimens in neonates. *Clin Pharmacokinet* 2004;**43**:417–40.

Gemmell CG, Edwards DI, Fraise AP, *et al.* Guidelines for the prophylaxis and treatment of methicillin-resistant *Staphylococcus aureus* (MRSA) infections in the UK. *J Antimicrob Chemother* 2006;**57**:589–608. [SR]

Lodha A, Furlan AD, Whyte H, *et al.* Prophylactic antibiotics in the prevention of catheter-associated bloodstream bacterial infection in preterm neonates: a systematic review. *J Perinatol* 2008;**28**:526–33. [SR]

Plan O, Cambonie G, Barbotte E, *et al.* Continuous-infusion vancomycin therapy for preterm neonates with suspected or documented gram-positive infections: a new dosage schedule. *Arch Dis Child* 2008;**93**:F418–21. (But see also 2009;**94**:F233–4.)

Use

Varicella-zoster immunoglobulin (VZIG or ZIG) is used to provide passive immunity to chickenpox.

Pharmacology

This product is prepared from the pooled plasma of HIV-, hepatitis B- and hepatitis C-negative blood donors in the UK with a recent history of chickenpox or shingles. The product has a minimum potency of 100 units of varicella-zoster (VZ) antibody per millitre. Supplies are limited. Normal immunoglobulin offers some protection. No comparable product is available for treating herpes simplex virus (HSV) infection.

Chickenpox

Primary infection with the VZ virus (or human herpes virus 3) causes chickenpox, and reactivation of the latent virus causes herpes zoster (shingles). Vesicles then appear in the skin area served by the spinal nerve ganglia where the virus has lain dormant. Spread is by droplets or contact causing infection after an incubation period of 10–21 (usually 14–17) days, subjects with chickenpox being infectious for about a week (from 1–2 days before until about 5 days after the rash first appears). Illness in childhood is usually less severe than illness in adults. 95% of women of child-bearing age in the UK have lasting immunity as a result of natural infection during childhood. Chickenpox during pregnancy can cause severe pulmonary disease (although selective reporting may have lead to the magnitude of the risk being exaggerated). Illness late in the first half of pregnancy also exposes the fetus to a 1–2% risk of embryopathy: lesions include cicatricial skin scarring and limb hypoplasia; CNS and eye lesions also occur. No technique has yet been developed for identifying whether the fetus has been affected or not, and it should not be assumed that exposure in the third trimester incurs no risk. Infection shortly before birth certainly exposes the baby to the risk of severe neonatal infection. The babies at greatest risk are those delivered 2–4 days before or after the onset of maternal symptoms; such babies have been exposed to massive viraemia but have not had time to benefit from placentally transferred maternal antibody. These babies are at risk of multiorgan involvement and death from necrotising pneumonia. They need *urgent* treatment with VZIG, and careful monitoring for the next 2 weeks. Try to delay labour for at least 3 days if the mother develops a typical rash shortly before delivery is due. Shingles during pregnancy presents little hazard to the baby.

An attenuated Oka strain live varicella vaccine (£29 per vial) is now available in the UK, and this should certainly be offered to non-immune children with leukaemia or a transplant because immunosuppressant drug use puts these children at risk of life-threatening infection. Even post-exposure vaccination seems to work if carried out within 2–3 days of exposure. The vaccine (two doses 6–8 weeks apart) is now also being offered to non-immune UK health care workers. Non-immune women contemplating pregnancy should also seek protection if there is a risk of exposure during pregnancy. Although the need to prevent childhood infection has been questioned and the utility cost of routine vaccination is marginal, all American children are now offered one dose of the vaccine when they are 12–18 months old and (because this does not always provide lasting immunity) a second dose when they are at least 4 years old.

Prophylaxis

Give an immediate dose of VZIG IM to:

- Women with no serological immunity to chickenpox who are exposed to the virus while pregnant.
- All babies born in the 7-day period before or after their mother first develops signs of chickenpox.
- Non-immune term babies exposed to anyone with chickenpox or shingles within a week of delivery.
- Preterm babies exposed to chickenpox or shingles before reaching a postmenstrual age of 40 weeks when it is not possible to obtain convincing serological evidence of immunity.

The neonatal dose of VZIG is 250 mg IM; the maternal dose is 1 gram.

It is also worth giving IV aciclovir (q.v.) to mothers developing chickenpox around the time of birth, as long as treatment is started within a day of the mother becoming symptomatic. Offer the baby early treatment if symptomatic, to limit the severity of the infection. Keep the mother and baby isolated but together.

Supply

VZIG is available from Health Protection Agency laboratories in England and Wales. 250 mg (1·7 ml) ampoules for IM use should be stored at 4°C, but are stable enough to withstand dispatch by post. Ampoules have a nominal shelf life of 3 years; they must not be frozen.

References

See also the Cochrane reviews and UK guideline on exposure in pregnancy

American Academy of Pediatrics, Committee on Infectious Diseases. Prevention of varicella: recommendations for use of varicella vaccines in children, including a recommendation for a routine 2-dose varicella schedule. *Pediatrics* 2007;**120**:221–31.

Chaves SS, Gargiullo P, Zhang JX, *et al.* Loss of vaccine-induced immunity to varicella over time. *N Eng J Med* 2007;**356**:1121–9.

Daley AJ, Thorpe S, Garland SM. Varicella and the pregnant woman: prevention and management. *Aust NZ J Obstet Gynaecol* 2008;**48**:26–33.

Farlow A. Childhood immunization for varicella zoster virus. *BMJ* 2008;**337**:419–20.

Grote V, von Kries R, Stringer W, *et al.* Varicella-related deaths in children and adolescents – Germany 2003–2004. *Acta Paediatr* 2008;**97**:187–92.

Heininger U, Seward JF. Varicella. [Seminar] *Lancet* 2006;**368**:1365–76. [SR]

Marchetto S, de Benedictis FM, de Martino M, *et al.* Epidemiology of hospital admissions for chickenpox in children: an Italian multicentre study in the pre-vaccine era. *Acta Paediatr* 2007;**96**:1490–3.

Smith CK, Arvin AM. Varicella in the fetus and newborn. *Semin Fetal Neonat Med* 2009;**14**:209–17.

VASOPRESSIN (and desmopressin)

Use
Vasopressin (AVP) and its long-acting analogue desmopressin (DDAVP) act to limit water loss in the urine. Artificially high levels of vasopressin given IV can cause arteriolar vasoconstriction.

Pharmacology
Vasopressin and oxytocin (q.v.) are natural hormones produced by the posterior lobe of the pituitary gland. Arginine-vasopressin is a nine peptide molecule first synthesised in 1958 with a structure very similar to that of oxytocin which acts to increase the reabsorption of solute-free water from the distal tubules of the kidney. It is also sometimes known as the antidiuretic hormone (ADH). High (supraphysiological) blood levels cause a rise in blood pressure due to arteriolar vasoconstriction – hence the name vasopressin. Evidence is accumulating that, in septic or postoperative shock with hypotension and vasodilatation resistant to treatment with catecholamines such as adrenaline (q.v.), natural AVP levels sometimes become depleted. In this situation even a modest dose of AVP can resensitise the vessels to catecholamine, raising blood pressure without threatening tissue perfusion.

DDAVP is a synthetic analogue of AVP with a longer functional half life, and enhanced diuretic potency but little vasoconstrictor potency. DDAVP (unlike AVP) is only partially inactivated when given by mouth, making oral treatment possible (although the dose required varies greatly). Treatment is usually only necessary once or twice a day. DDAVP stimulates factor VIII production, and a 0·4 microgram/kg IV dose is enough to produce a four-fold rise in patients with only moderately severe haemophilia (factor VIII levels ≥7%) within 30 minutes. Maternal treatment with AVP, which is inactivated by placental vasopressinase and destroyed by trypsin in the gut, is very unlikely to affect the baby, and reports show that DDAVP can also be used during pregnancy and lactation with confidence when clinically indicated.

Diabetes insipidus
The polyuria seen in diabetes mellitus is caused by loss of sugar in the urine (the word mellitus indicating that the urine is sweet or honey-like). Any failure of AVP production causes the kidney to pass large quantities of *un*sweet (insipid) urine – hence the term diabetes insipidus. Similar symptoms can be caused by hormone insensitivity (nephrogenic diabetes insipidus). Inappropriately dilute urine (a urine osmolality of <300 mosmol/kg when plasma osmolality exceeds this value) makes diabetes insipidus likely, and the response to a dose of DDAVP clinches the diagnosis. Midline cranial anomalies, infection and haemorrhage account for most cases of neonatal intracranial diabetes insipidus. Most mild cases are best managed by merely altering fluid intake. Insufficiency is sometimes only transient.

Treatment
Vasopressin: Treat severe vasodilatory shock (i.e. hypotension resistant to 200 nanograms/kg per minute of adrenaline with adequate vascular filling and peripheral perfusion and a good cardiac output) with 0·02 units/kg per hour of vasopressin (0·2 ml/hour of a solution made up as described below). Increase this if hypotension persists, by stages, to no more than 0·1 units/kg per hour (1 ml/hour). One-tenth of this dose is enough to control the diabetes insipidus sometimes triggered by brain injury.
Desmopressin: The impact of treatment is difficult to predict, and it is very important to give a low dose to start with. Babies with cranial diabetes insipidus should be given 1–4 micrograms orally, 0·1–0·5 micrograms into the nose or 0·1 micrograms IM, irrespective of body weight. A second dose should only be given when the impact of the first has been assessed. Monitor fluid balance with great care and adjust the size (and timing) of further doses as necessary. Avoid changing the route of administration unnecessarily. Get expert endocrine advice, especially if there is coexistent hypoadrenalism.

Supply and administration
Vasopressin: A 1 ml 20 unit (49 micrograms) ampoule of synthetic vasopressin (argipressin (rINN)) for IV use costs £17. Store at 4°C. To give 0·01 units/kg per hour take 0·1 ml of this fluid for each kg the baby weighs, dilute to 20 ml with glucose or glucose saline, and infuse at a rate of 0·1 ml/hour.
Desmopressin: 1 ml (4 micrograms) ampoules of desmopressin for subcutaneous, IM or oral use cost £1·10. Store ampoules at 4°C. To obtain a 1 microgram/ml solution for more accurate low-dose administration take the contents of this ampoule and dilute to 4 ml with 0·9% sodium chloride. If this dilute sugar-free solution is given into the nose or mouth it can be stored for up to a week at 4°C. 2·5 ml dropper bottles of a 100 microgram/ml multidose intranasal solution cost £10·40. These can be kept for 2 weeks at room temperature. Do *not* dilute further. 100 microgram dispersible tablets cost 52p each.

References
Cheetham TD, Baylis P. Diabetes insipidus in children. Pathophysiology, diagnosis and management. *Pediatr Drugs* 2002;**4**:785–96.
Landry DW, Oliver JA. The pathogenesis of vasodilatory shock. [Review] *N Engl J Med* 2001;**345**:588–95.
Masutani S, Senzaki H, Ishido H, *et al*. Vasopressin in the treatment of vasodilatory shock in children. *Pediatr Int* 2005;**47**:132–6.
Ray JG. DDAVP use during pregnancy: an analysis of its safety for mother and child. *Obstet Gynecol Survey* 1998;**53**:450–5.
Stapleton G, DiGeronimo RJ. Persistent central diabetes insipidus presenting in a very low birth weight infant successfully managed with intranasal dDAVP. *J Perinatol* 2000;**2**:132–34.
Wolf A. Vasopressin in paediatric practice. [Review] *Pediatr Anesth* 2008;**18**:579–81.

Use

Vigabatrin has been used to treat focal (partial) seizures since 1989, and infantile spasms since 1994. While sustained use often causes progressive peripheral visual field damage, this should not inhibit short-term use.

Pharmacology

Vigabatrin is an anticonvulsant that is currently only licensed for use as a secondary *additional* drug in the management of seizures resistant to other antiepileptic drugs. It is certainly of value in the management of partial seizures with, or without, secondary generalisation, and in infantile epileptic encephalopathy (Ohtahara syndrome). There does not appear to be any very clear dose–response relationship, and the plasma level seems to bear no relationship to the concentration in the CNS. It is not, therefore, either necessary or helpful to monitor drug levels. Vigabatrin has also been used on its own in the management of infantile spasms (West syndrome) and is now accepted as the treatment of choice if a child developing infantile spasms has Down syndrome, or is found to have tuberous sclerosis. The first UKISS trial suggested that most other children show a better short-term response to prednisolone, but assessment a year later was unable to detect any long-term advantage to the adoption of this approach. If prednisolone *is* used, many would start by giving 2 mg/kg by mouth four times a day and some would then increase this, if necessary, to as much as 5 mg/kg four times a day, before then tailing treatment off over the next 3–4 weeks. A further trial (www.iciss.org.uk) is currently looking to see whether the best approach is to *start* treatment with both drugs.

Vigabatrin is an amino acid with a structure similar to gamma amino butyric acid (GABA), a potent inhibitory neurotransmitter. It acts as an irreversible inhibitor of GABA-transaminase, the enzyme responsible for degrading GABA. It is rapidly absorbed when given by mouth, achieving good bioavailability because of limited first pass metabolism in the liver. It is excreted, mostly in the urine, with a plasma elimination half life of 5–10 hours both in infancy and in adult life. Vigabatrin is given as a racemic mixture, but only the S(+) enantiomer is pharmacologically active. The drug penetrates the central nervous system where levels seem to stabilise after about 2 weeks. Because the drug is neither plasma-protein bound nor metabolised by the liver it does not interact with, or influence, the metabolism of other anticonvulsants.

Adverse effects in infancy (usually drowsiness, irritability and hypo- or hypertonia) are few and usually transient and mild. Sustained use has been shown to cause progressive, concentric, peripheral visual field damage, but seldom with use in the first year of life and only after continuous exposure for at least 6 months and more usually 2 years (the median time of onset being 5 years). It is almost always bilateral. While this can eventually be disabling, central vision is very seldom affected. Little is known about teratogenicity in man; high-dose treatment caused a slight increase in the incidence of cleft palate in rabbits but not in rats. The breastfed baby only ingests about 2% of the weight-adjusted maternal dose.

Treatment

Start by giving 50 mg/kg twice a day by mouth, and increase this, if necessary, after 3–6 days, to no more than 75 mg/kg twice a day. Double the dosage interval if there is renal failure. Stop treatment if meaningful benefit is not seen after 12 weeks. Sustained benefit is most often seen in children with tuberous sclerosis.

Monitoring treatment

Organise baseline age-appropriate visual field testing if benefit seems to make sustained use appropriate, and repeat this every 3 months, and subsequently every 6 months, looking, in particular, for nasal field changes.

Supply

Vigabatrin is available as a white sugar-free powder in 500 mg sachets costing 34p each. The powder dissolves immediately in water, juice or milk giving a colourless and tasteless solution which is stable for at least 24 hours after reconstitution if kept at 4°C. It can be given into the rectum if oral treatment is temporarily not possible. Dissolve the sachet in 20 ml of water to obtain a solution containing 25 mg/ml.

References

See also the relevant Cochrane reviews

Curatolo P, D'Argenzio L, Cerminara C, *et al*. Management of epilepsy in tuberous sclerosis complex. *Expert Rev Neurother* 2008;**8**:457–67.

Desguerre I, Nabbout R, Dulac O. The management of infantile spasms. *Arch Dis Child* 2008;**93**:462–3.

Dunin WD, Kasprzyk OJ, Jurkiewicz E, *et al*. Infantile spasms and cytomegalovirus infection: antiviral and antiepileptic treatment. *Dev Med Child Neurol* 2007;**49**:684–92.

Gaily E, Jonsson H, Lappi M. Visual fields in school-age children treated with vigabatrin in infancy. *Epilepsia* 2009;**50**:206–16.

Kroll-Seger J, Kaminska A, Moutard ML, *et al*. Severe relapse of epilepsy after vigabatrin withdrawal: for how long should we treat symptomatic infantile spasms. *Epilepsia* 2007;**48**:612–13.

Lux AL, Edwards SW, Hancock E, *et al*. The United Kingdom Infantile Spasms Study (UKISS) comparing hormone treatment with vigabatrin: on developmental and epilepsy outcomes to age 14 months: a multicentre randomised trial. *Lancet Neurol* 2005;**4**:712–17. [RCT]

Parisi P, Bambardieri R, Curatolo P. Current role of vigabatrin in infantile spasms. *Eur J Paediatr Neurol* 2007;**11**:331–6.

Tran A, O'Mahoney T, Rey E, *et al*. Vigabatrin: placental transfer in vivo and excretion into breast milk of the enantiomers. *Br J Clin Pharmacol* 1998;**45**:409–11.

Vanhatalo S, Nousiainen I, Eriksson K, *et al*. Visual field constriction in 91 Finnish children treated with vigabatrin. *Epilepsia* 2002;**43**:748–56.

Vauzelle-Kervroëdan FR, Rey E, Pons G, *et al*. Pharmacokinetics of the individual enantiomers of vigabatrin in neonates with uncontrolled seizures. *Br J Clin Pharmacol* 1996;**42**:779–81.

Willmore LJ, Abelson MB, Ben-Menachem E, *et al*. Vigabatrin: 2008 update. *Epilepsia* 2009;**50**:163–73.

VITAMIN A (Retinol)

Use
Large IM doses can marginally reduce the risk of chronic oxygen dependency in the ventilator-dependent preterm baby, but there is no other good evidence that postnatal supplementation is ever beneficial.

Nutritional factors
Vitamin A is the generic name given to a group of fat-soluble compounds exhibiting the same biological activity as the primary alcohol, retinol. Deficiency, first recognised in 1912, can damage the epithelial cells lining the respiratory tract. It can also affect immunocompetence, reproductive function, growth and vision (the vitamin being responsible for the formation of the retina's photosensitive visual pigment).

Green vegetables, carrots, tomatoes, fruit, eggs and dairy produce all provide vitamin A. Deficiency is rare in the UK but is still a common cause of blindness due to xerophthalmia ('dry eye') in the Third World, increasing the mortality associated with pregnancy and with measles in the first 2 years of life. Weekly supplements reduced maternal mortality in a trial in Nepal, and eliminated anaemia in women also taking iron in one trial in Indonesia, but this finding could not be replicated during trials in Malawi. A 50,000 unit dose at birth by mouth seemed to reduce infant mortality in recent trials in Indonesia and south India, but a systematic review of the data from all the trials that have been done to date failed to show that such supplements generally reduce either infant mortality or serious morbidity.

However, vitamin A is toxic in excess and also teratogenic, and women planning to become pregnant should avoid an intake in excess of 8000 units per day. Inappropriate and excessive multivitamin supplementation can be unwittingly hazardous, and women are advised not to eat liver during pregnancy because of its high vitamin A content (650 units per gram). The anti-acne drugs tretinoin and isotretinoin are also teratogenic when taken by mouth around the time of conception. Topical use may be safe, but many will not wish to take any such risk. Toxicity might also (in theory) develop in a breastfed baby whose mother was taking an excess of any of these retinoids. The dietary antioxidant precursors of vitamin A, including β-carotene, are not teratogenic.

Human milk contains 100–250 units of vitamin A per 100 ml, and the term baby requires no further supplementation whether artificially or breast fed. However, the fetal liver only accumulates vitamin A in the last third of pregnancy, and plasma levels are low in the preterm baby at birth. While overt clinical deficiency has not been detected, additional supplementation has been widely recommended for the very preterm baby. Those fed IV are often given a 900 unit/kg daily supplement with their Intralipid® (q.v.). Most orally fed preterm babies are also supplemented – often with a multi-vitamin product (q.v.). A trial involving 807 babies weighing 1 kg or less has recently shown that an even larger dose IM (5000 units three times a week from birth) slightly reduces the number of babies who are still oxygen dependant at a postmenstrual age of 36 weeks (odds ratio 0·85). Mortality was not reduced. Some will consider the benefit marginal, given the number of injections required. No benefit was detected in a trial where 157 babies were given a similar dose daily by mouth. IV prophylaxis remains unexplored.

Prophylaxis
Prematurity: A daily 4000 unit oral supplement normalises blood levels in the very preterm baby, but whether this is of any functional benefit is less clear.

Preventing lung damage: Ventilator-dependent babies of less than 28 weeks' gestation may derive some benefit from 5000 units (0·1 ml) of vitamin A given IM three times a week for 4 weeks.

Liver disease: Counteract malabsorption due to prolonged cholestasis by giving 4000 or 5000 units once a day by mouth. Give babies with complete biliary obstruction 50,000 IU once a month IM.

In communities where dietary deficiency is common: The WHO has long recommended that such women should receive a single 200,000 unit dose by mouth shortly after delivery, and that their babies should be given a 100,000 unit dose at 9 months and a 200,000 unit dose 3 months later. In communities where severe deficiency is common babies should be given 50,000 units at birth.

Supply
2 ml ampoules containing 50,000 units of vitamin A palmitate per ml cost £4·10 (1 unit is equivalent to 0·3 micrograms of preformed retinol). Store ampoules at less than 15°C, and protect from light. Do not dilute, or use if the yellowish opalescent solution shows signs of flocculation. An unlicensed oral preparation containing 5000 units per drop can be imported on request. For information on Dalivit® (which contains 5000 units of vitamin A in 0·6 ml) see the monograph on multiple vitamins.

References
See also the relevant Cochrane reviews

Ambalavanan N, Tyson JE, Kennedy KA, et al. Vitamin A supplementation for extremely low birth weight infants: outcome at 18 to 22 months. *Pediatrics* 2005;**115**:e249–54. [RCT]

Benn CS, Diness BR, Roth A, et al. Effect of 50,000 IU vitamin A given with BCG vaccine on mortality in infants in Guinea-Bissau: a randomized placebo controlled trial. *BMJ* 2008;**336**:1416–20. [RCT] (See also pp. 1385–6.)

Gogia S, Sachdev HS. Neonatal vitamin A supplementation for prevention of mortality and morbidity in infancy: systematic review of randomised controlled trials. *BMJ* 2009;**338**:b919. [SR]

Klemm RSW, Labrique AB, Christian P, et al. Newborn vitamin A supplementation reduced infant mortality in rural Bangladesh. *Pediatrics* 2008;**122**:e242–50. [RCT] (See also pp. 180–1.)

Rothman KJ, Moore LL, Singer MR, et al. Teratogenicity of high dose vitamin A intake. *N Engl J Med* 1995;**333**:1369–73.

Use

The breastfed babies of mothers with unrecognised pernicious anaemia occasionally become B$_{12}$ deficient, as do a few on a deficient vegetarian diet, and older children occasionally become deficient because of malabsorption. Pharmacological doses are beneficial in several rare (autosomal recessive) disorders of cobalamin (vitamin B$_{12}$) transport and metabolism.

Nutritional factors

Vitamin B$_{12}$ is a water-soluble vitamin that is actively transported across the placenta. Babies have high serum levels and significant liver stores at birth. Meat and milk are the main dietary sources. Toxicity has not been described. Absorption requires binding to intrinsic factor (a protein secreted by the stomach), recognition of the complex by receptors in the terminal ileum and release into the portal circulation bound to transcobalamin II. Ileal absorption can be affected by surgery for necrotising enterocolitis (NEC), while congenital transcobalamin II deficiency can also affect tissue delivery. The first sign of deficiency is neutrophil hypersegmentation. Megaloblastic anaemia develops, and severe deficiency causes neurological damage that can be irreversible. A high folic acid intake can mask the haematological signs of vitamin B$_{12}$ deficiency. Intrinsic factor failure causes pernicious anaemia which Whipple was first able to cure in 1926 with a liver diet. The active ingredient (cyanocobalamin) was finally isolated in 1948, and a bacterial source of production developed the following year.

Pharmacology

Cobalamin is released from transcobalamin II within target cells and converted to adenosylcobalamin or methylcobalamin, cofactors respectively for methylmalonyl mutase and methionine synthase. Rare genetic defects can impair cobalamin metabolism at various stages. Patients can present at any age from 2 days to 5 years with symptoms ranging from vomiting and encephalopathy to developmental delay and failure to thrive. Investigations may show a megaloblastic anaemia, methylmalonic aciduria and/or homocystinuria, depending on the precise defect. A trial of vitamin B$_{12}$ should be undertaken in all patients with methylmalonic aciduria, whether or not this is accompanied by homocystinuria. It needs to be conducted when the patient is well and on a constant protein intake. Hydroxocobalamin (1 mg IM) is given daily for five consecutive days and methylmalonate excretion measured before, during and after the intervention. Patients with isolated homocystinuria and low or normal plasma methionine concentrations are also likely to have a cobalamin defect and should have a similar trial of vitamin B$_{12}$. Patients with these conditions who are acutely unwell should be started on vitamin B$_{12}$ at once and a formal trial deferred until later. Patients who respond should be started on a 1 mg dose IM daily. Treatment should be accompanied by other measures appropriate to the specific defect, such as protein restriction, metronidazole, carnitine and/or betaine under the guidance of a consultant experienced in the management of metabolic disease.

Treatment

Dietary deficiency: Give a single IM injection of between 250 micrograms and 1 mg, and then ensure that the diet remains adequate (1 microgram/kg a day is sufficient).
Absorptive defects: Malabsorption is treated with 1 mg of hydroxocobalamin IM at monthly intervals, but 1 mg IM three times a week is usually given in transcobalamin II deficiency during the first year of life, later reducing to 1 mg once a week with haematological monitoring.
Metabolic disease: The initial maintenance dose is 1 mg IM daily irrespective of weight, but this can often be reduced later to 1–3 injections a week, with biochemical monitoring to ensure that there is no deterioration. Oral hydroxocobalamin (1–20 mg/day) is sometimes substituted, but is usually less effective because the intestinal tract's absorptive capacity becomes saturated.

Supply

1 ml ampoules containing 1 mg of hydroxocobalamin for IM use cost £2·50.

References

Andersson HC, Shapira E. Biochemical and clinical response to hydroxocobalamin versus cyanocobalamin treatment in patients with methylmalonic acidemia and homocystinuria (cblC). *J Pediatr* 1998;**132**:121–4.

Korenke GC, Hunneman DH, Eber S, *et al*. Severe encephalopathy with epilepsy in infant caused by subclinical maternal pernicious anaemia: case report and review of the literature. *Eur J Pediatr* 2004;**163**:196–201.

Kuhne T, Bubl R, Baumgartner R. Maternal vegan diet causing a serious infantile neurological disorder due to vitamin B$_{12}$ deficiency. *Eur J Pediatr* 1991;**150**:205–8.

Marble M, Copeland S, Khanfar N, *et al*. Neonatal vitamin B$_{12}$ deficiency secondary to maternal subclinical pernicious anemia: identification by expanded newborn screening. *J Pediatr* 2008;**152**:731–3.

Monagle PT, Tauro GP. Long term follow up of patients with transcobalamin II deficiency. *Arch Dis Child* 1995;**72**:237–8.

Roschitz B, Plaeko B, Huemer M, *et al*. Nutritional infantile vitamin B$_{12}$ deficiency; pathobiological considerations in seven patients. [Letter] *Arch Dis Child* 2005;**90**:F281–2.

Rosenblatt DS, Fenton WA. Inherited disorders of folate and cobalamin transport and metabolism. In: Scriver CR, Beaudet AL, Sky WS, *et al*., eds. *The metabolic and molecular bases of inherited disease*, 8th edn. New York: McGraw-Hill, 2001: pp. 3897–934.

Rosenblatt DS, Fowler B, Disorders of cobalamin and folate transport and metabolism. In: Fernandes J, Saudubray J-M, van den Berghe G, *et al*., eds. *Inborn metabolic diseases. Diagnosis and treatment*, 4th edn. Berlin: Springer-Verlag, 2006: pp. 341–56.

VITAMIN D (special formulations)

Use

These formulations should only be used for babies unable to metabolise dietary vitamin D into alfacalcidol or calcitriol because of renal damage (although some babies with congenital hypoparathyroidism also benefit from taking the more potent active substance). Prematurity does not, in itself, make such use appropriate.

Pharmacology

A range of closely related sterol compounds possess vitamin D-like properties, as outlined in the main monograph on vitamin D. Most have to be hydroxylated before becoming metabolically active. Toxicity is more likely with vitamin D than with any other vitamin, and it seems particularly common in infancy. It first manifests as hypercalcaemia, with muscle weakness, nausea and vomiting, pain and even cardiac arrhythmia and, if persistent, with generalised vascular calcification and a progressive deterioration in renal function. Because the metabolically active products have a shorter biological half life, they need to be given daily but this also means that any toxicity also resolves rather more quickly. Because patients vary quite widely in the amount of calcitriol or alfacalcidol they require, it is important to monitor the total (and, if possible, the ionised) plasma calcium concentration regularly. Such limited information as there is suggests that, if use is necessary to keep the mother well during pregnancy, it will keep the fetus well too, but high-dose maternal use during lactation should only be attempted if the baby is monitored with some care.

Pathophysiology

Renal disease: Patients with severe renal disease, and on long-term renal dialysis, often become hypocalcaemic. Many develop secondary hyperparathyroidism if the plasma phosphate level remains high, and some develop renal rickets (osteodystrophy). Management is outlined in the website entry for vitamin D, but all such children need to be managed by an experienced paediatric nephrologist. Use just enough alfacalcidol or calcitriol to keep the ionised plasma calcium concentration in the upper half of the normal range (1·18−1·38 mmol/l in late infancy).
Parathyroid disorders: Deficient parathyroid production (as, for example in the DiGeorge and CATCH 22 syndromes) causes hypocalcaemia best controlled by giving a metabolically active form of vitamin D. Adjust the dose used to keep the plasma calcium level in the low normal range (2·0−2·25 mmol/l). Patients with receptor insensitivity to parathyroid hormone (pseudohypoparathyroidism) should be managed in the same way.
Pseudovitamin D-deficiency rickets: This is a recessively inherited condition in which the kidney's 1α-hydroxylase enzyme system is inactivated, causing hypocalcaemia, rickets and secondary hyperparathyroidism. All symptoms can be abolished by giving a physiological dose of one of the metabolically active forms of vitamin D.

Treatment

Alfacalcidol (1α-hydroxycholecalciferol): Start babies on 25 nanograms/kg by mouth or IV once a day and optimise the dose as outlined above by measuring the plasma calcium level twice a week. Monitoring needs to continue every 2−4 weeks even after treatment seems to have stabilised.
Calcitriol (1,25-dihydroxycholecalciferol): Start babies on 15 nanograms/kg by mouth or IV once a day, and monitor treatment regularly as indicated above.

Supply

Alfacalcidol: 1 microgram 0·5 ml ampoules for IV or IM use cost £2·20. They contain 207 mg of propylene glycol. 10 ml bottles of a sugar-free oral liquid (100 nanograms/drop) cost £22. This liquid cannot be further diluted, so the only way to give a really low dose is to give treatment less than daily.
Calcitriol: 1 microgram (1 ml) ampoules for IV or IM use cost £5·10. No low-dose oral formulation is available in the UK because no manufacturer has yet sought a licence to market the product for use in children. This is, however, the product used in the US (where no manufacturer markets alfacalcidol).

References

Caplan RH, Beguin EA. Hypercalemia in a calcitriol-treated hypoparathyroid woman during lactation. *Obstetr Gynecol* 1990;**76**:485−9.
Chan JCM, McEnery PT, Chinchilli VM, *et al*. A prospective double-blind study of growth failure in children with chronic renal insufficiency and the effectiveness of treatment with calcitriol versus dihydrotachysterol. *J Pediatr* 1994;**124**:520−8. [RCT]
Hochberg Z, Tiosano D, Even L. Calcium therapy for calcitriol-resistant rickets. *J Pediatr* 1992;**121**:803−8.
Hodson EM, Evans RA, Dunstan CR, *et al*. Treatment of childhood osteodystrophy with calcitriol or ergocalciferol. *Clin Nephrol* 1985;**24**:192−200.
Holick MF. Vitamin D deficiency. [Review] *N Engl J Med* 2007;**357**:266−81.
Rigden SPA. The treatment of renal osteodystrophy. *Pediatr Nephrol* 1996;**10**:653−5.
Seikaly MG, Browne RH, Baum M. The effect of phosphate supplementation on linear growth in children with X-lined hypophosphatemia. *Pediatrics* 1994;**94**:478−81.
Thomas BR, Bennett JD. Symptomatic hypocalcaemia and hypoparathyroidism in two infants of mothers with hyperparathyroidism and familial benign hypercalcemia. *J Perinatol* 1995;**15**:23−6.

Use

Irrespective of weight, babies need 10 micrograms (400 IU) of vitamin D a day for optimal bone growth. While all artificial milks provide this, breast milk will not do this if the mother herself is subclinically deficient. The case for prophylactic supplementation is widely acknowledged and just as widely ignored.

Pharmacology

Vitamin D (calciferol) is the generic term used to describe a range of compounds that control calcium and phosphate absorption from the intestine, their mobilisation from bone, and also possibly their retention by the kidneys. Vitamin D_2 (ergocalciferol) and vitamin D_3 (colecalciferol) are the main dietary sources. Both have to be hydroxylated to 25-hydroxyvitamin D (25(OH)D) by the liver and finally activated by further hydroxylation to 1,25-hydroxy D by the kidney and placenta. D_3 is more effectively hydroxylated than D_2. Microgram for microgram, D_3 is also more than three times as effective in raising plasma 25(OH)D levels than is D_2. After a single, high-dose IM injection of D_3, levels take 3 months to respond; and even longer after IM D_2. Somewhat surprisingly the response is much faster (days) if either IM preparation is taken orally.

Nutritional factors

Most breakfast cereals and spreading margarines provide dietary vitamin D, as do oily fish. Exposure to ultraviolet summer sunlight is, however, the main reason why most people avoid becoming vitamin D deficient and clothing can block this, as can the excessive use of sunblock cream. Maternal deficiency severe enough to cause congenital rickets or craniotabes is rare, but many women have suboptimal levels rendering their children, if breastfed, vulnerable to the hazards of overt rickets. There is also increasing evidence that subclinical deficiency during pregnancy and the first year of life can have a permanently damaging impact on bone growth in later childhood (see web commentary).

The amount of vitamin D required in infancy is influenced by the adequacy of the stores built up during fetal life, and by subsequent exposure to sunlight. If neither can be guaranteed the case for a regular supplement is overwhelming, and there is no reason not to start this at birth. Many weaning foods are fortified, while all formula milks (q.v.) contain at least 10 micrograms/l but, because breast milk usually contains less than 1 microgram/l even in women with good nutritional reserves, many breastfed babies continue to become covertly deficient if they are not supplemented, especially in winter.

Maternal prophylaxis

The optimum strategy is to get all women to take a 10 microgram supplement daily throughout pregnancy and, in the UK, the 'Healthy Start' women's vitamin tablets now make this possible. An alternative strategy, adopted in some parts of Europe, is to give all women suspected of having suboptimal vitamin D stores (including all veiled women) a 2·5 mg IM dose of vitamin D_3 early in the third trimester of pregnancy, though taking the IM preparation by mouth is much more effective at raising 25(OH)D levels.

Prophylaxis after birth

Breastfed babies: Give 7·5 micrograms once a day until mixed feeding is established.
Preterm babies: Give all preterm babies 7·5 micrograms once a day until they weigh at least 3 kg.
Malabsorption: Give babies with complete biliary obstruction 750 micrograms IM once a month.
Renal disease: Give *alfacalcidol* instead by mouth or IV to babies unable to hydroxylate calciferol, as outlined in the monograph on special formulations of vitamin D.

Supply

Prophylaxis during pregnancy: 'Healthy Start' women's vitamin tablets, costing 1–2p each and containing 10 micrograms of D_3, 70 mg of vitamin C and 400 micrograms of folic acid (but no vitamin A), became available in the UK to all women who are pregnant or breastfeeding in March 2007. For details, and for more general advice on diet during pregnancy and infancy, see www.healthystart.nhs.uk.
Prophylaxis during the first year of life: See the multivitamin monograph for various alternatives.
Treatment of established vitamin deficiency: 1 ml (7·5 mg, 300,000 units) ampoules of D_2 for IM use cost £5·90. 10 microgram (400 units) tablets, containing redundant calcium, cost 3p each. A 3000 unit/ml oral liquid is available from Martindale; 100 ml costs £37.

References

See also the relevant Cochrane reviews

Armas LAG, Hollis BW, Heaney RP. Vitamin D_2 is much less effective than vitamin D_3 in humans. *J Clin Endocrinol Metab* 2004;**89**:5387–91.
Backström MC, Mäki R, Kuusela A-L, *et al*. Randomised controlled trial of vitamin D supplementation on bone density and biochemical indices in preterm infants. *Arch Dis Child* 1999;**80**:F161–6. [RCT]
Dawodu A, Wagner CL. Mother–child vitamin D deficiency: an international perspective. [Review] *Arch Dis Child* 2007;**92**:737–40.
Dimitri P, Bishop N. Rickets. *Paediatr Child Health* 2007;**17**:279–87.
Holick MF. Vitamin D deficiency. [Review] *N Engl J Med* 2007;**357**:266–81.
Misra M, Pacaud D, Petryk A, *et al*. Vitamin D deficiency in children and its management: review of current knowledge and recommendations. *Pediatrics* 2008;**122**:398–417.
Pearce SHS, Cheetham TD. Diagnosis and management of vitamin D deficiency. *BMJ* 2010;**340**:142–7.
Romagnoli E, Mascia ML, Cipriani C, *et al*. Short and long-term variations in serum calcitropic hormones after a single very large dose of ergocaliferol (D2) or cholecalciferol (D3) in the elderly. *J Clin Endocrinol Metab* 2008;**93**:3015–20.
Taylor SN, Wagner CL, Hollis BW. Vitamin D supplementation during lactation to support infant and mother. *J Am Coll Nutr* 2008;**27**:690–71.

Use

Vitamin E is used to prevent haemolytic anaemia in vitamin E-deficient babies, and in babies with malabsorption due to cholestasis. Pharmacological doses are used in abetalipoproteinaemia.

Pharmacology

Vitamin E is the name given to a group of fat-soluble antioxidant tocopherols of which α-tocopherol shows the greatest activity. The natural vitamin, first isolated in 1936, is concentrated from soya bean oil. Excessive intake (100 mg/kg daily) is toxic to the newborn kitten. Plasma levels in excess of 100 mg/l caused hepatomegaly and levels over 180 mg/l were sometimes lethal. The effect of excessive medication in man is unknown. Vitamin deficiency was first identified as causing fetal death and resorption in the laboratory rat. It is now known to cause enhanced platelet aggregation and is also thought to cause a haemolytic anaemia, probably as a result of peroxidation of the lipid component of the red cell membrane (a problem that seems to be exacerbated by giving artificial milk containing extra iron).

Various studies in the 1980s looked to see whether early high-dose IV or IM use reduced the risk of intraventricular haemorrhage, bronchpulmonary dysplasia or retinopathy of prematurity, but the benefits achieved were marginal, and no study ever looked to see how much long-term benefit such treatment delivered. The preparations used in those studies have, in any case, now been withdrawn from general sale because of concern about one of the stabilisation agents used, while high-dose oral administration has been linked to an increased incidence of necrotising enterocolitis that may (or may not) have been related to the product's high osmolarity. Interest in the vitamin's prophylactic use as an antioxidant has now declined, and one recent meta-analysis has suggested that sustained high-dose use to limit the risk of cardiovascular disease and cancer in older people may actually be harmful. Neither does high-dose supplementation with vitamins C and E in pregnancy seem to reduce the risk of pre-eclampsia as much as early studies had suggested.

High doses of vitamin E can prevent neuromuscular problems in abetalipoproteinaemia, an autosomal recessive disorder associated with fat malabsorption and acanthocytosis. Such babies should also be treated with a low fat diet and supplements of vitamins A (7 mg) and K (5–10 mg) once a day by mouth irrespective of weight.

Nutritional factors

Human milk contains an average of 0·35 mg α-tocopherol per 100 ml (some four times as much as cows' milk) and commercial feeds between 0·5 and 4·0 mg/100 ml. Babies are relatively deficient in vitamin E at birth, and plasma levels (2·5 mg/l) are less than a quarter those in the mother. Plasma levels rise rapidly after birth in the breastfed term baby but remain low for several weeks in artificially fed preterm babies (especially those weighing <1·5 kg at birth). No significant anaemia develops, however, with artificial feeds that provide a daily intake of 2 mg/kg of d-α-tocopherol (approximately 3 units/kg vitamin E) as long as the ratio of vitamin E to polyunsaturated fat in the diet is well above 0·4 mg/g even if the milk contains supplemental iron. Haemolytic anaemia, when it does occur, usually becomes apparent 4–6 weeks after birth and is usually associated with a reticulocytosis (>8%), an unusually high platelet count and an abnormal peroxide-induced haemolysis test (>30%).

Treatment

Prophylaxis in the preterm baby: Only a minority of units now offer routine oral supplementation. The optimum IV dose for a parenterally fed baby is probably about 2·8 mg/kg per day.
Nutritional deficiency: 10 mg/kg by mouth once a day will quickly correct any nutritional deficiency.
Malabsorption: Babies with cholestasis may benefit from a 50 mg supplement once a day by mouth. Give babies with complete biliary obstruction 10 mg/kg twice a month IM.
Abetaliproteinaemia: Give 100 mg/kg by mouth once a day.

Supply

An oral suspension of α-tocopherol acetate (£17·20 per 100 ml) containing 100 mg/ml of vitamin E can be obtained by the pharmacy on request: some say it should be diluted before use with syrup BP because of its hyperosmolarity (see above). 2 ml vials of Ephynal® costing £1·30 and containing 50 mg/ml suitable for IM use are obtainable from Roche in the UK on a 'named patient' basis but no licensed parenteral preparation is commercially available either in the UK or North America.

References

See also the relevant Cochrane reviews

Brion LP, Bell EF, Raghuveer TS, et al. What is the appropriate intravenous dose of vitamin E for very-low-birth-weight infants? *J Perinatol* 2004;**24**:205–7.

Greer FR, Vitamins A, E, and K. In: Tsang RC, Uauy R, Zlotkin S, et al., eds. *Nutrition in the preterm infant. Scientific basis and practical guidelines*, 2nd edn. Cincinnati, OH: Digital Educational Publishing, 2005; pp. 141–72.

Low MR, Wijewardene K, Wald NK. Is routine vitamin E administration justified in very low-birthweight infants? *Dev Med Child Neurol* 1990;**32**:442–50.

Miller ER, Pastor-Barriuso R, Dalal D, et al. Meta-analysis: high-dosage vitamin E supplementation may increase all-cause mortality. *Ann Intern Med* 2005;**142**:37–46. [SR] (See also pp. 75–6.)

Raju TNK, Lagenberg P, Bhutani V, et al. Vitamin E prophylaxis to reduce retinopathy of prematurity: a reappraisal of published trials. *J Pediatr* 1997;**131**:844–50. [SR]

Use
Vitamin K is required for the hepatic production of coagulation factors II, VII, IX and X.

Nutritional factors
The term vitamin K refers to a variety of fat-soluble 2-methyl-1,4-naphthoquinone derivatives. Vitamin K_1 (isolated in 1939) occurs in green plants, while vitamin K_2 (menaquinone) is synthesised by microbial flora in the gut. Human milk contains about 1·5 μg of vitamin K per litre, while cows' milk contains about three times as much as this. Most artificial milks contain over 50 μg/l. Vitamin K crosses the placenta poorly, and babies are relatively deficient at birth. Any resultant vitamin-responsive bleeding used to be called 'haemorrhagic disease of the newborn' but is now, more informatively, called 'vitamin K deficiency bleeding' (VKDB) because it can occur at any time in the first 3 months of life. Any unexplained bruise or bleed in a young baby calls for *immediate* attention (see below) if catastrophic cerebral bleeding is to be avoided.

Pharmacology
Bleeding in the first week of life is usually mild, except in the babies of mothers on some anticonvulsants. Later VKDB can, however, cause potentially lethal intracranial bleeding, and there is a 1:6000 risk of this in the unsupplemented breastfed baby. Malabsorption, usually due to unrecognised liver disease, accounts for most of this increased risk. A single 1 mg IM dose provides *almost* complete protection, probably by providing a slow release IM 'depot', but a dose this large causes some liver overload in the very preterm baby. In North America a single IM dose at birth is the preferred preventive strategy, but in Europe the breastfed baby is more commonly given at least three 2 mg oral doses at intervals (see web commentary). Britain is somewhere in 'mid-Atlantic', but the UK Government is committed to ensuring that all families are allowed to choose which strategy they would prefer. A 50 microgram oral daily supplement approximates what 'formula' fed babies get and this is what the recently introduced commercial Neokay® drops provide.

Prophylaxis
IM prophylaxis: 1 mg is the dose traditionally given IM to every baby at birth. IV administration does ***not*** give the *sustained* protection provided by IM injection. For babies below 2·5 kg, give 0·3 mg/kg to a maximum dose of 1 mg (and then give those later offered breast milk an oral supplement from 4 weeks).

Oral option: Babies born to mothers on carbamazepine, phenobarbital, phenytoin, rifampicin or warfarin, and those too ill for early feeding, should be offered IM prophylaxis at birth, but all other babies can, with parental consent, be given a 1 or 2 mg dose by mouth instead. This is *just* as effective provided all exclusively breastfed babies are then started on a daily 50 microgram oral supplement, or given either two further oral doses each of 2 mg over the next 6–8 weeks or, preferably, 1 mg a week for 12 weeks.

Babies with obstructive liver disease: These need a 1 mg protective IM dose once every 2 weeks.

Diagnosis of vitamin K deficiency
Changes in the prothrombin time and international normalised ratio (INR) are poor indicators of vitamin K deficiency. Low vitamin K states lead to production of abnormal prothrombin (PIVKA-II). In vitamin K replete neonates PIVKA-II levels are below 0·2 AU/ml. Levels >1 AU/ml indicate subclinical deficiency and >5 AU/ml a clinically relevant deficiency. As PIVKA-II has a half life of about 60 hours deficiency can be confirmed by finding high levels even if the test is done a couple of days after vitamin K treatment.

Treatment
Where bleeding may be due to vitamin K deficiency give 100 micrograms/kg IV (or subcutaneously).

Supply and administration
A concentrated colloidal (mixed micelle) preparation (Konakion MM®) designed to make IV use safe, and containing 2 mg in 0·2 ml, has been the only product available in Europe since 2006. Ampoules cost £1 each. This can be given IV, IM or by mouth, although the manufacturer originally designed the product for administration by a health professional, cautions against further dilution, and advises (without giving any reason) that 0·4 mg/kg IM is better than oral prophylaxis for babies under 2·5 kg. The IM formulation still used in North America is a 1 mg (0·5 ml) ampoule containing some benzyl alcohol.

A recently licensed oral preparation of K_1 (Neokay® Capsules 1 mg) provides an easier option in Europe for use at birth. Oral supplementation must be continued for the first 3 months of life in exclusively breastfed infants, either with a once *weekly* 1 mg oral dose or alternatively with a *daily* lower dose oral supplement using a convenient multidose dropper-bottle product (Neokay® Drops 200 micrograms/ml). A 0·25 ml daily dose provides 50 micrograms of vitamin K_1 and a 25 ml bottle, enough for 3 months, costs £3.

UK midwives can, under the 1968 Medicines Act, give licensed vitamin K products on their own authority.

References
See also the relevant Cochrane reviews

Clarke P, Mitchell S, Wynn R, *et al*. Vitamin K prophylaxis for preterm infants: a randomized, controlled trial of three regimens. *Pediatrics* 2006;**118**:e1657–66. [RCT]

Clarke P. Vitamin K prophylaxis for preterm infants. [Review] *Early Hum Dev* 2010;**86**(suppl 1):17–20.

Hansen KN, Minousis M, Ebbesen F. Weekly oral vitamin K prophylaxis in Denmark. *Acta Paediatr* 2003;**92**:802–5.

Van Hasselt PM, de Koning TJ, Kvist N, *et al*. Prevention of vitamin K deficiency bleeding in breastfed infants: lessons from the Dutch and Danish biliary atresia registries. *Pediatrics* 2008;**121**:e857–63. (See also pp. 1048–9.)

von Kries R, Hachmeister A, Göbel U. Oral mixed micellar vitamin K for prevention of late vitamin K deficiency bleeding. *Arch Dis Child* 2003;**88**:F109–12. (See also pp. F80–3.)

Use

Children with malabsorption often develop subclinical fat-soluble vitamin deficiency, and babies on sustained IV nutrition are at similar risk. All breastfed babies benefit from being offered additional vitamins D and K.

Nutritional factors

The UK 'Welfare Food' scheme, as originally introduced in 1940, included liquid milk, national dried milk, concentrated orange juice and cod liver oil, and few disputed Winston Churchill's claim that there could be 'no finer investment for any country than putting milk into babies'. Mothers also received special supplements. Because the scheme was generally credited with actually improving the health of children during the war years, the relevant regulations were never repealed, although infant vitamin drops (and maternal tablets) replaced cod liver oil and orange juice in 1975, and commercial formula milks replaced National Dried Milk in 1977. Uptake has, however, declined in recent years. By 2000, less than 5% of babies were getting a vitamin supplement in the first 6 months of life, and only 10% of babies 8–9 months old.

The scheme was eventually revised in 2006 and pregnant women and children under 4 years in the UK in families on income support, income-based job-seekers allowance or child tax credit and an income of below £15,575 a year, are now legally entitled to vouchers that can be obtained from midwives and health visitors and exchanged for fresh fruit, vegetables and milk worth £3·10 a week. For details see www.healthystart.nhs.uk. Children 6 months to 4 years old in these families are also entitled to free 'Healthy Start' vitamin A and D drops, while pregnant women are entitled to free vitamin D tablets (as outlined in the vitamin D monograph).

Unfortunately the programme has not offered clear guidance on the needs of babies less than 6 months old. While artificially fed babies seldom have problems because all formula milks are fortified, this does not cover the need of preterm babies on a total intake of less than 500 ml a day. Many breastfed babies across the world also suffer subclinical vitamin D deficiency – in part because their mothers are, themselves, unknowingly deficient – and serious vitamin D deficiency can cause hypocalcaemic seizures, rickets and even, occasionally, death from cardiomyopathy. It is, therefore, best to give all breastfed babies additional vitamin D *from birth*.

Oral vitamins

The following three options differ very little. It is, however, important to realise that ***none*** contain vitamin K.

'Healthy Start' children's vitamin drops: One 5-drop dose each day provides 233 micrograms of vitamin A and 7·5 micrograms of D_3 (and also a small amount of C).

Abidec® drops: The usual dose is 0·3 ml once a day by mouth throughout the first year of life. Very preterm babies, and children with cystic fibrosis and other forms of malabsorption, are often given 0·6 ml once a day, a dose that provides 400 micrograms (1333 units) of vitamin A, 10 micrograms (400 units) of D_2, 40 mg of C and some B_1, B_2, B_6 and nicotinamide (but no E or K).

Dalivit® drops: Normally given in the same way, and in the same dose, as Abidec. The vitamin content is almost the same as for Abidec, but a 0·6 ml dose contains an excess (1·5 mg (5000 units)) of A.

Intravenous vitamins

Water-soluble vitamins: Amino acid solutions used to provide parenteral nutrition (q.v.) will have usually had all the more important vitamins added (as Solivito N®) prior to issue by the pharmacy.

Fat-soluble vitamins: The manufacturers say that babies weighing under 2·5 kg should have 4 ml/kg of Vitlipid N® *infant* added to their Intralipid® (q.v.) each day so that they get the D_2 and K_1 they need, but this strategy reduces calorie intake (since Vitlipid is formulated in 10% Intralipid); a quarter of this dose normally suffices. A dose of 10 ml/day is recommended for all children weighing >2·5 kg, but such supplements are only important when sustained IV feeding becomes necessary.

Supply

Oral preparations: 10 ml bottles of the UK Government's 'Healthy Start Children's Drops' (which should last 2 months) are at present only easily available from maternity and child health clinics. They cost £1.93 but are available free to certain families (see above). 25 ml bottles of Abidec and Dalivit are also available without a prescription and cost £2 and £3 respectively. Both products contain sucrose.

IV preparations: 10 ml ampoules of Vitlipid N *infant*, designed for adding to Intralipid, contain 690 micrograms (2300 units) of vitamin A, 10 micrograms (400 units) of D_2, 7 mg of E, and 200 micrograms of K_1. They cost £1·70. Any amino acid solution designed for IV use will have normally had a vial of Solivito N (containing small amounts of B_1, B_2, B_6, B_{12}, nicotinamide, sodium pantothenate, C and folic acid) added prior to issue. Such vials also cost £1·70 each. Supplements of Solivito N can, alternatively, be added to Intralipid, or to a plain infusion of IV glucose.

References

Committee on Medical Aspects of Food and Nutrition Policy Panel on Child and Maternal Nutrition. *Scientific review of the welfare food scheme*. Report on Health and Social Subjects, Department of Health No. 51. London: The Stationery Office, 2002.

Ferenchak AP, Sontag MK, Wagener JS, *et al*. Prospective long-term study of fat-soluble vitamin status in children with cystic fibrosis identified by newborn screen. *J Pediatr* 1999;**135**:601–10.

Leaf A. Vitamins for babies and young children. [Review] *Arch Dis Child* 2007;**92**:160–4.

Use
Warfarin is used in the long-term control of thromboembolic disease. Heparin (q.v.) is better for short-term treatment. There is limited experience of use in the neonatal period.

Pharmacology
Warfarin is an oral coumarin anticoagulant that works, after a latent period of 1–2 days, by depressing the vitamin K-dependent synthesis of a range of plasma coagulation factors, including prothrombin, by the liver. It was developed as a rat poison in 1948 before later coming into clinical use. Because the half life is about 36 hours, blood levels only stabilise after a week of treatment. Babies need a higher weight-related dose than adults. Those with chronic atrial fibrillation, dilated cardiomyopathy or certain forms of reconstructive heart surgery benefit from prophylactic warfarin, and it has occasionally been used to manage intravascular or intracardiac thrombi. Treatment could initially precipitate purpura fulminans (a form of tissue infarction) in patients with thromboses due to homozygous protein C or S deficiency.

Warfarin crosses the placenta, but is not excreted in breast milk. Exposure at 6–9 weeks' gestation can cause a syndrome simulating chondrodysplasia punctata, and drug use may not be entirely safe even in later pregnancy because of the risk of fetal and neonatal haemorrhage. Problems are minimised by not letting the dose exceed 5 mg/day. The small risk of congenital optic atrophy, microcephaly and mental retardation (possibly caused by minor recurrent bleeding) may be of more concern than the commoner, but less serious, defects associated with exposure in early pregnancy. Unfortunately, while heparin provides reasonable prophylaxis for most women at risk of thromboembolism during pregnancy, it does not provide adequate protection for mothers with pulmonary vascular disease, atrial fibrillation or an artificial heart valve. Here the balance of risk is such that warfarin should be given until delivery threatens or the pregnancy reaches 37 weeks, and then restarted 2 days after delivery. Always cover the intervening period with enoxaparin (q.v.) or heparin. Babies of mothers taking warfarin at the time of delivery need immediate prophylaxis with at least 100 micrograms/kg of IM vitamin K (q.v.).

Drug interactions
Many drugs increase the anticoagulant effect of warfarin including amiodarone, some cephalosporins, cimetidine, erythromycin, fluconazole, glucagon, metronidazole, miconazole, phenytoin, ritonavir and the sulphonamide drugs; L-carnitine, ciprofloxacin and some penicillins can sometimes have a similar effect. So can high-dose paracetamol. Other drugs, including barbiturates, carbamazepine, rifampicin, spironolactone and vitamin K, decrease warfarin's anticoagulant effect.

Treatment
Initial anticoagulation: Give 200 micrograms/kg by mouth on day 1, and half this dose on the next 2 days (unless the international normalised ratio (INR) is still <1·5). Always seek expert advice before starting anticoagulation.
Maintenance: Laboratory monitoring is essential to determine long-term needs. Most children need 100–300 micrograms/kg once a day, but babies under 1 year old often need 150–400 micrograms/kg a day, especially if bottle fed (possibly because of the high vitamin K intake that this provides).

Dose monitoring
Collect 1 ml of blood into 0·1 ml of citrate, avoiding any line that has *ever* contained heparin. Testing is only needed every few weeks once treatment has stabilised but, because many drugs affect the half life of warfarin, additional checks are needed each time other treatment is changed. An INR of between 2 and 3 seems to be the best level to aim for in most adults (Fig. 1), but slightly higher values have often been recommended for adults after heart valve replacement. Parents must be told about the need for monitoring, given an anticoagulant book with a note of all treatment, and have the book's importance explained.

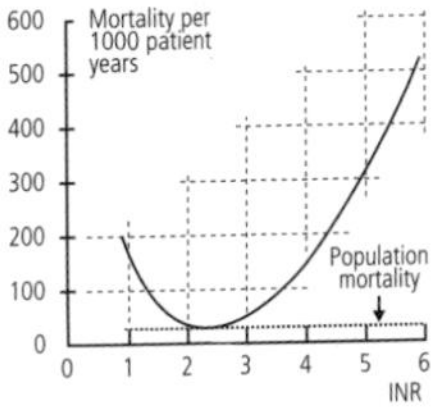

Fig. 1

Antidote
Stop treatment if the INR exceeds 4·5. Give fresh frozen plasma (q.v.) if the INR exceeds 7, and 1 mg of IV vitamin K if there is overt bleeding.

Supply
Warfarin can be provided as a 1 mg/ml sugar-free suspension. This is stable for 2 weeks. 500 micrograms (white), 1 mg (brown) and 3 mg (blue) tablets are available costing a few pence each.

References
Bradbury MJE, Taylor G, Short P, *et al.* A comparison of anticoagulant control in patients on long-term warfarin using home and hospital monitoring of the international normalised ratio. *Arch Dis Child* 2008;**93**:303–6.
Odén A, Fahlén M. Oral anticoagulation and risk of death: a medical record linkage study. *BMJ* 2002;**325**:1073–5.
Streif W, Andrew M, Marzinotto V, *et al.* Analysis of warfarin therapy in pediatric patients: a prospective cohort study of 319 patients. *Blood* 1999;**94**:3007–14.
Vitali N, de Feo M, de Santo LS, *et al.* Dose dependent fetal complications of warfarin in pregnant women with mechanical heart valves. *J Am Coll Cardiol* 1999;**33**:1637–41. (See also pp. 1642–5.)

Use

An understanding of neonatal fluid balance, and of the limits of neonatal homeostasis, is essential to the management of any baby on IV fluids. See also the monograph on sodium chloride.

Physiology

Babies lose about 30 ml/kg of water through the skin and nose each day ('insensible' water loss). Babies born more than 10 weeks early may lose twice as much as this for the first few days of life, and very immature babies may lose three times as much in the first week of life, especially if the skin is damaged (cf. the monograph on skin care). These losses can be reduced by the use of a humidified incubator and there is no evidence that this need increase the risk of infection. Compressed oxygen contains no water vapour so babies in >40% oxygen also need supplemental humidity to stop their nasal and tracheal secretions becoming excessively dry. Some water is lost in the stools, and mature babies also sweat intermittently so, as a useful rule of thumb, babies should be allowed 60 ml/kg of water a day to balance these insensible losses even when anuric.

Babies require a further 60 ml/kg of water a day to provide the kidney with an appropriate 'vehicle' for the excretion of waste products. The **minimum** basic requirement of a baby with normal renal function is, therefore, 100–120 ml/kg of water a day, and there is a strong case for giving 130 ml/kg because, if this is given as 10% glucose this delivers the 9 mg/kg per minute of glucose needed (in the absence of marked hyperinsulinism) to minimise any risk of the blood glucose level falling below 2 mmol/l. Use 10% glucose when giving any continuously infused drug to sustain calorie intake and minimise unnecessary water intake. The **maximum** safe intake in most stable non-surgical babies more than 48 hours old is probably almost double the minimum requirement, even if the baby is both immature and ventilator dependent. With total intake in the range 120–200 ml/kg of water a day, most clinically stable babies more than 2 days old can autoregulate their own fluid balance making it quite unnecessary to adjust for clinical factors such as gestation, postnatal age, insensible loss, phototherapy, etc. Recent studies have undermined earlier controlled trial evidence suggesting that ventilator-dependent babies offered liberal fluids are more likely to develop necrotising enterocolitis and patent ductus arteriosus.

Hydration decreases after delivery. The amount of water in the body's interstitial tissues (that fraction of all body water not in the intravascular space or in body cells) normally falls by about 50 ml/kg irrespective of fluid intake during the first 3–5 days of life once hydration is no longer under placental control. Many have argued that early intake ought be restricted to assist this normal postnatal adjustment (at a time when oral intake is usually low anyway) especially in any preterm or ventilator-dependent baby, but there is no evidence that keeping early fluid intake below 90 ml/kg a day is beneficial unless renal function is abnormally compromised, and a low intake leaves many babies in negative calorie balance for many days after birth. The belief that babies who are not fed should not be given more than 60 ml/kg of fluid IV on the first day of life seems to have been derived from the widely accepted view that it is unwise to give vulnerable babies more than 60 ml/kg of fluid **by mouth** in the first day of life, but that is to falsely equate the gut's limited ability to cope with fluid soon after birth with the kidney's much less limited ability to cope with fluid within a day or two of birth.

Management

Shocked, ill babies: Post-asphyxial, post-hypotensive, septicaemic and hydropic babies should be started on 60 ml/kg of 10% glucose with 0·18% sodium chloride a day once any initial fluid deficit has been corrected, and blood glucose levels should be monitored until renal function can be assessed.

Other babies <32 weeks' gestation: Aim for an intake of 130 ml/kg a day from some combination of milk and 10% glucose by the time the baby is a day old. Fluid (and calorie) intake can then be increased fairly rapidly, unless daily weighing suggests that renal function is poor, aiming for an intake of 170–200 ml/kg by 1 week. Use IV 10% glucose with 0·18% sodium chloride to supplement oral intake in babies ≥1 week old.

Other babies in special care: A total oral and/or IV intake of 200 ml/kg a day is perfectly safe after the first 2–3 days, and continued IV supplementation can sometimes help optimise early calorie intake.

Babies in renal failure: If output does not respond to a single 5 mg/kg dose of IV furosemide or (unless there is already clinical evidence of fluid overload) a 10 ml/kg IV 'bolus' of 0·9% sodium chloride, insert a central long line and give 2 ml/kg per hour of 20% glucose to avert hypoglycaemia without giving more water than is being lost insensibly, adding an inotrope to this infusate if necessary. Replace all other loss (and its electrolyte content) with further 20% glucose containing added sodium chloride, or bicarbonate, from a second line as appropriate. Dialysis can usually be avoided unless the plasma potassium becomes very high.

Supply

0·5 litre bags of 10% anhydrous glucose with 0·18% sodium chloride cost 70p, 60 ml syringes cost 25p, and a simple IV giving set extension set and T tap costs £1·90. Avoid using any product containing a bacteriostatic such as benzyl alcohol when using an ampoule of sterile water to 'flush' any line in a preterm baby.

References

See also the relevant Cochrane reviews

Coulthard MG, Hey EN. Effect of varying water intake on renal function in healthy preterm babies. *Arch Dis Child* 1985;**60**:614–20. [RCT]
Coulthard MG, Vernon S. Managing acute renal failure in very low birthweight infants. *Arch Dis Child* 1995;**73**:F187–92.
Kavvadia V, Greenough A, Dimitriou G, *et al.* Randomised trial of two levels of fluid input in the perinatal period – effect on fluid balance, electrolyte and metabolic disturbances in ventilated VLBW infants. *Acta Paediatr* 2000;**89**:237–41. [RCT]

Use

Whooping cough (or 'pertussis'), due to *Bordetella pertussis*, remains a potentially devastating illness in children 3–6 months old and, because passive maternal immunity is relatively weak, it is very important to start immunisation 2 months after birth. Babies with lung problems are at particular risk. Toxoids that also provide protection against diphtheria and tetanus have long been employed in a range of combined vaccines. Diphtheria, tetanus and whooping cough are all notifiable illnesses in the UK (and in many other countries).

Clinical factors

More than 100,000 cases of whooping cough were notified every year in the UK prior to the introduction of a vaccine in 1956. Notifications fell 50-fold after that, but severe infection still occurs in young unimmunised children. Death is now rare, but severe non-fatal infection in early infancy is not that uncommon. Indeed the problem seems to have become commoner in the last 10 years (there was one notified case for every 2000 births in one recent US study). Serology, and polymerase chain reaction (PCR) tests, can often reveal evidence of infection even when direct culture fails. Vaccines made from a suspension of dead bacteria were the products first produced, but acellular vaccines have since been developed. They were, at one time, of variable potency, but are now preferred in Europe and North America because they trigger fewer hypotonic-hyporesponsive episodes and other adverse reactions. However, serious problems are uncommon with any product in babies less than 6 months old. No vaccine provides complete lasting immunity, and whooping cough is a commoner cause of troublesome cough in school-age children than is generally recognised.

Diphtheria was an even more dreaded disease before the introduction of an effective vaccine in 1940. Only 1–2 cases are now recognised each year in the UK but there is no doubt that a policy of universal immunisation remains appropriate, as with polio. Tetanus is an even more common and extremely dangerous condition that can strike at any time. Protection requires a personal immunisation programme with boosters (covered, where necessary, by tetanus immunoglobulin) following any injury if there is any risk that the wound has been contaminated with tetanus spores. Tetanus due to poor attention to umbilical cord care still kills 100,000 babies in the world each year. Skilled care, as outlined in the monograph on diazepam, will save a few lives, but the problem could be totally eliminated by ensuring that all pregnant women are fully immunised.

Indications

Immunisation should be started, as transplacental immunity starts to wane, 8 weeks after delivery. Six weeks might be even better since many babies have little maternally acquired passive immunity at birth. Give diphtheria, pertussis and tetanus toxoids and offer simultaneous protection from *Haemophilus influenzae* type b and polio (using a five-in-one vaccine where this is available). Give the meningococcal (MenC) vaccine (q.v.) at the same time. A personal or family history of allergy is not a contraindication to the use of any of these vaccines. Nor is a congenital abnormality (such as Down syndrome or a cardiac abnormality). While immunisation should not be delayed because of prematurity, it is *never* too late to immunise someone who was not immunised at the optimum time. Because efficacy wins over time, it may also be worth offering a booster dose to parents about to go home with a particularly vulnerable baby. Some would also give flu vaccine.

Contraindications

Anaphylaxis, stridor, bronchospasm, prolonged unresponsiveness, persistent unconsolable crying lasting ≥3 hours, an otherwise unexplained temperature of ≥40°C within 48 hours, or seizure within 72 hours of immunisation suggest a general reaction. Redness and induration involving much of the thigh or upper limb are evidence of a serious local reaction. Such events are very rare. If a problem of this nature is encountered it may be better to complete immunisation using a product that does not protect against whooping cough (or use an acellular product if treatment was started using a whole-cell product). A *brief* period of hypotonia or unresponsiveness is not a reason to withhold further treatment.

The one important relative contraindication to immunisation is the existence of an evolving cerebral abnormality of perinatal origin. Should any such child develop new signs or symptoms shortly after immunisation starts, diagnostic difficulties might occur and the possibility of litigation might arise. In this situation the perceived risk of immunisation needs to be balanced against the risk of whooping cough (a very real risk if there are coexisting pulmonary problems) and a decision on timing reached with the parents that allows immunisation to proceed as soon as the child's neurological condition has stabilised.

Immunisation against whooping cough should also be delayed in any child who is acutely unwell, but the specific contraindications associated with the administration of live vaccines (such as the oral polio vaccine) do not apply, and minor infections unassociated with fever or systemic symptoms are not a reason to delay immunisation even if the child is on an antibiotic or other medicine.

A personal history of seizures (or, more doubtfully, a history of seizures in a brother, sister or parent) was for some years considered a 'relative' contraindication to pertussis immunisation in the UK (but not in the USA). Such children may be at increased risk of a febrile seizure if immunised when more than 6 months old, but there is no evidence that such an untoward effect carries with it any long-term risk. Primary care and community staff should *not*, therefore, advise against pertussis immunisation without first discussing the issues with a consultant paediatrician familiar with all the issues and circumstances.

Administration

General guidance: Give 0·5 ml deep into the anterolateral thigh muscle using a 25 mm, 23 gauge needle. Stretch the skin taught, and insert the needle, up to its hilt, at right angles to the skin surface. Use deep *subcutaneous* injection for

Continued on p. 278

children with haemophilia. A combined five-in-one vaccine that also offers protection against diphtheria, *H. influenza* type b (Hib), polio and tetanus is the product now used in the UK. Simultaneous vaccination against type C meningococcal infection (MenC) is normally undertaken at the same time. Babies given BCG do not need to have the timing of these other procedures modified. The normal vaccine schedule is as laid out in the monograph on immunisation, where brief guidance on documentation and on parental consent is also given.

Prematurity: Immunisation should start 8 weeks after birth even in babies not yet discharged home from hospital. Some preterm babies only develop a limited response to the Hib vaccine and probably merit a dose of the monovalent Hib vaccine (q.v.), or another dose of the five-in-one vaccine at a year.

Systemic steroids: While inactivated vaccines (unlike live virus vaccines) are safe when given to patients on high-dose steroid treatment, such exposure can blunt the immune response. Even brief high-dose treatment shortly before, or after, birth can sometimes reduce the response to vaccine administration at 2 months. However, it would seem that this effect is probably only serious enough for a further 1-year booster dose to be merited in those countries where diphtheria remains endemic.

Abnormal reactions: Fever is uncommon when vaccination is undertaken in the first 6 months of life, and usually responds to a single 30 mg/kg dose of paracetamol (q.v.). Such reactions are of no lasting consequence, even when associated with a febrile fit, but parents should be told to seek medical advice if fever persists for more than 12 hours. Anaphylaxis (which is extremely rare) should be managed as laid out in the monograph on immunisation. Sudden limpness, with pallor and brief loss of consciousness, can occur in young children especially in the hours after they receive their first dose of vaccine. These babies recover without treatment, and such reactions, though alarming, should not result in further doses of the whooping cough vaccine being withheld. Parents can be told that the episode is not unlike a fainting attack, is unlikely to recur and is of no lasting significance.

Documentation

Tell the family doctor every time a child is immunised in hospital, and record what was done in the child's own personal health booklet. Community-based registers of vaccine uptake also need to be informed.

Supply

A range of vaccines are now in use round the world, and a new five-in-one vaccine (Pediacel©), in 0·5 ml ampoules, containing purified diphtheria, pertussis and tetanus toxoids, *H. influenzae* type b polysaccharide and inactivated polio virus (types 1–3), came into use in the UK in 2004.

A vaccine that only contains diphtheria and tetanus toxoids (but also contains thiomersal) can be used for the rare infant who suffers a severe reaction to the pertussis component of the five-in-one vaccine. The best available advice on when such a product might be indicated is currently provided by the section on pertussis in the 'Red Book' published by the American Academy of Pediatrics in 2003.

Vaccines must be stored in the dark at 2–8°C, and shaken well before use. Ampoules should be used as soon as possible once they have been opened. Frozen ampoules must be discarded.

References

See also the relevant Cochrane reviews and UK guidelines **DHUK**

Cortese MM, Baughman AL, Zhang R, *et al*. Pertussis hospitalizations among infants in the United States, 1993 to 2004. *Pediatrics* 2008;**121**:484–92.

Dylag AM, Shah SI. Administration of tetanus, diphtheria, and acellular pertussis vaccine to parents of high-risk infants in neonatal intensive care unit. *Pediatrics* 2008;**122**:e550–5.

Grant CC, Roberts M, Scragg R, *et al*. Delayed immunisation and risk of pertussis in infants: unmatched case–control study. *BMJ* 2003;**326**:852–3. (See also comment on p. 853.)

Harnden A, Grant C, Harrison T, *et al*. Whooping cough in school age children with persistent cough: prospective cohort study in primary care. *BMJ* 2006;**333**:174–7. (See also pp. 159–60.)

Hoppe JE. Neonatal pertussis. *Pediatr Infect Dis J* 2000;**19**:244–9.

Le Saux N, Barrowman NJ, Moore DL, *et al*. Decrease in hospital admissions for febrile seizures and reports of hypotonic-hyporesponsive episodes presenting to hospital emergency departments since switching to acellular pertussis vaccine in Canada: a report from IMPACT. *Pediatrics* 2003;**112**:e348–53.

Lim SS, Stein DB, Charrow A, *et al*. Tracking progress towards universal childhood immunisation and the impact of global initiatives: systematic analysis of three-dose diphtheria, tetanus and pertussis immunization coverage. *Lancet* 2008;**372**:2013–46. [SR]

Omeñaca F, Garcia-Sicilia J, Garcia-Corbeira P, *et al*. Response of preterm newborns to immunization with a hexavalent diphtheria-tetanus-acellular pertussis-hepatitis B-inactivated polio and *Haemophilus influenae* type B vaccine: first experiences and solutions to a serious and sensitive issue. *Pediatrics* 2005;**116**:1292–8.

Rank C, Quinn HE, McIntyre PB. Pertussis vaccine effectiveness after mass immunization of high school students in Australia. *Pediatr Infect Dis J* 2009;**28**:152–3.

Robbins JB, Schneerson R, Trollfors B. Pertussis in developed countries. [Commentary] *Lancet* 2002;**360**:657–8.

Shiball MC, Peters TR, Zhu H, *et al*. Potental impact of acceleration of the pertussis vaccine primary series for infants. *Pediatrics* 2008;**122**:1021–6.

Surridge J, Segedin ER, Grant CC. Pertussis requiring intensive care. *Arch Dis Child* 2007;**92**:970–5.

Theilen U, Johnson ED, Robinson PA. Rapidly fatal invasive pertussis in young infants – how can we change the outcome. *BMJ* 2008;**337**:a343.

Use
Zidovudine inhibits the replication of the human immunodeficiency virus (HIV), reducing feto-maternal transmission and slowing the progression of the resultant acquired immune deficiency syndrome (AIDS).

HIV infection
AIDS is a notifiable disease caused by one of two closely related human retroviruses (HIV-1 and HIV-2) that target T-helper (CD4) lymphocytes and macrophages, rendering the patient immunodeficient and vulnerable to a range of chronic infectious illnesses that are not normally lethal. Infection is generally by sexual contact or the use of contaminated needles. Babies of infected mothers have a 1 in 5 chance of becoming infected around the time of birth if avoiding action is not taken. Contaminated blood infected many haemophiliacs before the nature of the condition was understood. The risk of infection after needlestick exposure is <0·5%.

Care of HIV-infected women during pregnancy
Since chemoprophylaxis and Caesarean delivery before the membranes rupture can almost eliminate risk of materno-fetal transmission, there is an overwhelming case for routine screening in pregnancy, as long as this has the mother's full informed consent. Seek experienced local advice to supplement the guidance provided by the US website (www.AIDSinfo.nih.gov) and UK websites (www.bhiva.org and www.aidsmap.com).

Pharmacology
Zidovudine or azidothymidine (AZT) is a thymidine analogue that acts intracellularly, after conversion to triphosphate, to halt retrovirus DNA synthesis by competitive inhibition of reverse transcriptase and incorporation into viral DNA. It inhibits the replication of the HIV virus, but does not eradicate it from the body. It is not, therefore, a cure for the resultant AIDS, but it can delay the progression of the disease, and the drug's arrival in 1987 did much to transform the management of this previously untreatable condition. The most common adverse effects are anaemia and leucopenia (which make regular haematological checks essential), but myalgia, malaise, nausea, headache and insomnia have also been reported. Zidovudine is well absorbed by mouth but first pass liver uptake reduces bioavailability. The half life is 1 hour, but 3 hours in term babies and 6 hours in preterm babies in the first week of life. Concurrent treatment with ganciclovir (q.v.) increases the risk of toxicity while fluconazole increases the half life. Tissue levels exceed plasma levels (neonatal V_D ~2 l/kg). Zidovudine crosses the blood:brain barrier and the placenta with ease, but there is no human evidence of teratogenicity. Excretion occurs into breast milk, but has not been studied in any detail.

Intrapartum prophylaxis
Mothers: Start giving 300 mg twice a day by mouth, as soon after 28 weeks' gestation as possible. Give this dose once every 3 hours as soon as labour starts (or give 2 mg/kg over an hour IV and then 1 mg/kg every hour) until delivery is over. Virus transmission is reduced by also giving nevirapine (q.v.).
Term babies: Give 4 mg/kg by mouth twice a day for 4 weeks. Start this within 8 hours of birth.
Preterm babies: Give babies of 30–36 weeks' gestation 2 mg/kg twice a day for 2 weeks, and then 3 mg/kg twice a day for 2 weeks. Give babies under 30 weeks' gestation 2 mg/kg twice a day for 4 weeks. If oral treatment is not possible give 1·5 mg/kg IV once every 12 hours (or every 6 hours if a term baby).

Sustained prophylaxis when bottle feeding seems inadvisable
In situations where hygiene and cost combine to make bottle feeding hazardous *exclusive* breastfeeding for 6 months reduces the risk of the baby becoming infected after birth. Risk can also be reduced by giving the baby nevirapine once a day by mouth until mixed feeding can be established.

Treatment after birth
See the monographs on lamivudine, nevirapine and lopinavir with ritonavir for advice on how to treat babies with known infection. Only give prophylactic co-trimoxazole (q.v.) to babies at serious risk of overt infection.

Case notification
Register all pregnant HIV-positive women and their babies in the UK anonymously with the linked RCOG and RCPCH surveillance programmes (e-mail: j.masters@ich.ucl.ac.uk; tel: 020 7829 8686).

Supply
Dilute the content of a 200 mg (20 ml) ampoule (costing £11) to 50 ml with 5% glucose to produce an IV solution containing 4 mg/ml, and give any IV dose slowly (over 30 minutes). 100 and 250 mg capsules cost £1·10 and £2·70 respectively. A sugar-free oral syrup (10 mg/ml) is also available (100 ml costs £11).

References
See the Cochrane review and UK guideline on managing HIV in pregnancy

Committee on Pediatric AIDS, American Academy of Pediatrics. HIV testing and prophylaxis to prevent mother-to-child transmission in the United States. *Pediatrics* 2008;**122**:1127–34.
Coovadia HM, Rollins NC, Bland RM, *et al*. Mother-to-child transmission of HIV-1 infection during exclusive breastfeeding in the first 6 months of life: an intervention cohort study. *Lancet* 2007;**369**:1107–16. (See also pp. 1065–6 and 2073–5.)
Gray GE, Saloojee H. Breast-feeding, antiretroviral prophylaxis, and HIV. [Editorial] *N Engl J Med* 2008;**359**:189–91.
Pilwoz EG, Humphrey JH, Tavengwa NV, *et al*. The impact of safer breastfeeding practices on postnatal HIV-1 transmission in Zimbabwe. *Am J Public Health* 2007;**97**:1249–54.

Use

Oral zinc sulphate is used, both diagnostically and therapeutically, to supplement the dietary intake of babies with clinical signs of zinc deficiency. Routine supplementation in infancy seems beneficial in some community settings, but trials of *multiple* micronutrient use in pregnancy have not yet delivered consistent outcomes.

Nutritional factors

Zinc is an essential nutrient, being a constituent of many enzymes. It is also a constituent of the DNA and RNA polymerases involved in cell replication and growth. Overt deficiency causes perioral and perianal dermatitis, symmetrical blistering and pustular lesions on the hands and feet, alopecia, irritability, anorexia, diarrhoea and growth failure. The features are the same as for acrodermatitis enteropathica (a rare, and potentially lethal, condition caused by a recessively inherited abnormality of zinc absorption, first recognised in 1973). Enterostomy loss, and renal loss due to the use of a thiazide diuretic, both make zinc deficiency more likely. While the serum zinc level is usually, but not always, below the normal range (7·6–15 µmol/l at 1–3 months), the diagnosis is clinched by the response to a direct trial of supplementation. Debilitating subclinical deficiency is still common in Central and southern Africa and in South East Asia, particularly where soil zinc levels are low and cereal foods account for much of the daily diet.

An intake of at least 700 micrograms/kg of zinc per day may be necessary for healthy growth in some babies during early infancy, but all the artificial formula milks commercially available in the UK currently provide more than this minimum amount. Human milk initially contains more zinc than cows' milk (0·2 mg/100 ml) and, because much of this is present as zinc citrate rather than bound to casein, absorption may be better, but the zinc content of human milk falls 10-fold during the first 6 months of lactation. Reserves of zinc accumulate in the skeleton and liver before birth help to tide the baby over the unexplained period of negative zinc balance normally seen in the first month of life. Nevertheless a small number of cases of overt zinc deficiency have been seen in exclusively breastfed babies of less than 33 weeks' gestation 2–4 months after birth that responded to zinc supplementation. Deficiency was due to the milk containing little zinc, rather than a defect of absorption or utilisation. Overt symptoms of acrodermatitis take some time to appear.

Subclinical dietary deficiency is less easily recognised, but the consequences can be equally devastating. A small daily supplement (10 mg of elemental zinc a day) reduced the incidence of pneumonia and of malaria by 40% among babies in one at-risk population. Mortality fell 60% among supplemented light for dates children in another trial in India, while immediate supplementation in those developing diarrhoea halved the risk of death for any reason other than trauma in another trial in Bangladesh. Babies with severe pneumonia recovered quicker when given a 20 mg dose once a day from the day of admission. African children with HIV also fare better with supplementation. Recent trials not yet included in the Cochrane Collaboration's overview also show that maternal supplementation (30 mg daily from 12–16 weeks) can increase birth weight and reduce the risk of subsequent illness among children in areas where subclinical deficiency is common.

Treatment

As little as 1 mg/kg of zinc a day will rapidly cure any symptoms due to simple dietary deficiency. A regular daily 5 mg/kg oral supplement may be necessary in babies with acrodermatitis enteropathica.

Supply

125 mg effervescent zinc sulphate monohyrate tablets contain 45 mg (0·7 mmol) of zinc, and cost 15p each. One tablet dissolved in 4·5 ml of water gives a 10 mg/ml solution for accurate low-dose administration. Accurate dosing is not important when correcting acute dietary deficiency; here it suffices to give most babies and toddlers half of a 45 mg tablet once a day for 2 weeks. Orphan Europe market 25 mg capsules designed for use in Wilson disease costing 50p each; open and add the contents to water.

The use of 1 ml/kg per day of Peditrace® will meet the elemental zinc requirement of most babies on parenteral nutrition. 10 ml vials for IV use cost £4·20.

References

See also the relevant Cochrane reviews

Aggarwal R, Sentz J, Miller MA. Role of zinc administration in prevention of childhood diarrhea and respiratory illnesses: a meta-analysis. *Pediatrics* 2007;**119**:1120–30. [SR] (For a meta-analysis of use to treat diarrhoea see *Pediatrics* 2008;**121**:326–36.)

Bobat R, Coovadia H, Stephen C, *et al.* Safety and efficacy of zinc supplementation for children with HIV-1 infection in South Africa: a randomised double-blind placebo-controlled trial. *Lancet* 2005;**366**:1862–7. [RCT]

Brooks WA, Santosham M, Naheed A, *et al.* Effect of weekly zinc supplements on incidence of pneumonia and diarrhoea in children younger than 2 years in an urban, low-income population in Bangladesh: randomised controlled trial. *Lancet* 2005;**366**:999–1004. [RCT]

Obladen M, Loui A, Kampmann E, *et al.* Zinc deficiency in rapidly growing preterm infants. *Acta Paediatr* 1998;**67**:685–91.

Osendarp SJM, van Raaij JMA, Darmstadt GL, *et al.* Zinc supplementation during pregnancy and effects on growth and morbidity in low birthweight infants: a randomised placebo controlled trial. *Lancet* 2001;**357**:1080–5. [RCT]

Shrimpton R, Gross R, Darnton-Hill I, *et al.* Zinc deficiency: what are the most appropriate interventions? *BMJ* 2005;**330**:347–9. (Review advocating multimicronutrient trials.)

Stephens J, Lubitz L. Symptomatic zinc deficiency in breast-fed term and premature infants. *J Paediatr Child Health* 1998;**34**:97–100.

SUMMIT Trial Study Group. Effect of maternal multiple micronutrient supplementation on fetal loss and infant death in Indonesia: a double-blind cluster-randomised trial. *Lancet* 2008;**371**:215–27. [RCT] (See also pp. 450–2 and 492–9.)

Tielsch JM, Khatry SK, Stoltzfus RJ, *et al.* Effect of daily zinc supplementation on child mortality in southern Nepal: a community-based, cluster-randomised placebo-controlled trial. *Lancet* 2007;**370**:1230–9. [RCT] (See also pp. 1194–5.)

Part 3

Maternal medication and its effect on the baby

This section of NNF6 provides information on most drugs commonly used during pregnancy and lactation that do *not* have a full monograph to themselves in Part 2 of this book.

Introduction

No attempt has been made to review the extensive literature that now exists on the impact of medication during early pregnancy on the growing fetus. However, a summary of what is known about placental transfer, teratogenicity (the propensity to cause a malformation), fetal toxicity, and use in the lactating mother, is included in the section labelled 'Pharmacology' for each drug listed in the main body of this book. Where the text merely says that treatment during lactation is safe it can be taken that the dose ingested by the baby is almost certain to be less than 10% of that being taken by the mother on a weight-for-weight basis, and that no reports have appeared suggesting that the baby could be clinically affected. The purpose of this short addendum is to summarise what is known about the impact on the baby of those drugs that do **not** receive a mention in the main body of this compendium even though they are commonly given to mothers during pregnancy, labour or the puerperium. Information is also given on a range of other drugs that are often taken illicitly. A small number of entries review groups of drugs (such as the antihistamines) offering a general comment rather than information on one specific drug.

Advice to parents has, in the past, often been too authoritarian. While there are a small number of drugs whose use makes breast feeding extremely unwise, for most drugs it is more a matter of balancing the advantages and the disadvantages, and of being alert to the possibility that the baby might conceivably exhibit a side effect of maternal medication. It is not enough to just say that a particular drug will appear in the mother's milk – that is true of almost every drug ever studied. Mothers will also question why it should be thought unwise to expose their baby to a low level of a drug during lactation when no reservation was voiced over much greater exposure during pregnancy. Much of the advice offered to UK clinicians in the *British National Formulary* and in its paediatric counterpart simply reflects, of necessity, the advice offered by the manufacturer in the Summary of Product Characteristics. Such statements are always cautious, seldom very informative and often merely designed to meet the minimum requirement laid down by the licensing authority. The same is true of drug use in pregnancy – the arbitrary classification of drugs into one of five 'risk' categories currently used by the Federal Drugs Agency in America is increasingly seen to be an over simple approach to a complex issue.

The task of the clinician, in most of these situations, is to provide parents with the information they need to make up their own minds on such issues. To that end, each statement in this section is backed by at least one or two published references. In certain cases readers may also wish to refer to the more comprehensive overviews provided in the books by Bennett (1996), Briggs *et al.* (2008), Schaefer *et al.* (2007) and Hale (2008) (see p. 283).

The dose the breastfed baby is likely to receive has been calculated, wherever this is possible, as a percentage of the maternal dose (both calculated on a mg/kg basis) using the approach first recommended in Bennett's authoritative text. Particular caution should be observed when this fraction exceeds 10% because drug elimination will initially be much slower in the baby than in the mother. The human milk:plasma (M:P) ratio is also given, where known. However, while this shows the extent to which the drug is concentrated in breast milk, it does not, on its own, reveal how much drug the baby will receive because some drugs achieve a therapeutic effect even when the blood level is very low. Unfortunately there are still some commonly used drugs for which no reliable information yet exists. Mothers who are breastfeeding and who are already taking one of these drugs are usually more than willing to help with the collection of some steady-state milk and plasma samples if approached, and the analysis of these would soon diminish many of the residual gaps in our knowledge as long as some care is taken to exclude the residual effect of earlier *in utero* exposure.

It is often said that risks can be minimised if the mother takes any necessary medication immediately after completing a breastfeed so that the baby avoids being exposed to peak maternal plasma levels. This is something of a counsel of perfection, however, for any mother feeding frequently and on demand, and the sort of advice usually offered by someone with more theoretical knowledge than practical bedside experience. In many situations,

the question is not whether a medicated mother should be allowed to nurse, but whether a nursing mother needs to be medicated.

(Sumner Yaffe)

Further reading

Many reviews of the issues that need to be considered when prescribing medication to a mother who is pregnant or breastfeeding have been published in the last 10 years and these should be turned to for information on drugs not included in this brief overview. Much high-quality epidemiological work has also been done to define the risks of drug use during pregnancy. A lot of information on use during lactation is, by contrast, still anecdotal. Isolated reports recording apparent complications of use during lactation need to be interpreted with caution (especially where these relate to drugs that have been used by large numbers of other mothers uneventfully). Reports published before 1990, in particular, frequently lacked any documentary evidence that significant quantities of the offending drug were actually present in the baby's blood.

Reference texts on drug use during pregnancy and lactation

Twelve relatively recent, comprehensively referenced, texts are:

American Academy of Pediatrics, Committee on Drugs. The transfer of drugs and other chemicals into human milk. *Pediatrics* 2001;**108**:776–89.

Bennett PM, ed. *Drugs and human lactation*, 2nd edn. Amsterdam: Elsevier, 1996.

Briggs GG, Freeman RK, Yaffe SJ. *Drugs in pregnancy and lactation*, 8th edn. Philadelphia: Lippincott, Williams & Wilkins, 2008. (CD-ROM and PDA versions and web updates are available.)

Friedman JM, Polifka JE. *Teratogenic effects of drugs. A resource for clinicians*, 2nd edn. Baltimore: Johns Hopkins University Press, 2000.

Hale TW. *Medications and mothers' milk*, 13th edn. Amarillo, TX: Pharmasoft Publishing, 2008.

Koren G, ed. *Maternal-fetal toxicology. A clinician's guide*, 3rd edn. New York: Marcel Dekker, 2001.

Lee, A, Inch S, Finnigan D. *Therapeutics in pregnancy and lactation*. Abingdon, UK: Radcliffe Medical Press, 2000.

Little BB. *Drugs and pregnancy: a handbook*. London: Hodder Education, 2006. (With web updates.)

Rubin R, Ramsay M, eds. *Prescribing in pregnancy*, 4th edn. Oxford: Blackwell Publishing, 2008.

Schaefer C, Peters P, Miller RK, eds. *Drugs during pregnancy and lactation. Treatment options and risk assessment*, 2nd edn. Amsterdam: Elsevier, 2007.

Weiner CP, Buhimschi C. *Drugs for pregnant and lactating women*. New York: Churchill Livingstone, 2004. (CD-ROM and PDA versions are available.)

Yankowitz J, Niebyl JR. *Drug therapy in pregnancy*, 3rd edn. Philadelphia: Lippincott, Williams and Wilkins, 2001.

The publishers of the book by Briggs *et al*. update this with a quarterly bulletin, and the book by Hale is reissued every 1–2 years. Up-to-date information is available from the Organisation of Teratogen Information Specialists (OTIS) in North America (www.otispregnancy.org) and the European Network of Teratology Information Services (ENTIS) in Europe and Latin America (www.entis-org.com). The UK Breast Feeding Network (www.breastfeedingnetwork.org.uk) have a help line that mothers can ring if they have worries on such issues (tel: 0300 100 0212); leave a phone number where you can be contacted during the evening.

Further information

The information given in the *British national formulary* (BNF), and in the version giving advice on drug use in children (BNFC), is generally authoritative, but this is *not* always true of the advice it offers on drug use during pregnancy and lactation. Further useful information on safe drug use in ***pregnancy*** can be obtained in the UK through local hospital pharmacies and from the Specialist Advisory and Information Service provided by the Northern and Yorkshire Drug and Therapeutics Centre at the Wolfson Unit, 24 Claremont Place, Newcastle upon Tyne NE2 4HH (tel: 0191 232 1525). This unit also maintains the UK's main teratology data base (see www.ncl.ac.uk/pharmsc/entis.htm). More detailed information on drugs in ***breast milk*** can be obtained from the Trent Drug Information Centre, Leicester Royal Infirmary, Leicester LE1 5WW (tel: 0116 255 5779) or the West Midlands Drug Information Service, Good Hope General Hospital, Sutton Coldfield B75 7RR (tel: 0121 311 1974). Details of how to contact other similar advice centres in Europe and in North and South America are provided in the excellent book edited by Christof Schaefer.

Maternal medication and the baby

Acebutolol M:P ratio 9–12 (metabolite ratio 25)
While there is no evidence of teratogenicity, this drug (and other β blockers) can cause neonatal bradycardia, mild hypotension and transient hypoglycaemia when prescribed to a mother immediately before delivery. No complications have been reported following use during lactation but the drug and its metabolite, diacetolol, accumulate in breast milk, making labetalol or propranolol (q.v.) a better drug to use during lactation, especially if the dose exceeds 400 mg a day.
Rubin: *N Engl J Med* 1981;**305**:132.
Yassen: *Arch Fr Pediatr* 1992;**49**:351.

Acenocoumarol = Nicoumalone (former BAN) M:P ratio <0·01
As for the monograph on warfarin in Part 2. Breastfeeding is safe.
Barbour: *Obstet Gynecol Clin North Am* 1997;**24**:499.
Pauli: *Dev Brain Dysfunc* 1993;**6**:229.

Acitretin
Vitamin A, in excess, is a known teratogen and, although this oral vitamin A derivative is rapidly excreted from the body, some is metabolised to etretinate (q.v.) and this can still be detected in the body for 50 months after treatment is stopped. Use is not generally recommended during lactation either, although the baby would only receive weight-for-weight about 2% of the maternal dose when breastfed.
Maradit: *Dermatology* 1999;**198**:3.
Pilkington: *Drugs* 1992;**43**:597.

Alcohol M:P ratio 0·9; infant dose 4–19%
There is no good evidence that taking one or 2 'units' of alcohol once or twice a week during pregnancy increases the risk of miscarriage, stillbirth, malformation or preterm birth but, because drinking more than this is certainly harmful, several governments now say that women should not drink *any* alcohol while pregnant. Half a pint of beer, lager or cider contains about 1 'unit' (8 grams) of alcohol, and one small glass of wine about 1·5 'units'. High consumption during pregnancy can certainly result in the baby have a characteristic cluster of features at birth, and even moderate intake may also have an effect on later behaviour and cognition. Breast milk contains almost as much alcohol (90%) as maternal blood so, while there are few reports of drinking during lactation affecting the baby, some drowsiness is probably more common than is generally appreciated.
Gray: *BJOG* 2007;**114**:243 (See also p. 778).
Little: *N Engl J Med* 1989;**321**:425. (See also **322**:338.)

Alimemazine = Trimeprazine (former BAN)
There is no evidence that this long-established antihistamine is hazardous in pregnancy. While use (either as a sedative or to control itch and pruritis) is not now recommended in children less than 2 years old, use during lactation has not been reported to cause problems. Little appears in animal milk. The content in human milk does not seem to have been studied.
O'Brien: *Am J Hosp Pharm* 1974;**31**:844.

Allergic rhinitis
The use of nasal decongestants, of sodium cromoglicate, and of nasal corticosteroids is entirely safe during pregnancy and during lactation. See also the entry on the use of systemic antihistamines.

Amantadine
This antiviral drug used in Parkinsonism is teratogenic in animals and its use is not recommended in pregnancy. Mothers should probably be advised against breastfeeding, although only a little appears in breast milk.
Nora: *Lancet* 1975; **2**:607 and 1044.
Rosa: *Reprod Toxicol* 1994;**8**:531.

Amitriptyline M:P ratio 1·5; infant dose ~1%
There is no good evidence that this tricyclic antidepressant and its metabolite, nortriptyline, are teratogenic. They are excreted in breast milk, but no hazardous neonatal consequences have been documented.
Bader: *Am J Psychiatr* 1980;**137**:855.
Breyer-Pfaff: *Am J Psychiatr* 1995;**152**:812.

Angiotensin-converting enzyme (ACE) inhibitors
All the ACE inhibitors are known to be fetotoxic, interfering, sometimes lethally, with fetal kidney function in the second and third trimester of pregnancy. There is also one, as yet uncorroborated, report that exposure in the first trimester of pregnancy is also teratogenic, causing a modest but significant increase in the number of babies born with at least some (often minor) congenital malformation. Captopril (q.v.), cilazapril, enalapril, fosinopril, imidapril, lisinopril, mosexipril, perindopril, quinapril, ramipril and trandolapril are among the more commonly used drugs in this class. Captopril and enalapril are safe to use during lactation because the baby will not be exposed to even 1% of the weight-related maternal dose, but it is not yet known whether this is true of other drugs in this class.
Cooper: *N Eng J Med* 2006;**354**:2443. (See also p. 2498.)
Devlin: *J Clin Pharmacol* 1981;**21**:110.

Angiotensin-II receptor antagonists
There is accumulating evidence that the recently introduced drugs in this group (including candesartan, cilexetil, eprosartan, irbesartan, losartan potassium, medoxomil, olmesartan, telmisartan and valsartan) cause the same problems as the more widely studied ACE inhibitors (see above). Nothing is known about use during lactation. Time may show that they are as safe then as the ACE inhibitor drugs.
Serrreau: *Br J Obstet Gynaecol* 2005;**112**:710.

Antidepressants
Most tricyclic antidepressants are safe during both pregnancy and lactation, and studies of later preschool development have been equally reassuring. Blood levels may need monitoring once each trimester if treatment is to be optimised, and neonatal withdrawal symptoms are sometimes seen for a few days shortly after birth. Monoamine oxidase inhibitors are generally avoided in pregnancy because they can increase the risk of hypertension. See also the separate entry on selective serotonin reuptake inhibitors (SSRIs), where there are growing concerns over first trimester use.
Nulman: *Am J Psychiatry* 2002;**159**:1889.
Simon: *Am J Psychiatry* 2002;**159**:2055.

Antiemetics
Vomiting in pregnancy causes much alarm and distress. The alarm is largely misplaced since vomiting is not a sign that the pregnancy is 'in trouble', and the nausea is generally treatable. The antihistamine doxylamine (q.v.) is probably the best studied and most effective product but, because of the pressure

caused by (unsuccessful) litigation, it was withdrawn from sale in most parts of the world in the early 1980s. Meclozine (q.v.) is a widely recommended alternative that is available without prescription. Other antihistamines (see next entry) are probably equally safe. A short course of vitamin B$_6$ (10 mg three times a day) helped, but did not abolish the nausea, in two small trials. Chlorpromazine (q.v.) or prochlorperazine will usually control severe nausea and vomiting when simpler remedies fail. Metoclopramide (q.v.) may be appropriate where there is also reflux or heartburn.

Mazzota: *Drugs* 2000;**59**:781.

Oates-Whitehead: *Clin Evid* 2004;**12**:1966 (and updates). [SR]

Antihistamines

A wide range of prescribed products are used to treat allergy and hay fever, travel sickness and nausea in early pregnancy. Many 'over the counter' remedies for coughs and colds contain antihistamines, and some of these also cause drowsiness. None seem to be a hazard during pregnancy but it is probably best to try and avoid the frequent use of any formulation that carries the warning *'may cause drowsiness: do not drive or operate machinery'* while breastfeeding. Many such products also contain a sympathomimetic such as ephedrine (q.v.). Alimemazine (q.v.), though sedating, has been used uneventfully for many years. Loratadine (q.v.) causes less sedation and excretion into breast milk is minimal.

Kallen: *J Matern Fetal Neonatal Med* 2002;**11**:146.

Mazzotta: *Drug Saf* 1999;**20**:385.

Antipsychotics

Chlorpromazine (q.v.) seems safe to use during pregnancy and lactation. Less is known about the safety of most other antipsychotic drugs, but little clinical evidence of teratogenicity seems to have emerged. American guidelines support the use of high-potency agents such as fluphenazine, haloperidol, perphenazine or trifluoperazine (as listed elsewhere in this overview) because they minimise maternal anticholinergic, hypotensive and antihistaminergic effects even though they may cause troublesome, if self-limiting, extrapyramidal reactions in the neonate.

American Academy of Pediatrics: *Pediatrics* 2000;**105**:880.

McElhatton: *Reprod Toxicol* 1992;**6**:475.

Asthma

Drugs taken by inhalation to control asthma can and should be taken as usual during pregnancy and lactation as outlined in the monograph on salbutamol in Part 2. Studies looking at the use of oral steroids to control asthma have, to date, been equally reassuring, but there is some evidence that oral corticosteroid use for other indications in the first trimester of pregnancy may marginally increase the risk of the baby being born with a cleft lip and/or palate.

Tata: *Thorax* 2008;**63**:981.

Atenolol M:P ratio 1·1–6·8; infant dose 8–19%

While many cardioselective β-adrenergic blocking agents (β blockers) have been used to control hypertension in pregnancy, methyldopa may be a better option when treatment needs to be started early, because there seems to be less risk of fetal growth retardation. There is not enough experience with use in the first trimester for all risk of teratogenicity to be excluded. β blockers occasionally cause a generally benign fetal bradycardia, and can cause transient neonatal bradycardia and hypoglycaemia. Glucagon (q.v.) can be used if the side effects are severe. Alternatives to atenolol, such as labetalol or propranolol are preferable during lactation because the uptake of these drugs by the breastfed baby is much lower.

Marlettini: *Curr Ther Res* 1990;**48**:684.

Schmimmel: *J Pediatr* 1989;**114**:476. (See also **115**:336.)

Auranofin

As for aurothiomalate.

Aurothiomalate M:P ratio 0·0–0·2; infant dose ~10%

Auranofin is said to be teratogenic in animals (although the clinical significance of these findings is uncertain) but there is no good reason, on the basis of the published evidence, to avoid the use of aurothiomalate during pregnancy or lactation if other treatments for rheumatoid arthritis have proved unsatisfactory.

Bennett: *Br J Clin Pharmacol* 1990;**29**:777.

Tarp: *Arthritis Rheum* 1985;**28**:235.

Azathioprine Infant dose ~0·1%

There is no evidence that this drug is teratogenic. Used frequently as an immunosuppressant during pregnancy in mothers with an organ transplant, it has occasionally been associated with transient neonatal lymphopenia and thrombocytopenia, but treatment is usually well tolerated. Average birthweight may be marginally decreased , but this could be due to the disease process itself, or to co-treatment with a glucocorticosteroid. Only very small amounts of azathioprine appear in breast milk, and oral absorption is limited. Parents can be advised that, although lactation is not generally advised, no overt problem or haematological sign of immunosuppression has yet been reported in any of the babies who have been breastfed.

Kallen: *Scand J Rheumatol* 1998;**27**(suppl 107):119.

Wu: *Clin Transplant* 1998;**12**:454.

Baclofen M:P ratio 0·7; infant dose ~1%

There are few reports of the use of this muscle spasm-relieving drug in pregnancy. Exposure to normal doses is not teratogenic in animals. Sudden treatment cessation can precipitate seizures, and there is one report of a baby developing fits after birth that failed to respond to anticonvulsant treatment but did stop as soon as a tapered dose of baclofen was started. While there is only one report of short-term use during lactation, the dose ingested would seem to be small.

Eriksson: *Scand J Clin Lab Invest* 1981;**41**:185.

Moram: *Pediatrics* 2004;**114**:e267.

Benzodiazepines

Concerns about the use of any benzodiazepine during pregnancy or lactation are the same as for diazepam, as outlined in Part 2. Studies looking for evidence of teratogenicity have produced inconsistent findings. Neonatal withdrawal symptoms are not uncommon with sustained use in late pregnancy. Products with a short half life may pose less of a problem.

Dolovich: *BMJI* 1998;**317**:839. (See also 1999;**319**:918.)

Hägg: *Drug Saf* 2000;**22**:425.

Beta-adrenoceptor blocking drugs

For a comment on the use of 'β blockers' to manage hypertension see the entry on atenolol.

Bromide salts

Teratogenicity has not been seen, but use during lactation can cause a rash and neonatal sedation. Most drugs containing bromide have now been withdrawn, but some mothers still face exposure from photographic chemicals.

Tyson: *J Pediatr* 1938;**13**:91.

Buprenorphine

This long-acting analgesic (with both opioid agonist and antagonist properties that are only partially reversible with naloxone) is probably safe in pregnancy although sustained use can cause addiction. Only small amounts of the drug appear in human milk, but there is one report that sustained extradural use after delivery can depress lactation (or the vigour with which the baby feeds) in the first few days of life. There is

no good reason why women who have become addicted to buprenorphine should not breastfeed.
Hirose: *Br J Anaesth* 1997;**79**:120.
Marquet: *Clin Pharmacol Ther* 1997;**62**:569.

Busulfan = Busulphan (former BAN)
This alkylating antineoplastic drug is used in the treatment of chronic myeloid leukaemia. Use in the second and third trimester of pregnancy seems reasonably safe. Use during lactation has never been studied.
Wiebe: *Crit Rev Oncol Hematol* 1994;**16**:75.

Carbimazole M:P ratio 1–1·2; infant dose 3–12%
There is no evidence of teratogenicity, but there is a theoretical risk of neonatal goitre or hypothyroidism especially when a dose in pregnancy exceeds 30 mg a day. Most authorities consider propylthiouracil preferable to carbimazole, especially during lactation, because of the risk of neonatal hypothyroidism.
Cooper: *Am J Obstet Gynecol* 1987;**157**:234.
Low: *Lancet* 1979;**2**:1011.

Carisoprodol M:P ratio 2–4; infant dose ~4%
There have been no reports of teratogenicity, or of problems associated with use during lactation, to date. This muscular relaxant is, however, concentrated in breast milk and might conceivably make the baby drowsy. Baclofen may be a rather better drug to use during lactation.
Nordeng: *Therap Drug Monitor* 2001;**23**:298.

Celecoxib
A number of second-generation, non-steroidal, anti-inflammatory agents (NSAIDs) have recently come on the market. They are thought to selectively inhibit the inflammatory (COX-2) role of cyclo-oxygenase without inhibiting gastric, platelet or renal prostaglandin (COX-1) production. Too little is yet known about the effect of these new drugs to recommend use during pregnancy or lactation. There is no evidence of teratogenicity, but the risk of miscarriage could be increased by use in early pregnancy (as with other NSAIDs), and could make conception less likely. Reservations over use in the third trimester are the same as those outlined in the monograph on ibuprofen.
Dawood. *Am J Obstet Gynecol* 1993;**169**:1255.

Chlorpropamide
See the comments on tolbutamide. Both drugs were once quite widely used in patients where the problem is resistance to endogenous insulin secretion (type 2 diabetes) rather than inadequate secretion (type 1 diabetes).
Towner: *Diabetes Care* 1995;**18**:1446.
Zucker: *Arch Dis Child* 1970;**45**:696.

Ciclosporin = Cyclosporin (former BAN) M:P ratio 0·3; infant dose ~2%
There is no evidence that this immunosuppressant is teratogenic, and the fetal growth retardation sometimes seen could be due to the condition under treatment. More data are needed before the reproductive risk can be assessed accurately. Authorities have advised against lactation (citing neutropenia, immunosuppression, renal toxicity, a possible effect on growth and the carcinogenic risk associated with any form of immuno-supression), but a recent report found neonatal blood levels to be immeasurably low, in keeping with calculations based on known drug milk levels. Mothers should, therefore, be allowed to make their own informed choice.
Bar-Oz: *Teratology* 1999;**59**:440.
Nyberg: *Transplantation* 1998;**65**:253.

Cisplatin Infant dose ~35%
There is, as yet, little information on the use of this anticancer drug during pregnancy, although a normal outcome has been

documented after treatment in the second or third trimester. Severe transient neonatal leukopenia has been reported after maternal treatment shortly before delivery. Conflicting reports regarding the drug's excretion in breast milk make it difficult to advise on the safety of lactation while on treatment.
Ben-Baruch: *J Natl Cancer Inst* 1995;**84**:451.
Egan: *Cancer Treat Rep* 1985;**69**:1387.

Citalopram M:P ratio 1·8; infant dose ~4%
Information on the use of this serotonin reuptake inhibitor (SSRI) antidepressant in pregnancy is, as yet, less than for several other SSRI drugs. Transient symptoms suggestive of serotonergic overstimulation may be seen in the baby at birth if looked for carefully, but no complications have been reported as a result of use during lactation, and the amount of citalopram and demethylcitalopram ingested is small. See also the entry commenting on the use of any SSRI during pregnancy.
Laine: *Arch Gen Psychiatry* 2003;**60**:730.
Lee: *Am J Obstet Gynecol* 2004;**190**:218.

Clemastine M:P ratio 0·25–0·5
Authorities have advised, because of a single anecdotal report of irritability, that this drug should only be used with caution during lactation, but infant intake is low – since breast milk levels are modest – making this product as safe as most other antihistamines (q.v.).
Kok: *Lancet* 1982;**1**:914.
Moretti: *Reprod Toxicol* 1995;**9**:588.

Clomifene = Clomephine (former BAN)
The use of clomifene to induce ovulation can cause a multiple pregnancy but does not increase the risk of congenital malformation. A few reports of inadvertent use in the first trimester of pregnancy have generated continuing, as yet un-substantiated, concern that continued use after conception could be teratogenic.
Greenland: *Fertil Steril* 1995;**64**:936.

Clomipramine Infant dose <2%
Most tricyclic antidepressants are considered safe to use during pregnancy although the dose needed may need adjustment to optimise care, but there is one report that first trimester exposure to clomipramine may increase the risk of a cardiac malformation. Use during lactation certainly seems safe.
Källén: *Reprod Toxicol* 2004;**21**:221.
Weissman: *Am J Psychiatry* 2004;**161**:1066.

Clormethiazole = Chlormethiazole (former BAN) M:P ratio 0·9; infant dose 0·1–1·6%
The potential teratogenicity of this drug in early pregnancy remains unknown. Use by IV infusion as a hypnotic in the man-agement of toxaemia can cause severe neonatal hypotonia requiring ventilatory support, because clormethiazole crosses the placenta easily and is only slowly metabolised by the baby. Breastfeeding, in contrast, seems safe.
Johnson: *BMJ* 1976;**1**:943.
Tunstall: *Br J Obstet Gynaecol* 1979;**86**:793.

Clotrimazole
There is no evidence that this widely used topical 'over the counter' antifungal agent is teratogenic. It is not known whether the drug appears in breast milk, but absorption is minimal and topical use by the mother to treat vaginal candidiasis during pregnancy or lactation has not been associated with either fetal or neonatal toxicity.
Siffel: *Teratology* 1997;**55**:161.

Clozapine M:P ratio 2·8–4·3; infant dose ~1%
Women with schizophrenia taking this drug because of a failure to respond to other standard forms of treatment require

regular monitoring for agranulocytosis, but there is, as yet, no evidence of teratogenicity. Experience of use during lactation is very limited, but women keen to breastfeed can be told that there is a study of one baby showing uptake to be only about 1% of the weight-adjusted maternal dose.

Barnas: *Am J Psychiatry* 1994;**151**:945.
Walderman: *Am J Psychiatry* 1993;**150**:168.

Cocaine (crack)

The consequences of use during pregnancy are hard to establish because many addicts take a range of drugs. There may also be a bias towards reporting those studies where a positive association has been found. There is a belief that use can cause a variety of birth defects by disrupting blood flow but two recent studies found no such evidence. There is some increased risk of fetal growth retardation, reduced head size and preterm birth. Increased irritability 2–3 days after birth usually settles without treatment. Some cocaine persists in breast milk for 24 hours after maternal use, but the effect of use during lactation does not seem to have been studied in any detail. There seems to be an associated increase in the risk of sudden infant death (cot death).

Bauer: *Arch Pediatr Adolesc Med* 2005;**159**:824.
Behnke: *Pediatrics* 2001;**107**:e74.

Colchicine M:P ratio ~1; infant dose 2–8%

Colchicine is mostly used to treat familial Mediterranean fever and gout. Amniocentesis or chorion villus biopsy should be offered to mothers on colchicine at conception because of possible cytogenicity. The few reports of use during lactation suggest that only modest amounts of colchicine reach the baby, although there is one unconfirmed report of neonatal toxicity.

Ben-Chetrit: *Semin Arthritis Rheum* 1998;**28**:48.
Rabinovitch: *Am J Reprod Immunol* 1992;**28**:245.

Co-phenotrope

Lomotil® (which contains 100 parts of diphenoxylate hydrochloride to 1 part of atropine sulphate) is widely used in many parts of the world to control diarrhoea. Very little is known about use during pregnancy or lactation – loperamide (q.v.) is a much better studied alternative. Excessive Lomotil use in young children is potentially extremely hazardous, the diphenoxylate causing a delayed opiate collapse.

Corticosteroids

Pregnancy-associated hypertension is more likely to develop in women who take oral steroids during pregnancy, but this does not seem to happen to those taking an inhaled corticosteroid. For a comment on the fetal consequences of taking steroids during pregnancy see the entry under prednisolone.

Bracken: *Obstet Gynecol* 2003;**102**:739.
Martel: *BMJ* 2005;**330**:230.

Cough and cold remedies

Many compound proprietary medicines are available 'over the counter'. Avoid formulations with ingredients of the type mentioned in the commentary on antihistamines (q.v.). Pseudoephedrine use reduces prolactin levels, and might therefore impair lactation.

Cyclophosphamide

This anticancer drug would seem to be teratogenic when given in the first trimester, but there is less risk of fetotoxicity later in pregnancy. Treatment can affect subsequent fertility, and unconfirmed reports of problems following occupational exposure have resulted in strict guidelines being issued for the way staff should handle this drug. Breastfeeding would seem unwise. Enough of the drug seems to appear in breast milk to cause some degree of neonatal neutropenia.

Mutchinick: *Teratology* 1992;**45**:329.
Wiernik: *Lancet* 1971;**1**:912.

Danazol

This synthetic androgen used in the management of a range of conditions including endometriosis can cause marked female virilisation if exposure to a dose of 200 mg or more a day persists beyond the eighth week of pregnancy. Male fetuses are unaffected, and the risk of other non-genital anomalies does not seem to be increased. Use during lactation does not seem to have been studied but is generally discouraged.

Brunskill: *Br J Obstet Gynaecol* 1992;**99**:212.

Dapsone M:P ratio 0·4; infant dose ~20%

No problems emerged when the drug was used to prevent or treat malaria, often in combination with pyrimethamine (q.v.), although the baby ingests a significant amount of the drug during lactation. Dapsone is now more widely used in the management of leprosy. It can cause haemolytic anaemia, particularly in patients with G6PD deficiency.

Edstein: *Br J Clin Pharmacol* 1986;**2**:733.
Keuter: *BMJ* 1990;**301**:466.

Dexamfetamine = Dexamphetamine (former BAN) M:P ratio 2·8–7·5; infant dose ~6%

Amphetamines have been widely abused for their euphoric effect, but evidence of teratogenicity has not been established and neonatal symptoms are usually mild, even with sustained maternal use, when this is the only drug taken. Tolerance can develop, but physical dependence has not been documented. An acute overdose can cause symptoms similar to those seen with methylene dioxymethamfetamine (ecstasy). Most authorities deprecate any exposure of a baby to this CNS stimulant because of dexamfetamine's concentration in breast milk, but documentary evidence of harm is hard to find.

Steiner: *Eur J Clin Pharmacol* 1984;**27**:123.

Diethylstilbestrol = Stilboestrol (former BAN)

After this synthetic non-steroidal oestrogen had been given to 6 million women during early pregnancy to prevent miscarriage, prematurity and intrauterine death between 1940 and 1971 it was found to have caused later vaginal adenocarcinoma in over 400 of the girls born to these mothers. A range of serious reproductive disorders have since been documented in male and female offspring, while controlled studies have shown that diethylstilbestrol does nothing to prevent the problems for which it was originally given (see Cochrane review CD 004353). There are no recognised hazards associated with treatment during lactation.

Mittendorf: *Teratology* 1995;**51**:435.
Robboy: *JAMA* 1984;**252**:2979.

Disopyramide M:P ratio 0·5–1·0; infant dose ~15%

The teratogenic or fetotoxic potential of this antidysrrhythmic drug has not been well studied. Use during lactation has not been reported to cause problems, but the baby does ingest a very significant weight-adjusted quantity of the drug (and its active anticholinergic metabolite). The drug has a demonstrable oxytocic effect, and could increase the risk of preterm labour.

Ellsworth: *Ann Pharmacother* 1989;**23**:56.
Tadmor: *Am J Obstet Gynecol* 1990;**162**:482.

Dosulepin = Dothiepin M:P ratio 0·8-1·6; infant dose ~5%

There are few published data on the risks associated with exposure to this sedative tricyclic antidepressant during pregnancy. An overdose is sufficiently dangerous to make non-expert prescription unwise. Use during lactation has not been reported as causing a problem. Amitriptyline (q.v.) is a better studied alternative.

Ilett: *Br J Clin Pharmacol* 1993;**33**:635.

Doxepin M:P ratio 0·7–1·7; infant dose 1–3%

Very little is known about the use of this sedative tricyclic antidepressant during pregnancy, but there is no reason to suspect teratogenicity. Calculations suggest that breastfeeding should only expose the baby to a small amount of this drug and its slowly cleared active metabolite (N-desmethyldoxepin), but there are two reports of a breastfed baby becoming seriously hypotonic. In the first case the baby had a blood level of the metabolite that was inexplicably high if the child's only exposure to the drug was from maternal milk. The onset of symptoms also seemed very sudden. In the second the blood level was much lower and the drowsiness rather less clearly related to maternal medication. Uncertainties over use during lactation clearly remain worryingly unresolved.
Frey: *Ann Pharmacother* 1999;**22**:690.
Kemp: *Br J Clin Pharmacol* 1985;**20**:497.

Doxylamine

Doxylamine is an antihistamine that was widely used for many years to control nausea in pregnancy. It was marketed (as Debendox® in the UK and as Bendectin® in the USA) as a compound tablet with pyridoxine, but was withdrawn in 1983 as a result of the adverse publicity generated by litigation, even though there was more evidence of efficacy and better evidence of safety than for any other product. It still remains on sale in Canada (as Diclectin®).
Brent: *Reprod Toxicol* 1995;**59**:337.
McKeigue: *Teratology* 1994;**50**:27.

Ephedrine (and pseudoephedrine)

There is some suggestion that ventricular septal defects may be commoner after first trimester self-medication with 'over the counter' products containing pseudoephedrine. Although there is a single anecdotal report suggesting that the maternal use of ephedrine during lactation could cause the baby to become irritable, studies of pseudoephedrine and terbutaline (the only two sympathomimetics studied in any detail), suggest that the amount ingested is usually much too small to affect the baby. There is, however, limited evidence from one study to suggest that pseudoephedrine use may sometimes reduce milk production.
Aljazaf: *Br J Clin Pharmacol* 2003;**56**:18.
Werler: *Birth Defects Res A* 2006;**76**:445.

Escitalopram

For a comment on this SSRI antidepressant see the entry on citalopram, of which it is the active enantiomer.

Ergotamine

There is no known teratogenic effect, but the risk of ergotism should be borne in mind if this drug is used to treat migraine in pregnancy. Significant exposure in the breastfed baby could also cause ergotism, and repeated medication could inhibit lactation.
Hosking: *Aust NZ Obstet Gynaecol* 1996;**36**:159.
Raymond: *Teratology* 1995;**51**:344.

Ethambutol M:P ratio 1; infant dose 1–2%

This drug can be safely used to treat tuberculosis during pregnancy and lactation. There are no reports of any adverse effect from use during lactation. Calculations, however, suggest that the plasma level in a young breastfed baby might approach therapeutic levels, and ethambutol is not generally used in children less than 6 years old because it could be difficult to detect the onset of optic neuritis (an occasional but important adverse effect).
Medcill: *Obstet Gynecol Surv* 1989;**44**:81.
Snider: *Am Rev Respir Dis* 1980;**122**:65.

Ethosuximide M:P ratio 0·8–1·0; infant dose >50%

There is relatively little evidence that this anticonvulsant is teratogenic in man. The drug enters breast milk freely. While there is no evidence that this is of any clinical significance, there have been anecdotal reports of disturbed neonatal behaviour, and it is known that plasma levels in the breastfed baby sometimes approach those seen in the mother.
Kuhnz: *Br J Clin Pharmacol* 1984;**18**:671.
Samren: *Epilpsia* 1997;**38**:981.

Etodolac

For a comment see the entry on celecoxib.

Etretinate

This oral vitamin A derivative used to treat severe psoriasis and congenital ichthyosis is a serious teratogen, and pregnancy should not be contemplated until at least 3 years after treatment is stopped. Use during lactation is also generally considered unwise.
Geiger: *Dermatology* 1994;**189**:109.
Gollnick: *Br J Dermatol* 1996;**135**(suppl 49):6.

Fluoxetine M:P ratio 0·3–0·5; infant dose 6–13%

Some evidence is accumulating that fetal exposure to this antidepressant in the first trimester of pregnancy may increase the risk of congenital heart defects in the fetus from a background of 1/100 to less than 2/100 – as does paroxetine (q.v.) and possibly other selective serotonin reuptake inhibitors (SSRIs) (q.v.). Significant amounts are ingested in breast milk, the drug has a long half life, and irritability and somnolence have now been reported in several babies who had been exposed to fluoxetine both before and after delivery. Sertraline (q.v.) is less studied, but it may turn out to be a better antidepressant to use in late pregnancy where the mother wishes to breastfeed after delivery.
Gjerdingen: *J Am Board Fam Pract* 2003;**16**:273. [SR]
Mattson: *Teratology* 1999;**59**:376.

Fluphenazine

There is no evidence of teratogenicity but treatment with this antipsychotic drug during pregnancy may result in the baby showing hyperactivity for some weeks after delivery. Use during lactation has not been studied.
Auerbach: *Neurotoxicol Teratol* 1992;**14**:399.

Flurbiprofen M:P ratio <0·1; infant dose <1%

The use of this anti-inflammatory analgesic is safe during lactation. For a comment on use during pregnancy see the monograph on ibuprofen.
Smith: *J Clin Pharmacoll* 1989;**29**:174.

Fluvoxamine maleate M:P ratio 0·3; infant dose ~1%

There is no evidence, as yet, that this selective serotonin reuptake inhibitor (SSRI) (q.v.) is teratogenic, but the general comments on SSRIs probably apply. Minimal quantities are ingested from breast milk.
Hendrick: *Br J Psychiatr* 2001;**179**:163.
Wright: *Br J Clin Pharmacol* 1991;**31**:209.

Gabapentin

Very little is yet known about the safety of using this new anticonvulsant during pregnancy or lactation and there is some suggestion that use during pregnancy could carry some risk.
Chambers: *Birth Defects Res A* 2005;**73**:316.

Glibenclamide = Glyburide (USAN)

This sulphonylurea is widely used in the treatment of type 2 (insulin-resistant) diabetes and, unlike tolbutamide (q.v.), it only seems to cross the human placenta in trace quantities. While insulin (q.v.) is usually considered the better strategy for controlling both type 1 and type 2 diabetes during pregnancy, there is an accepted role for glibenclamide in 'gestational'

diabetes. The amount appearing in breast milk is too small to be detectable.
Feig: *Diabetes Care* 2005;**28**:1851.
Langer: *N Engl J Med* 2000;**343**:1134.

Griseofulvin
Itraconazole (q.v.) has now largely replaced griseofulvin in the treatment of fungal skin infections. Griseofulvin is known to be teratogenic and embryotoxic in some animals and has, as a result, been little used during pregnancy. The manufacturers advise men to avoid conceiving a child for 6 months after receiving treatment (advice reiterated in the BNF) because there is some evidence of genotoxicity in mice. No information exists on use during lactation.
Anon: *Med Lett Drugs Ther* 1976;**18**:17.

Halofantrine
Little is known about the use of this drug to treat chloroquine-resistant falciparum malaria during pregnancy or lactation. The manufacturers warn against its use because extremely high doses are teratogenic in animals, but such information is of limited clinical relevance.
Phillips-Howard: *Drug Safety* 1996;**14**:131.

Haloperidol M:P ratio 2–4; infant dose ~3%
There is no evidence that this antipsychotic is teratogenic. Maternal treatment during lactation only results in the baby ingesting a small amount of this drug, and there are no reports of this sedating the baby or affecting developmental progress.
Whalley: *BMJ* 1981;**282**:1746.
Yoshida: *Psychol Med* 1998;**28**:81.

Headache
See under migraine and headache.

Herbal remedies
The use of herbal remedies during pregnancy has been poorly studied, but 14 get a mention in the latest edition of the book by Briggs et al. (2008), while the book by Hale (2008) summarises the information available on the use of some 20 herbal medicines during lactation. It would seem that the use of blue cohosh (blue ginseng) is definitely contraindicated, and uncertainties exist over the use of chamomile, comfrey and kava-kava. St John's wort seems safe, but may interact with other medications.
Hale: *Medications and mothers' milk*, 13th edn, 2008. (See bibliography.)
Howard: *Clin Perinatol* 1999;**26**:447.

Imipramine M:P ratio 0·7; infant dose <2%
There is no evidence of teratogenicity in man, but neonatal withdrawal symptoms have sometimes been reported after delivery. A little of the drug appears in breast milk, but there is no evidence that use is unwise during lactation. Plasma levels are best monitored during pregnancy to optimise treatment.
McElhatton: *Reprod Toxicol* 1996;**10**:285.
Nulman: *Am J Psychiatry* 2002;**159**:1889.

Iodine
While iodine deficiency during pregnancy can cause cretinism and other problems (as outlined in the web-archived monograph on potassium iodate), excessive intake can cause fetal goitre and hypothyroidism. Even the use of an iodine-containing expectorant, topical antiseptic or vaginal gel in late pregnancy or after delivery may alter maternal and fetal thyroid function and increase the iodine content of the mother's breast milk. The danger to the baby during lactation can be exaggerated, however, because T_4 and TSH levels are usually normal even when neonatal serum and urinary iodine levels are grossly elevated. Extended exposure could be more hazardous however. Premature babies seem at greatest risk.
Linder: *J Pediatr* 1997;**131**:434.
Watanabe: *J Obstet Gynecol Res* 1998;**24**:285.

Isotretinoin
Isotretinoin is an isomer of the acid form of vitamin A. Topical and oral preparations are available. The hazards associated with maternal use are the same as for tretinoin (q.v.).

Itraconazole
There is evidence of dose-related toxicity and teratogenicity in animals. Brief exposure to this antifungal during early pregnancy is certainly compatible with a normal pregnancy outcome, but other azoles are known to be capable of inducing malformations in man. Systemic use during lactation has not been studied, but it can be predicted that sustained exposure would cause widespread tissue drug accumulation in a child. Fluconazole (q.v.) is probably the antifungal of choice when systemic treatment is necessary during lactation (or after the first trimester of pregnancy), and is virtually unabsorbed when applied topically.
Bar-Oz: *Am J Obstet Gynecol* 2000;**183**:617.
Briggs *et al.*: *Drugs in pregnancy and lactation*, 8th edn, 2008: p. 994. (See bibliography.)

Ketoconazole
Little specific information exists, but the concerns about the use of the related azole, itraconazole (q.v.), probably apply.
Moretti: *Am J Obstet Gynecol* 1995;**173**:1625.

Ketorolac M:P ratio <0·1; infant dose <1%
The use of this anti-inflammatory analgesic is safe during lactation. For a comment on use during pregnancy see the monograph on ibuprofen.
Wischnik: *Eur J Clin Pharmacol* 1989;**36**:521.

Levonorgestrel
There is no evidence of teratogenicity if the 'morning after' pill is taken in error during early pregnancy, and there is no contraindication to its use during lactation.

Lithium M:P ratio 0·3–0·7; infant dose ~20%
Treatment with lithium has transformed the management of manic-depressive illness, but use during pregnancy calls for careful judgement, and it may be possible to stabilise mood with lamotrigine (q.v.). While use in the first trimester carries enough risk to warrant a detailed cardiac anomaly scan, the risk of a major malformation is low as long as the mother's plasma level is carefully monitored, and discontinuing treatment may cause a relapse. Aim for a level of 0·5–0·8 mmol/l 12 hours after ingestion, remembering that renal clearance increases 50% during early pregnancy and decreases again abruptly soon after delivery (which may account for the fact that neonatal toxicity is commonest shortly after birth). Serum levels in the breastfed baby are only a fifth of those in the mother – a level that does not seem to affect neonatal development. It is probably advisable to monitor thyroid function at intervals.
Kozma: *Am J Med Genet* 2005;**132A**;441.
Viguera: *Am J Psychiatry* 2007;**164**:342.

Loperamide M:P ratio 0·4; infant dose <0·1%
Malformation was marginally commoner after use to control diarrhoea in early pregnancy in one recent study. No one pattern of defect predominated, and no causal link has yet been established. Use during lactation seems safe. Imodium® can currently be purchased in the UK without a prescription.
Einarson: *Can J Gastroenterol* 2000;**14**:185
Källén B: *Acta Paediatr* 2008;**97**:541.

Loratadine M:P ratio 1·2; infant dose ~1%
There is no evidence that this non-sedating antihistamine, which is often used to treat allergic rhinitis, is a teratogen, and maternal use during lactation will only result in the baby ingesting minimal amounts of the drug.
Hilbert: *J Clin Pharmacol* 1988;**28**:234.
Moretti: *J Allergy Clin Immunol* 2003;**111**:479.

Lysergic acid (LSD)
There are no published epidemiological studies of LSD use in pregnancy. While there is no evidence that *pure* LSD harms the fetus when taken on its own (in the absence of maternal toxicity), the long-term effect of fetal exposure has not been studied. Drug transfer into breast milk has not been studied either but can be expected to occur and, since even low doses can be hallucinogenic, use during lactation seems most unwise.
Aase: *Lancet* 1970;**2**:100.
Long: *Teratology* 1972;**6**:75.

Maprotiline M:P ratio 1·4; infant dose <2%
There is no animal evidence of teratogenicity, but little experience of use during human pregnancy. The increased risk of seizures may make it more appropriate to choose some other tricyclic antidepressant during pregnancy. Little is ingested from breast milk.
Lloyd: *J Int Med Res* 1997;**5**(suppl 4):122.
Mendalis: *ADR Highlights* 1983;**83**:1.

Marijuana (cannabis) M:P ratio 8
There is very little evidence that this widely used illicit drug jeopardises fetal development or affects the behaviour of the baby after birth, but case–control studies have shown that maternal use is associated with an increased risk of sudden infant death (even after allowing for the even stronger correlation with tobacco use during and after pregnancy). Use by the mother's partner also remained an independent risk factor. No consistent effects have been seen when marijuana is used during lactation even though the drug and its metabolites appear to be concentrated in breast milk. Traces will persist in the urine for many weeks.
Blair: *BMJ* 1996;**313**:195.
Dreher: *Clin Pediatr* 1994;**93**:254.

Mebendazole
This poorly absorbed antihelminthic is widely used to treat hookworm, roundworm, threadworm and whipworm infection. The drug is embryotoxic in rats but there are no reports of teratogenicity in man, and treating serious intestinal helminth infection can improve pregnancy outcome. Intake from breast milk is likely to be negligible.
Diav-Citrin: *Am J Obstet Gynecol* 2003;**188**:282.

Meclozine = Meclizine (USAN)
Meclozine is an oral antihistamine with anticholinergic activity. It is available without prescription and widely used to control travel sickness. There is no evidence of teratogenicity, and its efficacy in controlling nausea and vomiting in pregnancy was established as early as 1962. The half life is just 3 hours, but one dose often provides symptomatic relief for 24 hours.
Broussard: *Gastroenterol Clin North Am* 1998;**27**:123.
Milkovich: *Am J Obstet Gynecol* 1976;**125**:244.

Medroxyprogesterone (Depo-provera®)
There is no evidence that inadvertent use of this long-acting contraceptive is hazardous during pregnancy, and no evidence that use after delivery will affect lactation, particularly if the administration of the first injection is delayed until at least 3 days after delivery. Indeed there is some evidence that it raises prolactin levels and increases milk production. See also the entry under oral contraceptives.
Kennedy: *Contraception* 1997;**55**:347.

Meloxicam
For a comment see the entry on celecoxib.

Meprobamate M:P ratio 2–4
This drug was, at one time, quite widely used in the management of anxiety states. Little is known about its teratogenic potential. It accumulates in breast milk and is probably best avoided during pregnancy and lactation.
Belafsky: *Obstet Gynecol* 1969;**34**:378.
Wilson: *Clin Pharmacokinet* 1980;**5**:1.

Mercaptopurine (6-MP)
Miscarriage, stillbirth and low birthweight have all occurred when this anticancer drug is used in pregnancy, but it is difficult to know if this is the result of drug treatment or not. A few congenital malformations have been seen, but no pattern of abnormality has emerged after monotherapy. Several babies have, however, shown transient bone marrow depression at birth. Breastfeeding while on treatment does not seem to have been reported. Azathioprine (q.v.), which is transformed into mercaptopurine in the body, has occasionally been taken during lactation without apparent ill effect. Pregnancy *after* treatment for choriocarcinoma with mercaptopurine has generally been uneventful.
Green: *Arch Pediatr Adolesc Med* 1997;**151**:379.
Song: *Am J Obstet Gynecol* 1988;**158**:538.

Mesalazine Infant dose (of metabolite) ~7%
Mesalazine (5-aminosalicylic acid), the prodrug balsalazide and the dimer olsalazine can all be used with safety to treat women with inflammatory bowel disease during pregnancy. Use during lactation also seems safe although diarrhoea has been reported in a few babies.
Christensen: *Acta Obstet Gynecol Scand* 1994;**74**:399.
Marteau: *Aliment Pharmacol Ther* 1998;**12**:1101.

Metformin Infant dose <1%
There is no good reason not to use of this biguanide to control blood sugar levels during pregnancy in women with type 2 diabetes (i.e. some residual pancreatic islet cell function), although insulin was, until recently, thought to provide a better strategy for minimising the fetal risks (except in a Third World setting). Metformin is as effective as insulin in women with gestational diabetes (although glyburide (see the monograph on insulin) may offer better control). First trimester use also seems safe in women with polycystic ovary syndrome. Use in late pregnancy does not seem to increase the risk of neonatal hypoglycaemia, and exposure to metformin in breast milk is minimal.
Gilbert: *Fertil Steril* 2006;**86**:658.
Swaminathan: *J R Coll Physicians Edinb* 2009;**39**:10.

Methamfetamine (speed)
Most of the comments made about dexamfetamine (q.v.) probably apply. There is, however, some suggestion of an excess of babies with gastroschisis or intestinal atresia (suggesting brief fetal vascular disruption).
Oro: *J Pediatr* 1987;**111**:571.
Sherman: *Pediatr Res* 2001;**49**:364A.

Methotrexate M:P ratio <0·1; infant dose 0·3%
This folic acid antagonist is used in the treatment of rheumatic disease and some cancers. Use in early pregnancy (8–10 weeks after the last menstrual period) is known to be teratogenic, and there may be an increased risk of miscarriage, but most children born to mothers on low-dose treatment (<10 mg/week) seem normal at birth. While most standard texts advise mothers taking methotrexate not to breastfeed, and few seem to have done so, the amount ingested by the baby seems to be less than 1% of the lowest antineoplastic dose.

Chakravarty: *J Rheumatol* 2003;**30**:241.
Johns: *Am J Obstet Gynecol* 1972;**112**:978.

Methylenedioxymethamfetamine (ecstasy)

This stimulant drug, structurally related to dexamfetamine (q.v.) and mescaline, is subject to abuse although dependence has not been reported. The response to a fixed dose varies greatly. Hyperthermia, hyponatraemia (possibly due to inappropriate ADH secretion) and convulsions are amongst the more severe complications, making experimental intake during pregnancy potentially hazardous for the fetus. It can be predicted that the drug would transfer into breast milk, so exposure should be avoided during lactation.
Henry: *Lancet* 1992;**340**:384.
McElhatton: *Lancet* 1999;**354**:1441.

Migraine and headache

The aim should be to control attacks both during pregnancy and lactation by early treatment with paracetamol in combination, if necessary, with codeine and/or caffeine. It is said that aspirin (q.v.) should be avoided during lactation, but occasional use is harmless. The nausea associated with migraine may need treating with metoclopramide (q.v.) to enable one of the above analgesics to be given by mouth. Parenteral chlorpromazine (q.v.) or prochlorperazine may rarely be necessary. Products containing ergotamine should probably be avoided. Sumatriptan (q.v.) is the only newer remedy to have received enough study as yet for use to be recommended if other strategies fail.
Goadsby: *BMJ* 2008;**336**:1502.
Spigset: *Paediatr Drugs* 2000;**2**:223.

Mirtazapine Infant dose ~1%

Mirtazapine is a tetracyclic antidepressant, chemically unrelated to most of the other antidepressants currently in common use. It only came onto the market in 1996 and because there are, as yet, no reports of its use in pregnancy such use is currently being monitored by the Canadian Motherisk programme (tel: +01 800 670 6126). It is, however, known that the breastfed baby only ingests about 1% of the weight-adjusted maternal dose.
Djulus: *J Clin Psychiatry* 2006;**67**:1280.
Kristenson: *Br J Pharmacol* 2007;**63**:322.

Moclobemide M:P ratio ~0·7; infant dose <1%

This drug, a *reversible* inhibitor of monoamine oxidase, has a valued place in the second line management of major depression and social phobia. While the problems seen with most monoamime oxidase inhibitor (MAOI) drugs are seldom encountered with this particular product, similar dietary restrictions apply, and treatment should only be started a variable time after other antidepressants have been withdrawn. No problems have been reported with use during lactation. There seem to be no published reports of use during pregnancy.
Buist: *Hum Pyschopharmacol Clin Exp* 1998;**13**:579.

Montelukast

This leukotreine receptor antagonist is used to stabilize airway tone in selected patients with asthma serious enough to require long-term prophylactic management with an inhaled corticosteroid. It has a molecular weight low enough to make transplacental passage likely, but animal studies detected no evidence of teratogenicity, and the limited evidence available in the manufacturer's prospective case register of use during pregnancy has not, as yet, revealed any cause for concern. Nothing is yet known about use during lactation, but only limited quantities of the related drug zafirlukast (q.v.) appear in breast milk.
Bakhireva: *J Allergy Clin Immunol* 2007;**119**:618.

Mycophenolate mofetil

This new drug is increasingly used to enhance immunosuppression in patients who have had a solid organ transplant, and it also seems to have some advantages over cyclophosphamide in the management of some autoimmune diseases. It is, however, a recognised human teratogen, affecting in particular structures derived from the frontonasal prominence and first pharyngeal arch. Therefore any such treatment should be stopped at least 6 weeks before the start of any pregnancy. Use would seem to be equally unwise during lactation.
Vento: *Pediatrics* 2008;**122**:184.

Nadolol M:P ratio 4·6; infant dose ~5%

While there is no evidence of teratogenicity, little is known about the use of nadolol to control hypertension in pregnancy, and other β blockers have been much better studied. Alternatives are also preferred during lactation.
Devlin: *Br J Clin Pharmacol* 1981;**12**:393.
Fox: *Am J Obstet Gynecol* 1985;**152**:1045.

Nalidixic acid M:P ratio 0·06; infant dose <0·1%

This antibiotic has damaged growing cartilage in animals but its use to treat urinary infection during pregnancy does not seem to have caused detectable fetal damage. Many texts warn that this drug could cause haemolysis in a baby with G6PD deficiency but, in the one published case report on which this warning is based, the baby did not have G6PD deficiency! Other strategies for treatment can usually be found. Use in the neonatal period has been reported to cause a metabolic acidosis.
Belton: *Lancet* 1965;**2**:691.
Murray: *BMJ* 1981;**282**:224.

Naproxen M:P ratio <0·1; infant dose ~2%

The use of this anti-inflammatory analgesic is safe during lactation. For a comment on use during pregnancy see the monograph on ibuprofen.
Jamili: *Drug Intell Clin Pharmacol* 1983;**17**:910.

Nausea and vomiting in pregnancy

See under antiemetics.

Nicotine

The effects of smoking during pregnancy are well known. Nicotine, and its metabolite cotinine, also appear in breast milk. The amount present in the urine of a breastfed baby is ten times as high as the amount present in a baby whose mother smokes but gives her baby bottle milk. Nicotine patch use will cause less exposure than heavy smoking (unless it delivers more than 14 mg of nicotine per 24 hours), but that will not always be true with gum use. The effectiveness of patch replacement treatment in pregnancy remains very unclear, but mothers can certainly be advised that the advantages of breastfeeding greatly outweigh the hazards of nicotine exposure from breast milk. Parents should avoid smoking in the presence of their baby.
Ilett: *Clin Pharmacol Ther* 2003;**74**:516.
Moore: *BMJ* 2009;**338**:867. [SR]

Nitrazepam M:P ratio 0·3; infant dose ~2%

As for the monograph on diazepam in Part 2.
Matheson: *Br J Clin Pharmacol* 1990;**30**:787.

Nitrofurantoin M:P ratio 6; infant dose ~6%

There is as yet only one study suggesting that first trimester use can increase the risk of malformation, but there is also a theoretical risk that the baby could develop haemolytic anaemia when the drug is given in late pregnancy, during labour or while the mother is breastfeeding (especially in the presence of G6PD deficiency).
Crider: *Arch Pediatr Adolesc Med* 2009;**163**:978.
Gerk: *Pharmacotherapy* 2001;**21**:669.

Maternal medication and the baby

Non-steroidal anti-inflammatory drugs (NSAIDs)

See the monograph on ibuprofen in Part 2. Paracetamol (q.v.) is generally considered a safer product to recommend to anyone seeking 'over the counter' pain relief during pregnancy. Diclofenac (which requires a prescription) may be a good option during lactation because the short serum half life will limit transfer into milk (although no formal studies of uptake by the baby have yet been published). For a comment on the new second-generation NSAID drugs see the entry on celecoxib.
Neilsen: *BMJ* 2001;**308**:266.

Nortriptyline M:P ratio 0·9−3·7; infant dose ~2%

As for amitriptyline.
Wisner: *Am J Psychiatry* 1991;**148**:1234.

Oral contraceptives

Most oral contraceptives contain an oestrogen and a progestogen. There is very little evidence of teratogenicity, although some synthetic oestrogens like diethylstilbestrol (q.v.) can have a profound effect on genital tract development. Oestrogens can depress lactation, so mothers wishing to breastfeed should, where possible, use a progestogen-only pill (mini-pill) starting 3 or more weeks after birth for the first 6 months after delivery. If there is evidence that this has proved unreliable in the past, depot medroxyprogesterone (q.v.) should be considered. For authoritative advice see the UK Faculty of Family Planning website: www.ffprhc.org.uk.
Koetsawang: *Int J Gynecol Obstet* 1987;**25**(suppl):115. (See also p. 129.)
Martinez-Frias: *Teratology* 1998;**57**:8.

Oral hypoglycaemic agents

There is no clear evidence of teratogenicity, but also no established consensus over the use of such drugs during pregnancy. Chlorpropamide, glibenclamide and tolbutamide (q.v.) can all cause serious early neonatal hypoglycaemia, but this has not been reported with metformin (q.v.). Other oral hypoglycaemic agents have not yet received much study. The use of these drugs during lactation has not been studied, but is probably safe.

Panic disorder

Fluoxetine (q.v.) is probably the best preventative drug to use when cognitive-behavioural techniques prove inadequate. If a benzodiazepine (q.v.) is indicated for acute symptoms, lorazepam has the advantage of a relatively short half life, although the baby may show withdrawal symptoms.
American Academy of Pediatrics, Committee on Drugs: *Pediatrics* 2000;**205**:880.

Paroxetine M:P ratio 0·1; infant dose ~2%

This popular antidepressant is increasingly used for panic attacks and for obsessive-compulsive disorder. There seems to be a definite slight increase in the risk of miscarriage, and recent evidence suggests that malformation is commoner after maternal use during the first trimester – particularly after high-dose (> 25 mg/day) exposure. Most documented defects have been of a minor nature, but cardiac defects predominate and a few have been severe. Transient neonatal withdrawal symptoms are quite often seen after maternal use during pregnancy, as outlined in the general entry on selective serotonin reuptake inhibitor (SSRI) use (q.v.). Use during lactation exposes the baby to less than 2% of the weight-adjusted maternal dose, and no problems have yet been reported following such exposure (although no major long-term follow-up study has yet been done).
Berle: *J Clin Psychiatry* 2004;**65**:1228.
Einanarson: *Am J Psychiatry* 2008;**165**:749.

Perphenazine M:P ratio 1; infant dose <1%

This antipsychotic does not seem to be teratogenic, but the baby may show hyperactivity and extrapyramidal signs (as with fluphenazine). Lactation is considered safe.
Olesen: *Am J Psychiatry* 1990;**147**:1378.
Stone: *Am J Obstet Gynecol* 1977;**128**:486.

Phencyclidine (PCP or angel dust) M:P ratio >10

This illicit hallucinogen is a potent analgesic and anaesthetic related to ketamine. Despite placental transfer most newborns are healthy, but some show toxic irritability alternating with lethargy. Teratogenicity is not suspected and no prolonged neurobehavioural abnormalities have been documented. Because the drug is concentrated in breast milk, exposure should be avoided during lactation.
Nicholas: *Am J Obstet Gynecol* 1982;**143**:143.
Wachsman: *Am J Drug Alcohol Abuse* 1989;**15**:31.

Phenindione Infant dose ~15%

This drug, like warfarin, should be avoided in pregnancy. Heparin (q.v.) is the drug of choice where anticoagulation is called for during pregnancy because it does not cross the placenta. Anticoagulation with phenindione in pregnancy carries fetal risks similar to those seen with warfarin treatment. Although there is only one report of maternal treatment causing a breastfed baby to bleed after surgery, warfarin is undoubtedly a safer drug to use during lactation.
Goguel: *Rev Fr Gynecol Obstet* 1970;**65**:409.
Phenybutvon-Kries: *Monatsschr Kinderheilkd* 1993;**141**:505.

Phenylbutazone

This drug is not now as widely prescribed as other non-steroidal anti-inflammatory drugs (NSAIDs) (q.v.) and there is only limited evidence as to safety during pregnancy or lactation. Animal evidence suggests that use could decrease fertility by blocking blastocyst implantation. The drug is excreted in breast milk producing serum levels in the baby a fifth to a half of those found in the mother.
Dawood: *Am J Obstet Gynecol* 1993;**169**:1255.
Leuxner: *Munch Med Wschr* 1956;**98**:84.

Piroxicam M:P ratio <0·1; infant dose ~4%

The use of this anti-inflammatory analgesic is safe during lactation. For a comment on use during pregnancy see the monograph on ibuprofen.
Østensen: *Eur J Clin Pharmacol* 1988;**36**:567.

Praziquantel

There is no animal evidence that this drug is teratogenic or causes infertility, but there are virtually no reports of use during pregnancy or lactation to treat tapeworm (cestode) or fluke (trematode) generated illness. Praziquantel is also the drug of choice for schistasomiasis (bilharziasis). All these parasitic infections are sometimes endemic enough to require population-based treatment from which pregnant or lactating mothers should not be excluded. Any theoretical hazard to the child from brief maternal treatment during lactation is almost completely eliminated by taking the child off the breast for 1 day.
Olds: *Acta Tropica* 2003;**86**:185.

Prednisolone M:P ratio 0·16; infant dose ~3%

Corticosteroid administration can cause facial clefting in animals, and systemic use in the first trimester of pregnancy can also marginally increase the risk of this happening to the human baby. Prolonged and repeated use can also cause some degree of fetal growth retardation, but this is not a problem with short-term use. While betamethasone and dexamethasone readily cross the placenta, 90% of prednisolone is inactivated. Even moderately high-dose systemic treatment with prednisolone during lactation (60–80 mg a day) does not seem to depress endogenous cortisol production in the baby. Whether this also holds true for other corticosteroids is less clear.

Greenberger: *Clin Pharmacol Ther* 1993;**53**:324.
Park-Wyllie: *Teratology* 2000;**62**:385.

Primaquine

Rather surprisingly there have still been no published studies of the use of this antimalarial drug either during pregnancy or lactation. The CDC in America believes that use (to eliminate dormant liver organisms) should always be delayed until after delivery, but the balance of risk may not always make such dogmatism appropriate. Haemolysis is, however, a real risk with high-dose treatment in patients with the Mediterranean and Asian (B⁻) but not the milder African (A⁻) variants of G6PD deficiency. There are no reports of haemolysis in the baby of a mother taking primaquine while breastfeeding but it remains a theoretical risk in a baby whose G6PD status is unknown. Nevertheless because plasma drug levels are low, milk levels are also likely to be fairly low.
Anon: *MMWR* 1978;**27**:81.
Diro M. *South Med J* 1982;**75**:959.

Primidone M:P ratio 0·5–0·8; infant dose 15–25%

This anticonvulsant can be teratogenic in mice, but there are no convincing reports of teratogenicity in man. Studies are difficult to interpret because epilepsy itself may increase the risk of malformation, and many epileptic patients are on more than one drug. The risk of neonatal haemorrhage (as for phenobarbital) is easily corrected by giving vitamin K at birth. Treatment during lactation has been associated with reports of transient drowsiness.
Kaneko: *Jpn J Psychiatry Neurol* 1993;**47**:306.
Olafsson: *Epilepsia* 1998;**39**:887.

Procainamide M:P ratio 4; infant dose ~7%

Use to treat a maternal arrhythmia poses no recognised risk to the baby. The drug has also been used with (some) success for fetal supraventricular tachycardia. While the amount ingested by the baby is relatively small the long-term effect of maternal use during lactation has not yet been properly documented.
Allen: *Clin Pharm* 1993;**12**:58.
Itto: *Clin Perinatol* 1994;**21**:543.

Prochlorperazine

Originally used, like chlorpromazine (q.v.), to manage schizophrenia, this drug is now mainly used to control severe nausea and vomiting. There is no evidence that it is hazardous in pregnancy. Use during lactation does not seem to have been studied – high-dose maternal treatment might well make the baby drowsy.
Slone: *Am J Obst Gynecol* 1977;**128**:486.

Promethazine

Promethazine has been widely used for nausea in pregnancy without hazard. Ondansetron (q.v.) may be a less sedating alternative when symptoms are very severe. There is one report of use during labour causing neonatal respiratory depression but no other study has found any such association. While some antihistamines (q.v.) could conceivably cause neonatal drowsiness if given to the lactating mother, promethazine has never been reported to cause such a problem. It can have a sedative effect in children (which parents often appreciated) but, because some children ended up oversedated, the authorities no longer recommend use in children under 2 years.
Vella: *BMJ* 1985;**290**:1173.

Propylthiouracil M:P ratio 0·6; infant dose 0·3%

Propylthiouracil is used to control maternal thyrotoxicosis during pregnancy. It can also be given with safety to the lactating mother (despite earlier reports to the contrary). Other thiouracil drugs seem to be less safe.

Atkins: *Drug Saf* 2000;**23**:229.
O'Doherty: *BMJ* 1999;**318**:5.

Radiopharmaceuticals

Breastfeeding should normally be suspended, at least briefly, if the mother has to be prescribed a radioactive drug. The appropriate period of suspension varies. For some radio-nuclides, such as chromium-51, indium-111 and thallium-201, it is generally only thought necessary to express and discard milk for 4 hours. With iodine-123 and orthoiodohippuric acid-labelled iodine-125 and -131, an interval of 2 days is usually necessary. For other products labelled with iodine-131, and with phosphorus-32, galium-67 and selenium-75, the period of significant radioactivity may exceed 2 weeks, making any attempt at continued lactation generally inappropriate. Technetium-labelled radiopharmaceuticals (⁹⁹ᵐTc) are currently used for 75% of all radioactive imaging procedures. With many of these products it is only necessary to express and discard milk for 4 hours, but with sodium pertechnetate milk may need to be expressed and discarded for a day if the dose to the infant is to be kept below 1 mSv. The same is true after the technetium labelling of red and white blood cells and of human serum albumin microaggregates. See also the separate comment on X-ray contrast media.
Bennett: *Drugs and human lactation*, 2nd edn, 1996, pp. 609–77. (See bibliography.)
US Nuclear Regulatory Commission. *Regulatory guide 8.39*, April 1997, table 3.

Selective serotonin reuptake inhibitors (SSRIs)

Several of these widely used antidepressants have now been subject to careful study (cf. citralopram, escitalopram, fluoxetine, fluvoxamine, paroxetine and sertraline). SSRI use in the first trimester does seem to be associated with an increased risk of miscarriage and to double the chance that the baby will have a cardiac defect at birth (usually, but not always, a minor septal defect). It would, however, be wrong to leave serious maternal depression untreated if it does not respond to a tricyclic antidepressant. Use later in pregnancy does not seem to cause any long-term problems, but it can cause transient cardiac QT prolongation, and often causes signs of acute withdrawal with neonatal agitation and irritability shortly after birth. However, while this can cause much unnecessary distress if symptoms are wrongly interpreted as indicating that the baby has suffered asphyxial stress during delivery, the symptoms are rarely severe and seldom last more than a week. More rarely use during pregnancy may be associated with a slightly increased risk that the baby will exhibit signs of persistent pulmonary hypertension at birth. There is little logic in avoiding the further low-dose exposure that will result from letting the baby breastfed if the fetus has already experienced high-dose exposure throughout pregnancy.
Cipriani: *Lancet* 2009;**373**:746. (See also p. 700.)
Greene: *N Engl J Med* 2007;**356**:2732.

Senna Infant dose <7%

See the monograph on enemas, stool softeners and laxatives.

Sertraline M:P ratio 1·5–2 ; infant dose <2%

This antidepressant does not seem to be a serious teratogen, but the general comments about selective serotonin reuptake inhibitor (SSRI) use (q.v.) probably apply. There may also be a marginally increased risk of omphalocele, although the absolute risk is certainly small. Use during lactation exposes the baby to only 1% of the weight-adjusted maternal dose, but some babies display what were thought to be withdrawal symptoms shortly after delivery following maternal use during pregnancy.
Berle: *J Clin Psychiatry* 2004;**65**:1228.
Louik: *N Engl J Med* 2007;**356**:2675.

Solvent abuse

A wide range of products including adhesives (containing toluene and xylenes), aerosols (containing butane and halons), lighter fuel (containing *n*-butane), typewriter correcting fluid (containing trichloroethane) and solvents have been associated with abuse. Other sources include petrol, paint stripper and nail varnish remover. Excitement and euphoria can be followed by headache, dizziness, blurred vision, ataxia and coma. Toluene, in particular, can be toxic to the kidneys and to the central nervous system. Solvent abuse in pregnancy seems to be associated with an increased risk of prematurity and perinatal death, and there are suggestions that toluene exposure could be teratogenic. Withdrawal symptoms have been described in babies of such mothers 1–2 days after birth. A tell-tale odour may sometimes be present.

Pearson: *Pediatrics* 1994;**93**:211. (See also p. 216.)
Tenenbein: *Arch Dis Child* 1996;**74**:F204.

Statins

Statins reduce serum cholesterol levels and are used in the primary and secondary prevention of coronary heart disease. Licensed UK preparations include atorvastatin, fluvastatin, pravastatin and simvastatin. There is only limited evidence that any of these products are teratogenic in man, but a related drug, lovastatin, is teratogenic in rats and mice. Since there is no evidence that suspending use during pregnancy is likely to have any long-term impact on maternal health it is hard to justify continued use during pregnancy. Pravastatin might be the safest to use in pregnancy since it is not lipophilic. Only minimal amounts of pravastatin appear in breast milk (<1% of the weight-related dose) but too little is known to recommend the use of any other statin during lactation.

Eddison: *N Engl J Med* 2004;**350**:1579. (See also **352**:2759.)
Pan: *J Clin Pharmacol* 1988;**28**:942.

Steroids

See under corticosteroids and under prednisolone.

Streptomycin

Ototoxicity is a potential problem, as it is with every aminoglycoside. Deafness has been seen after fetal exposure, but seems rare. There are, nevertheless, good grounds for choosing a different, less ototoxic, antibiotic during pregnancy except when treating severe drug-resistant tuberculosis. Streptomycin is excreted into breast milk but poorly absorbed by the gut, making maternal treatment compatible with lactation.

Donald: *Cent Afr J Med* 1991;**37**:268.
Rubin: *Am J Dis Child* 1951;**82**:14.

Sulfasalazine = Sulphasalazine (former BAN) M:P ratio 0·3–0·6; infant dose 6–10%

This was the main drug used in the management of ulcerative colitis and Crohn disease until mesalazine (q.v.) came on the market. There is no evidence that it is teratogenic, or that maternal use increases the risk of kernicterus in the baby after birth, even though one of the metabolic breakdown products is a sulphonamide (and these drugs are known to interfere with the binding of bilirubin to plasma albumin). This remains, nevertheless, a theoretical possibility. While some sulfasalazine appears in breast milk, most authorities consider treatment fully consistent with continued breastfeeding although one breastfed baby is reported to have developed chronic bloody diarrhoea which ceased 2 days after maternal treatment was stopped. Haemolysis is a theoretical hazard in the G6PD-deficient infant.

Connell: *Drug Saf* 1999;**21**:311.
Esbjorner: *Acta Paediatr Scand* 1987;**76**:137.

Sulpiride Infant dose 8–18%

Some authorities caution mothers on this antipsychotic

drug to avoid breastfeeding because significant amounts appear in breast milk. Little is yet known about use during pregnancy.

Polatti: *Clin Exp Obstet Gynecol* 1982;**9**:144.

Sumatriptan M:P ratio 5; infant dose ~3%

Experience with the use of this new treatment for migraine is limited, but no evidence of teratogenicity has yet emerged. Breastfeeding is likely to be hazard free since, as a result of poor oral absorption, the baby will only absorb a fifth of the weight-adjusted maternal dose quoted above.

Evans: *Ann Pharmacother* 2008;**42**:543.
Wojnar-Horton: *Br J Clin Pharmacol* 1996;**41**:217.

Tacrolimus M:P ratio 0·09; infant dose <0·1%

This oral immunosuppressant drug is often used to prevent tissue rejection after organ transplantation. While there is some evidence of dose-related embryotoxicity and teratogenicity in animals, most women taking 10–15 mg a day have had a normal pregnancy outcome. Pre-eclampsia and transient neonatal hyperkalaemia have been the most common problems encountered. Immunosuppression increases the risk of cytomegalovirus (CMV) infection. There are only two reports of use during lactation – the babies did well and calculated post-delivery exposure was minimal.

Gardiner: *Obstet Gynecol* 2006;**107**:453.
Jain: *Transplantation* 1997;**64**:559.

Tamoxifen

This non-steroidal anti-oestrogen, related to clomifine, is quite widely used in the treatment of breast cancer. It is genotoxic and fetotoxic in animals and, while there is little experience of its use during human pregnancy, there are suggestions that fetal exposure could induce genital abnormalities and fears that, like diethylstilbestrol (q.v.), it could be a possible cause of genital cancers some decades later. Because of the drug's very long half life the risk of fetal exposure can only be avoided by stopping treatment 2 months before conception. Tamoxifen is known to inhibit lactation.

Masala: *Br J Obstet Gynaecol* 1978;**85**:134.
Tewari: *Lancet* 1990;**350**:183.

Tazarotene

This drug, which is effective in the topical treatment of psoriasis or acne, should be avoided during pregnancy because it is effectively a 'prodrug' for vitamin A (q.v.). Only trace amounts appear in breast milk.

Tolbutamide M:P ratio 0·1–0·4; infant dose ~15%

Congenital malformations are common in diabetic pregnancy, especially when early glucose control is poor, and this makes it impossible to say whether chlorpropamide or tolbutamide are potential teratogens. There are several reports of prolonged neonatal hypoglycaemia after the use of these drugs during pregnancy even when the mother was changed onto insulin several weeks before delivery. Glibenclamide (q.v.) is an alternative sulphonylurea that does *not* cross the placenta that is sometimes used in patients with type 2 (insulin-resistant) diabetes. However, most obstetricians now believe that treatment with insulin (q.v.) is the only way to optimise control over blood glucose in all diabetic patients during conception and pregnancy. The use of tolbutamide during lactation is probably safe, but has been little studied.

Coetzee: *South Afr Med J* 1984;**65**:635.
Moiel: *Clin Pediatr* 1967;**6**:480.

Topiramate Infant dose 10–20%

Very little is yet known about the safety of using this new anticonvulsant during pregnancy or lactation.

Öhman: *Epilepsia* 2002;**43**:1157.

Tretinoin

See the monograph on vitamin A (tretinoin is the acid form of vitamin A) for a comment on this drug's serious teratogenic potential. Limited topical use is probably safe during pregnancy, and is almost certainly safe during lactation, although this has not been properly studied.

Jick: *J Am Acad Dermatol* 1998;**39**:S118.

Trifluoperazine

As for fluphenazine.

Vaccines

While there is no evidence that any commonly used vaccine is embryotoxic or teratogenic, elective use should be avoided in the first 3 months of pregnancy. Although this is particularly true for attenuated live vaccines, protection from rabies and yellow fever should not be withheld where administration would otherwise be justified simply because the woman is pregnant. There is no contraindication to vaccination during lactation.

Briggs *et al*.: *Drugs in pregnancy and lactation* 8th edn, 2008: pp. 1885–1922. (See bibliography.)
Schaefer *et al*.: *Drugs during pregnancy and lactation*, 2nd edn, 2007: pp. 178–89 and 674–8. (See bibliography.)

Venlafaxine M:P ratio 2·5; infant dose ~6%

There is no evidence that this antidepressant (a serotonin and noradrenaline reuptake inhibitor) is teratogenic. The non-significant increase in early miscarriage in the only large study to date (12% *v.* 7%), if not a chance finding, may relate to the depression for which the women were being treated. The babies of such mothers often seem restless for 1–3 days after birth but such withdrawal symptoms seldom last long and no other adverse consequences have been seen. Modest amounts are ingested by the baby when the drug is taken during lactation.

Einarson: *Am J Psychiatry* 2001;**158**:1728.
Illett: *Br J Clin Pharmacol* 2002;**53**:17.

Volatile substance abuse

See under solvent abuse.

X-ray (and MRI) contrast media

The risk of childhood leukaemia after maternal exposure to X-rays during pregnancy is now well known. In particular, none of the commonly used non-ionic radio-opaque contrast agents should be used during pregnancy except for the most exceptional reasons, however these agents only appear in breast milk to a minimal extent. The use of meglumine gadopentetate in a MRI scan exposes the breastfed baby to about 1% of the weight-adjusted maternal dose. Exposure after gadoteridol is probably similar. The iodine in iohexol, iopanoic acid, metrizamide and metrizoate is so inert that these X-ray contrast agents can also be administered without exposing the baby to more than 0·5% of the maternal dose. Barium studies can also be undertaken during lactation with complete safety.

Kubik-Huch: *Radiology* 2000;**216**:555.
Nielsen: *Acta Radiol* 1987;**28**:523.

Zafirlukast Infant dose probably ~1%

Little is yet known about use in pregnancy, but use of the related product montelukast (q.v.) has not yet caused concern. Only trace amounts seem to be present in the milk of mothers taking a high dose while breastfeeding, but the product is not yet licensed for use in children less than 6 years old.

Zolpidem tartrate M:P ratio 0·1–0·2; infant dose <2%

Too little is yet known about this new hypnotic ('sleeping tablet') to recommend use during pregnancy. Use during lactation is unlikely to be a problem given the very small amount present in breast milk.

Pons: *Eur J Clin Pharmacol* 1989;**37**:245.

Zopiclone M:P ratio 0·5; infant dose <4%

As for zolpidem. One prospective study of 40 women found no evidence of teratogenicity.

Diav-Citrin: *Am J Perinatol* 1999;**16**:15.
Matheson: *Br J Clin Pharmacol* 1990;**30**:267.

Index

Including synonyms and abbreviations

Note
Drug names beginning with an upper case letter are proprietary (trade) names.
Where several page references are given, the most important entry is printed in **bold**.
The letter **W** after a page number denotes a linked website guideline or commentary.
Page numbers in *italics* refer to figures and tables.
'WEB archive' indicates that a monograph on this drug is available on the book's website, but not in the current print version of the text.